Oral Healthcare and Dentistry

Oral Healthcare and Dentistry

Edited by Dave Clark

hayle medical
New York

Hayle Medical,
750 Third Avenue, 9th Floor,
New York, NY 10017, USA

Visit us on the World Wide Web at:
www.haylemedical.com

ISBN: 978-1-63241-456-4

The publisher's policy is to use permanent paper from mills that operate a sustainable forestry policy. Furthermore, the publisher ensures that the text paper and cover boards used have met acceptable environmental accreditation standards.

Printed in China.

Cataloging-in-Publication Data

Oral healthcare and dentistry / edited by Dave Clark.
p. cm.
Includes bibliographical references and index.
ISBN 978-1-63241-456-4
1. Mouth--Care and hygiene. 2. Mouth--Diseases--Case studies. 3. Mouth--Diseases--Diagnosis.
4. Dentistry. I. Clark, Dave.

RK60.7 .O73 2017
617.601--dc23

Table of Contents

Preface......IX

Chapter 1 **An Insight into the Genesis of Hypohidrotic Ectodermal Dysplasia in a Case Report**......1
Kiran Kumar, Devi Charan Shetty, Mahima Dua, Amit Dua, and Raghu Dhanapal

Chapter 2 **A Case of Old Calcifying Epithelioma Processed Symptomless over 40 Years**......5
Shinji Yamaguchi, Madoka Inui, Takashi Takeoka, Kenya Okumura, and Toshiro Tagawa

Chapter 3 **Modified Bluegrass Appliance: A Nonpunitive Therapy for Thumb Sucking in Pediatric Patients—A Case Report with Review of the Literature**......10
Amish Diwanji, Preet Jain, Jigar Doshi, Prakash Somani, and Dhaval Mehta

Chapter 4 **Refractory Pigmentation Associated with Laugier-Hunziker Syndrome following Er:YAG Laser Treatment**......14
Sertan Ergun, Alp Saruhanoğlu, Dante-Antonio Migliari, Ilay Maden, and Hakki Tanyeri

Chapter 5 **Recurrent Ameloblastic Fibroma: Report of a Rare Case**......18
Ravikumar S. Kulkarni, Amitabh Sarkar, and Sandeep Goyal

Chapter 6 **An Innovative Approach to Treat Incisors Hypomineralization (MIH): A Combined use of Casein Phosphopeptide-Amorphous Calcium Phosphate and Hydrogen Peroxide**......22
Stefano Mastroberardino, Guglielmo Campus, Laura Strohmenger, Alessandro Villa, and Maria Grazia Cagetti

Chapter 7 **Supraorbital Blowin Fracture Presenting as an Ocular Dystopia in a Nine-Year-Old Girl**......27
Ranganadh Nallamothu, Shanmukha Reddy Kallam, Srikanth Gunturu, Sukumar Singh, and Vijay Kumar Rachalapally

Chapter 8 **Cone Beam Computed Tomography Evaluation of the Diagnosis, Treatment Planning, and Long-Term Followup of Large Periapical Lesions Treated by Endodontic Surgery**......32
Vijay Shekhar, and K. Shashikala

Chapter 9 **Restoration of Strip Crown with a Resin-Bonded Composite Cement in Early Childhood Caries**......44
Mi-ae Jeong, Ah-hyeon Kim, Youn-soo Shim, and So-youn An

Chapter 10 **Dual Lesions: A Diagnostic Dilemma**......50
M. P. V. Prabhat, Prasannasrinivas Deshpande, Sarat Gummadapu, Suresh Babburi, Raja Lakshmi Chintamaneni, and Bhavana Sujanamulk

Chapter 11 **Use of Zirconia to Restore Severely Worn Dentition**.....55
Manish Agrawal, Banashree Sankeshwari, and Channaveer V. Pattanshetti

Chapter 12 **Management and Followup of Complicated Crown Fractures in Young Patients Treated with Partial Pulpotomy**.....59
Francisco Ojeda-Gutierrez, Brenda Martinez-Marquez, Soraya Arteaga-Larios, M. Socorro Ruiz-Rodriguez, and Amaury Pozos-Guillen

Chapter 13 **Neuroleptic Malignant Syndrome in a Patient with Tongue Cancer**.....64
Osamu Baba, Kenji Yamagata, Yasushi Tomidokoro, Akira Tamaoka, Hiroyuki Itoh, Toru Yanagawa, Kojiro Onizawa, and Hiroki Bukawa

Chapter 14 **Endodontic Management of aMaxillary FirstMolar with Two Palatal Canals and a Single Buccal Canal**.....69
Leila Atash biz Yeganeh,Mamak Adel, Reza Vahedi, and Maryam Tofangchiha

Chapter 15 **An Unusual Case Report of Erupted Odontoma**.....73
Dhaval Mehta, Nilesh Raval, Sneha Udhani, Viral Parekh, and ChintanModi

Chapter 16 **Multiple Pulp Stones in Primary and Developing Permanent Dentition**.....76
MohitaMarwaha, Radhika Chopra, Payal Chaudhuri, Atul Gupta, and Jayna Sachdev

Chapter 17 **A Clinical Report of Nonsyndromic Concomitant Hypo-Hyperdontia**.....80
Siddarth Gupta and Hashmat Popat

Chapter 18 **Management of Complex Root Canal Curvature of Bilateral Radix Entomolaris: Three-Dimensional Analysis with Cone Beam Computed Tomography**.....84
Muktishree Mahendra, Anand Verma, Sanjeev Tyagi, Santosh Singh, Kapil Malviya, and Ramit Chaddha

Chapter 19 **Hutchinson-Gilford Progeria Syndrome: A Rare Genetic Disorder**.....88
Rajat G. Panigrahi, Antarmayee Panigrahi, Poornima Vijayakumar, Priyadarshini Choudhury, Sanat K. Bhuyan, Ruchi Bhuyan, G. Maragathavalli, and Abhishek Ranjan Pati

Chapter 20 **Management of Root Fracture: A Novel, Noninvasive Treatment Approach**.....92
M. S. Rangareddy, Archana Daga, Y. Vishnu Vardhan, and M. Daneswari

Chapter 21 **Orthokeratinized Odontogenic Cyst: A Report of three Clinical Cases**.....98
María del Carmen González Galván, Abel García-García, Eduardo Anitua-Aldecoa, Rafael Martinez-Conde Llamosas, and José Manuel Aguirre-Urizar

Chapter 22 **Multiple Supplemental Supernumerary Premolars: Unusual Presentation in a Nonsyndrome Patient**.....102
Ashwini Ramakrishna and Kiran B. Rajashekarappa

Chapter 23 **Transmigration of Mandibular Canines**.....105
N. Umashree, Avinash Kumar, and Tejavathi Nagaraj

Chapter 24 **Dentinal Dysplasia Type I: A Case Report with a 6-Year Followup**.....112
Sezin Ozer, Bora Ozden, Feyza Otan Ozden, and Kaan Gunduz

Chapter 25 **Computer Guided Implantology Accuracy and Complications**.....115
Vincenzo Bruno, Mauro Badino, Francesco Riccitiello, Gianrico Spagnuolo, and Massimo Amato

Chapter 26 **Multidisciplinary Management of a Fused Tooth**.....121
Derya Demircioglu Guler, Emine Sen Tunc, Nursel Arici, and Nilüfer Ozkan

Chapter 27 **Sinus Lift and Transantral Approach to Root Fragment Removal**.....126
Andrea Enrico Borgonovo, Federica Rizza, Adele Dudaite, Rachele Censi, and Dino Re

Chapter 28 **Idiopathic Orofacial Granulomatosis with Varied Clinical Presentation**.....131
Rathy Ravindran and Anila Karunakaran

Chapter 29 **Intraductal Papilloma: Atypical Presentation**.....134
P. Ramaswamy, Tanya Khaitan, A. Anuradha, B. Praveen Kumar, and S. Sudhakar

Chapter 30 **Dental Treatments under the General Anesthesia in a Child with Keratitis, Ichthyosis, and Deafness Syndrome**.....137
Sera Sımsek Derelioglu, Yücel Yılmaz, and Sultan Keles

Chapter 31 **True Generalized Microdontia and Hypodontia with Spondyloepiphyseal Dysplasia**.....143
Anita Singhal, Parul Singhal, Ranjan Gupta, and Kush Dev Jarial

Chapter 32 **Nonsyndromic Facial Asymmetry with Unilateral Condylar Aplasia**.....147
Ranganadh Nallamothu, Rama Mohan Kodali, N. Koteswara Rao, Leela krishna Guttikonda, and U. Vijayalakshmi

Chapter 33 **Papilliferous Keratoameloblastoma: An Extremely Rare Case Report**.....151
Neeta Mohanty, Varun Rastogi, Satya Ranjan Misra, and Susant Mohanty

Chapter 34 **Histological Features and Biocompatibility of Bone and Soft Tissue Substitutes in the Atrophic Alveolar Ridge Reconstruction**.....155
Carlo Maiorana, Mario Beretta, Davide Rancitelli, Giovanni Battista Grossi, Marco Cicciù, and Alan Scott Herford

Chapter 35 **Management of Grossly Decayed Mandibular Molar with Different Designs of Split Cast Post and Core**.....162
Rashmi Bansal, Nakul Mehrotra, Priyanka Chowdhary, and Anuraag Gurtu

Chapter 36 **Management of Oehler's Type III Dens Invaginatus using Cone Beam Computed Tomography**.....168
Jaya Ranganathan, Mohan Kumar Rangarajan Sundaresan, and Srinivasan Ramasamy

Chapter 37 **Implant-Prosthetic Rehabilitation in Bilateral Agenesis of Maxillary Lateral Incisors with a Mini Split Crest**.....174
M. M. Figliuzzi, A. Giudice, S. Pileggi, D. Pacifico, M. Marrelli, M. Tatullo, and L. Fortunato

Chapter 38 **Adalimumab: Another Medication Related to Osteonecrosis of the Jaws?................................180**
Andrea Cassoni, Umberto Romeo, Valentina Terenzi, Marco Della Monaca, Oriana Rajabtork Zadeh, Ingrid Raponi, Maria Teresa Fadda, Antonella Polimeni, and Valentino Valentini

Chapter 39 **Mucoepidermoid Carcinoma in a Minor Salivary Gland in a Child..186**
Fatih Sengul, Sera Simsek, and Binali Cakur

Chapter 40 **Complex Odontoma: A Case Report with Micro-Computed Tomography Findings..190**
L. A. N. Santos, L. J. Lopes, G. D. Roque-Torres, V. F. Oliveira, and D. Q. Freitas

Chapter 41 **A New Multi-Ingredient Recipe for the Treatment of Localized Advanced Periodontal Disease following the Surgical Removal of Impacted Wisdom Teeth..196**
Nabil Khzam, Adam Fell, Anthony Fisher, Paul Kim, Usman A. Khan, and Mahmoud M. Bakr

Chapter 42 **Radiographic Follow-up during Orthodontic Treatment for Early Diagnosis of Sequential Supernumerary Teeth...200**
Selma Sano Suga, Paula de Castro Kruly, Talissa Mayer Garrido, Marise Sano Suga Matumoto, Uhana Seifert Guimarães Suga, and Raquel Sano Suga Terada

Chapter 43 **Clinical and Radiological Findings of Autosomal Dominant Osteopetrosis Type II..206**
Priyanka Kant, Neelkamal Sharda, and Rahul R. Bhowate

Chapter 44 **Recurrent Monostotic Fibrous Dysplasia in the Mandible..214**
Nilton Alves, Reinaldo José de Oliveira, Denise Takehana and Naira Figueiredo Deana

Chapter 45 **Treatment of Class II Division 2 Malocclusion using the Forsus Fatigue Resistance Device and 5-Year Follow-up...220**
Ezgi Atik, and Ilken Kocadereli

Permissions

List of Contributors

Index

Preface

This book has been a concerted effort by a group of academicians, researchers and scientists, who have contributed their research works for the realization of the book. This book has materialized in the wake of emerging advancements and innovations in this field. Therefore, the need of the hour was to compile all the required researches and disseminate the knowledge to a broad spectrum of people comprising of students, researchers and specialists of the field.

Dentistry is the branch of medicine that studies and treats diseases of the oral cavity. It also encompasses the disorders of the maxillofacial area. The advancement in science and technology has resulted in a better understanding of oral diseases and new and improved methods for treatment which have been discussed herein. This book on oral healthcare and dentistry is a compilation of various specialties that fall under the broader category of dentistry. It aims to provide an extensive elaboration of the various treatments available and used across the world to treat oral disorders. It aims to serve as a resource guide for students and experts alike and contribute to the growth of the discipline.

At the end of the preface, I would like to thank the authors for their brilliant chapters and the publisher for guiding us all-through the making of the book till its final stage. Also, I would like to thank my family for providing the support and encouragement throughout my academic career and research projects.

Editor

1

An Insight into the Genesis of Hypohidrotic Ectodermal Dysplasia in a Case Report

Kiran Kumar,[1] Devi Charan Shetty,[1] Mahima Dua,[2] Amit Dua,[3] and Raghu Dhanapal[1]

[1] *Department of Oral & Maxillofacial Pathology, I.T.S-CDSR, Muradnagar, Ghaziabad 201206, India*
[2] *Department of Oral & Maxillofacial Pathology, Inderprastha Dental College, Sahibabad, Ghaziabad 201010, India*
[3] *Department of Prosthodontics, Krishna Dental College, Mohannagar, Ghaziabad 201206, India*

Correspondence should be addressed to Mahima Dua, mahima.dua@gmail.com

Academic Editors: S. Anil and M. A. Polack

Hypohidrotic (anhidrotic) ectodermal dysplasia (HED) is a congenital syndrome characterized by sparse hair, oligodontia, and reduced sweating. It is estimated to affect at least one in 17000 people worldwide. We report a rare case of HED in a 14-year-old male child patient which extraorally manifested as alopecia, scanty eyebrow and eye lashes, frontal bossing, depressed nasal bridge, and full and everted lips. Intraoral examination revealed complete anodontia of the deciduous teeth and partial anodontia of the permanent teeth. It is usually inherited as an X-linked recessive trait caused by mutation in any of the three EDA pathway genes. X-linked and autosomal recessive forms are phenotypically similar; thus, identification of carriers of partial forms of the disorder in their families is the key to clarifying intrafamilial genetic transmission.

1. Introduction

Ectodermal dysplasia (ED) syndrome is a rare heterogeneous group of inherited disorders that share primary defects in the development of two or more tissues derived from ectoderm. These tissues primarily are the skin, hair, nails, eccrine glands, and teeth [1, 2]. Charles Darwin first documented the earliest accessible account of ectodermal dysplasia in English as early as 1840s. However, in the mid-19th century, it appeared that nobody understood the sex-linked inheritance and it was not until 1910 that this began to be understood [3]. To date, more than 150 distinctive syndromes have been described with all possible modes of inheritance. The most common syndromes within this group are hypohidrotic (anhidrotic) ED and hidrotic ED [1, 2].

Hypohidrotic ED (also known as Christ-Siemens-Touraine syndrome) is the most common phenotype [4]. Hypohidrotic (anhidrotic) ectodermal dysplasia (HED) is a congenital syndrome characterized by sparse hair, oligodontia, and reduced sweating [5]. Dental manifestations include conical or pegged teeth, hypodontia or complete anodontia, and delayed eruption of permanent teeth.

It is usually inherited as an X-linked recessive trait [4]. It is caused by mutations in any of the three EDA pathway genes: ectodysplasin (EDA), EDAR, and EDARADD which encode a ligand, a receptor, and an intracellular signal mediator of a single linear pathway, respectively. In rare cases, HED is associated with immune deficiency caused by mutations in further downstream components of the EDA pathway that are necessary for the activation of the transcription factor NF-kappa b [5].

Morbidity and mortality are related to the absence or presence of eccrine and mucous glands [4]. Children with decreased sweating may have a mortality rate of up to 30% in infancy or early childhood because of intermittent hyperpyrexia [6]. No definite pharmacological treatment is available, and the management of affected patients depends on which structures are involved [4]. Patients with HED are advised light clothing, a cool-water spray bottle, air conditioning for environment, use of artificial tears, and application of petrolatum jelly for nasal mucosa protection [7]. Orthodontic treatment may be indicated for cosmetic reasons and to ensure adequate nutritional intake [7–9].

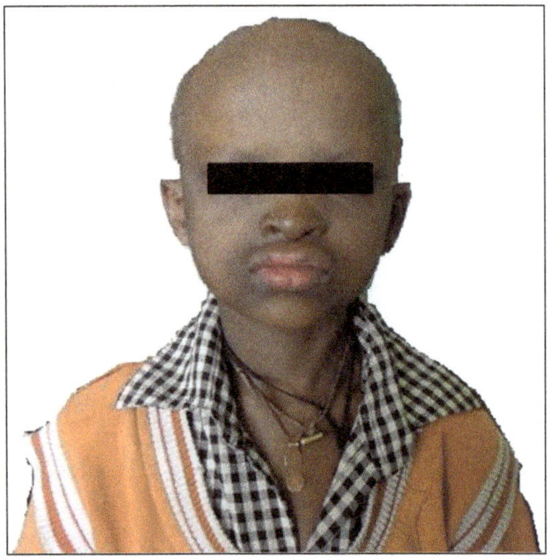

Figure 1: Photomicrograph showing fine, sparse scalp hair, scanty eyebrow and eye lashes, frontal bossing or depressed nasal bridge, and full and everted lips.

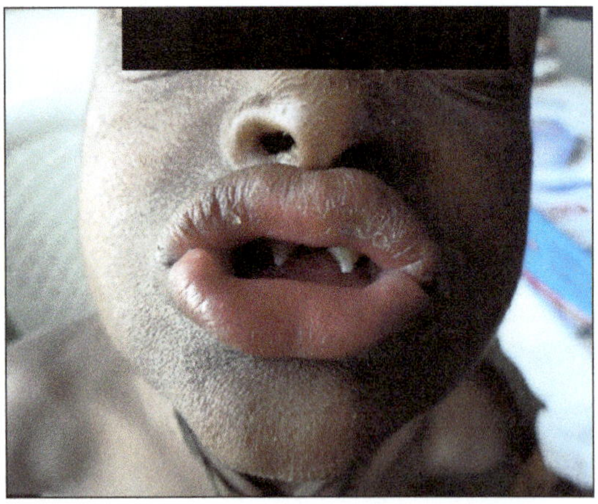

Figure 2: Photograph showing extraorally dry and eczematous rash on skin and intraorally conical shaped maxillary central incisors and a wide midline diastema and hypoplastic labial frenum.

2. Case Report

A 14-year-old male child patient reported to the department of Oral & Maxillofacial Pathology with a chief complaint of absence of teeth since birth. His parents stated that he had difficulty in speaking and eating. He also had repeated episodes of unexplained hyperpyrexia. No contributory medical, family, or personal history was elucidated.

On extraoral examination, patient presented with fine, sparse scalp hair, scanty eyebrow and eye lashes, frontal bossing, depressed nasal bridge, and full and everted lips (Figure 1), Dry eczematous (atopic) rash was seen on the face (Figure 2).

Intraoral examination revealed complete anodontia of the deciduous teeth and partial anodontia of the permanent. There was complete absence of mandibular teeth and partial anodontia in the maxillary arch. Teeth that were present were 11, 16, 21, and 26, widely spaced and pointed. Maxillary central incisors were conical shaped (Figure 2).

Soft tissue examination revealed a wide midline diastema and hypoplastic labial frenum (Figure 2).

Laboratory investigation shows that HED is diagnosed after infancy on the basis of physical features in most affected individuals. Carrier detection for X-linked HED was done by assessing the distribution and mosaic patterns of sweat pore function by the use of an iodine solution to assess sweat gland function or impression materials to assess number and distribution of sweat pores. The carriers for X-linked HED show this pattern, and 60% to 80% of carriers display some degree of hypodontia.

The mode of inheritance was further determined by family history. Diagnosis was confirmed by skin biopsy, which revealed thin and flattened epidermis, reduction in the number, and presence of rudimentary eccrine sweat glands.

Molecular genetic testing is clinically available for all three genes. Other newer methods are preimplantation genetic diagnosis (PGD) which is a means of detecting a specific genetic mutation within an embryo before it is transferred to the womb and forms a pregnancy. As the risk of having a child with a serious chromosomal abnormality increases significantly as you get older and this can be performed earlier, around the 11th week of pregnancy, CVS is preferred over amniocentesis

Treatment plan was emollient with topical steroid for his eczematous rash. Neither soap nor any perfumed bath additives, including baby bath products, were advised as these all have a drying effect and are irritating to the skin which may be sensitive. During the summer months individuals with fair skin should use a high factor sun block at all times, preferably one for sensitive skin. Cotton clothes next to the skin and cotton bedclothes were advisable.

3. Discussion

HED or anhidrotic ectodermal dysplasia is the most common syndrome among this large group of hereditary disorders. Hypohidrosis, hypotrichosis and hypodontia constitute the main symptoms of the syndrome [10]. HED affects at least one in 17000 people worldwide [10]. In the hypohidrotic form, the skin is soft, thin, and dry. The sebaceous glands are also defective or absent [11, 12]. Palms and soles are hyperkeratotic; pseudorhagades are present around the eyes. In the oral cavity, the most striking feature is oligodontia. The teeth that are present have abnormal crown form. Teeth in the anterior region of maxilla and mandible are conical in shape [12, 13]. There are a wide midline diastema and hypoplastic labial frenum in autosomal recessive condition where there is a total absence of permanent teeth with or without taurodontism of primary molars [14]. The characteristic facial features are frontal bossing, depressed nasal bridge, prominent supraorbital ridges, prominent and obliquely set ears, midface is depressed, the lower third of the face appears small due to lack of alveolar bone development, and lips are protuberant [11, 15]. A cephalometric study by Vierucci and coworkers [16] has shown that children with hypohidrotic type ectodermal dysplasia showed maxillary retrusion due to sagittally under developed maxilla, forward and upward displacement of the mandible, and collapsed lower anterior facial height [16]. The presentation of thin eyebrows, fine, stiff, and short scalp hair, scanty eyelashes and eyebrows, and partial anodontia observed in our case is in agreement with the existing literature.

The gene responsible for X-linked HED is localized at Xq12-q13.1 and affects a transmembrane protein expressed by keratinocytes, hair follicles, and sweat glands, possibly having a key role in epithelial-mesenchymal signaling [17]. Two different ways of transmission of the disorder are known. Along with the more common X-linked recessive modality of transmission, a less frequent autosomal recessive one has been demonstrated [18]. In X-linked HED, the affected patients are most often hemizygous male subjects. Autosomal recessive HED is similar to the hemizygous form of X-linked HED from the clinical point of view except that males and females are equally affected. A gene responsible for autosomal HED has recently been mapped to chromosome 2q11-q13 [18].

The molecular pathogenesis of hypohidrotic ectodermal dysplasia (HED) is poorly understood. The gene responsible for X-linked HED, EDA, produces ectodysplasin-A, a protein that is important for normal development of ectodermal appendages including hair, teeth, and sweat glands. Evidence is accumulating that ectodysplasin-A is important in several pathways that involve ectodermal-mesodermal interactions during embryogenesis. Defects in the molecular structure of ectodysplasin-A may inhibit the action of enzymes necessary for normal development of the ectoderm and/or its interaction with the underlying mesoderm [19].

The protein encoded by *EDARADD* is similar to the death domain, MyD88, a cytoplasmic transducer of Toll/interleukin receptor signaling [20]. It also contains a Traf-binding consensus sequence. It is coexpressed with tumor necrosis factor receptor superfamily member EDAR in epithelial cells during the formation of hair follicles and teeth. It interacts with the death domain of EDAR and links the receptor to signaling pathways downstream [19].

Abnormal gene product: *EDARADD* mutations alter the charge of an amino acid in the resultant gene, rendering it incapable of performing its function [19].

Even though X-linked and autosomal recessive forms are phenotypically similar, identification of the way of transmission is mandatory to give reliable genetic counseling to the family and to address molecular studies. Complete examination of relatives of patients with HED and identification of carriers of partial forms of the disorder in their families are the key to clarifying intrafamilial genetic transmission [21]. No similar case of ectodermal dysplasia has been identified among the relatives, which suggests that the propositus was probably a fresh mutation or due to translocation of genes as was suggested in a few other literature [22].

DNA, being the prime source for diagnosis, should be stored (typically extracted from white blood cells) for possible future use which is known as DNA banking. It is likely that testing methodology and our understanding of genes, mutations, and diseases will improve in the future, and consideration should be given to banking DNA of affected individuals [19].

4. Conclusion

In developed countries diagnosis pertains to laboratory identification of genes [23] and mode of inheritance of mutant genes associated with recessively X chromosome or autosomal dominant or recessive. It is to be considered that an absence of a positive family history should not be a factor in causing any diagnostic dilemmas with respect to ectodermal dysplasia, a condition that shows multiple modes of inheritance.

References

[1] A. A. Weech, "Hereditary ectodermal dysplasia (congenital ectodermal defect)," *American Journal of Diseases of Children*, vol. 37, pp. 766–790, 1929.

[2] L. M. Solomon and E. J. Keuer, "The ectodermal dysplasias. Problems of classification and some newer syndromes," *Archives of Dermatology*, vol. 116, no. 11, pp. 1295–1299, 1980.

[3] D. Perry, Living with x-linked hypohidrotic ectodermal Dysplasia. Ectodermal Dysplasia Society, 108 Charlton Lane, Cheltenham, Glos. GL53 9EA. England.

[4] A. Ul Bari and S. B. Rahman, "Hypohidrotic ectodermal dysplasia: a case report and literature review," *Journal of Pakistan Association of Dermatologists*, vol. 17, no. 1, pp. 52–55, 2007.

[5] M. L. Mikkola, "Molecular aspects of hypohidrotic ectodermal dysplasia," *American Journal of Medical Genetics A*, vol. 149, no. 9, pp. 2031–2036, 2009.

[6] D. Berg, D. H. Weingold, K. G. Abson, and E. A. Olsen, "Sweating in ectodermal dysplasia syndromes. A review," *Archives of Dermatology*, vol. 126, no. 8, pp. 1075–1079, 1990.

[7] P. J. Dhanrajani and A. O. Jiffry, "Management of ectodermal dysplasia: a literature review," *Dental Update*, vol. 25, no. 2, pp. 73–75, 1998.

[8] M. J. Till and A. P. Marques, "Ectodermal dysplasia: treatment considerations and case reports," *Northwest Dentistry*, vol. 71, no. 3, pp. 25–28, 1992.

[9] I. P. Sweeney, J. W. Ferguson, A. A. Heggie, and J. O. Lucas, "Treatment outcomes for adolescent ectodermal dysplasia patients treated with dental implants," *International Journal of Paediatric Dentistry*, vol. 15, no. 4, pp. 241–248, 2005.

[10] G. Varghese and P. Sathyan, "Hypohidrotic ectodermal dysplasia—a case study," *Oral & Maxillofacial Pathology Journal*, vol. 2, article 1, 2011.

[11] B. S. Suprabha, "Hereditary ectodermal dysplasia: a case report," *Journal of the Indian Society of Pedodontics and Preventive Dentistry*, vol. 20, no. 1, pp. 37–40, 2002.

[12] P. J. M. Crawford, M. J. Aldred, and A. Clarke, "Clinical and radiographic dental findings in X linked hypohidrotic ectodermal dysplasia," *Journal of Medical Genetics*, vol. 28, no. 3, pp. 181–185, 1991.

[13] S. N. Ramraje, M. Wasnik, and Y. A. Momin, "Anhidrotic ectodermal dysplasia—a report of two cases," *Bombay Hospital Journal*, vol. 5, article 12, 2009.

[14] R. Rajendran and B. Sivapathasundaram, *Shafer's Textbook of Oral Pathology*, Saunders, Philadelphia, Pa, USA, 5th edition, 1983.

[15] R. M. Shaw, "Prosthetic management of hypohydrotic ectodermal dysplasia with anodontia. Case report," *Australian Dental Journal*, vol. 35, no. 2, pp. 113–116, 1990.

[16] S. Vierucci, T. Baccetti, and I. Tollaro, "Dental and craniofacial findings in hypohidrotic ectodermal dysplasia during the primary dentition phase," *The Journal of Clinical Pediatric Dentistry*, vol. 18, no. 4, pp. 291–297, 1994.

[17] J. Kere, A. K. Srivastava, O. Montonen et al., "X-linked anhidrotic (hypohidrotic) ectodermal dysplasia is caused by mutation in a novel transmembrane protein," *Nature Genetics*, vol. 13, no. 4, pp. 409–416, 1996.

[18] F. Munoz, G. Lestringant, V. Sybert et al., "Definitive evidence for an autosomal recessive form of hypohidrotic ectodermal dysplasia clinically indistinguishable from the more common X-linked disorder," *American Journal of Human Genetics*, vol. 61, no. 1, pp. 94–100, 1997.

[19] J. T. Wright, D. K. Grange, and M. K. Richter, *Hypohidrotic Ectodermal Dysplasia*, University of Washington, Seattle, Wash, USA, 1993.

[20] D. J. Headon, S. A. Emmal, B. M. Ferguson et al., "Gene defect in ectodermal dysplasia implicates a death domain adapter in development," *Nature*, vol. 414, no. 6866, pp. 913–916, 2001.

[21] S. Cambiaghi, L. Restano, K. Pääkkönen, R. Caputo, and J. Kere, "Clinical findings in mosaic carriers of hypohidrotic ectodermal dysplasia," *Archives of Dermatology*, vol. 136, no. 2, pp. 217–224, 2000.

[22] J. Sharma and G. P. Mamatha, "Hereditary ectodermal dysplasia: diagnostic dilemmas," *Revista de Clínica e Pesquisa Odontológica*, vol. 4, no. 1, pp. 35–40, 2008.

[23] A. Kumar, M. T. Eby, S. Sinha, A. Jasmin, and P. M. Chaudhary, "The ectodermal dysplasia receptor activates the nuclear factor-κB, JNK, and cell death pathways and binds to ectodysplasin A," *Journal of Biological Chemistry*, vol. 276, no. 4, pp. 2668–2677, 2001.

2

A Case of Old Calcifying Epithelioma Processed Symptomless over 40 Years

Shinji Yamaguchi, Madoka Inui, Takashi Takeoka, Kenya Okumura, and Toshiro Tagawa

Department of Oral and Maxillofacial Surgery, Department of Clinical Sciences, Medical Life Sciences, Mie University, Graduate School of Medicine, 2-174 Edobashi, Tsu, Mie 514-8507, Japan

Correspondence should be addressed to Shinji Yamaguchi; sy1016-1984@clin.medic.mie-u.ac.jp

Academic Editors: S. R. Watt-Smith, E. F. Wright, and K. H. Zawawi

Calcifying epithelioma, a benign tumor derived from the hair apparatus and consisted of hair matrix cells, is relatively prevalent in females. We report a case of right preauricular calcifying epithelioma that was incidentally detected at the examination of multiple facial fractures and became an old lesion without symptoms for 40 years. The patient who was a 42-year-old male visited our department for the first time in October 2011 with a chief complaint of multiple facial fractures. Radiographic imaging demonstrated fracture lines at the anterior and posterior walls of the left maxillary sinus and zygomatic arch and revealed a mass at a right preauricular area. The extraction was performed under general anaesthesia. No recurrence has been observed 15 months after surgery. We also reviewed the literature of calcifying epithelioma.

1. Introduction

Calcifying epithelioma, a benign tumor derived from the hair apparatus and consisted of hair matrix cells, is relatively prevalent in females. It often develops on the face, neck, and upper limbs in the youth and is palpable as a hard nodule under the skin. Pathologically, it is mostly consisted of eosinophils and shadow cells, and the proportion of shadow cells increases over time, which leads to calcification and osteogenesis [1].

Although there are a number of reports on this tumor from the dermatology, reporting from the oral and maxillofacial region is relatively rare. We here report a case of calcifying epithelioma that was incidentally detected at the examination of multiple facial fractures and became an old lesion without symptoms for 40 years.

2. Case

A 42-year-old male visited our department for the first time in October 2011 with a chief complaint of multiple facial fractures. He had no past history or family history. As for the present history, he fell down from a bicycle and was hit severely in his left face in October 2011. He visited a nearby general hospital and was diagnosed with facial fractures. Then, he was referred to our department.

Radiographic imaging demonstrated fracture lines at the anterior and posterior walls of the left maxillary sinus and zygomatic arch and revealed a mass at a right preauricular area, well delineated radiopaque (Figure 1).

History taking revealed that his mother had noticed the mass when he was three years old, but there was no symptom. Since he hoped extraction, the right preauricular mass was resected at the same time with reduction and fixation of multiple facial fractures under general anesthesia.

General physical examination revealed average body constitution with excellent nutritious status and no abnormality. Extraoral findings revealed a depression at the cheek on the left, anesthesia, and palpebral subconjunctival hemorrhage on the left, but there was no motility disorder of the left eyeball, double vision, or occlusal deviation. A bone-like hard mass about 10 mm in size was palpable subcutaneously at the right preauricular area. The mass was well delineated without adhesion to the adjacent tissue. The surface of the skin

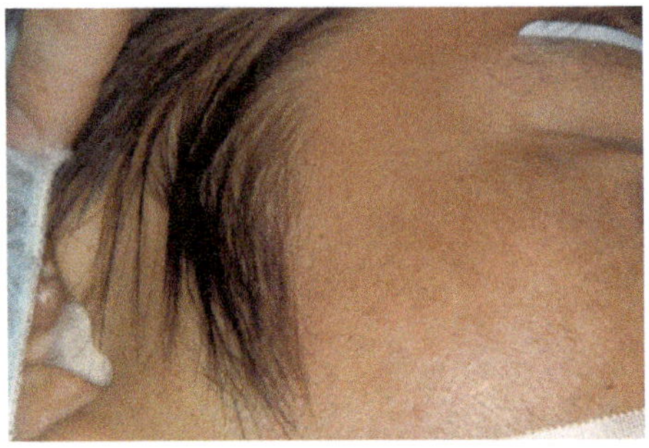

Figure 1: Revealed mass at the right preauricular area.

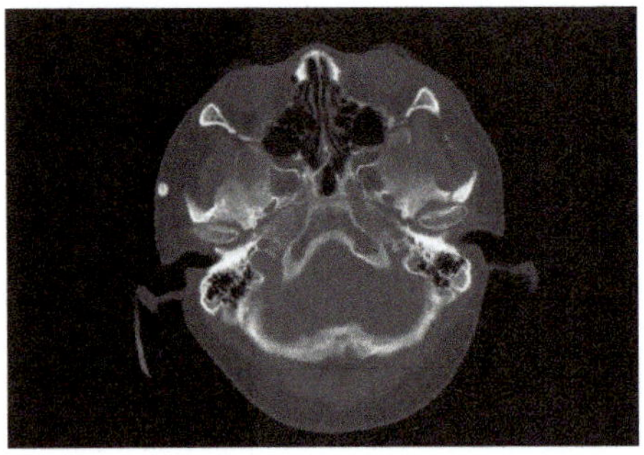

Figure 2: A bone-like hard mass about 10 mm in size was palpable subcutaneously at the right preauricular area.

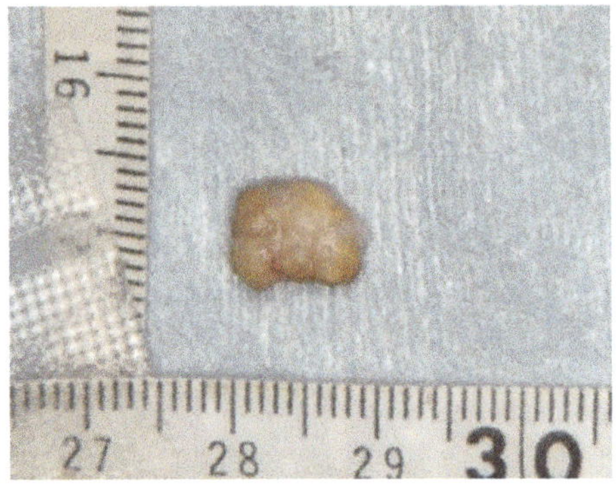

Figure 3: The excised specimen was hard and yellowish white 10 × 9 mm in size, and the cross section showed a coarse and bone-like surface.

Figure 4: Dental X-rays showed an image of patchy calcification in the mass.

showed a healthy color, and the mass developed no symptom or growing tendency from the childhood (Figure 2).

In the oral cavity, there was no abnormal finding, and the excretion and nature of saliva were normal.

Tentative diagnosis of maxillary fracture and preauricular benign tumor was made, and the right preauricular mass was resected at the same time with open reduction and fixation of multiple left facial fractures. A horizontal skin incision was made about 1 cm from the top of the mass, and the mass was dissected from the adjacent tissue. The mass had no adhesion with the adjacent tissue, and it was resected *en bloc*.

The resected specimen was hard and yellowish white 10 × 9 mm in size, and the cross section showed a coarse and bone-like surface (Figure 3). Dental X-rays showed an image of patchy calcification in the mass (Figure 4).

3. Pathological Findings

Aggregation of shadow cells and surrounded bone tissue were observed. At the stroma, multinuclear giant cells are sparsely observed, and there was no infiltration of eosinophils. Old calcifying epithelioma with ossification was diagnosed (Figures 5(a) and 5(b)).

4. Discussion

Calcifying epithelioma, mostly consisted of eosinophils, shadow cells, and transitional cells, exhibits a variety of images of calcareous deposits, bone formation, foreign-body giant cells, and melanin deposits. It is known that the component ratio of eosinophils to shadow cells in this tumor changes as disease stages advance and tumor parenchyma is rich in eosinophils at the early stage, whereas shadow cells are predominant in the old tumor with almost no eosinophil infiltration [2, 3]. Moreover, the tumor is characterized by calcification, but calcification is not always accompanied. Calcification is mostly observed in shadow cells, and it is considered dystrophic calcification associated with degeneration and necrosis of shadow cells [1].

We experienced a case of calcifying epithelioma that was incidentally detected as a circle-like radiopaque finding by CT in a patient with multiple facial fractures and diagnosed by history taking as an old lesion without symptoms for about 40 years. The prognosis of the tumor is generally excellent, but recurrent cases have been reported [1, 4], and malignant change after repeated recurrences has also been reported [5, 6]. In our case, despite a short postoperative follow-up period of about fifteen months, no recurrence has been observed.

Moehlenbeck [7] mentioned that this tumor occurred at younger than 10 years old in more than 40% of 900 cases examined at the dermatology department, and patients developed symptoms in their 30s or at younger age in more than 60% with an average period of 4.4 years from appearance to extraction. Cases without symptoms for a long time, such as this case for 40 years, are rare.

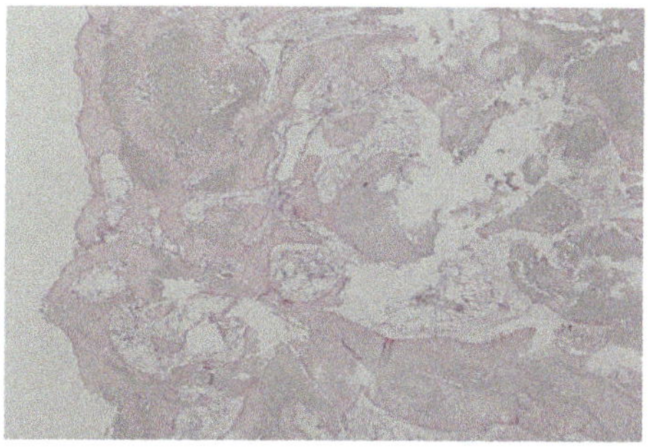

(a)

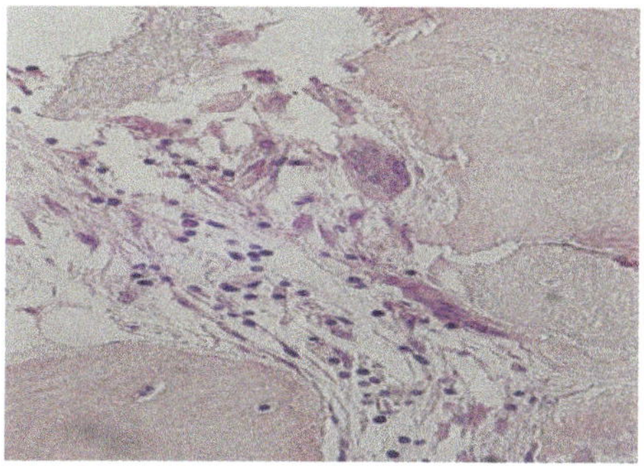

(b)

FIGURE 5: Pathological findings 1 (H-E, ×40 and 400): aggregation of shadow cells and surrounded bone tissue were observed. At the stroma, multinuclear giant cells are sparsely observed, and there was no infiltration of eosinophils. Old calcifying epithelioma with ossification was diagnosed.

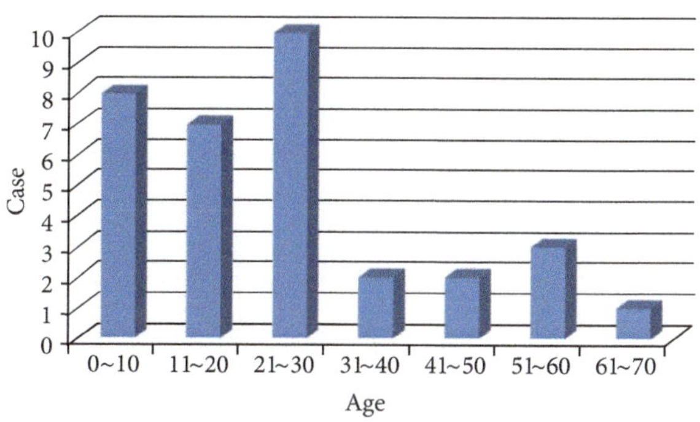

FIGURE 6

In Japan, 33 cases of calcifying epithelioma in the oral and maxillofacial region were reported between 1978 and 2012 including our case [2–4, 8–24]. The age distributed from 4 to 68 years old, and the average age was 23.8 years. The most frequent site of occurrence is periauricular in 18 cases, followed by the cheek in 8, neck in 5, and angle of the mandible in 2. Disease duration ranged from 1 month to 40 years with the average of 5.8 years. The tumor diameter ranged from 4 mm to 50 mm with the average of 22.1 mm (Table 1, Figures 6 and 7).

Pathologically, there were 9 cases with only shadow cells without eosinophils, 13 with bone formation, and 17

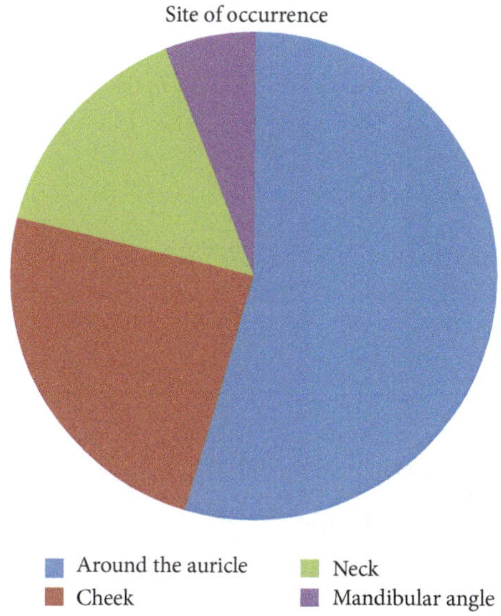

FIGURE 7

with giant cells, while there were only 3 cases with only shadow cells accompanied by bone formation and giant cells, including our case.

Then, we focused on the occurrence of the tumor and the period of its presence *in vivo*. However, since it is impossible to clearly determine the period of its presence *in vivo*, it was examined how the duration from the time when a mass was noticed to extraction (disease duration) was associated with the proportion of eosinophils to shadow cells and the presence or absence of bone formation and giant cells. The average disease duration was 13.9 years in cases with only shadow cells, while it was 2.7 years in cases with both eosinophils and shadow cells, and it was significantly longer in the former cases ($P < 0.01$). With regard to osteogenesis, the average disease duration was 11.5 years in cases with bone formation, while it was 0.8 years in cases without it, and it was significantly longer in the former cases ($P < 0.001$). The average disease duration was 4.0 years in cases with giant cells, while it was 7.1 years without them, and there was no significant difference between the former and latter cases.

Taken together, the present case with only shadow cells and bone formation was considered an old one. Bone formation is thought to appear subsequent to calcification [1], and Anneroth and Sigurdson mentioned that giant cells were osteoclast-type cells without phagocytic capacity in giant cell epulis and the stroma was rich in fibroblasts and osteoblasts, which differentiated into bone and osteoid tissue, eventually forming bone [25].

Since dye affinity changed from eosinophilic to basophilic properties in the parenchyma just beneath the osteoclast-like multinuclear giant cells around the edge of the calcified tumor parenchyma, Miyahara et al. reported that the edge of the calcified layer was decalcified and subsequently osteoblasts were induced to form bone, and a mechanism similar to general bone remodeling was present even in ectopic osteogenesis [24].

TABLE 1

Case	Reporter	Reported year	Age	Sex	Region	Duration that the patients lived with symptoms (year)	Pathological findings	Bone formation	Giant cells	Tumor diameter (mm)
1	Suzuki	1978	12	F	Around the right auricle	1.67	Eosinophils + shadow cells	−	+	45 × 25 × 30
2	Goto	1983	6	M	Around the left auricle	0.5	Eosinophils + shadow cells	−	+	28 × 25 × 5
3	Daito	1985	27	M	Left parotid masseteric	0.17	Eosinophils + shadow cells	−	+	70 × 45 × 25
4	Aoki	1987	8	F	Right cheek	0.5	Eosinophils + shadow cells	−	+	11 × 17 × 13
5	Kurachi	1989	4	M	Right cheek	1	Shadow cell only	−	+	4 × 5 × 8
6	Hasegawa	1992	5	M	Left cheek	1	Eosinophils + shadow cells	−	+	20 × 15 × 9
7	Katsuyama	1995	7	F	Left mandibular angle	0.67	Shadow cell only	−	−	22 × 16
8	Ashiyama	1995	7	M	Right cheek	5	Eosinophils + shadow cells	−	+	20 × 12 × 12
9	Nishimura	1996	52	M	Left neck	0.08	Eosinophils + shadow cells	−	−	10 × 8
10	Nobumori	2002	5	F	Left cheek	0.08	Eosinophils + shadow cells	−	−	5 × 5
11	Suzuki	2004	56	M	Right mandibular angle	1	Eosinophils + shadow cells	−	+	20 × 10 × 10
12	Fujita	2005	24	M	Around the right auricle	0.08	Eosinophils + shadow cells	−	+	12 × 10
13	Fujita	2005	29	M	Left cheek	0.08	Eosinophils + shadow cells	−	+	20 × 20
14	Fujita	2005	13	M	Left neck	0.08	Eosinophils + shadow cells	−	+	15 × 10
15	Fujita	2005	21	M	Around the right auricle	0.17	Eosinophils + shadow cells	−	+	39 × 32
16	Miyahara	2007	68	F	Right cheek	0.5	Eosinophils + shadow cells	−	−	18 × 18
17	Miyahara	2007	20	F	Left neck	0.67	Eosinophils + shadow cells	−	+	21 × 22
18	Miyahara	2007	12	F	Around the right auricle	1	Eosinophils + shadow cells	−	−	15 × 13 × 6
19	Miyahara	2007	4	F	Left neck	1	Eosinophils + shadow cells	−	−	15 × 20
20	Miyahara	2007	21	F	Left mandibular angle	1.5	Eosinophils + shadow cells	−	−	25 × 15
21	Hasegawa	1983	30	M	Right neck	20	Eosinophils + shadow cells	+	−	15 × 13 × 6
22	Kawaguchi	1983	22	F	Around the right auricle	4	Shadow cell only	+	+	7 × 7 × 6
23	Tanaka	1985	41	F	Around the right auricle	20	Eosinophils + shadow cells	+	−	19 × 22 × 7
24	Kamakura	1991	23	F	Around the right auricle	13	Shadow cell only	+	+	40 × 28 × 15
25	Takano	1993	59	F	Left parotid masseteric	30	Shadow cell only	+	−	30 × 20
26	Takano	1993	38	M	Left parotid masseteric	30	Shadow cell only	+	−	20 × 13 × 7
27	Tsukamoto	1994	12	F	Left parotid masseteric	0.25	Eosinophils + shadow cells	+	+	50 × 28
28	Nishimura	1996	11	F	Around the left auricle	8	Shadow cell only	+	−	10 × 8 × 7
29	Fujita	2005	23	F	Around the left auricle	0.08	Eosinophils + shadow cells	+	−	7 × 8
30	Fujita	2005	27	F	Around the left auricle	5	Eosinophils + shadow cells	+	−	14 × 20
31	Maejima	2006	37	M	Around the right auricle	0.08	Shadow cell only	+	−	26 × 26 × 15
32	Miyahara	2007	20	F	Around the right auricle	4	Eosinophils + shadow cells	+	−	20 × 13
33	Our patient	2011	43	M	Around the right auricle	40	Shadow cell only	+	+	10 × 9

In the present case, disease duration and formation of giant cells and bone were discussed with references, but no giant cell was observed in any case at the early stage. Therefore, it was speculated that the component proportion of eosinophils to shadow cells changed as disease stages advanced, and as shadow cells became predominant, giant cells appeared in the stroma, which promoted osteogenesis subsequently to calcification.

In conclusions, we reported a case of calcifying epithelioma that became an old lesion without symptoms for 40 years. In 33 cases reported in our country from the oral and maxillofacial region, including our case, pathological characteristics and disease duration were compared by clinical statistics.

References

[1] R. Forbis and E. B. Helwig, "Pilomatrixoma (calcifying epithelioma)," *Archives of Dermatology*, vol. 83, no. 4, pp. 606–618, 1961.

[2] K. Fujita, H. Harada, S. Hasegawa, H. Imai, Y. Kabasawa, K. Morita et al., "Clinicopathological study of calcifying epithelioma in the head and neck region," *Journal of Oral and Maxillofacial Surgery*, vol. 51, pp. 285–290, 2006 (Japanese).

[3] N. Nishimura, S. Iida, M. Takeda, T. Sakai, H. Yamaoka, and T. Kimura, "Two cases of calcifying epithelioma arising at the periauricular region," *Journal of Oral and Maxillofacial Surgery*, vol. 42, pp. 693–695, 1996 (Japanese).

[4] K. Suzuki, K. Fujita, T. Nakashima, T. Tomikawa, K. Miyake, M. Masuda et al., "Case of calcifying epithelioma in the right subauricular region," *Journal of Oral and Maxillofacial Surgery*, vol. 24, pp. 619–622, 1978 (Japanese).

[5] S. Lopansri and M. C. Mihm, "Pilomatrix carcinoma or calcifying epitheliocarcinoma of Malherbe. A case report and review of literature," *Cancer*, vol. 45, no. 9, pp. 2368–2373, 1980.

[6] J. D. Van Der Walt and B. Rohlova, "Carcinomatous transformation in a pilomatrixoma," *American Journal of Dermatopathology*, vol. 6, no. 1, pp. 63–69, 1984.

[7] F. W. Moehlenbeck, "Pilomatrixoma (calcifying epithelioma) a statistical study," *Archives of Dermatology*, vol. 108, no. 4, pp. 532–534, 1973.

[8] M. Maejima, Y. Sato, and K. Masumoto, "Calcifying epithelioma arising in the subauricular region," *Journal of Oral and Maxillofacial Surgery*, vol. 19, no. 2, pp. 339–344, 2006 (Japanese).

[9] S. Suzuki, T. Takemoto, Y. Ishida, H. Inamoto, and Y. Kameyama, "A case of calcifying epithelioma due to traumatic injury in the submandibular region," *Journal of Japanese Society for Oral Mucous Membrane*, vol. 10, no. 2, pp. 36–40, 2004 (Japanese).

[10] M. Takano, K. Tominaga, H. Furusawa, Y. Kuga, A. Mizuno, Y. Shibata et al., "Two cases of calcifying epithelioma arising in the parotid-masseteric region," *Journal of Oral and Maxillofacial Surgery*, vol. 39, no. 12, pp. 88–90, 1993 (Japanese).

[11] S. Kamakura, R. Sato, Y. Fujita, K. Motegi, and K. Ohya, "Pilomatrixoma (calcifying epithelioma of Malhebe) in the right subauricular region," *Journal of Oral and Maxillofacial Surgery*, vol. 37, no. 5, pp. 1002–1006, 1991 (Japanese).

[12] M. Ashihara, K. Komatsu, R. Fukui, K. Nakayama, T. Akitaya, A. Narita et al., "Calcifying epithelioma in the right cheek region: report of a case," *Pediatric Oral and Maxillofacial Surgery*, vol. 5, pp. 105–108, 1995 (Japanese).

[13] T. Kazuyama, Y. Hayatsu, T. Tsuji, J. Hirayama, and F. Shinozaki, "A case of calcifying epithelioma in the cheek region," *Pediatric Oral and Maxillofacial Surgery*, vol. 5, pp. 80–83, 1995 (Japanese).

[14] T. Nobumori, Y. Itoh, K. Ohta, H. Tohmori, S. Inoue, M. Sugiyama et al., "A case of calcifying epithelioma of the cheek in a childhood," *Pediatric Oral and Maxillofacial Surgery*, vol. 12, pp. 29–32, 2002 (Japanese).

[15] G. Tsukamoto, A. Sasaki, and T. A. Matsumura, "Case of rapidly growing calcifying epithelioma in the parotidomasseteric region," *Journal of Oral and Maxillofacial Surgery*, vol. 40, no. 1, pp. 215–217, 1994.

[16] Y. Kurachi, H. Sakamaki, M. Manabe, R. Kamijo, M. Nagumo, Y. Kohno et al., "A case of calcifying epithelioma in the cheek region," *Journal of Oral and Maxillofacial Surgery*, vol. 35, pp. 176–182, 1989 (Japanese).

[17] H. Hasegawa and Y. Matsuzaki, "Calcifying epithelioma in the left cheek region: report of a case," *Journal of Oral and Maxillofacial Surgery*, vol. 38, no. 4, pp. 699–700, 1992.

[18] S. Aoki, M. Osada, R. Kawabe, S. Ono, and K. Fujita, "Calcifying epithelioma in the right cheek region: report og a case," *Journal of Oral and Maxillofacial Surgery*, vol. 33, no. 3, pp. 609–614, 1987 (Japanese).

[19] M. Tanaka, Y. Sangu, T. Takeuchi, H. Ogiuchi, and I. Kawanishi, "Calcifying epithelioma in the right subauricular region: report of a case," *Journal of Oral and Maxillofacial Surgery*, vol. 31, no. 6, pp. 1483–1486, 1985 (Japanese).

[20] T. Kawaguchi, K. Kodama, and A. Taen, "Calcifying epithelioma in the left subauricular region: report of a case," *Journal of Oral and Maxillofacial Surgery*, vol. 29, no. 9, pp. 1661–1666, 1983 (Japanese).

[21] Y. Daito, Y. Takayama, H. Yamanoi, M. Miyake, T. Misaki, I. Kudo et al., "A case of calcifying epithelioma which was doubted a parotid gland origin tumor," *Journal of Oral and Maxillofacial Surgery*, vol. 31, no. 5, pp. 1099–1103, 1985 (Japanese).

[22] H. Hasegawa, T. Kawai, M. Shirakawa, A. Ikai, and H. Tanabe, "Calcifying epithelioma in the lateral neck," *Journal of Oral and Maxillofacial Surgery*, vol. 29, pp. 1579–1583, 1983 (Japanese).

[23] K. Goto, K. Mogi, A. Takeuchi, Y. Yokoyama, M. Yokobori, T. Shiba et al., "A case of calcifying epithelioma in the left preauricular region," *Journal of Oral and Maxillofacial Surgery*, vol. 29, no. 5, pp. 969–974, 1983 (Japanese).

[24] M. Miyahara, J. Tanuma, K. Kawashima, E. Nozoe, I. Semba, and K. A. Sugihara, "Case of calcifying epithelioma with marked calcification and ossification," *Journal of Oral and Maxillofacial Surgery*, vol. 53, no. 8, pp. 499–503, 2007 (Japanese).

[25] G. Anneroth and A. Sigurdson, "Hyperplastic lesions of the gingiva and alveolar mucosa. A study of 175 cases," *Acta Odontologica Scandinavica*, vol. 41, no. 2, pp. 75–86, 1983.

3

Modified Bluegrass Appliance: A Nonpunitive Therapy for Thumb Sucking in Pediatric Patients—A Case Report with Review of the Literature

Amish Diwanji,[1] Preet Jain,[2] Jigar Doshi,[3] Prakash Somani,[2] and Dhaval Mehta[4]

[1] *Department of Pedodontics and Preventive Dentistry, Faculty of Dental Science, Nadiad, Gujarat, India*
[2] *Department of Prosthodontics, Pacific Dental College, Udaipur, India*
[3] *Department of Orthodontics and Dentofacial Orthopedics, Darshan Dental College, Udaipur, India*
[4] *Department of Oral Medicine and Radiology, Karnavati School of Dentistry, Gandhinagar, Gujarat, India*

Correspondence should be addressed to Amish Diwanji; amishdiwanji@yahoo.co.in

Academic Editors: P. G. Arduino and D. Ram

Oral habits in form of digit/thumb sucking are common phenomenon and part of childhood behavior. They are normally associated with oral pleasure, hunger, anxiety, and sometimes psychological disturbances. Chronic practice can cause major orthopedic alterations to the skeletal structures of the oral cavity and lower face. Aversive approaches in form of punitive therapy have been moderately effective. Modified bluegrass appliance is nonpunitive therapy to treat sucking habits. It acts as a habit reversal technique and installs positive reinforcement in children. Modified blue grass appliance proved to be very comfortable to patients and encourages neuromuscular stimulations.

1. Introduction

Oral habit is a part of normal development in children. Habits are learned patterns of muscle contraction with complex nature. Oral habits are repetitive act seen commonly from infancy and should finish automatically as age advances. Common repetitive behavior seen in infants is hand or figure sucking [1]. Sucking is one of the most common reflexes seen in infants. It manifests when they are in womb around 29 wk of age [2]. This is the first pattern of behavior observed in infant. Infants and young children may use finger, thumb, pacifiers, or other objects to feel secure and learn the outside world. This is commonly seen when the child is anxious, insecure or surrounded by strangers and in families when they are separated from their parents. Sucking habit induces sleep and hence makes infant and child calm and relaxed [3].

Hand sucking is naturally developed in 89% of infants in the second month and increases by first year of life [1]. It is normal up to 2–4 years of age. It becomes a concern when continued for longer time and even seen in mixed dentition phase. This is the first sign for child to manifest future malocclusion or discrepancy during mixed dentition. The prevalence of oral habit has been reported up to 88% and 30% in high school girls and boys, respectively [4]. 34% of prevalence has been reported in other literature [5]. It has been documented that parental education, child's nutrition, and sucking habits are associated with each other [6]. However, higher prevalence rate has been claimed with high stress level among children in recent time [7].

When child performs sucking habit in the first year of life, parents can move away his/her thumb smoothly and attract the child to other things. After second year of age, sucking habit should start decreasing and should appear only when child goes to sleep [1]. When it continues in mixed and permanent dentition, it becomes a parental concern, as it is believed to affect growth of maxilla palate leading to skeletal changes, showing side effects on developing occlusion and resulting in malocclusion and constriction of skeletal structures [8, 9].

The effect of prolonged sucking habit in children can affect development of occlusion. It may result in anterior open bite, increased over jet, lingual inclination of lower incisor and labial inclination of maxillary anterior, posterior crossbite, deep palate, compensatory tongue thrust, and sometimes speech defect [10, 11]. The changes in dentition depend upon duration and frequency of habit being performed. During active eruption phase of permanent teeth, children who perform sucking habit for longer duration (more than 6 hrs in a day), especially during sleep, tend to develop minor skeletal abnormalities and sever dentoalveolar changes [12].

Historically, correction of habit revolves around direct counseling of child, encouragement to improve self-confidence by rewarding the child, appliance therapy, and, in case of more complex dental changes, orthodontic therapy along with habit breaking appliances [1]. The use of pacifier may cause severe and harmful effects on dentition if used for more than 5-year-old child [13]. Tongue, Cribs, Hay rakes and other sharp points employ an aversive negative stimulus to cease the undesirable oral habits. They are moderately effective and may trigger unexpected behavior sometimes. In 1991, Haskell and Mink introduced Blue grass appliance, also known as habit correction roller which gained universal attention and acceptance [14]. It is userfriendly, nondestructive, easy to wear appliance replacing the common destructive habits. It is useful in avoiding traditional physical barriers of appliance in form of cribs and helping child with positive reinforcement. Later, similar appliance called Lingual Pearl was used as a habit breaking and for multiple clinical applications [15]. Further, Baker modified blue grass appliance with multiple rollers/beads and thus expanding its use from primary to permanent dentition [16].

2. Management

Management of sucking habit depends upon the age. Many questions arise in parents' mind and among pediatricians regarding intervention by specific therapy to break the habit. Counseling by pediatric dentist and pediatrician is important. If habit is stopped by 4-5 years of age, However, when they persists during eruption of permanent teeth child should be motivated to stop the habit [17, 18].

Appliance therapy involves use of either fixed or removable design in form of palatal crib or spurs. It is reminder therapy for child to make the habit unpleasant and difficult to practice. However, it causes difficulty in speech and eating and can cause iatrogenically inflicted wound and make child emotionally disturbed [14, 19]. Here, we present a case of thumb sucking habit where habit was corrected using Bluegrass appliance as a non punitive therapy.

2.1. Case Report. We present a case of an 8-year-old child, gir,l whose parents reported proclination of maxillary teeth and also complained of thumb sucking habit since birth. The patient used to suck her thumb regularly, 8-9 hrs/day, unconsciously in sleep or when idle from the primary dentition period. Callous formation was seen over her digits (Figure 1). The patient reported with proclination of teeth, increased overjet and overbite with high palatal vault (Figures 2(a) and 2(b)). Management was started by counseling the parent and the child regarding the ill effects of digit sucking on the developing dentition during the first visit. On the second visit, the patient was willing to discontinue the habit by treatment. A modified blue grass appliance was planned. Molar bands were fabricated and adapted on maxillary molars. Alginate impression was taken and casts were poured with dental stone over which molar bands were transferred. Stainless steel wire (0.9 mm) was adapted over the palate extending from either side of molars. Acrylic beads were made in laboratory using dental monomer and polymer. Later, beads were inserted into stainless steel wire over palatal rugae area. No contact was established by beads with palatal tissues. The wire was soldered to molar bands by protecting the beads. The appliance was cemented using luting cement (Figure 3). The patient was instructed to roll the bead with tongue whenever she feels like sucking her thumb. The patient was kept on followup every month for checkup. The child was comfortable with the appliance and played by rolling the beads with the tongue. By end of 4 months, callous formation had almost disappeared. Patient was asked to wear appliance for almost 6 months after correction to avoid relapse of the habit. Appliance was removed after the discontinuation of habit.

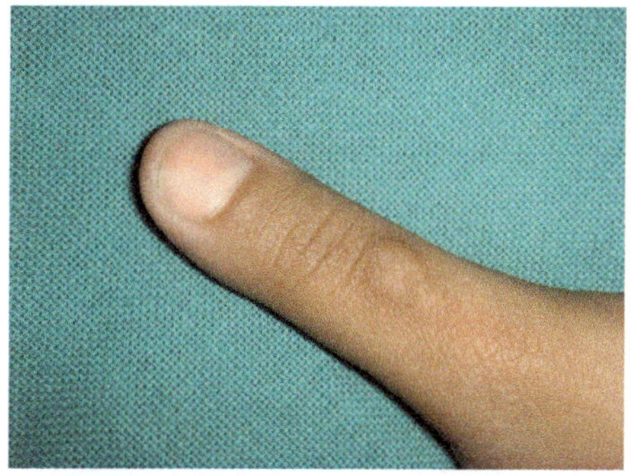

FIGURE 1: Callous formation was seen over digits of patient.

3. Discussion

Digit sucking is common phenomenon in pediatric age group that reflects the earliest form of habitual manipulation of body. Many questions arise in the minds of general dentist, pediatricians, pediatric dentists and psychiatrists regarding impact of sucking habits on developing dentition.

When should an attempt be made to break the habit? How does it disturb the child psychologically? In case of major orthopedic alterations to the skeletal structures of the oral cavity and lower face, intervention of orthodontist may require correct malocclusion. Since years, habit breaking appliances in form of palatal cribs, spurs, palatal bars, hay rakes, and cage type appliances have been given to pediatric age group. However, emotional disturbances, difficulty in speech and eating, and iantrogenically self-inflicted wounds can occur with such appliances. Hay rake and cage type appliances tend to get mutilated or destroyed while eating or due to habitual sucking habit. It reminds the child as punitive

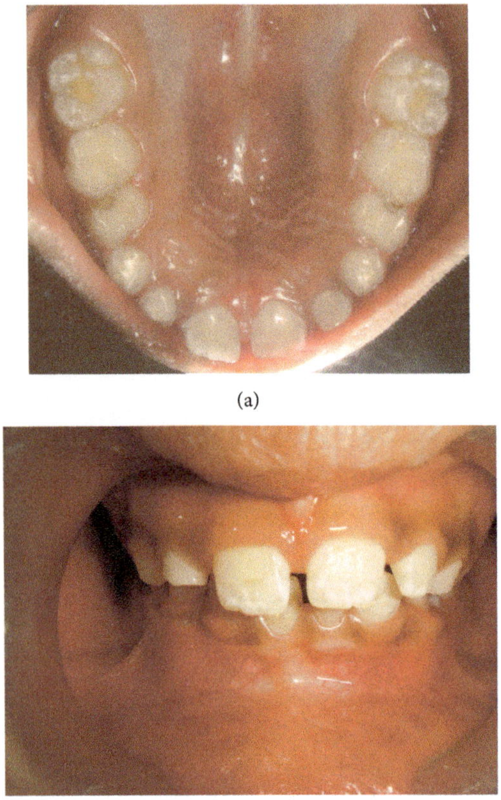

(a)

(b)

FIGURE 2: Proclination of teeth and increased overjet and overbite with high palatal vault.

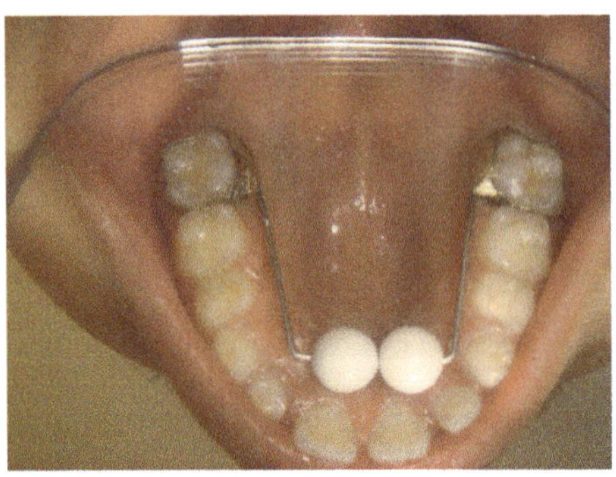

FIGURE 3: Modified blue grass appliance.

therapy to cease the habit [19]. Haskell and Mink described that blue grass appliance which is easy to wear, and did not have problems associated with traditional palatal cribs. The design consisted of hexagonal Teflon roller on a cross-palatal wire which was effective to ending the sucking habit in several days [14].

In the present study, modified blue grass appliance was used using 3 mm acrylic beads as per recommended by Baker [16]. It encourages neuromuscular stimulations by using multiple beads as per what was the principles of Castillo-Morales [20]. Between 4–6-year-old children can be instructed to play with the beads with the tongue immediately after placement. This allows the child to accept the appliance and learn the neuromuscular activity to normalize the tongue position. When a spinning roller is placed in close proximity to the tip of the tongue, "fascinating" response is quickly implemented due to neuromuscular and sensitive nature of tongue. Since Teflon rollers are not in contact with palatal tissues, children can roll them with their tongues. Within few days, the tongue establishes new nonharmful habit of playing with roller. Hence, this appliance works through counter conditioning response to the original conditioned stimulus for thumb sucking.

Psychologically, it is acceptable for parents also as they can encourage the child to play with beads instead of instructing the child to cease the habit all the time and thus making him/her anxious. Reduced bulk of bead does not obstruct while eating, presents minimum disturbances with speech, and stimulates tongue movement. It is esthetic and child becomes comfortable quickly. The patient believes to have acquired a new toy in mouth to play with tongue.

On the other side, direct relationship between age and time of appliance placement has been observed. The younger the patients are, the more quickly and completely the tongue position becomes normalized and the lesser the time required for cessation of the habit is. Limbrock et al. [20] suggested the appliance design even for toddler group to 12 year old child. Cessation of habit was reported on very 1st day in toddlers, whereas it takes few weeks in case of 10–12-year-old children. Hence, in early mixed detention or even in younger group, appliance could be used comfortably. If habit persists for longer time exhibiting posterior cross bite, modified blue grass appliance can be given with Quad Helix [21] to expand arch. Hence, two stage treatments can be completed with single appliance with correction of habit.

4. Conclusion

Hence, modified blue grass appliance is a non punitive appliance and esthetic and child can wear it comfortably. It can be given as a supportive therapy as it requires no reminding or bribing, and parents can be freed of anxiety and frustration. It does not interfere with child's growth and eliminates the habit with limited complications.

References

[1] J. A. Maguire, "The evaluation and treatment of pediatric oral habits," *Dental Clinics of North America*, vol. 44, no. 3, pp. 659–669, 2000.

[2] L. Davidson, "Thumb and finger sucking," *Pediatrics in Review*, vol. 29, no. 6, pp. 207–208, 2008.

[3] JADA, vol.138: 1176, 2007.

[4] S. Yassaei, M. Rafieian, and R. Ghafari, "Abnormal oral habits in the children of war veterans," *Journal of Clinical Pediatric Dentistry*, vol. 29, no. 3, pp. 189–192, 2005.

[5] R. Quashie-Williams, O. O. daCosta, and M. C. Isiekwe, "The prevalence of oral habits among 4 to 15 yr old school children in Lagos," *Journal of Health and Biomedical Sciences*, vol. 17, no. 2, pp. 113–117, 2010.

[6] N. M. A. Farsi, "Sucking habits in Saudi children: prevalence, contributing factors and effects on the primary dentition," *Pediatric Dentistry*, vol. 19, no. 1, pp. 28–33, 1997.

[7] N. Shahraki, S. Yassaei, and M. Goldani, "Abnormal oral habits: a review," *Journal of Dentistry and Oral Hygiene*, vol. 4, no. 2, pp. 12–15, 2012.

[8] T. M. Graber, "Thumb- and finger-sucking," *American Journal of Orthodontics*, vol. 45, no. 4, pp. 258–264, 1959.

[9] A. T. Ruttle, W. Quigley, J. T. Crouch, and G. E. Ewan, "A serial study of the effects of finger-sucking," *Journal of Dental Research*, vol. 32, no. 6, pp. 739–748, 1953.

[10] E. N. Gale and W. A. Ager, "Thumb sucking revisited," *American Journal of Orthodontics*, vol. 55, no. 2, pp. 167–170, 1979.

[11] T. A. Yemitan, O. O. daCosta, O. O. Sanu, and M. C. Isiekwe, "Effects of digit sucking on dental arch dimensions in the primary dentition," *African Journal of Medicine and Medical Sciences*, vol. 39, no. 1, pp. 55–61, 2010.

[12] M. B. Moore and J. P. McDonald, "A cephalometric evaluation of patients presenting with persistent digit sucking habits," *British Journal of Orthodontics*, vol. 24, no. 1, pp. 17–23, 1997.

[13] J. Poyak, "Effects of pacifiers on early oral development," *International Journal of Orthodontics*, vol. 17, no. 4, pp. 13–16, 2006.

[14] B. S. Haskell and J. R. Mink, "An aid to stop thumb sucking: the "Bluegrass" appliance," *Pediatric Dentistry*, vol. 13, no. 2, pp. 83–85, 1991.

[15] A. K. Ritto and P. Leitão, "The lingual pearl," *Journal of Clinical Orthodontics*, vol. 32, no. 5, pp. 318–327, 1998.

[16] C. Baker, "The modified blue grass appliance," *Journal of Clinical Orthodontics*, vol. 17, no. 9, pp. 535–537, 2000.

[17] J. J. Warren, S. E. Bishara, K. L. Steinbock, T. Yonezu, and A. J. Nowak, "Effects of oral habits' duration on dental characteristics in the primary dentition," *Journal of the American Dental Association*, vol. 132, no. 12, pp. 1685–1693, 2001.

[18] J. J. Warren and S. E. Bishara, "Duration of nutritive and nonnutritive sucking behaviors and their effects on the dental arches in the primary dentition," *American Journal of Orthodontics and Dentofacial Orthopedics*, vol. 121, no. 4, pp. 347–356, 2002.

[19] M. Massler and A. W. Wood, "Thumb-sucking," *Journal of Dentistry for Children*, vol. 16, no. 1, pp. 1–9, 1949.

[20] G. J. Limbrock, H. Hoyer, and H. Scheying, "Regulation therapy by Castillo-Morales in children with Down syndrome: primary and secondary orofacial pathology," *ASDC Journal of Dentistry for Children*, vol. 57, no. 6, pp. 437–441, 1990.

[21] B. S. Haskell, "Construction of a habit correction roller with arch expansion: chair side application of a new 2 piece bondable "Bluegrass" appliance," *Journal of Southeastern Society of Pediatric Dentistry*, vol. 8, no. 1, pp. 22–26, 2002.

4

Refractory Pigmentation Associated with Laugier-Hunziker Syndrome following Er:YAG Laser Treatment

Sertan Ergun,[1] Alp Saruhanoğlu,[1] Dante-Antonio Migliari,[2] Ilay Maden,[3] and Hakkı Tanyeri[1]

[1] *Department of Oral Medicine and Surgery, Faculty of Dentistry, Istanbul University, 34093 Istanbul, Turkey*
[2] *Department of Oral Diagnosis, School of Dentistry, University of Sao Paulo, 05508-900 Sao Paulo, SP, Brazil*
[3] *Department of Periodontology, Istanbul Faculty of Medicine, Istanbul University, 34093 Istanbul, Turkey*

Correspondence should be addressed to Alp Saruhanoğlu; saruhanoglualp@yahoo.com

Academic Editors: R. A. de Mesquita and C. S. Farah

The present report describes a case of Laugier-Hunziker syndrome (LHS), a rare benign condition. A patient with LHS develops acquired melanotic pigmentation of the lips and buccal mucosa, often with pigmentation of the nails occurring. No systemic symptoms are associated with this syndrome. Normally, no treatment is required for this condition, unless for aesthetic reason, mainly due to pigmentation on the lip mucosa. We present a case of LHS, 37-year-old female, whose pigmentations on her lip and in the oral cavity were treated with an Er:YAG laser. At the postoperative 12th month followup, the lesions recurred. The effects of any surgical attempt to treat pigmentations associated with LHS were discussed.

1. Introduction

The Laugier-Hunziker syndrome (LHS) is a rare benign condition, characterized by acquired pigmentation of the nails and melanotic pigmentation of the parts of the oral cavity such as lips, buccal, and palatal mucosa, [1]. Oral pigmentation is either focal or diffuse. Lip lesions and mucosa present as multiple, flat, smooth, discrete or confluent pigmented macules of variable size and color, ranging from grey to brown or blue-black [2].

Focal lesions may be more worrying, and require an examination of a biopsy specimen for an accurate diagnosis and, mainly, for excluding melanoma. Histopathological examination of oral pigmentation associated with LHS is not a diagnosis in itself; it only shows a significant increase in melanin or melanocytes in the basal layer. Diagnosis of LHS should be made on a clinical basis, by excluding other similar disorders such as Peutz-Jeghers syndrome and adrenal insufficiency [3].

It has been reported that very few patients actually receive treatment for LHS because it is a benign condition. We present a case of LHS treated with Er:YAG laser to remove the oral pigmentations which were cleared after four sessions but recurred twelve months later.

2. Case Report

A 37-year-old Turkish woman was referred to the department of oral surgery because of pigmented areas in her mouth. She had noticed the pigmented lesions in her oral cavity 3 years ago and till the beginning of the treatment no major change in the oral cavity was observed by the patient. Oral examination revealed multiple, painless brown-black pigmentation, on the buccal mucosa, lower lip and posterior of the palate, bilaterally (Figure 1). No cutaneous or fingernail lesions were observed. She was systemically healthy and was not on any medication. She was neither a smoker nor a habitual drinker of alcohol. There was no family history of abnormal mucocutaneous pigmentation.

Laboratory investigation results, including a full blood count, hematinic levels, serum chemistry and inflammatory markers, were all within normal range. The patient underwent an upper gastrointestinal endoscopy, as well as

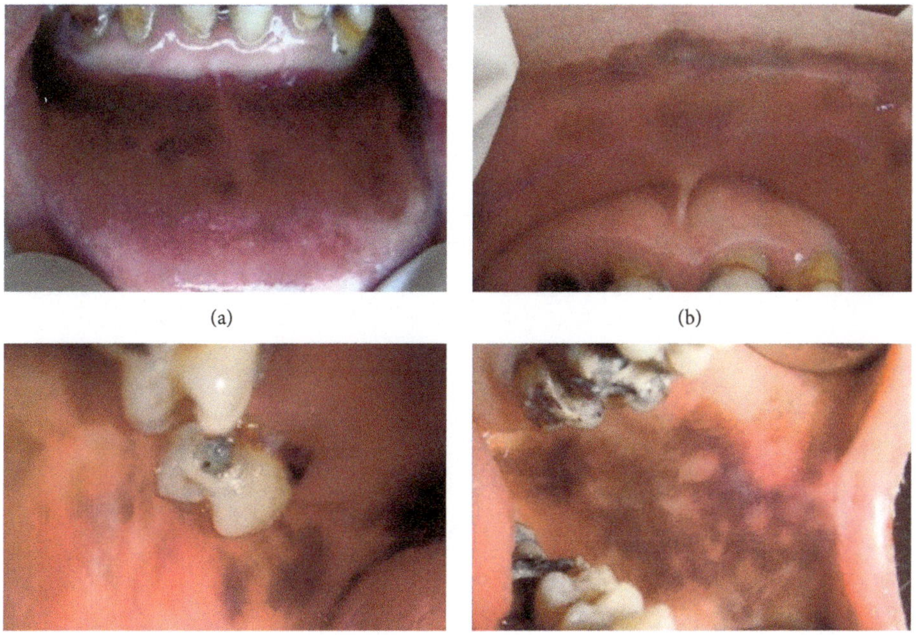

(a) (b) (c) (d)

FIGURE 1: Multiple, painless brown-black pigmentation, on the buccal mucosa, lower lip, and posterior of the palate, bilaterally.

a colonoscopy, which revealed no evidence of polyps. To rule out Addisons disease, the serum cortisol and adrenocorticotrophic hormone (ACTH) levels were measured and the values were normal. A biopsy was taken from the buccal mucosa with the aim of excluding melanoma. Histopathological examination revealed lentiginous proliferation of melanocytes. Inflammatory changes or malignant features were not noted in any area. A diagnosis of LH syndrome was made based on the clinical presentation of lesions coupled with the absence of systemic findings.

An Er:YAG laser with a wavelength of 2940 nm (Fotona Fidelis Plus III, Slovenia) was used because of its capability of superficially ablating oral soft tissues to treat oral pigmentation, especially on the lips, soft palate, and buccal mucosa, bilaterally. The parameters used were 120 mJ output energy, 10 Hz frequency, 1000 μs pulse duration, and a 0.8 mm spot size with the noncontact hand-piece. The fluence was 25 J/cm^2 and the lasing was continued until the pigmentation on the intervention area was visibly ablated as there is no accumulation of energy or heat by Er:YAG lasers. The treatment was performed under local anesthesia with no water and air spray. No sutures or other means of bleeding control were needed at the end of the procedure. Postoperative healing was uneventful, only mild "burning" sensation was reported by the patient for a few hours postoperatively. The reason of the need for anesthetics is that the water spray was turned off in order to obtain hemostasis. The procedure was straightforward, scanning all the pigmented areas of the oral cavity and the lips, ablating the superficial layers of the tissues including the buccal mucosa and the soft palate.

As the area of pigmentation was rather large the surgical treatment was performed in 4 sessions. In each session one quadrant was chosen and cleared in order to reduce scarring. After the 4th session, the healing process occurred without any complication and the entire pigmentation had been cleared (Figure 2). Two months later, however, a small pigmented area was seen, and it was cleared again in one appointment. By the 12th month of followup, the pigmentation had recurred, being observed in an area close to half of the initial situation (Figure 3).

3. Discussion

Diagnosis of Laugier-Hunziker syndrome must be established to exclude underlying systemic pathologic conditions such as Addison's disease, Albright's syndrome, and Peutz-Jeghers syndrome [4]. Diffuse oral pigmentation may also be associated with systemic intake of drugs such as tetracyclines, antimalarials, amiodarone, chemotherapeutic agents, oral contraceptives, phenothiazines, azidothymidine, and ketoconazole [5]. A correct diagnosis will resolve the drug induced oral mucosal pigmentation following the suspension of the causative drug [6]. No drugs were being taken by our patient.

Smoking may produce oral pigmentation, although it is usually confined to the anterior attached gingival and not associated with pigmentation in other parts of the body [7]. The patient has been nonsmoker for her entire life.

The majority of pigmentations associated with LHS do not require any treatment, it necessary to reassure the patient of the benign behavior of the lesions. In the present case, the pigmentations were treated by laser because the patient was concerned about her appearance. She was unable to socialize

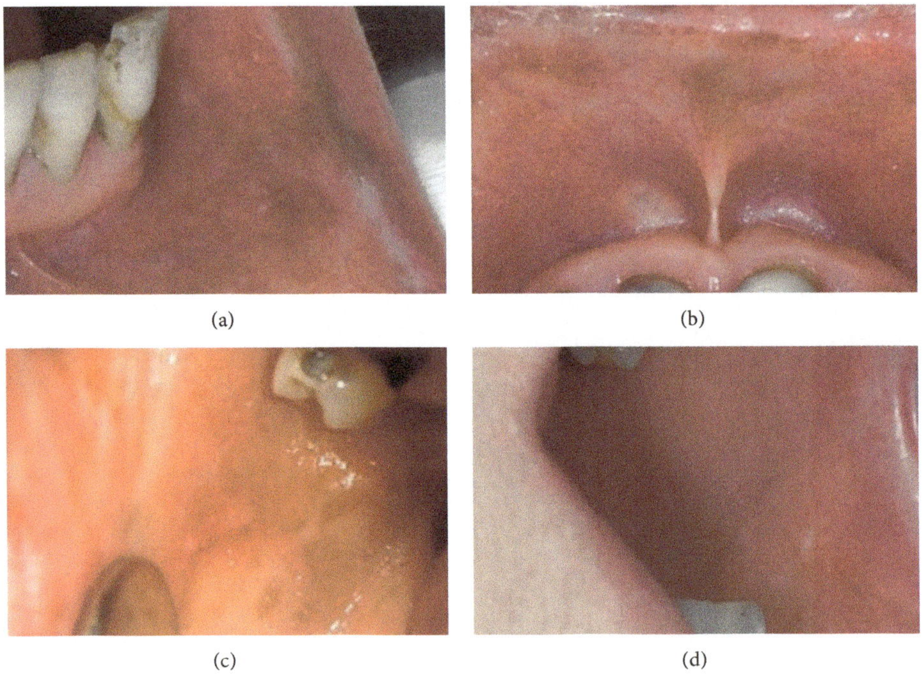

Figure 2: The healing process occurred without any complication and the entire pigmentation had been cleared (14th day postoperatively).

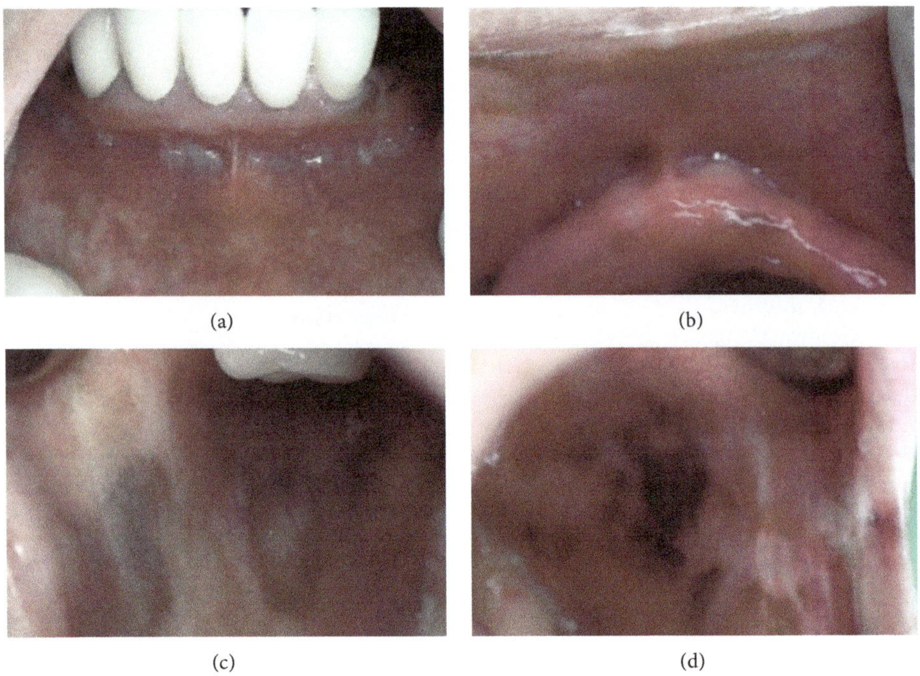

Figure 3: By the 12th month of follow-up, the pigmentation had recurred.

being unhappy with her "unhealthy look". The treatment was carried out in order to improve patient's quality of life as requested by the patient herself. Unfortunately, this treatment rendered only a transitory clearance of the pigmentations, as the lesions recurred later on, and no other attempt to treat the patient was made.

Treatment using the Q-switched neodymium: yttrium-aluminum-garnet (Nd:YAG) laser [5], Q-switched alexandrite laser (QSAL) [2, 8, 9], and cryosurgery [10] has been reported in only a small number of patients.

Er:YAG laser was the tool of choice as it is very superficially absorbed by the oral tissues, not risking the underlying structures. Even though the procedure required anesthetic solutions to be administered, the thermal effects of Er:YAG are minimal, thus not delaying the healing but maintaining hemostasis during the operation. Other wavelengths like Nd:YAG or diodes which are absorbed in hemoglobin and melanin could also be used in this case, however the thermal side effects are more, which may cause delayed wound healing [11]. This procedure may be very difficult or even not possible to be done by scalpel surgery while with the Er:YAG it is simple for an experienced laser user.

There seems to be no risk of induction of malignancy with Er:YAG laser ablation in this case because the diagnosis of the case was already known to be non-premalignant after the biopsy taken and there is no biomodulation effect of 2940 nm wavelength as it is highly absorbed by water, not letting the energy penetration into the tissues. Another biopsy after the treatment was not justified because of these reasons and was not done.

There are few report of treatment by surgical laser with no recurrence within 12-month follow-up [2, 9]. Further studies are therefore called for with long term follow-up in order to confirm whether the effects of the surgical treatment of pigmentations associated with LHS are permanent or not.

The main limitation of this case report was the lack of the related references. There were a few published LH cases who were treated with other types of lasers than Er:YAG laser whereas there was only one study evaluating the treatment of Laugier-Hunziker Syndrome with the Q-switched alexandrite laser whose study group was consisted of 22 Chinese patients [2]. For further investigations, there is a need for a study with higher study population which will compare the treatment outcomes of different types of lasers.

As recurrences were observed in the present case after 12 months of followup it may be reasonable to consider that this acquired pigmentation is to be persistent for life with a tendency to be refractory to a surgical intervention. It can be concluded that the reason of the recurrence in this case may be the superficial removal of tissue layers with Er:YAG which was thought to be advantageous as it is safe. The advantage of using the Er:YAG laser is being able to see the pigmented areas easily; however, the disadvantage is that it is only possible to see them clinically. The advantage of another laser could be that it could interact with the pigmentation on molecular scales which could prevent recurring. Other surgical tools or another laser with a different choice of wavelength to interact with the deeper pigment content of the lesions could be investigated for a longer term successful result.

Conflict of Interests

The authors declare that there is no conflict of interests regarding the publication of this paper.

References

[1] A. J. Kanwar, S. Kaur, C. Kaur, and G. P. Thami, "Laugier-Hunziker syndrome," *Journal of Dermatology*, vol. 28, no. 1, pp. 54–57, 2001.

[2] Y. Zuo, D. Ma, H. Jin, Y. Liu, H. Wang, and Q. Sun, "Treatment of Laugier-Hunziker syndrome with the Q-switched alexandrite laser in 22 Chinese patients," *Archives of Dermatological Research*, vol. 302, no. 2, pp. 125–130, 2010.

[3] P. Kosari and K. M. Kelly, "Asymptomatic lower lip hyperpigmentation from Laugier-Hunziker syndrome," *Cutis*, vol. 88, no. 5, pp. 235–236, 2011.

[4] L. Montebugnoli, I. Grelli, F. Cervellati, C. Misciali, and B. Raone, "Laugier-Hunziker Syndrome: an uncommon cause of oral pigmentation and a review of the literature," *International Journal of Dentistry*, vol. 2010, Article ID 525404, 4 pages, 2010.

[5] M. J. B. Ferreira, A. M. Ferreira, A. P. Soares, and J. C. F. Rodrigues, "Laugier-Hunziker syndrome: case report and treatment with the Q-switched Nd-Yag laser," *Journal of the European Academy of Dermatology and Venereology*, vol. 12, no. 2, pp. 171–173, 1999.

[6] O. Dereure, "Drug-induced skin pigmentation epidemiology, diagnosis and treatment," *American Journal of Clinical Dermatology*, vol. 2, no. 4, pp. 253–262, 2001.

[7] S. M. Mirbod and S. I. Ahing, "Tobacco-associated lesions of the oral cavity, part I: nonmalignant lesions," *Journal of the Canadian Dental Association*, vol. 66, no. 5, pp. 252–256, 2000.

[8] E. Papadavid and N. P. J. Walker, "Q-switched Alexandrite laser in the treatment of pigmented macules in Laugier-Hunziker syndrome," *Journal of the European Academy of Dermatology and Venereology*, vol. 15, no. 5, pp. 468–469, 2001.

[9] T. Ozawa, M. Fujiwara, T. Harada, M. Muraoka, and M. Ishii, "Q-switched alexandrite laser therapy for pigmentation of the lips owing to Laugier-Hunziker Syndrome," *Dermatologic Surgery*, vol. 31, no. 6, pp. 709–712, 2005.

[10] A. T. Sheridan and R. P. R. Dawber, "Laugier-Hunziker syndrome: treatment with cryosurgery," *Journal of the European Academy of Dermatology and Venereology*, vol. 13, no. 2, pp. 146–148, 1999.

[11] J. Jin, S. Lee, and H. Yoon, "A comparative study of wound healing following incision with a scalpel, diode laser or Er,Cr:YSGG laser in guinea pig oral mucosa: a histological and immunohistochemical analysis," *Acta Odontologica Scandinavica*, vol. 68, no. 4, pp. 232–238, 2010.

5

Recurrent Ameloblastic Fibroma: Report of a Rare Case

Ravikumar S. Kulkarni, Amitabh Sarkar, and Sandeep Goyal

Department of Oral Pathology, Surendera Dental College and Research Institute, H. H. Gardens, Sri Ganganagar, Rajasthan 335001, India

Correspondence should be addressed to Ravikumar S. Kulkarni; ravioralpathology@yahoo.com

Academic Editors: R. S. Brown, P. Lopez Jornet, and M. A. D. A. M. Machado

Ameloblastic fibroma (AF) is an uncommon mixed neoplasm of odontogenic origin frequently seen in the second decade of life. It mainly presents as an intrabony lesion but can even occur peripherally. Histologically, our case showed hypercellular areas, an uncommon feature seen in typical AF. Whether this benign lesion is treated by mode of enucleation and curettage or by extensive surgery is still a topic of debate. An extensive surgical treatment is suggested as the initial approach due to its high recurrence rate (18%) and the greater chances of recurrent AFs transforming into ameloblastic fibrosarcoma (45%), together with a long-term followup. We report a case of recurrent AF with hypercellular ectomesenchyme which developed a year after its conservative removal. We conclude that in recurrent AF sufficient sections of the pathological specimen are to be taken to rule out any malignant changes that might have begun in focal areas.

1. Introduction

Ameloblastic fibroma (AF) is a rare tumor of odontogenic origin comprising 1.5–4.5% of all odontogenic tumors [1]. It was first described by Kruse (1891) and later classified as a separate entity by Thoma and Goldman (1946) [1, 2].

Although reported in a wide age range (0.5–62 years), most AFs are seen in the first two decades of life with 77.7% of cases being diagnosed before the age of 20. Males show slightly higher prevalence (M : F = 1.4 : 1), and the posterior mandible is the most common anatomic location [2].

Small lesions are asymptomatic, whereas larger ones may cause painless swelling [2]. Approximately, 20% of cases are discovered accidentally on radiographs taken to detect the failure of tooth eruption [3–5]. Three-fourth cases are associated with impacted or unerupted teeth or at times develop in areas of congenitally missing teeth [2].

Radiologically, AF is a unilocular (when small) or multilocular (when large) radiolucent lesion often with a smooth, sclerotic border and may or may not produce bulging of bone [2, 6].

Grossly, it appears as a solid, soft tissue mass with a smooth surface. It may or may not be encapsulated [7]. Histologically, the ectomesenchymal portion is made up of primitive connective tissue, characterized by plump fibroblasts and delicate collagen fibrils closely resembling the dental papilla. The epithelial component which resembles embryonic dental lamina is arranged in various patterns—thin long strands, cords, nests, or islands. The strands show double or triple layer of cuboidal cells, in contrast to the nests which are surrounded by columnar ameloblast-like cells enclosing stellate reticulum-like cells. Cyst formation within the epithelium is uncommon [2, 6].

AF needs to be differentiated from ameloblastoma, odontogenic myxoma, dentigerous cyst, odontogenic keratocyst, central giant cell granuloma, and histiocytosis [8]. Presence of numerous mitotic cells or any atypical mitosis should suggest malignant entities such as AFS in the differential diagnosis [3, 4].

Treatment of AF in general is a conservative approach, such as enucleation with curettage of the surrounding bone along with the removal of the affected tooth [1, 3]. Long-term followup is necessary [4].

2. Case Report

In August 2011, an 18-year-old female patient reported with a complaint of gingival overgrowth in the left lower back region, which interfered with chewing. Growth was insidious,

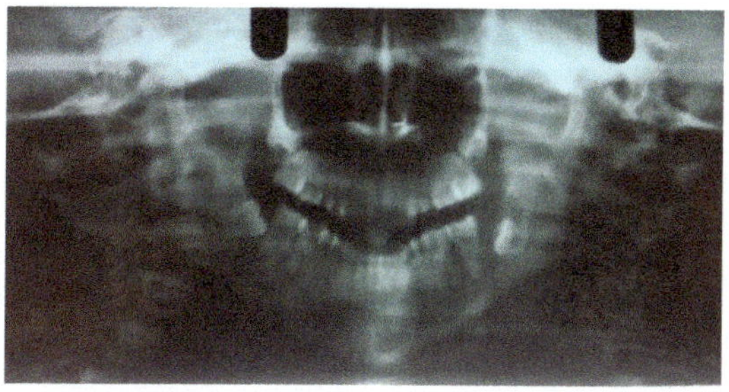

Figure 1: OPG showing well-defined radiolucency associated with an impacted mandibular left third molar (August 2011).

slowly progressing, and no history of associated pain. On intraoral examination, a huge exophytic growth measuring roughly 3 × 4 cms was noticed posterior to the mandibular left second molar. It extended anteroposteriorly from 37 to retromolar pad, buccally in the vestibule and inferiorly till the floor of the mouth. On radiographic examination, a well-defined radiolucency was found around impacted 38 (Figure 1). Surgical excision of the entire intraosseous and extraosseous mass along with the removal of the impacted 38 was performed. A histopathologic diagnosis of ameloblastic fibroma was made. The patient was kept on followup.

The patient reported again in August 2012 with a recurrent swelling in the same area. It was associated with difficulty in mastication. There was no history of pain, paresthesia, or discharge. Intraoral examination revealed a proliferative growth measuring 5 × 4 × 3 cms and extending from 35 to retromolar area (Figure 2). Submandibular lymph nodes on the ipsilateral side were enlarged. Orthopantomograph showed multilocular radiolucency involving the left side of the mandible and discontinuity of the lower border (Figure 3). Hemimandibulectomy was performed with primary reconstruction using titanium plate.

The excised specimen consisted of left half of the body and ramus of the mandible with the tumor mass measuring 7.5 × 6.5 × 6.5 cms (Figure 4). Histopathologic examination of hematoxylin and eosin-stained sections showed cords, interconnecting strands, and islands of odontogenic epithelium laid in a myxoid cell-rich stroma. The cords and strands consisted of a double layer of cuboidal cells (Figure 5). The islands showed the peripheral tall columnar cells having polarized nucleus, clear vacuolated cytoplasm, and central stellate reticulum-like cells (Figure 6). Juxtaepithelial hyalinization was noted around few islands. There was no hard tissue formation. The degree of cellularity varied in different areas of the lesion. Some areas were hypercellular (Figure 7), whereas others were sparsely cellular and myxoid. Atypia and mitotic activities were not evident. The lesion was partly covered by fibrous capsule (Figure 8). Sections were taken from different areas to look for any malignant changes. However, it was not appreciated. A final diagnosis of ameloblastic fibroma was made.

3. Discussion

World Health Organization (WHO 1992) classifies AF as a true mixed neoplasm of odontogenic origin with both

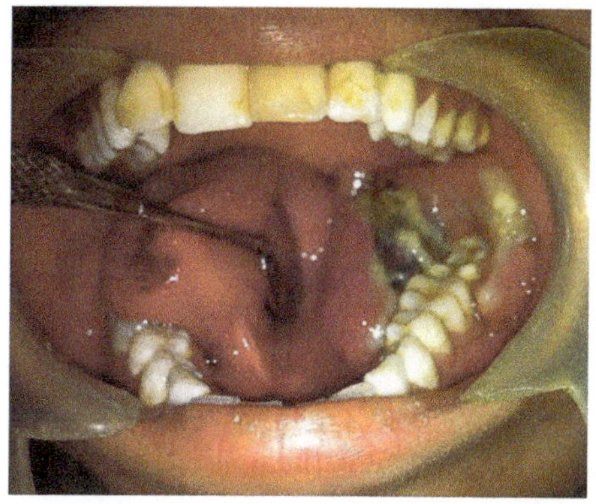

Figure 2: Intraoral view of tumor mass (August 2012).

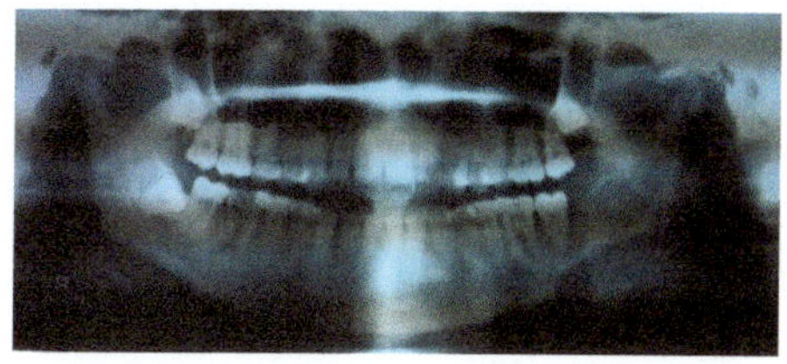

Figure 3: OPG showing multiocular radiolucency in the mandibular left molar-ramus area and discontinuity of the lower border (August 2012).

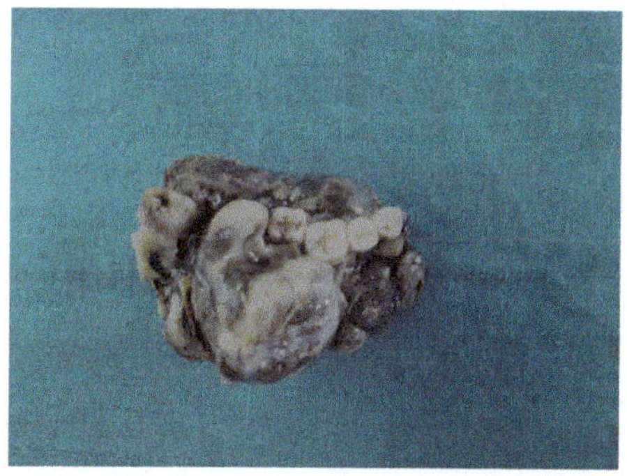

Figure 4: Gross photograph of the left half of the mandible with the tumor mass.

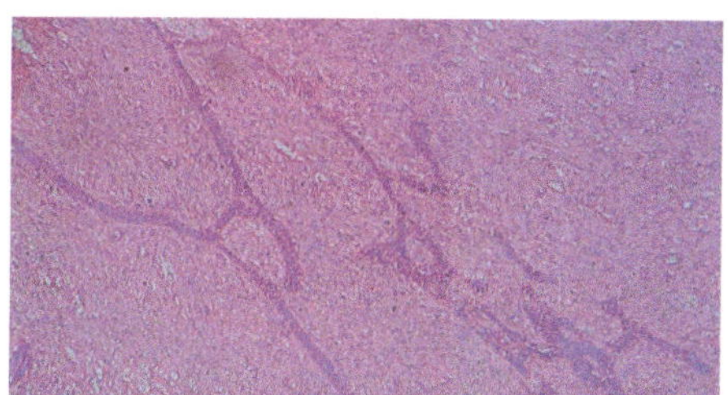

Figure 5: Photomicrograph showing interconnecting strands of odontogenic epithelium in a primitive connective tissue stroma (10x).

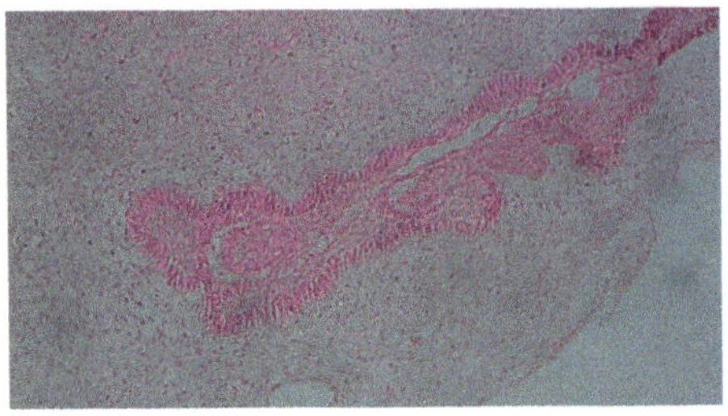

Figure 6: Photomicrograph showing odontogenic epithelial island with peripheral tall columnar cells and central stellate reticulum-like cells in a primitive ectomesenchyme (40x).

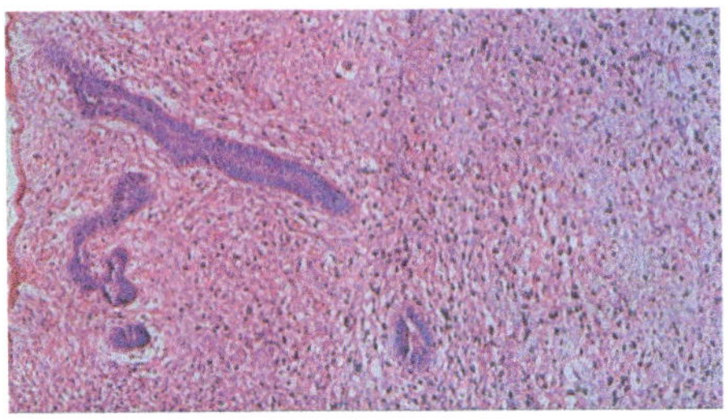

Figure 7: Photomicrograph showing cords and islands of odontogenic epithelium in hypercellular connective tissue stroma (10x).

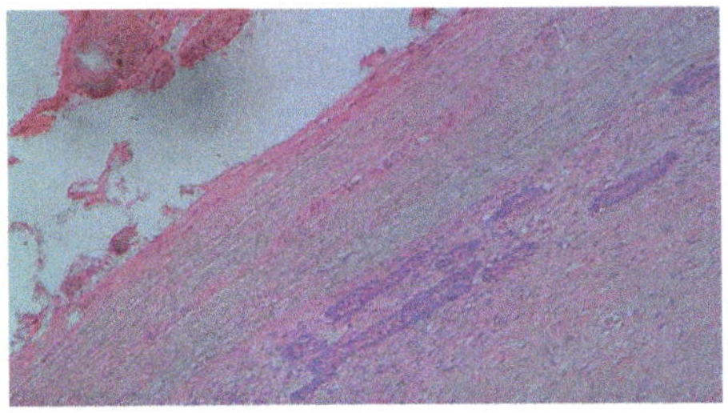

Figure 8: Photomicrograph showing strands of odontogenic epithelium near the capsule (10x).

epithelial and ectomesenchymal components, without hard tissue formation [2]. It mainly occurs as an intraosseous variant, and only few peripheral cases are reported [9].

Although AF is the most common in posterior mandible region of young adults, a case occurring in anterior mandible of a 45-year-old man with considerable extension and soft tissue involvement has been reported [10].

The exact pathogenesis is not clear. The tall columnar ameloblast-like cells in the epithelial component are too primitive to induce the cells of the ectomesenchyme, and only little is known about their interactions. It is also unknown why induction of odontoblastic differentiation is lacking in AF [2]. Immunohistochemical analysis shows positive staining of odontogenic epithelium for cytokeratin, mesenchymal tissue around the dental lamina-like epithelium for tenascin, focal areas of immature dental papilla-like cells, and basement membrane of the epithelium for vimentin. These findings suggest that AF develops at an early stage of tooth formation [1].

Histological variants of AF that have been described are granular cell AF, in which the ectomesenchyme is dominated by granular cells, papilliferous AF showing marked proliferation of the epithelium with plexiform arrangement [2], ameloblastoma in association with AF, and cystic AF [5]. The density of collagen fibers in AF was found to have an impact on the shape and direction of enlargement of the epithelial follicle. Its growth was found to be restricted in areas of dense collagen deposits, leading to its enlargement in planes of less resistance [11]. In the current case, strands, cords, and islands of odontogenic epithelium are seen in a cell-rich ectomesenchyme. Strands show double layer of cuboidal cells, and islands are lined by tall columnar cells with polarized nucleus surrounding stellate reticulum-like cells. Few islands were bordered by juxtaepithelial hyalinization. Our case presented with an uncommon feature of hypercellularity in few areas which are usually not seen in routine AF. There was no hard tissue formation, thus eliminating ameloblastic fibroodontoma/fibrodentinoma. Hence, it is important that sections are taken from different parts of the lesion especially in recurrent cases of AF to look for any malignant changes. In the present case, atypical features and mitotic activity were not observed.

MIB-1, a monoclonal antibody against proliferation-associated nuclear antigen, in AF ranged from 2.9 to 7.5% and from 1.5 to 13.5% in the epithelial and mesenchymal components, respectively. These indices were higher in recurrent AF and AFS [12]. Knowledge of malignant potential of ectomesenchyme in AF helps to understand its aggressiveness and to determine appropriate management of these benign tumors to prevent malignant transformation to AFS, which can occur years later [13].

Approximately, 45% of AFS is reported to arise from a recurrent AF [7]. Hence, sufficient sampling of the pathological specimen is needed to rule out malignant changes if any, which might have begun in focal areas. Cases undergoing malignant transformation show unequivocal changes in the ectomesenchymal component and complete disappearance of odontogenic epithelium [1]. Immunohistochemical markers could be helpful to distinguish AF and AFS. The mesenchymal component of AF is negative to Ki67, PCNA, and p53, in front of the positivity of AFS [14]. But in our case, no histological changes were noted in the stroma, and mitotic activity was not appreciated.

Whether AF is to be treated by conservative enucleation or by aggressive modality is still a topic of debate. A recurrence rate of 43.5% and 18% was reported by Trodahl and Zallen, respectively. Gundlach was of the opinion that simple enucleation would not be sufficient for AF [2]. Most of them agree for a conservative surgical approach initially, and a more aggressive excision for recurrent lesions, larger tumors, or those involving maxilla [2, 7]. A long-term followup is recommended [4]. Total excision of extraosseous AF with no recurrence is reported [9]. In our case, a conservative surgical approach was followed initially along with the removal of the impacted tooth. But the case reoccurred a year later after the first surgery. Aggressive treatment of hemimandibulectomy was performed for the second time. We recommend a more aggressive treatment in the initial step to prevent its recurrence and transformation to AFS.

Conflict of Interests

The authors declare that they have no conflict of interests.

References

[1] S. Gupta, A. Tandon, D. Mehrotra, and O. P. Gupta, "Ameloblastic fibroma: report of 3 cases and literature review," *International Journal of Oral and Maxillofacial Pathology*, vol. 2, no. 3, pp. 59–63, 2011.

[2] A. R. Peter and P. P. Hans, *Odontogenic Tumors and Allied Lesions*, Quintessence Publishing, Hanover Park, Ill, USA, 1st edition, 2004.

[3] B. L. Nelson and G. S. Folk, "Ameloblastic fibroma," *Head and Neck Pathology*, vol. 3, no. 1, pp. 51–53, 2009.

[4] D. O. Pereira da Costa, A. T. N. N. Alves, M. D. Calasans-Maia, R. L. da Cruz, and S. Q. C. Lourenço, "Maxillary ameloblastic fibroma: a case report," *Brazilian Dental Journal*, vol. 22, no. 2, pp. 171–174, 2011.

[5] N. J. McGuinness, T. Faughnan, F. Bennani, and C. E. Connolly, "Ameloblastic fibroma of the anterior maxilla presenting as a complication of tooth eruption: a case report," *Journal of orthodontics*, vol. 28, no. 2, pp. 115–118, 2001.

[6] R. Rajendran and B. Sivapathasundharam, *Shafer's Text Book of Oral Pathology*, Elsevier, Amsterdam, The Netherlands, 7th edition, 2012.

[7] B. W. Neville, D. D. Damm, C. M. Allen, and J. E. Bouquot, *Oral and Maxillofacial Pathology*, Elsevier, Amsterdam, The Netherlands, 3rd edition, 2011.

[8] J. A. Regezi, J. J. Sciubba, and R. C. Jordan, *Oral Pathology Clinical Pathologic Correlations*, Elsevier, Amsterdam, The Netherlands, 4th edition, 2003.

[9] M. R. Darling and T. D. Daley, "Peripheral ameloblastic fibroma," *Journal of Oral Pathology and Medicine*, vol. 35, no. 3, pp. 190–192, 2006.

[10] C. E. V. Belmiro, S. S. A. Emanuel, S. R. Nelson, H. A. M. Hecio, and W. F. C. Ricardo, "Treatment of large ameloblastic fibroma: a case report," *Journal of Oral Science*, vol. 51, no. 2, pp. 293–296, 2009.

[11] R. Hangelbroek, R. Vorster, and S. P. Ngwenya, "Collagen in odontogenic tumors: a histochemical and immunohistocheical study of 19 cases," *Medical Technology*, vol. 26, no. 1, pp. 28–32, 2012.

[12] K. Sano, S. I. Yoshida, H. Ninomiya et al., "Assessment of growth potential by MIB-1 immunohistochemistry in ameloblastic fibroma and related lesions of the jaws compared with ameloblastic fibrosarcoma," *Journal of Oral Pathology and Medicine*, vol. 27, no. 2, pp. 59–63, 1998.

[13] B. Marko and I. H. Natasa, "Ameloblastic fibroma," *Radiology and Oncology*, vol. 40, no. 1, pp. 35–38, 2006.

[14] P. Huguet, J. Castellví, M. Ávila et al., "Ameloblastic fibrosarcoma: report of a case. Immunohistochemical study and review of the literature," *Medicina Oral*, vol. 6, no. 3, pp. 173–179, 2001.

6

An Innovative Approach to Treat Incisors Hypomineralization (MIH): A Combined Use of Casein Phosphopeptide-Amorphous Calcium Phosphate and Hydrogen Peroxide

Stefano Mastroberardino,[1] Guglielmo Campus,[2] Laura Strohmenger,[1] Alessandro Villa,[1] and Maria Grazia Cagetti[1]

[1] *Dental Clinic, San Paolo Hospital, University of Milan, 20142 Milan, Italy*
[2] *Dental Institute, University of Sassari, 07100 Sassari, Italy*

Correspondence should be addressed to Stefano Mastroberardino, stefano.mastroberardino@hotmail.it

Academic Editors: Y.-K. Chen and A. V. Ritter

Molar Incisor Hypomineralization (MIH) is characterized by a developmentally derived deficiency in mineral enamel. Affected teeth present demarcated enamel opacities, ranging from white to brown; also hypoplasia can be associated. Patient frequently claims aesthetic discomfort if anterior teeth are involved. This problem leads patients to request a bleaching treatment to improve aestheticconditions. Nevertheless, hydrogen peroxide can produce serious side-effects, resulting from further mineral loss. Microabrasion and/or a composite restoration are the treatments of choice in teeth with mild/moderate MIH, but they also need enamel loss. Recently, a new remineralizing agent based on Casein Phosphopeptide-Amorphous Calcium Phosphate (CPP-ACP) has been proposed to be effective in hypomineralized enamel, improving also aesthetic conditions. The present paper presents a case report of a young man with white opacities on incisors treated with a combined use of CPP-ACP mousse and hydrogen peroxide gel to correct the aesthetic defect. The patient was instructed to use CPP-ACP for two hours per day for three months in order to obtain enamel remineralization followed by a combined use of CPP-ACP and bleaching agent for further two months. At the end of this five-month treatment, a noticeable aesthetic improvement of the opacities was observed.

1. Introduction

"Molar Incisor Hypomineralization" (MIH) is the term used to describe teeth, generally permanent incisors and first molars, characterized by a developmentally derived deficiency in mineral enamel. Affected teeth present demarcated enamel opacities, ranging from white to brown, according to the severity of the disease and the hypoplasia that can be associated.

Hypomineralized enamel is soft and porous and occasionally it undergoes to posteruptive breakdown, resulting in anomalous noncarious cavities [1]. Scanning electron microscope and semiquantitative analysis by Energy Dispersive X-ray Spectrometry showed that affected enamel is not organized in hydroxyapatite crystals and it is low in calcium and phosphate ions [2].

Patients affected by MIH present several clinical problems, including rapid wear, enamel loss, increased susceptibility to caries, and sensitivity [1]. Patients frequently claim aesthetics discomfort when anterior teeth are involved. This problem leads patients to request a bleaching treatment to improve aesthetic conditions. Nevertheless, hydrogen peroxide-based gels applied on enamel produce serious side-effects such as hardness decrease and increased roughness and morphologic alterations resulting from mineral loss [3]. Low concentration bleaching peroxides can change calcium and phosphate mineral content of bleached enamel [4]. These enamel changes may highlight the appearance of opacities. Therefore, enamel bleaching is not safe for hypomineralized enamel low in calcium and phosphate content.

Microabrasion and/or a composite restoration are the treatments of choice to improve aesthetic conditions in

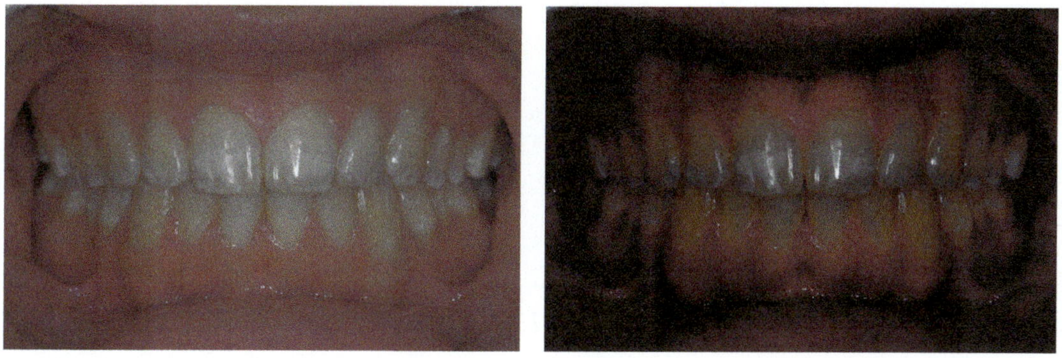

(a) (b)

Figure 1: (a) Initial frontal picture. (b) Software-modified initial frontal picture.

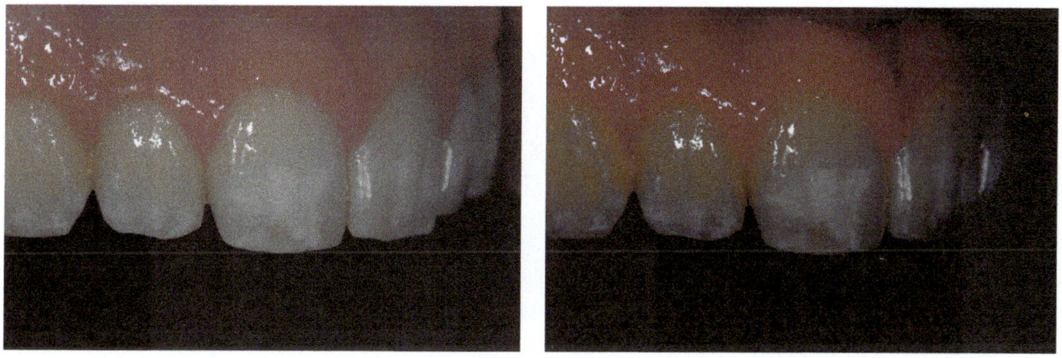

(a) (b)

Figure 2: (a) Initial right side picture. (b) Software-modified initial right side picture.

teeth with mild/moderate MIH, but this approach needs enamel removal. Furthermore, the adhesion of composite resins to hypomineralized tissue is critical [1]. A conservative approach to improve the conditions of teeth affected by mild/moderate MIH would be useful.

Recently, a new remineralizing agent based on Casein Phosphopeptide-Amorphous Calcium Phosphate (CPP-ACP) (GC Tooth Mousse, GC Corporation 76-1 HASUNUMA-CHO ITABASHI-KU, Tokyo, Japan) has been developed. CPP stabilizes high concentration of calcium and phosphate that bind themselves to pellicle and plaque. This reservoir of ions, under acid challenge, maintains a supersaturated mineral environment, reduces demineralization, and enhances remineralization of enamel [3]. CPP-ACP supplementation has been shown to be effective in remineralization of the enamel affected by MIH, resulting in an aesthetic improvement too [2]. However, this clinical approach requires a long-time treatment that could last months or years, requiring patients' cooperation.

The hypothesis tested in the present paper is that a combined use of CPP-ACP mousse and hydrogen peroxide gel may minimize the aesthetic defect caused by MIH opacities without requiring microabrasion or a composite restoration.

2. Case Presentation

The present paper shows a case report of a seventeen-year-old young man (M. N.) affected by moderate MIH. Superior central incisors show white-demarcated opacities in the incisal half of the labial surfaces. All the other teeth show less extensive incisal and occlusal opacities (Figures 1(a), 2(a), and 3(a)). Dental sensitivity is reported as normal. M. N. states a great aesthetic concern.

Consent was signed by M. N. and his parents: a combined CCP-ACP/hydrogen peroxide individualized protocol was used.

Pictures were captured under standardized conditions and, then, were edited using an imaging software (iPhoto, Apple, CA, USA) only increasing contrast and saturation exclusively in order to enhance the visualization of opacities (Figures 1(b), 2(b), and 3(b)).

Alginate impressions were realized to obtain custom trays using low-density polyethylene plates in a vacuum plasticizer.

The patient together with custom trays received a GC Tooth Mousse tube and he was instructed to use the trays two hours/day with CPP-ACP inside, after an accurate tooth-brushing. This first step lasted for three months, in order to obtain a noticeable remineralization of the enamel opacities.

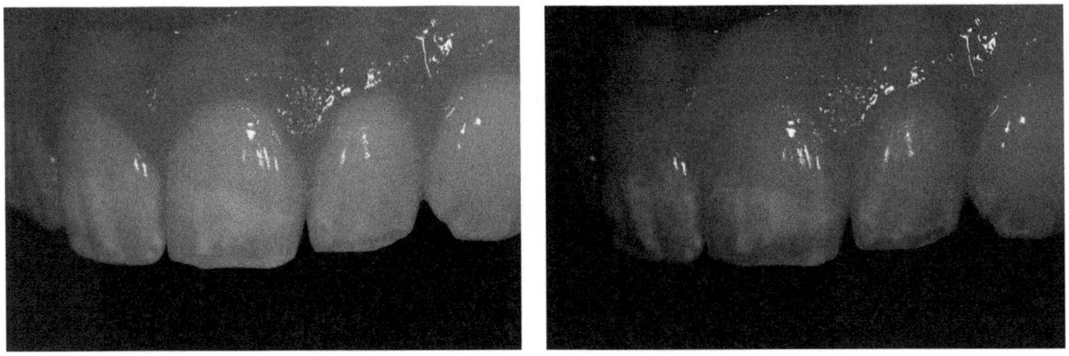

(a) (b)

FIGURE 3: (a) Initial left side picture. (b) Software-modified initial left side picture.

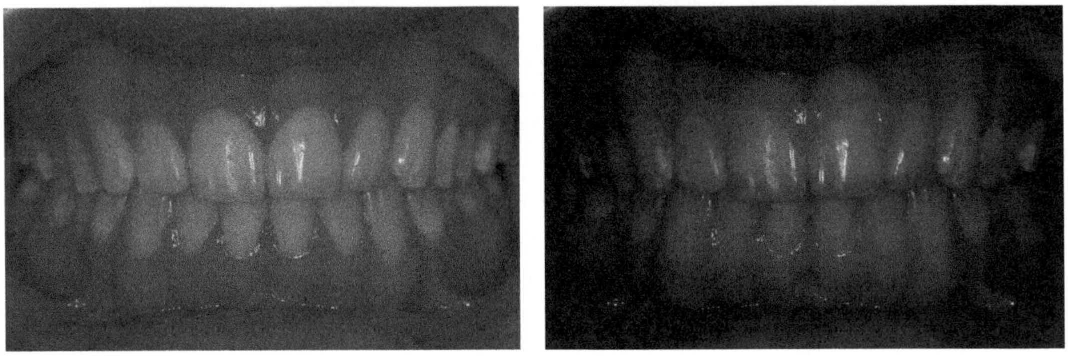

(a) (b)

FIGURE 4: (a) Final frontal picture. (b) Software-modified final frontal picture.

Dental examination was performed every month, in order to enhance M. N.'s motivation and take pictures.

After a three-month period, a combined use of CPP-ACP and bleaching agent was applied. A low-concentration hydrogen peroxide product was used. A 20% carbamide peroxide gel (Opalescence 20% Whitening gel, Ultradent Products, Inc. 505 West 10200 South, South Jordan, UT 84095, USA), approximately an equivalent to 6% of hydrogen peroxide, was provided.

The patient was instructed to wear trays with the bleaching agent for two hours on two consecutive days and for the remaining five days of the week the remineralizing agent. This protocol was repeated for two months in order to obtain 14 days of bleaching treatment (according to the manufactures instructions) (Table 1). During these two months, dental examinations were weekly performed to ensure safety and efficacy of the treatment and to early intercept any side-effects of hydrogen peroxide on MIH.

At the end of this five-month treatment, a noticeable aesthetic improvement of opacities was observed (Figures 4(a), 5(a), 6(a), 4(b), 5(b), and 6(b)).

TABLE 1: Scheme of the combined use of Casein Phosphopeptide-Amorphous Calcium Phosphate (CCP-ACP) and hydrogen peroxide.

	Month				
	I	II	III	IV	V
	Product utilization days/week				
CCP-ACP 2 hrs/day	7	7	7	5	5
Hydrogen peroxide 2 hrs/day	/	/	/	2	2

3. Discussion

MIH is a widespread dental condition; its prevalence ranges from 2.4% to 40.2% in different studies [5]. It is likely that MIH is not caused by one specific aetiological factor. An increased risk of MIH occurs if several agents or conditions act synergistically [5]. These factors act systemically and affect the developmental enamel during prenatal, perinatal, or the childhood period [1]. Particularly, pathogenic "noxae" during the first year of life are more frequent in children with MIH. Asthma, pneumonia, upper respiratory tract infections, otitis media, antibiotics, dioxins in mother's milk, tonsillitis and tonsillectomy, and exanthematous fevers during childhood were involved in the process [6]. Amoxicillin has been shown to affect enamel formation in animal model and a twofold increase in risk of MIH has been recorded

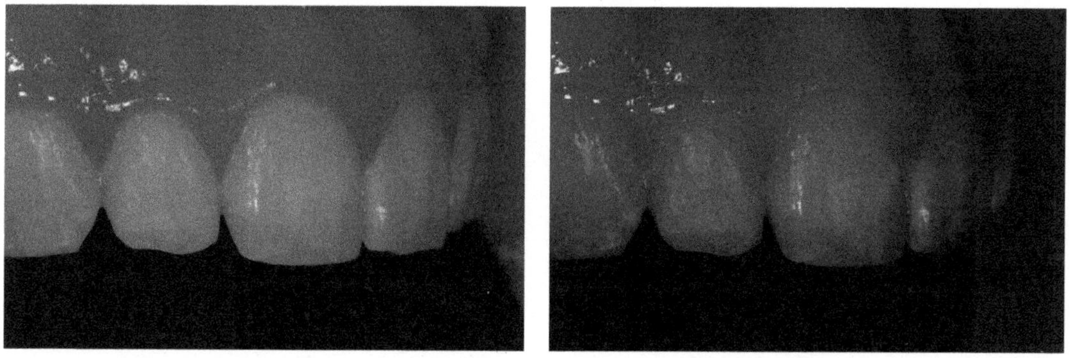

(a) (b)

FIGURE 5: (a) Final right side picture. (b) Software-modified final right side picture.

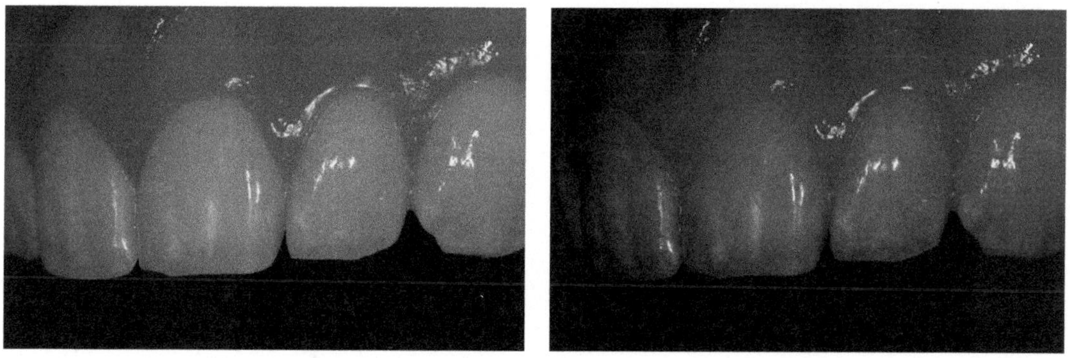

(a) (b)

FIGURE 6: (a) Final left side picture. (b) Software-modified final left side picture.

if amoxicillin was used during the first year [5]. So, at the present time, the aetiology of MIH still remains unclear.

Clinical problems associated with MIH regard function and aesthetics. Treatment approach for teeth affected by MIH is wide, ranging from prevention, restoration, to extraction [1]. MIH forms need a noninvasive treatment in order to preserve enamel integrity; nevertheless, simple and unambiguous clinical guidance is missing nowadays.

MIH opacities have a total reduced mineral content (about 20% of the weight) and a relative increase in organic substance [2, 7, 8]; its remineralization with conventional or new aids, like fluoride or CCP-ACP, is an arduous and slow proceeding. Microabrasion and/or composite resin restorations are the most used solutions to improve aesthetics of anterior teeth affected by opacities, but these approaches are quite invasive.

The use of bleaching systems on hypomineralized teeth is not recommended because of mineral changes caused by peroxides especially on enamel presenting an increase in carbon content and a decrease in calcium and phosphate content [2]. During a bleaching treatment, peroxides initiate oxide-reduction reaction that may lead to dissolution of both organic and inorganic matrices [9]. Enamel remineralization from saliva action is expected; nevertheless, an increase of enamel porosity, depression, superficial irregularities [10], roughness [11], and a decrease of hardness [12] are reported. This hardness reduction could be related to mineral loss resulting from demineralization [13].

CCP-ACP containing paste applied on teeth before and after the bleaching treatment [9], or mixed in similar proportion with the bleaching gel [3], has shown to be able to prevent roughness and hardness decrease of bleached teeth, without interfering with bleaching effect. CCP-ACP has, also, been shown to be effective in remineralization of MIH opacities *in vivo*, helping functional restorative techniques in MIH molars and aesthetics in untreated incisors [2]. Up to date it has never been investigated the possibility to treat MIH opacities using bleaching system combined with CCP-ACP mousse.

The protocol used in this paper has shown to be effective to improve aesthetics, although some weaknesses are to be considered. A long-term patient collaboration is required: two hours per day for five consecutive months. Furthermore, this protocol was applied to a patient affected by a moderate MIH; upper frontal incisors were the teeth mostly involved. White-demarcated opacities were wide, involving the incisal half of the labial surfaces and hypoplasia was not associated.

The short follow-up period (two months) could represent a limit. Results seem to be stable, but they have to be monitored for a longer period of time. In order to decrease the risk of recurrence of the defects, a maintenance therapy with CCP-ACP, (i.e., one time/week) should be considered.

This protocol has been described in the present paper for the first time and further corrections or revisions could be necessary. As recently described by de Vasconcelos et al. [3], in an *in vitro* study, the possibility to mix in similar proportion CCP-ACP mousse and the bleaching gel could be taken into account in enamel opacities treatment, decreasing the bleaching period to the usual two/three weeks.

An important aspect that must be considered is the need to personalize the protocol on the features of the opacities and the response of the defect to the treatment. The combined use of hydrogen peroxide and CCP-ACP, for example, could be performed with a ratio range from 1 : 6 to 3 : 4, depending on the opacity response to the bleaching agent.

The present protocol based on the combined use of CPP-ACP and hydrogen peroxide has shown to be effective and safe in bleaching teeth with enamel white opacities, allowing to preserve enamel integrity without recurring to restorative treatment or enamel abrasion.

References

[1] N. A. Lygidakis, "Treatment modalities in children with teeth affected by molar-incisor enamel hypomineralisation (MIH): a systematic review," *European Archives of Paediatric Dentistry*, vol. 11, no. 2, pp. 65–74, 2010.

[2] C. Baroni and S. Marchionni, "MIH supplementation strategies: prospective clinical and laboratory trial," *Journal of Dental Research*, vol. 90, no. 3, pp. 371–376, 2011.

[3] A. A. de Vasconcelos, A. G. Cunha, B. C. Borges et al., "Enamel properties after tooth bleaching with hydrogen/carbamide peroxides in association with a CPP-ACP paste," *Acta Odontologica Scandinavica*, vol. 70, no. 4, pp. 337–343, 2012.

[4] N. Efeoglu, D. Wood, and C. Efeoglu, "Microcomputerised tomography evaluation of 10% carbamide peroxide applied to enamel," *Journal of Dentistry*, vol. 33, no. 7, pp. 561–567, 2005.

[5] N. A. Lygidakis, F. Wong, B. Jälevik, A. M. Vierrou, S. Alaluusua, and I. Espelid, "Best clinical practice guidance for clinicians dealing with children presenting with molar-incisor-hypomineralisation (MIH): an EAPD policy document," *European Archives of Paediatric Dentistry*, vol. 11, no. 2, pp. 75–81, 2010.

[6] N. S. Willmott, R. A. Bryan, and M. S. Duggal, "Molar-incisor-hypomineralisation: a literature review," *European Archives of Paediatric Dentistry*, vol. 9, no. 4, pp. 172–179, 2008.

[7] B. Jälevik and J. G. Norén, "Enamel hypomineralization of permanent first molars: a morphological study and survey of possible aetiological factors," *International Journal of Paediatric Dentistry*, vol. 10, no. 4, pp. 278–289, 2000.

[8] R. A. Farah, M. V. Swain, B. K. Drummond, R. Cook, and M. Atieh, "Mineral density of hypomineralised enamel," *Journal of Dentistry*, vol. 38, no. 1, pp. 50–58, 2010.

[9] A. G. Gama Cunha, A. A. Meira de Vasconcelos, B. C. Dutra Borges et al., "Efficacy of in-office bleaching techniques combined with the application of a Casein Phosphopeptide-Amorphous Calcium Phosphate paste at different moments and its influence on enamel surface properties," *Microscopy Research and Technique*, vol. 75, no. 8, pp. 1019–1025, 2012.

[10] S. S. Ferreira, J. L. N. Araújo, O. N. Morhy, C. M. C. Tapety, M. N. Youssef, and M. A. P. Sobral, "The effect of fluoride therapies on the morphology of bleached human dental enamel," *Microscopy Research and Technique*, vol. 74, no. 6, pp. 512–516, 2011.

[11] J. M. Martin, J. B. de Almeida, E. A. Rosa et al., "Effect of fluoride therapies on the surface roughness of human enamel exposed to bleaching agents," *Quintessence International*, vol. 41, no. 1, pp. 71–78, 2010.

[12] A. B. Borges, L. Y. Samezima, L. P. Fonseca, K. C. K. Yui, A. L. S. Borges, and C. R. G. Torres, "Influence of potentially remineralizing agents on bleached enamel microhardness," *Operative Dentistry*, vol. 34, no. 5, pp. 593–597, 2009.

[13] J. D. Featherstone, J. M. ten Cate, M. Shariati, and J. Arends, "Comparison of artificial caries-like lesions by quantitative microradiography and microhardness profiles," *Caries Research*, vol. 17, no. 5, pp. 385–391, 1983.

7

Supraorbital Blowin Fracture Presenting as an Ocular Dystopia in a Nine-Year-Old Girl

Ranganadh Nallamothu,[1] Shanmukha Reddy Kallam,[2] Srikanth Gunturu,[3] Sukumar Singh,[4] and Vijay Kumar Rachalapally[5]

[1] *Department of Oral and Maxillofacial Surgery, Drs. Sudha & Nageswarao Siddhartha Institute of Dental Sciences, Chinoutpalli, Gannavaram 521 286, Krishna District, Andhra Pradesh, India*
[2] *Sri Sai College of Dental Surgery, Shiv Nagar, Kotherapally, Range Reddy District, Vikarabad 501101, Andhra Pradesh, India*
[3] *A B Shetty Memorial Institute of Dental Sciences Medical Sciences Complex, P.O. Nityanandanagar, Deralakatte 575018, India*
[4] *Subharati Dental College, Meerut Subharati Puram, NH-58, Delhi-Haridwar Bypass Road, Meerut 250005, Uttar Pradesh, India*
[5] *S.V.S. Institute of Dental Sciences, Mahabubnagar 509 001, Andhra Pradesh, India*

Correspondence should be addressed to Ranganadh Nallamothu; drranganadh@gmail.com

Academic Editors: L. Junquera and K. Seymour

A 9-year-old girl was referred to a trauma centre with severe head injury. 3D CT scan revealed depressed fracture involving the frontal bone on the right side, right parietal bone, and right superior orbital margin, right lamina papyracea. The frontal table was managed conservatively and open reduction and internal fixation was done for the supraorbital blow in to correct the ocular dystopia. The clinical course, possible mechanism, and management of the patient are discussed.

1. Introduction

Head injury is a common sequelae in the road traffic accident. Fractures of the supraorbital region are rare and are frequently associated with high-energy craniomaxillofacial trauma. When displacement of the orbital roof occurs, exploration and precise reconstruction are warranted to limit such ocular complications as exophthalmos, enophthalmos, proptosis, dystopia (ocular and orbital), diplopia, restricted ocular movement, altered vision, pain, and discomfort [1–13]. Fractures of the supraorbital rim can result in significant ophthalmologic and cosmetic morbidity. Isolated supraorbital rim fractures are rare [14, 15]. However, an estimated 1% to 9% of facial fractures can involve the supraorbital rims and the anterior table of the frontal sinus, and many supraorbital rim fractures are associated with other forms of craniomaxillofacial injury [1–6, 13]. Many of these patients have multisystem injuries, most of which are neurologic [16, 17]. These fractures are associated with high-energy impacts, motor vehicle collisions being the most frequently reported etiology [1, 18]. Many other causes have been identified, including tire explosions, ruptured garage door springs, chain saws, high-voltage electric shocks, swinging objects, and falls from high places [1, 3, 9, 10, 18, 19].

Patients with supraorbital rim fractures have characteristic physical signs and symptoms [1, 2, 12, 18]. If they are seen soon after the traumatic episode, then a cosmetic deformity consisting of depression or flattening of the supraorbital ridge can be visualized. Later, these injuries may present with intensely turgid periorbital ecchymosis, edema, soft tissue lacerations, and paresthesia over the area of distribution of the supraorbital and supratrochlear nerves. If the fracture is displaced, dystopia (ocular and orbital), enophthalmos, exophthalmos, and proptosis may be noted, along with diplopia [12]. Ocular discomfort, epiphora, limitation of eye movement, increased scleral show, and increased width of the palpebral fissure have all been reported [12].

A review of the literature reveals no uniform system for the classification of supraorbital rim fractures; most authors rely on descriptive terminology. A nondisplaced supraorbital rim fracture generally requires no surgical intervention [20, 21]. An orbital roof fracture, with undisplaced supraorbital

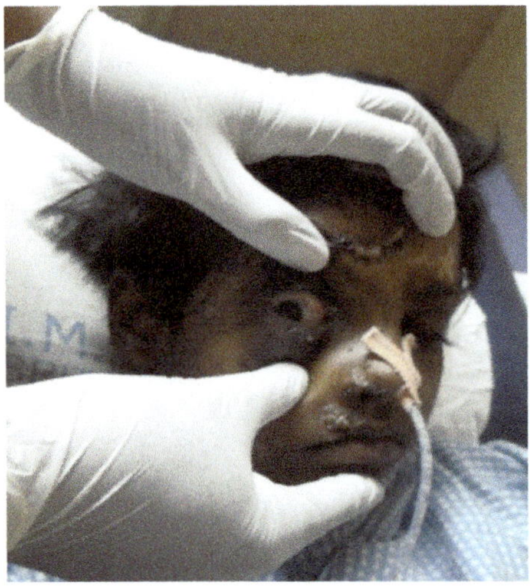

FIGURE 1: Subconjunctival hemorrhage, circumorbital ecchymosis, and horizontal ocular dystopia involving the right eye.

rim involvement and no frontal sinus fracture, is common in children [22]. When the fractured segments are displaced, surgical exploration, reduction, and stabilization are indicated. Supraorbital rim fractures frequently involve the frontal sinus. If the anterior table of the frontal sinus and the supraorbital rim was displaced, then operative treatment is required [14, 15].

A computed tomography (CT) scan can rule out damage to the posterior table of the frontal sinus. If there is a displaced fracture of the posterior table, then a dural tear is quite possible. However, treatment of such an injury is beyond the scope of this paper and must be carried out by a neurosurgeon of the team. The need for fixation in supraorbital rim fractures depends on the type of fracture encountered. The reduction is often stable once the fragments have been levered into position because of the absence of muscular displacing forces [14]. The introduction of rigid fixation into craniomaxillofacial fracture management revolutionized the treatment of orbital injuries [23].

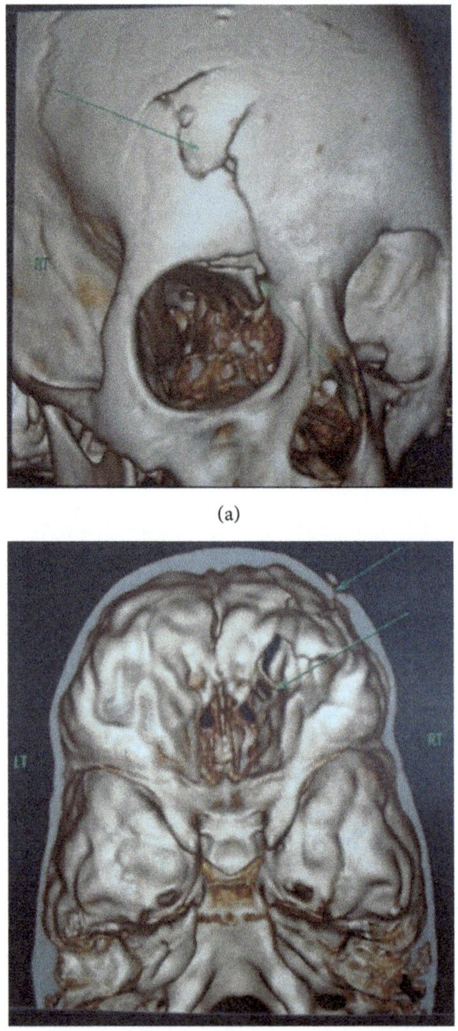

(a)

(b)

FIGURE 2: 3D CT scan revealed depressed fracture involving the frontal bone on the right side, right parietal bone, right superior orbital margin, right lamina papyracea, right maxillary, bilateral ethmoid, sphenoid sinusitis/hemosinus, and small posttraumatic encephalocele at anterior skull base from cribriform plate.

2. Case Report

A nine-year-old girl reported to a trauma centre with head injury with history of loss consciousness at the time of trauma and brought semiconscious to the hospital GCS-E1M5V2. On examination, she had a laceration on the frontal aspect of the face, right supraorbital region, and some abrasions on the chest. Subconjunctival hemorrhage, circumorbital ecchymosis, and horizontal ocular dystopia involving the right eye were observed (Figure 1). Right-eye ball was displaced to the lateral side of the orbit. 3D CT scan revealed depressed fracture involving the frontal bone on the right side, right parietal bone, right superior orbital margin, right lamina papyracea, right maxillary, bilateral ethmoid, sphenoid sinusitis/hemosinus, and small posttraumatic encephalocele at anterior skull base from cribriform plate.

Soft tissue swelling involving right orbitonasal and frontal region (Figures 2(a) and 2(b)). Frontal laceration was sutured primarily by a plastic surgeon at the primary stage. Later the patient was operated for the correction of the ocular dystopia. It was noticed that the supraorbital rim (medial 1/3) was pushing the globe from medial to lateral direction, and there was a step deformity on the right frontal aspect. Open reduction and internal fixation of supraorbital margin were planned under GA with nasal intubation. Supraorbital rim was approached through the existing scar with extension to the glabella region (Figures 3(a)–3(c)).

Dissection was carried out layerwise, the displaced supraorbital bony part was identified. It was noticed that a part of brain tissue was herniating between the two fracture segments; so an attempt was made to push the brain tissue,

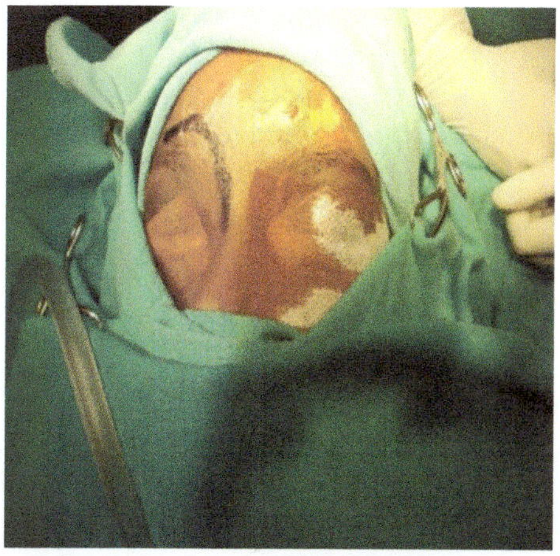

(a)

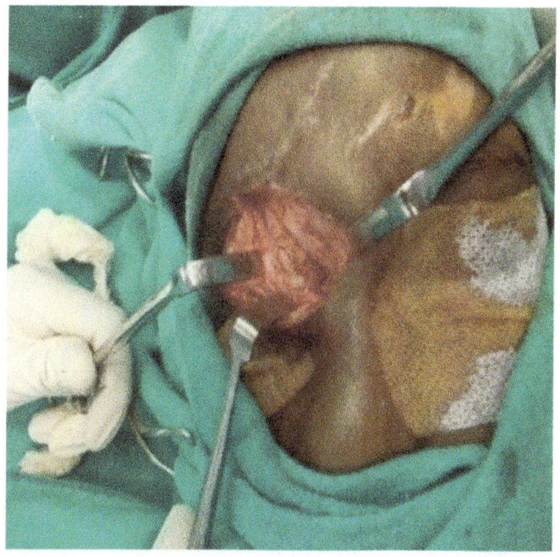

(b)

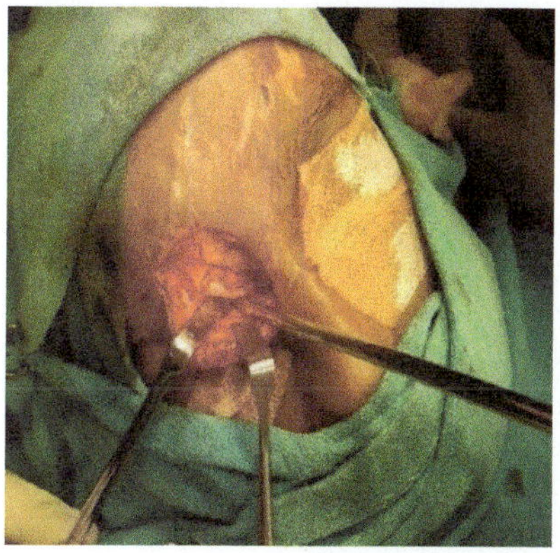

(c)

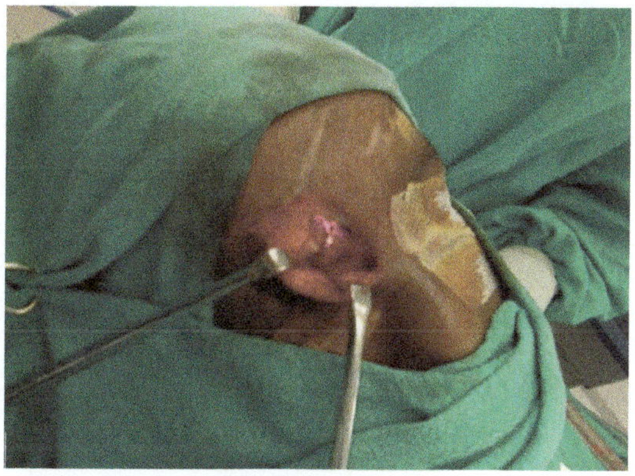

(d)

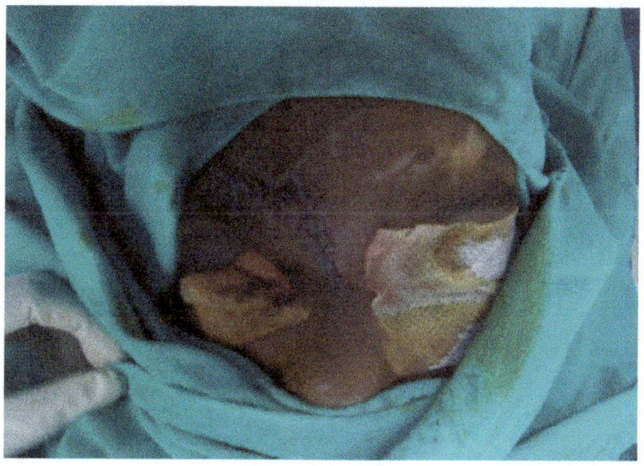

(e)

FIGURE 3: (a) Marking for the incision. (b) Fracture site exposed. (c) Reducing the segment manually with Howarth's periosteal elevator. (d) Open reduction and internal fixation with titanium plate and screws. (e) Layerwise closure done.

and the two fracture segments were reduced manually. A T-shaped titanium plate was bent according to contour of supraorbital roof and supraorbital ridge; horizontal bar of the plate was fixed on the supraorbital margin with 1.5 mm screws, and vertical bar was fixed to the roof with one 1.5 mm screw. Layerwise closure was done (3–0 vicryl for submucosal and 5–0 prolene for skin), and the recovery was uneventful. Frontal bone fracture was managed conservatively. Postoperative 3D CT scan was advised to confirm the reduction (Figure 4). Patient was discharged after 5 days and reviewed every 4 weeks. After one month postoperatively the patient was reviewed (Figure 5). Upon examination, it was found that the healing and the ocular dystopia were corrected satisfactorily.

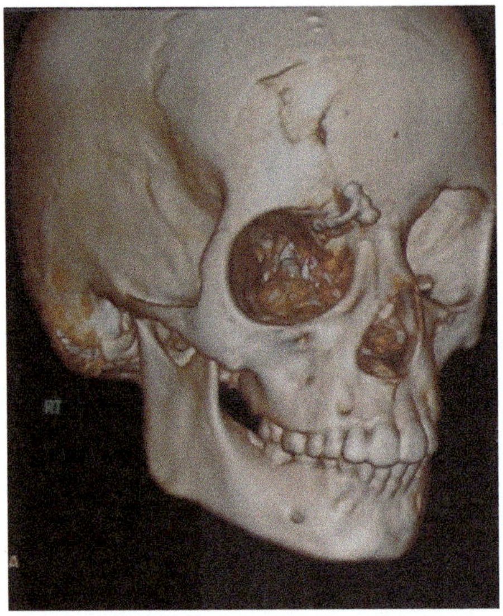

FIGURE 4: Postoperative 3D CT scan revealing titanium plate and screws intact at the fracture site.

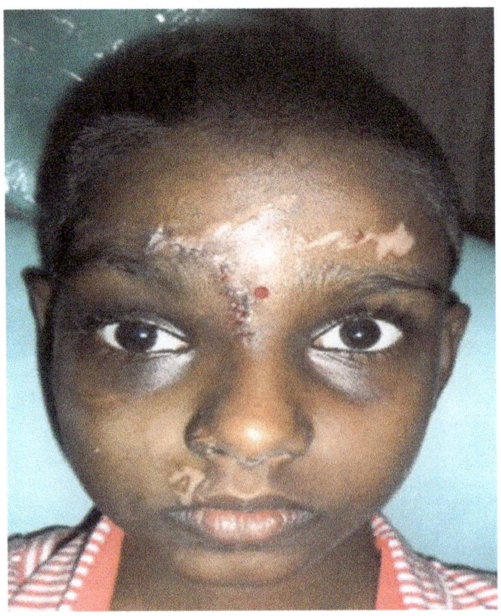

FIGURE 5: Two weeks after operation.

3. Discussion

3.1. Orbital Roof Fractures: Pathophysiology. There are several different configurations of orbital roof fractures including nondisplaced, isolated "blowin," isolated "blowout" (or "blowup"), supraorbital rim involvement (without frontal sinus), frontal sinus involvement, and combination fracture [24]. The common mechanism of injury for a superior orbital fracture is high-energy, blunt trauma to the orbit or forehead. The fracture is generally the result of direct extension of a force vector into the site of fracture, or due to a transient increase in orbital or intracranial pressure that results in fracture of the orbital roof.

The isolated orbital roof "blowup" fracture, also known as "blowout" fracture, is defined as superior displacement of the fracture fragment into the anterior cranial fossa without involvement of the supraorbital rim, with possible herniation of orbital contents outside of the orbital confines [24]. The isolated "blowup" fracture is thought to be the result of direct orbital blunt force with subsequent increased intraorbital pressure, hydraulic forces, and/or shear strain [24].

The isolated "blowin" fracture is defined as inferior displacement of the roof without involvement of the supraorbital rim or the frontal sinus and is thought to be the result of increased intracranial pressure, a shift of the cranium, and/or a shift of the intracranial contents [24]. The blowin fracture effectively reduces the volume of the orbit and can cause associated intraorbital injuries including extraocular muscle entrapment and optic nerve injury. Although the terms "blowin" and "blowup" fractures refer to isolated injuries of the internal superior orbit, these injuries occur far more commonly in conjunction with supraorbital rim and frontal sinus involvement [24].

When other craniofacial injuries are identified, it is thought that the mechanism of injury is direct transmission of force from displacement of the adjacent injury [24]. Very rarely, the orbital roof will fracture without displacement of fractures fragments, resulting in the nondisplaced orbital roof fracture [24].

4. Treatment

Orbital roof fractures are typically managed by otolaryngologists, ophthalmologists, neurosurgeons, plastic surgeons, and/or oral-maxillofacial surgeons depending on the individual case and associated imaging/clinical findings. Generally speaking, pediatric orbital roof fractures are less likely to require surgical repair than their adult counterpart [24, 25]. Currently, there is no specific consensus on the treatment of orbital fractures in the pediatric population [26].

Surgery is often performed if significant neurological, ophthalmologic, or aesthetic deficiency is clinically apparent or expected to eventually result from the injury, and the surgical intervention is likely to improve clinical outcomes. In general, surgical intervention is utilized only to repair displaced and comminuted fractures that will likely cause functional disability, cosmetic deformity, or both [27]. Pure "blowin" fractures, "blowout" fractures, and nondisplaced fractures that are asymptomatic generally have minimal clinical consequences and can be managed conservatively without surgery [26]. Fractures that extend beyond the orbital roof can generally be treated conservatively with diligent clinical and CT followup [26].

Surgical intervention is not an entirely benign solution with postoperative complications including enophthalmos, ocular dystopia, extraocular muscle entrapment, infection, orbital volume discrepancy, and blindness [24, 26].

References

[1] R. H. Haug, "Management of the trochlea of the superior oblique muscle in the repair of orbital roof trauma," *Journal of Oral and Maxillofacial Surgery*, vol. 58, no. 6, pp. 602–606, 2000.

[2] W. G. Sullivan, "Displaced orbital roof fractures: presentation and treatment," *Plastic and Reconstructive Surgery*, vol. 87, no. 4, pp. 657–661, 1991.

[3] C. N. Penfold, D. Lang, and B. T. Evans, "The management of orbital roof fractures," *British Journal of Oral and Maxillofacial Surgery*, vol. 30, no. 2, pp. 97–103, 1992.

[4] D. L. McLachlan, J. C. Flanagan, and G. M. Shannon, "Complications of orbital roof fractures," *Ophthalmology*, vol. 89, no. 11, pp. 1274–1278, 1982.

[5] R. C. Schultz, "Supraorbital and glabellar fractures," *Plastic and Reconstructive Surgery*, vol. 45, no. 3, pp. 227–233, 1970.

[6] R. R. Smith and R. L. Blount, "Blowout fracture of the orbital roof with pulsating exophthalmos, blepharoptosis, and superior gaze paresis," *American Journal of Ophthalmology*, vol. 71, no. 5, pp. 1052–1054, 1971.

[7] J. H. Horowitz, J. A. Persing, H. R. Winn, and M. T. Edgerton, "The late treatment of vertical orbital dystopia resulting from an orbital roof fracture," *Annals of Plastic Surgery*, vol. 13, no. 6, pp. 519–524, 1984.

[8] J. J. Bloem, J. C. Meulen, and J. M. Ramselaar, "Orbital roof fractures," *Modern Problems in Ophthalmology*, vol. 14, pp. 510–512, 1975.

[9] C. Ma and J. A. Nerad, "Orbital roof fracture with ocular herniation," *American Journal of Ophthalmology*, vol. 105, no. 6, pp. 700–701, 1988.

[10] I. A. Al-Qurainy, G. N. Dutton, K. F. Moos, S. T. Reynolds, and N. McMillan, "Orbital injury complicated by entrapment of the superior oblique tendon: a case report," *British Journal of Oral and Maxillofacial Surgery*, vol. 26, no. 4, pp. 336–340, 1988.

[11] F. L. McClurg Jr. and P. J. Swanson, "An orbital roof fracture causing diplopia," *Archives of Otolaryngology*, vol. 102, no. 8, pp. 497–498, 1976.

[12] M. A. P. Cabrini Gabrielli, E. H. Vieira, M. F. R. Gabrielli, and R. H. Barbeiro, "Orbital roof blow-in fracture: report of a case," *Journal of Oral and Maxillofacial Surgery*, vol. 55, no. 12, pp. 1475–1478, 1997.

[13] M. W. Ochs, "Management of the trochlea of the superior oblique muscle in the repair of orbital roof trauma," *Journal of Oral and Maxillofacial Surgery*, vol. 58, no. 6, p. 606, 2000.

[14] D. T. Lanigan and J. W. Stoelinga, "Fractures of the supraorbital rim," *Journal of Oral Surgery*, vol. 38, no. 10, pp. 764–770, 1980.

[15] R. H. Haug, J. E. Van Sickels, and W. S. Jenkins, "Demographics and treatment options for orbital roof fractures," *Oral Surgery, Oral Medicine, Oral Pathology, Oral Radiology, and Endodontics*, vol. 93, no. 3, pp. 238–245, 2002.

[16] J. C. Flanagan, D. L. McLachlan, and G. M. Shannon, "Orbital roof fractures. Neurologic and neurosurgical considerations," *Ophthalmology*, vol. 87, no. 4, pp. 325–329, 1980.

[17] D. J. Donahue, K. Smith, E. Church, and W. M. Chadduck, "Intracranial neurological injuries associated with orbital fracture," *Pediatric Neurosurgery*, vol. 26, no. 5, pp. 261–268, 1997.

[18] W. P. Piotrowski and J. Beck-Mannagetta, "Surgical techniques in orbital roof fractures: early treatment and results," *Journal of Cranio-Maxillo-Facial Surgery*, vol. 23, no. 1, pp. 6–11, 1995.

[19] M. Marchau, "Explosion of the orbital roof due to electrical current," *Neurosurgery*, vol. 23, no. 6, pp. 769–770, 1988.

[20] L. Manfre, G. Nicoletti, M. Lombardo, V. Consoli, G. Pero, and V. Albanese, "Orbital 'blow-in' fracture: MRI," *Neuroradiology*, vol. 35, no. 8, pp. 612–613, 1993.

[21] R. C. Schultz, "Supraorbital and glabellar fractures," *Plastic and Reconstructive Surgery*, vol. 45, no. 3, pp. 227–233, 1970.

[22] A. Hirano, K. Tsuneda, and G. Nisimura, "Unusual fronto-orbital fractures in children," *Journal of Cranio-Maxillo-Facial Surgery*, vol. 19, no. 2, pp. 81–86, 1991.

[23] H. G. Luhr, "Orbital fractures," in *Maxillofacial Traumatology*, vol. 1, pp. 319–348, Quintessence Publishing, Chicago, Ill, USA, 1982.

[24] R. H. Haug, J. E. Van Sickels, and W. S. Jenkins, "Demographics and treatment options for orbital roof fractures," *Oral Surgery, Oral Medicine, Oral Pathology, Oral Radiology, and Endodontics*, vol. 93, no. 3, pp. 238–245, 2002.

[25] V. M. Chapman, L. Z. Fenton, D. Gao, and J. D. Strain, "Facial fractures in children: unique patterns of injury observed by computed tomography," *Journal of Computer Assisted Tomography*, vol. 33, no. 1, pp. 70–72, 2009.

[26] J. E. Losee, A. Afifi, S. Jiang et al., "Pediatric orbital fractures: classification, management, and early follow-up," *Plastic and Reconstructive Surgery*, vol. 122, no. 3, pp. 886–897, 2008.

[27] A. Alcalá-Galiano, I. J. Arribas-García, M. A. Martin-Pérez, A. Romance, J. J. Montalvo-Moreno, and J. M. M. Juncos, "Pediatric facial fractures: children are not just small adults," *Radiographics*, vol. 28, no. 2, pp. 441–461, 2008.

8

Cone Beam Computed Tomography Evaluation of the Diagnosis, Treatment Planning, and Long-Term Followup of Large Periapical Lesions Treated by Endodontic Surgery: Two Case Reports

Vijay Shekhar and K. Shashikala

Department of Conservative Dentistry and Endodontics, D.A.P.M. R.V. Dental College and Hospital, Bangalore, Karnataka 560078, India

Correspondence should be addressed to Vijay Shekhar; vshekhar15@gmail.com

Academic Editors: D. W. Boston, A. C. B. Delbem, A. Markopoulos, and A. Milosevic

The aim of this case report is to present two cases where cone beam computed tomography (CBCT) was used for the diagnosis, treatment planning, and followup of large periapical lesions in relation to maxillary anterior teeth treated by endodontic surgery. Periapical disease may be detected sooner using CBCT, and their true size, extent, nature, and position can be assessed. It allows clinician to select the most relevant views of the area of interest resulting in improved detection of periapical lesions. CBCT scan may provide a better, more accurate, and faster method to differentially diagnose a solid (granuloma) from a fluid-filled lesion or cavity (cyst). In the present case report, endodontic treatment was performed for both the cases followed by endodontic surgery. Biopsy was done to establish the confirmatory histopathological diagnosis of the periapical lesions. Long-term assessment of the periapical healing following surgery was done in all the three dimensions using CBCT and was found to be more accurate than IOPA radiography. It was concluded that CBCT was a useful modality in making the diagnosis and treatment plan and assessing the outcome of endodontic surgery for large periapical lesions.

1. Introduction

The most common pathologic conditions that involve teeth are the periapical lesions, usually composed of solid soft tissue (granulomas) or semisolid, liquefied cystic area (cyst). They are the result of a localized inflammatory reaction to infection within the root canal system reducing mineral density of the affected periapical bone, resulting in resorption identified as radiolucencies in radiographs. It is essential to correctly diagnose these lesions as the choice of treatment is dependent on it [1]. Root canal therapy is accepted as the most effective conservative method for treating periapical lesions [2]. Periapical granuloma may heal without surgical treatment if given the opportunity; however, sometimes it may require surgical removal. It is controversial whether cysts heal with nonsurgical treatment because until a biopsy is taken, the clinician does not know the histologic diagnosis. Once a biopsy is taken, the treatment is no longer only nonsurgical. Periapical cyst usually requires surgical removal of the cyst.

The clinical, radiographic, and histological diagnosis of periapical lesions has been a challenge, and differentiating between the various periapical lesions remains an open research problem. Current diagnostic methods help in fair assessment of accurate size and nature of a periapical lesion which determine the treatment and prognosis of the tooth in question. Although, invasive post hoc biopsy is the only reliable method of diagnosis currently available, clinicians are aware of the difficulty in obtaining biopsies in routine clinical practice. Attempt to diagnose, the lesion before surgery with intraoral periapical (IOPA) radiographs, contrast media, Papanicolaou smears, and albumin tests have proven to be inaccurate. Thus, there is a need for a noninvasive method to diagnose lesions involving the periapical area. Recently with the advent of imaging modalities such as digital radiography, densitometry methods, computed tomography (CT), magnetic resonance imaging (MRI), ultrasound, and cone beam computed tomography (CBCT), differences in density may permit more accurate preoperative diagnosis [1, 3, 4].

The therapeutic protocol to treat diseases of endodontic origin is based on the evaluation of pathologic and clinical characteristics frequently complemented by radiographic findings using high-quality diagnostic radiographs. At present, IOPA radiography is the technique of choice for diagnosing, managing, and assessing endodontic diseases like periapical lesions. Radiographs provide bidimensional images of three-dimensional (3D) structures that do not permit the evaluation of bone thickness, determination of the size, and localization of periapical lesions. As a result of superimposition, IOPA radiographs reveal limited aspects of the 3D anatomy. In addition, there may also be geometric distortion of the anatomical structures being imaged. Limitations of IOPA radiographs for detecting periapical lesions include that, to be visible radiographically, cortical plate must be engaged. If confined within cancellous bone, they are usually not detected. A lesion of certain size can be detected in region covered by thin cortex but cannot be detected in region covered by thicker cortex. Many subsequent studies since that time have underscored the difficulty of detecting periapical lesions using IOPA radiographs. Therefore, considering some limitations on conventional radiography for detection of periapical bone lesions, advanced imaging methods such as CBCT might add benefits to endodontics and offer a higher quality for the diagnosis, treatment planning, and prognosis [1, 2, 4–9].

CBCT is a dentomaxillofacial imaging technique, which potentially provides dentistry with a practical tool for noninvasive and 3D reconstruction of teeth and their surrounding structures. CBCT exposes an object to multiple cone-shaped beams to acquire volume of the object, and later serial section images are obtained in coronal, sagittal, and axial planes, making possible the 3D interpretation. Thus, the clinician can visualize morphologic features and pathologies from different 3D perspectives [2]. Periapical disease may be detected sooner using CBCT compared with periapical views, and the true size, extent, nature, and position of periapical lesions can be assessed. Its other applications include visualization of root canal anatomy, assessment of true nature of the alveolar bone topography around teeth, treatment planning for periapical surgery, and the assessment of treatment outcomes. CBCT scans are desirable to assess teeth prior to periapical surgery, as the thickness of the cortical and cancellous bone and inclination of roots in relation to the surrounding jaw can be accurately determined, and the relationship of vital anatomical structures nerve to the root apices may also be clearly visualized [5, 10].

CBCT systems used in endodontics provide small field of view images at low dose with rapid scan time and sufficient spatial resolution. Various studies have found CBCT to be clinically superior to IOPA radiography for the detection of periapical lesions [1, 4–6, 11]. Thus, CBCT scan may provide safer, faster, and more accurate method for differential diagnosis of the periapical lesions. This allows clinician to decide, based on the type of periapical lesion, whether surgery is necessary or not, without the invasive biopsy procedure and waiting to see if healing has occurred (recall period). Evaluation of a periapical lesion with CBCT changes the estimation of size and choice of treatment among endodontists compared to IOPA radiography. Selecting the most appropriate choice of treatment using the most accurate imaging modality would ultimately reduce cost and morbidity significantly in patients undergoing endodontic therapy, and the lesion may be managed more effectively. However, scientific consensus maintains that true nature of a periapical lesion is accurately identified by histopathology only, which is considered to be the "gold standard" for achieving final confirmatory diagnosis of periapical lesions [1, 2, 4, 12].

A thorough history, clinical examination, and good quality radiographs are essential for preoperative diagnosis of teeth scheduled to undergo apical surgery [6]. In the currently available studies, no clear indications for the use of CBCT scans in diagnosis before apical surgery have been identified, and not as much emphasis has been placed on the applications of CBCT to endodontics, such as in the diagnosis, treatment planning, management, and followup of large periapical lesions requiring endodontic surgery [10].

The treatment outcome should be determined at follow-up examinations for at least 4 years, when it is established whether the preexisting periapical radiolucency has completely disappeared. IOPA radiographs have been widely used for root canal treatment followup [2]. Recently, CBCT has found to be useful in measuring the bone density before and after endodontic treatment [13]. Thus, CBCT can be used for the assessment of periapical healing following root canal treatment and endodontic surgery. CBCT provides an effective and safe way of producing 3D information of individual teeth and adjacent structures and may in time change the way in which the outcome of endodontic treatment is assessed [5].

The objective of this case report is to present two cases where CBCT was used for the diagnosis, treatment planning, and long-term followup of healing of large periapical lesions in relation to maxillary anterior teeth, treated by endodontic surgery, compared to IOPA radiographs.

2. Case Reports

2.1. History and Diagnosis

2.1.1. Case 1. A 27-year-old male patient reported with the chief complaint of swelling in the upper front right region of the mouth 1 month ago. He had a history of trauma to right upper anterior region 12 years back. The clinical examination revealed intraoral swelling in palatal region accompanied with salty discharge with respect to teeth 11, 12, and 21, and a sinus opening with respect to the apex on buccal aspect of 12 and 13 (Figures 1 and 2). The teeth were tender on percussion and nonvital with Ellis and Davey class 4 trauma. Palpation of right upper anterior region was painful. Teeth 11 and 12 had grade 1 mobility.

The IOPA radiographic examination revealed a large radiolucent lesion with a well-defined border in the periapical area of teeth 11, 12, and 21 suggestive of periapical

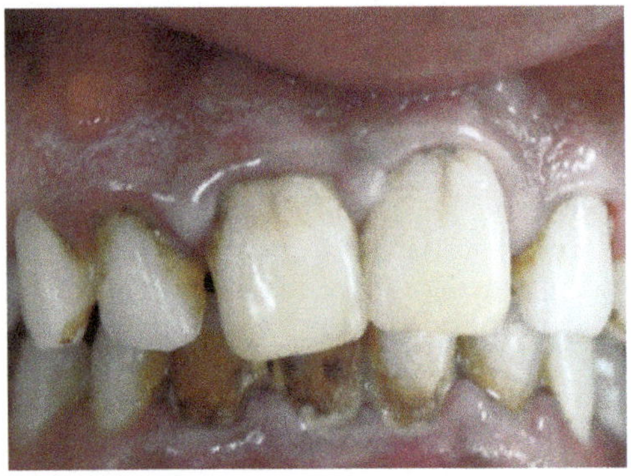

FIGURE 1: Preoperative photo showing presence of sinus tract with respect to 12 and 13.

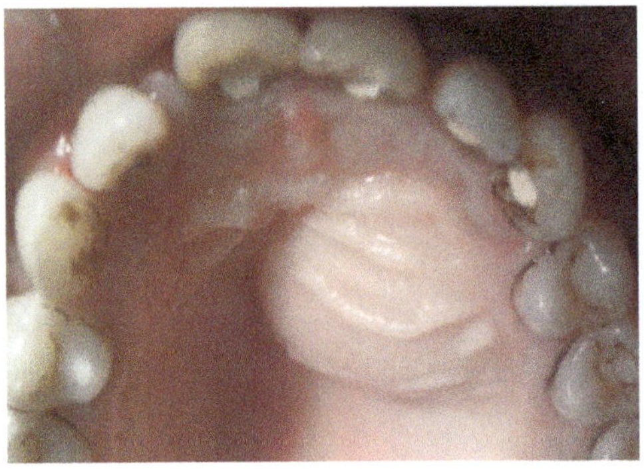

FIGURE 2: Pre-operative photo showing swelling of the palatal soft tissue.

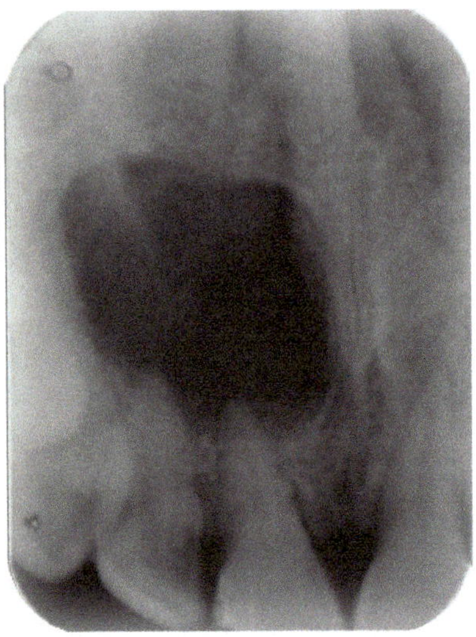

FIGURE 3: Pre-operative IOPA radiograph showing well-defined large periapical lesion.

cyst (Figure 3). CBCT examination revealed presence of periapical radiolucency with respect to 11, 12, 13, and 21 in sagittal, coronal, and axial planes and reconstructed three-dimensional image (Figures 4, 5, 6, and 7). Oral and maxillo-

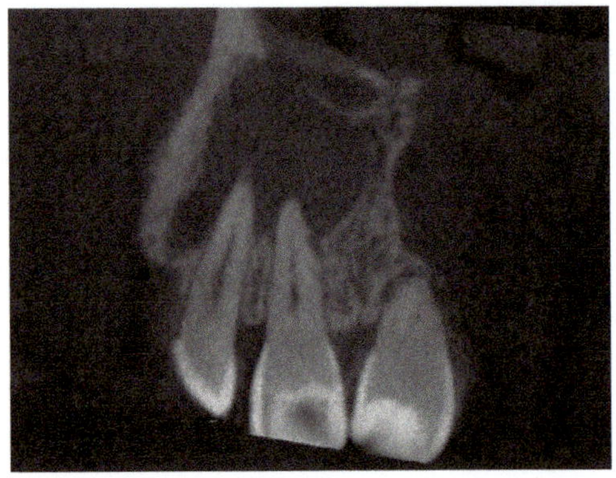

FIGURE 4: Pre-operative CBCT image in coronal plane showing presence of a large periapical lesion.

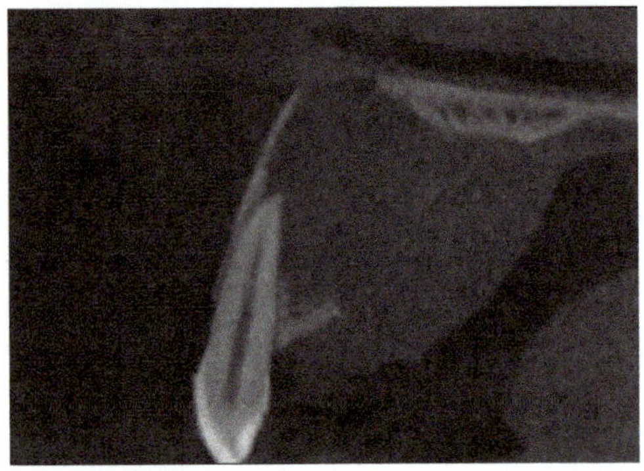

FIGURE 5: Pre-operative CBCT image in sagittal plane.

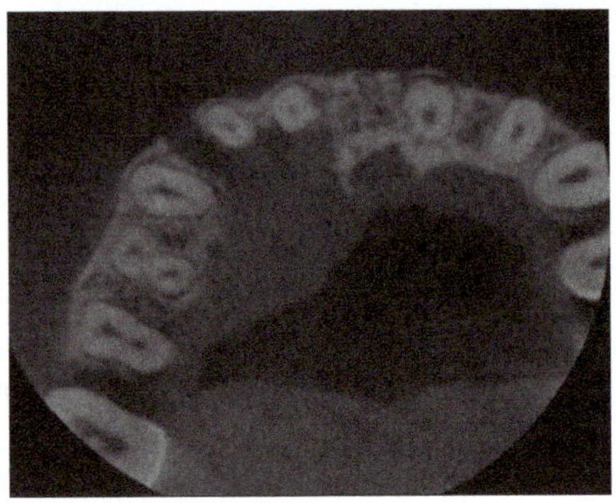

FIGURE 6: Pre-operative CBCT image in axial plane showing disruption of buccal and palatal cortex.

facial radiologist categorized the CBCT images, based on the radiodensity as periapical granuloma.

2.1.2. Case 2. A 22-year-old male patient reported with the chief complaint of pus discharge from upper right front region of mouth for 4-5 years. The clinical examination revealed discolored fractured crown fracture with respect to

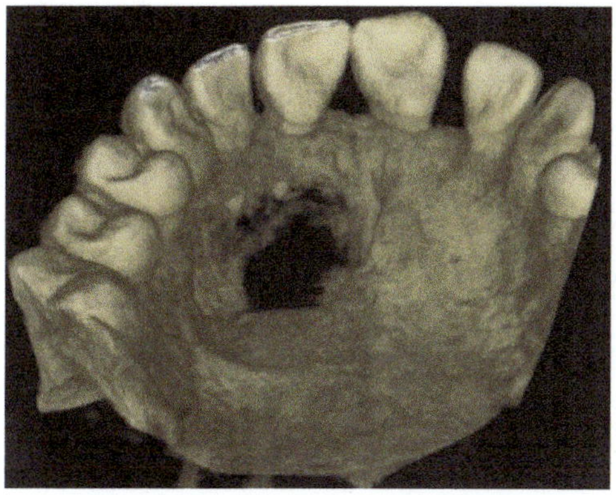

FIGURE 7: Reconstructed 3D CBCT image.

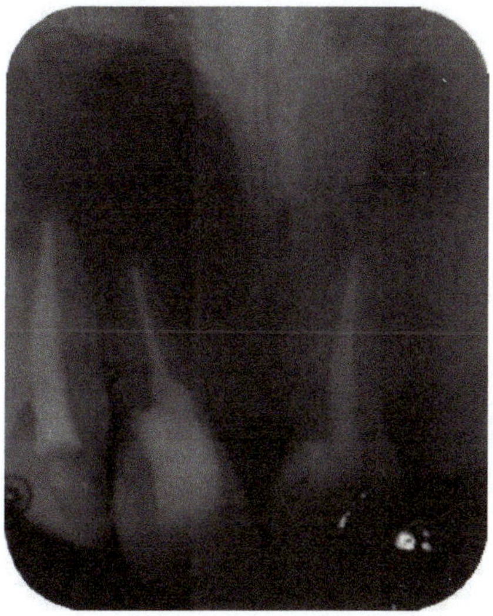

FIGURE 8: Postobturation IOPA radiograph.

tooth 11 while tooth 12 was displaced (Figure 27). Teeth 11 and 12 were nonvital with Ellis and Davey class 4 trauma.

The IOPA radiographic examination revealed large radiolucent lesion with a well-defined sclerotic border in the periapical area of teeth 11 and 12, along with displacement of these teeth suggestive of periapical cyst (Figure 28). CBCT examination revealed presence of periapical radiolucency with respect to 11 and 12 in sagittal, coronal, and axial planes and reconstructed three-dimensional image (Figures 29, 30, 31, and 32). Oral and maxillofacial radiologist categorized the CBCT images, based on the radiodensity as periapical cyst.

2.2. Management. The endodontic treatment was performed as per standard procedures in both cases under rubber dam isolation (Figures 8 and 33). All the canals were instrumented with hand K files and irrigated with 5.25% sodium hypochlorite. The root canals were obturated using gutta percha, and access cavity was sealed with temporary restorative material. This was followed by endodontic surgery (apicoectomy) (Figures 9, 10, 11, 12, 34, 35, 36, and 37), during which biopsy specimens were taken for histopathologic examination (Figures 13 and 38). Splinting with composite was done in the

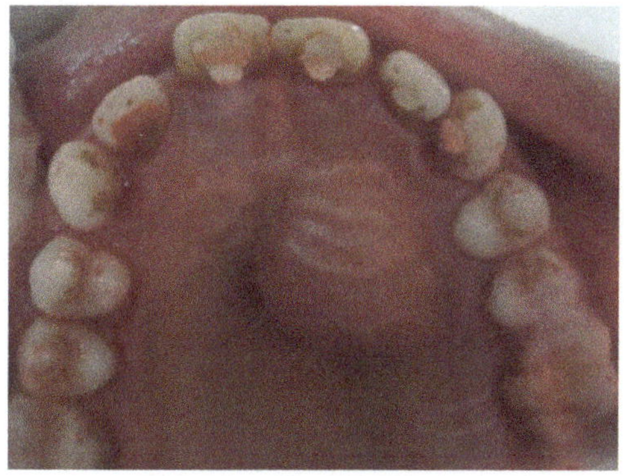

FIGURE 9: Surgical incision on palatal aspect.

first case of the mobile teeth for 4 weeks (Figure 14). Then tooth preparation was done followed by temporisation of the involved teeth with acrylic crowns (Figures 15, 16, 39, and 40). Finally, porcelain fused to metal (PFM) crowns were cemented on the involved teeth (Figures 17 and 41).

2.3. Histopathologic Examination. Histopathologic examination done in the first case revealed fibrous connective tissue which was inflamed, dense aggregate of chronic inflammatory cells, dilated and congested blood vessels and hemorrhagic foci, many Russell bodies, and few giant cells. No evidence of epithelium was present in the given sections. Oral pathologist diagnosed the specimen as periapical granuloma (Figure 18). Histopathologic examination done in the second case revealed cystic lining of nonkeratinized stratified squamous epithelium of varying thickness, an "arcading" pattern of proliferation, fibrovascular connective tissue wall which contained hemorrhagic areas and a dense inflammatory infiltrate of lymphocytes, plasma cells, and neutrophils. Oral pathologist diagnosed the specimen as infected periapical cyst (Figure 42).

2.4. Followup. The patient was recalled regularly for two years for followup done by clinical and radiographic examination using IOPA radiographs and CBCT. The IOPA radiographs at one month, six months, 12 months, 18 months, and 24 months showed a decrease in the size of periapical radiolucency (Figures 19, 20, 21, 22, 23, 43, 44, 45, 46, and 47). In both cases, at the end of two years, it was noted that at the periapex of the involved teeth, there was a small radiolucency termed as the periapical scar. Healing with periapical scar is acceptable and common with large periapical lesions. The CBCT examination done at the end of one year revealed a remarkably reduced size of the periapical radiolucency in all the three planes: coronal, sagittal, and axial in both cases (Figures 24, 25, 26, 48, 49, and 50). Thus, both clinical and radiographic examination revealed a complete healing of the periapical lesions at the end of two years.

3. Discussion

This case report used three study tools for the diagnosis of two large periapical lesions: 3D imaging by CBCT (9500 Cone

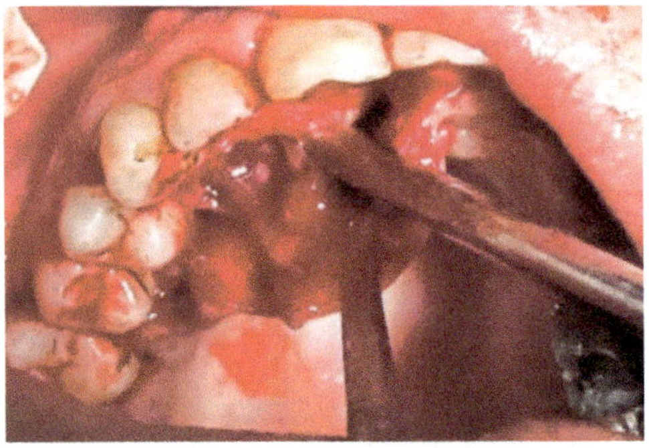

Figure 10: Flap reflection.

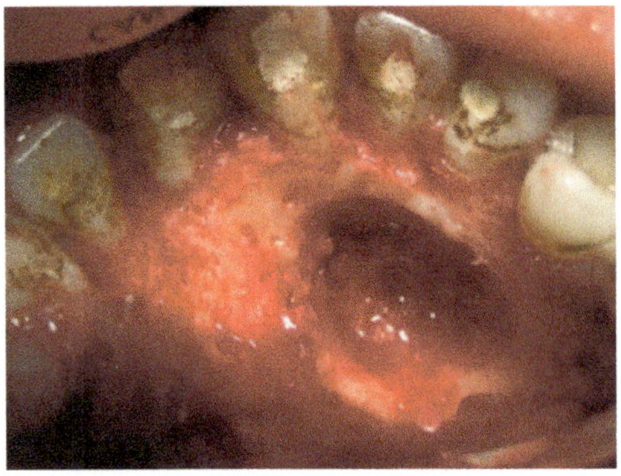

Figure 11: Flap retraction and exposure of bony defect.

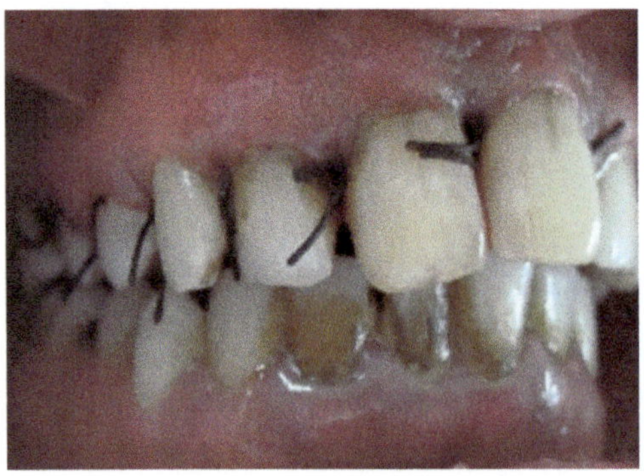

Figure 12: Suturing.

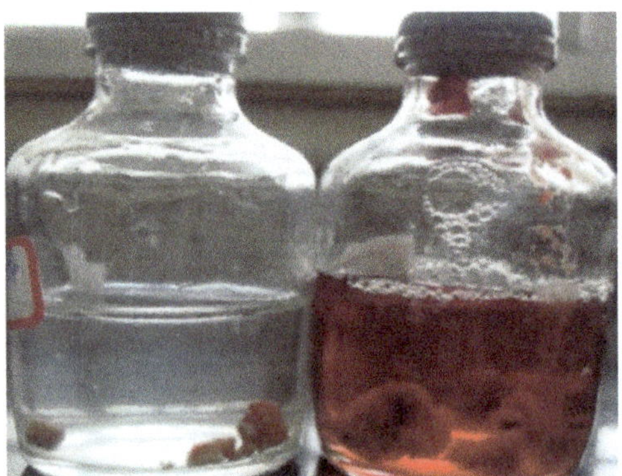

Figure 13: Lesional tissue stored in formalin for histopathological examination.

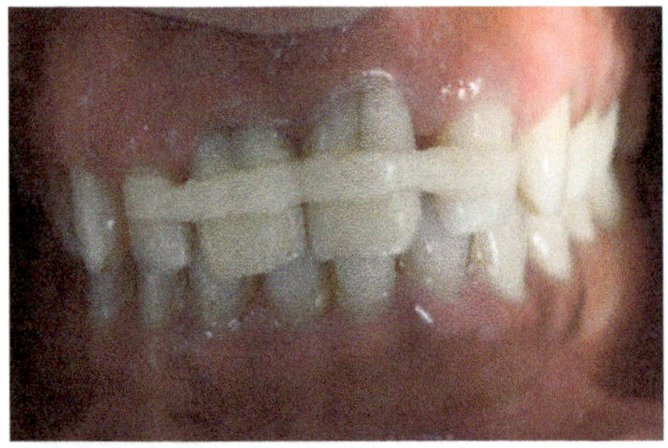

Figure 14: Splinting of mobile teeth using composite.

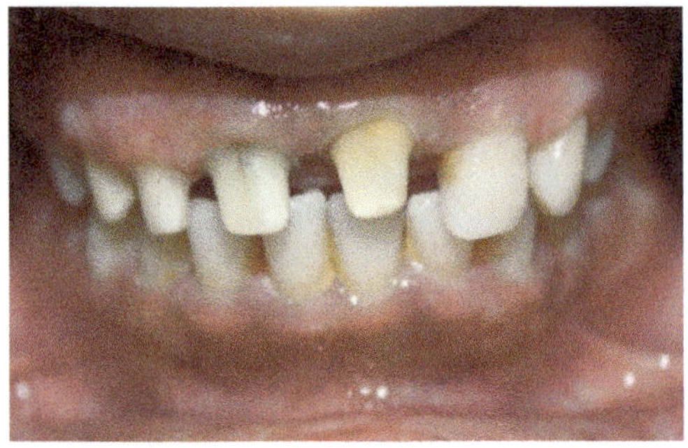

Figure 15: Tooth preparation.

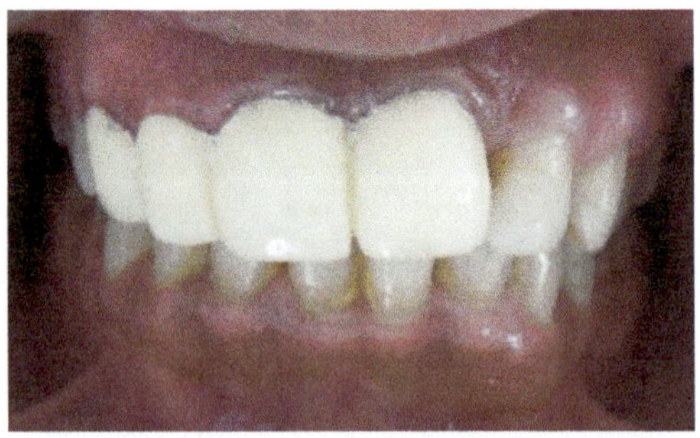

Figure 16: Temporization with acrylic crowns.

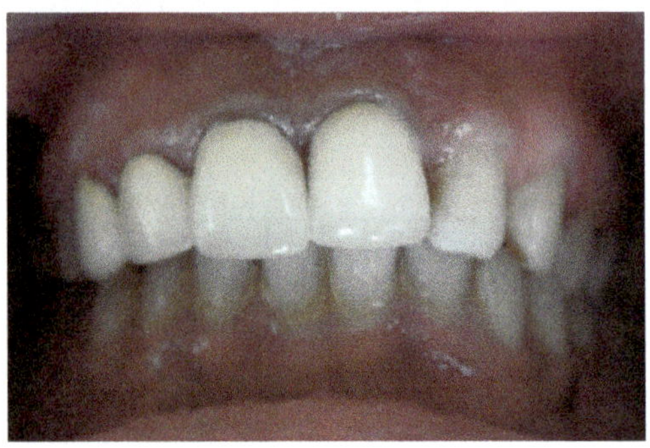

Figure 17: PFM crown cementation on 11, 12, 13, and 21.

Beam 3D System), conventional two-dimensional imaging by IOPA radiography, and histopathological examination by biopsy. The initial diagnosis and treatment planning for management of periapical lesions were done using IOPA

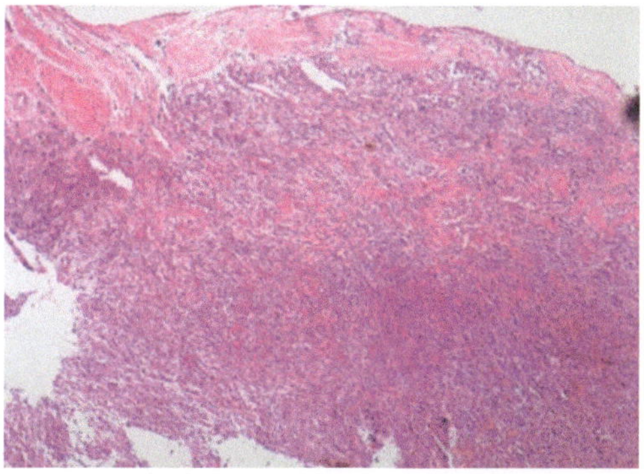

FIGURE 18: Histopathology report: periapical granuloma.

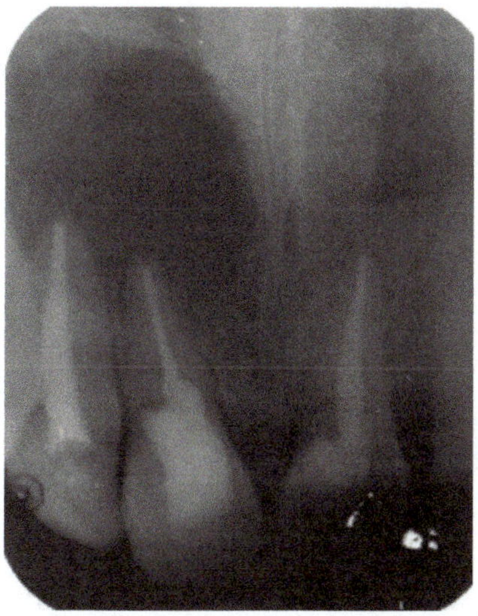

FIGURE 19: 1-month followup IOPA radiograph.

radiographs and gray scale value measurements with CBCT. For the management, endodontic treatment was performed for all cases followed by endodontic surgery. The radiographic findings were compared to surgical biopsy report which established the confirmatory histopathological diagnosis of the periapical lesions. Followup was done for the assessment of treatment outcome following surgery of the large periapical lesions, using CBCT and IOPA radiography.

A diagnostic test should exhibit validity and reliability if it is to be useful. Determining whether the periapical radiolucency is a cyst or granuloma cannot be done with IOPA radiographs alone. Until a biopsy is taken, the clinician does not know the confirmatory histopathologic diagnosis, but it is an invasive procedure requiring surgical intervention [1, 2, 4, 12]. Shortcomings in histological technique are that invasive surgery is mandatory to obtain specimen, lesion is curetted, often only small, multiple pieces are obtained, and false diagnosis is possible in lesions with epithelial lining that appears to be lining a lumen which is the histologic picture of bay/true cyst. To be accurate, serial sections through tooth with lesion attached are necessary. It is expensive, time consuming, and rarely done.

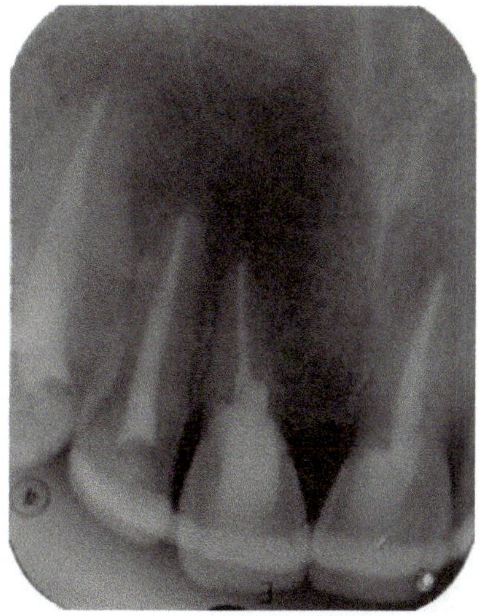

FIGURE 20: 6-month followup IOPA radiograph.

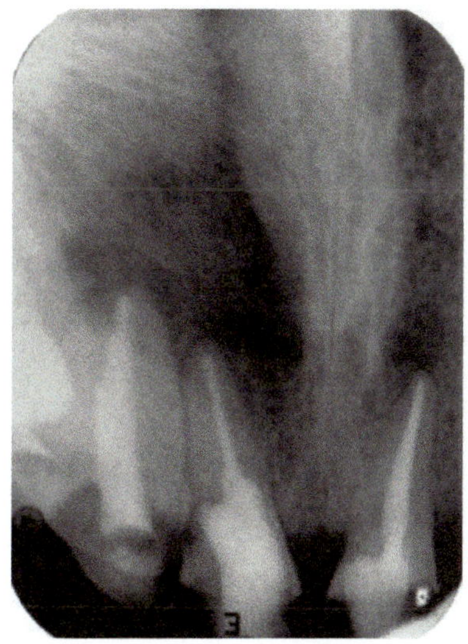

FIGURE 21: 12-month followup IOPA radiograph.

CBCT is a recent diagnostic modality whose software allows clinician to view reconstructed slices of data in 3D without the overlying cortical plate (anatomical noise). The reconstructed slices are geometrically accurate. The periapical lesions do not change size or disappear on reconstructed scans as can happen with IOPA radiography. CBCT gains an unabridged view of dental anatomy, thus eliminating some of the most prevalent problems, such as superimposition and distortion. CBCT reduces false diagnosis and is rapidly replacing other radiographic techniques in diagnosis, quality control of treatment methods and techniques, and outcome assessment.

A few studies have shown that CBCT imaging is not a reliable diagnostic method for differentiating radicular cysts from granulomas while histopathological evaluation by surgical biopsy remains the standard procedure [12]. The CBCT scan differentiates only a solid soft tissue lesion from

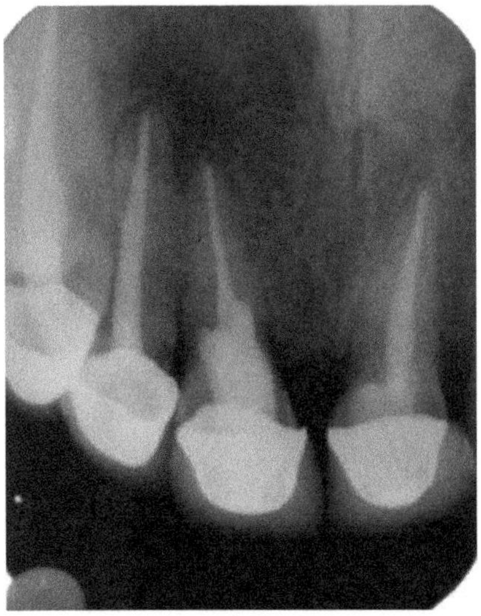

Figure 22: 18-month followup IOPA radiograph.

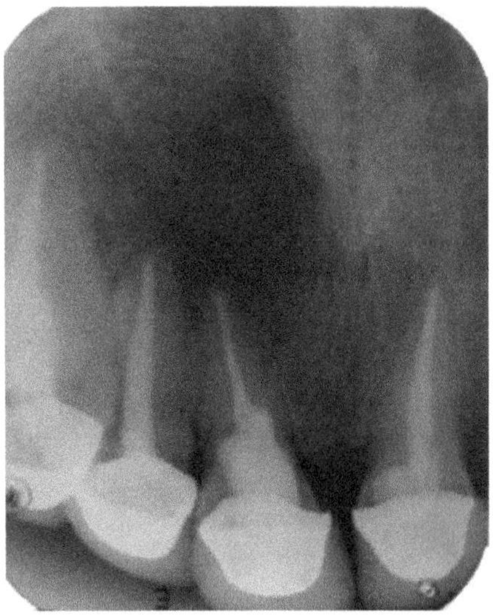

Figure 23: 24-month followup IOPA radiograph.

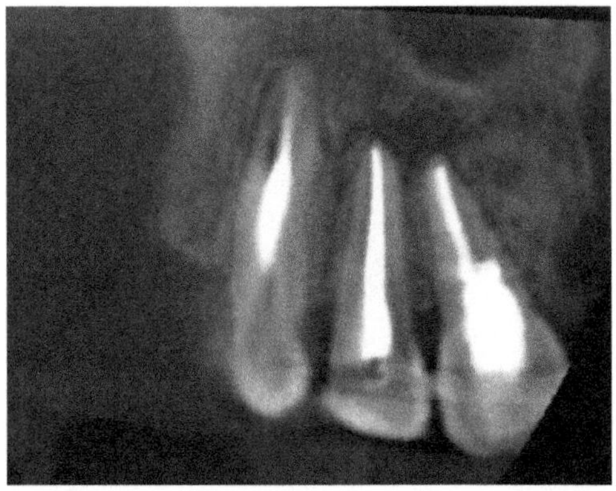

Figure 24: 1-year followup CBCT image in coronal plane.

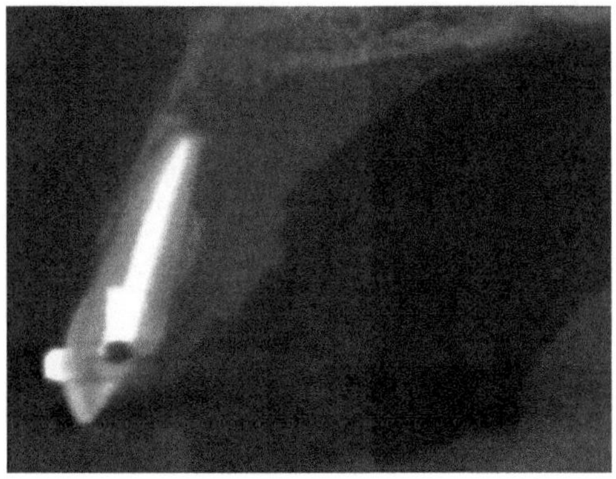

Figure 25: 1-year followup CBCT image in sagittal plane.

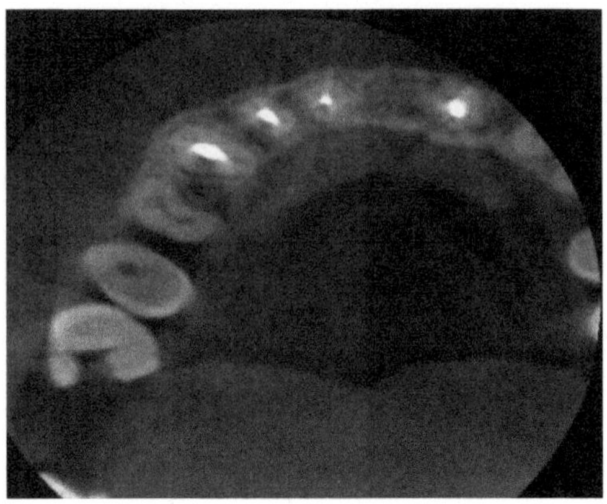

Figure 26: 1-year followup CBCT image in axial plane showing establishment of buccal and palatal cortical plates.

one that has soft tissue plus an area that is less dense, that is, cavity with fluid, semisolid substance in the lumen. However, one study revealed that CBCT may be clinically more accurate and more useful than the biopsy because of the shortcomings in histological technique. Other studies have concluded that the detection of periapical lesions was considerably higher with CBCT than with IOPA radiography. Not only can the presence of a periapical lesion be diagnosed with CBCT, but the specific root that it is associated with can also be confirmed, which influences treatment planning. Thus, CBCT was found to be an accurate diagnostic method to identify large periapical lesions based on the gray scale value and provide essential diagnostic information for the management of this complex endodontic problem as compared to IOPA radiographs [1, 8]. To get an accurate reading, the whole lucency should be scanned for the most lucent or least dense area. Negative grayscale value indicates lumen of a bay or true cyst (cavitated lesions). Positive grayscale value indicates epithelioid granuloma or a granuloma. However, it is not clear whether all CBCT scan-detected periapical lesions are true lesions [3].

Recently, limited field of view CBCT has proved to be useful in detecting periapical lesions in the maxillary region in a case report. The knowledge of the relationship of periapical lesions to the roots of maxillary teeth may be useful in treatment planning and in the prevention of complications

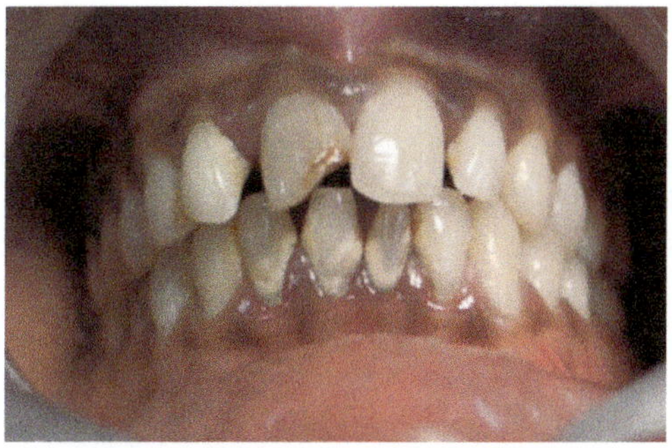

FIGURE 27: Pre-operative photo showing fractured and discolored 11 and displaced 12.

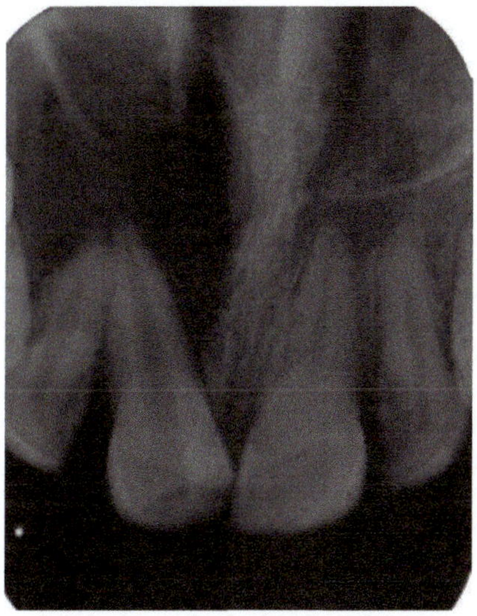

FIGURE 28: Pre-operative IOPA radiograph showing well-defined large periapical lesion.

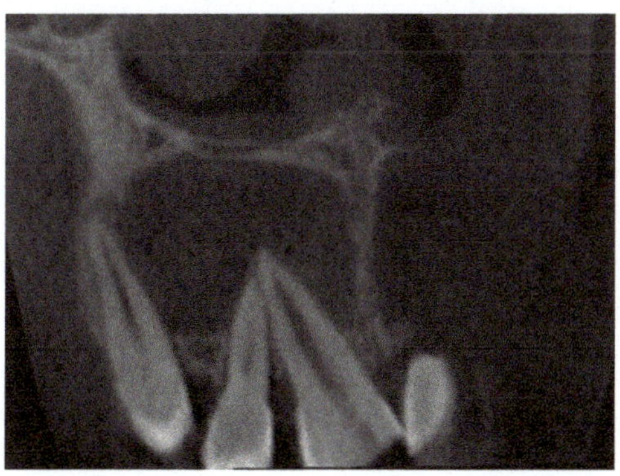

FIGURE 29: Pre-operative CBCT image in coronal plane.

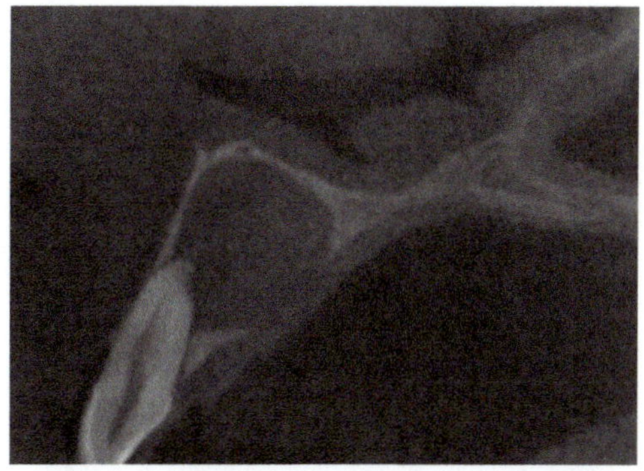

FIGURE 30: Pre-operative CBCT image in sagittal plane.

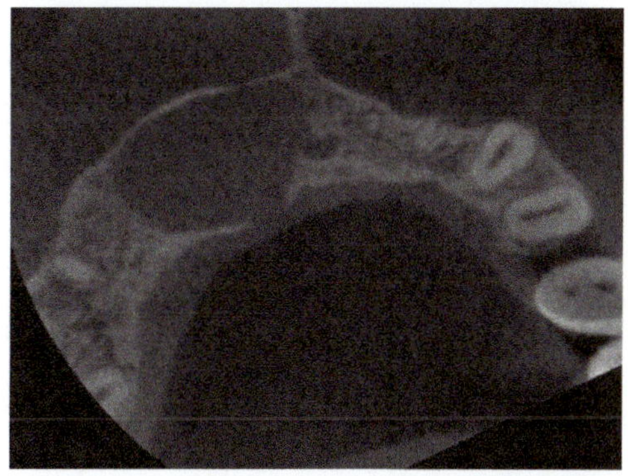

FIGURE 31: Pre-operative CBCT image in axial plane.

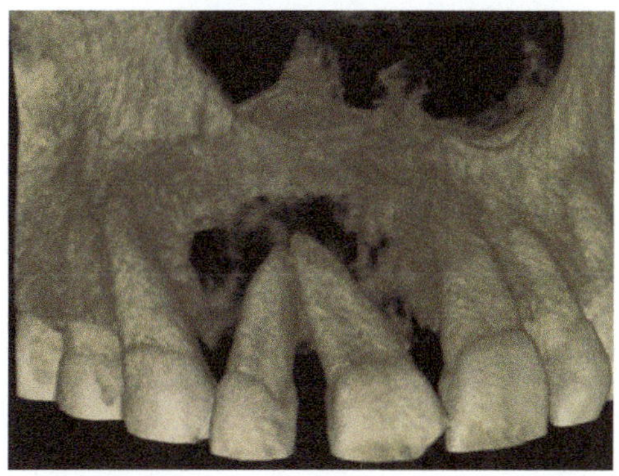

FIGURE 32: Reconstructed 3D CBCT image.

that may occur during apical surgery. A study revealed that 34% of the lesions detected with CBCT were missed with IOPA radiography in maxillary premolars and molars [6].

It is essential to understand which factors positively or negatively influence the outcome of endodontic treatment. IOPA radiographs were used in most previous outcome studies. However, periapical lesions could be radiographically undetectable when lesions are confined within the cancellous bone and covered by a thick cortex. A study compared the endodontic outcome predictors identified with IOPA radiography and CBCT revealed that CBCT was more sensitive than IOPA radiography in detecting extra canals and post-treatment periapical lesions [7]. The information obtained by CBCT evaluation of periapical repair following root canal treatment was comparable to histological analysis, whereas IOPA radiographs underestimated the size of the periapical lesion [2]. Absence of radiolucency in IOPA radiograph does not guarantee a healthy periapex. CBCT scan is better suited

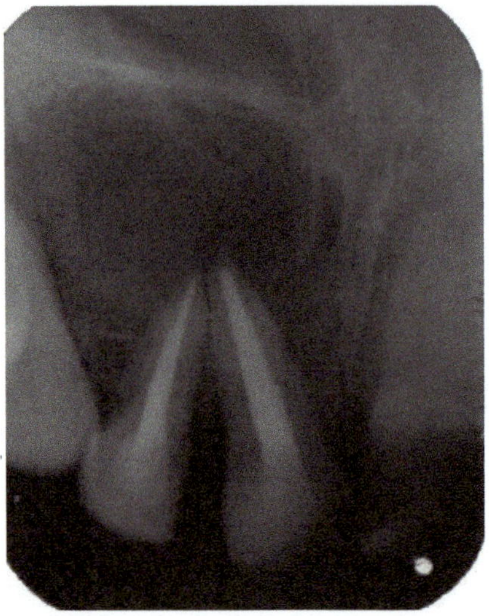

FIGURE 33: Postobturation IOPA radiograph.

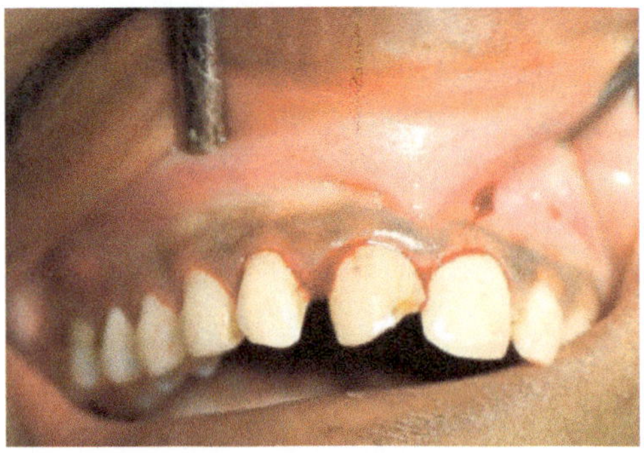

FIGURE 34: Surgical incision.

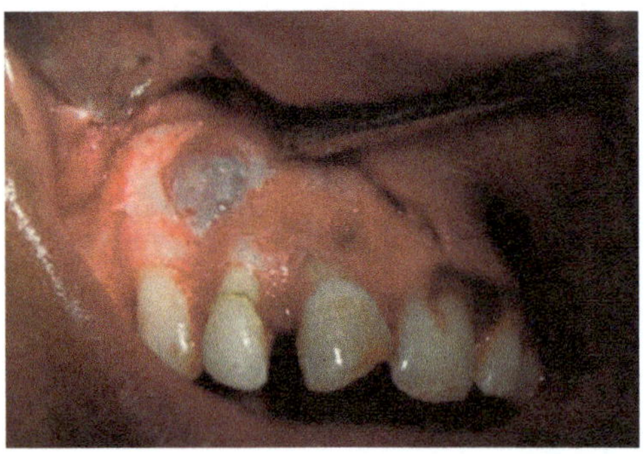

FIGURE 35: Flap retraction and exposure of the cyst.

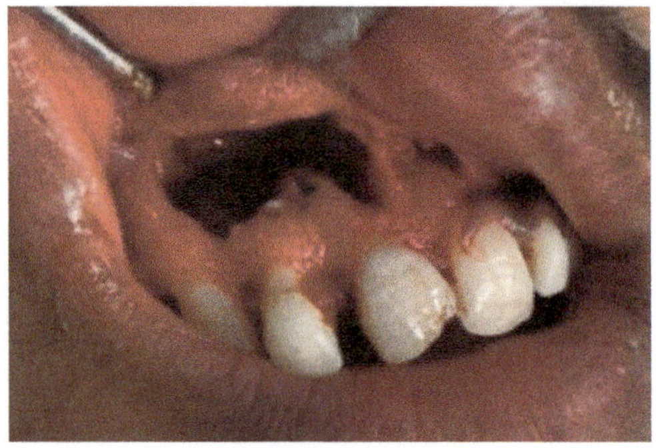

FIGURE 36: Apicoectomy.

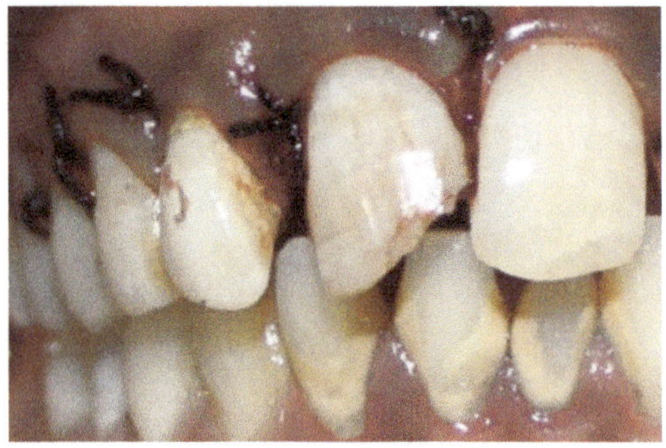

FIGURE 37: Suturing.

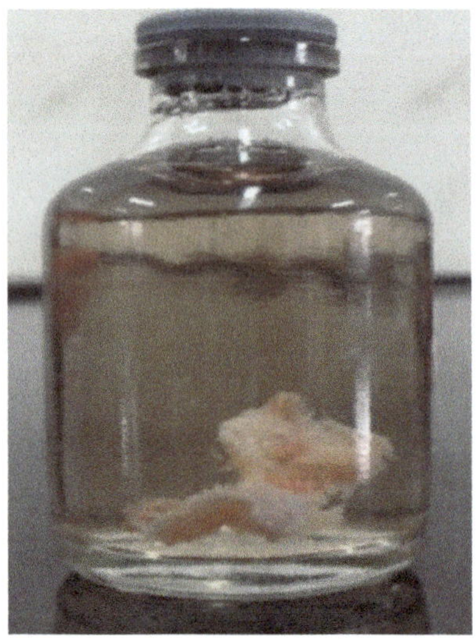

FIGURE 38: Lesional tissue stored in formalin.

for detection and diagnosis of periapical lesions. CBCT is a technology that has proven useful for localization and characterization of root canals and treatment planning of periapical surgery. This case report showed that CBCT is a good noninvasive modality towards the differential diagnosis of periapical lesions.

In both cases, the large lesions were treated by endodontic surgery (apicoectomy). Although CBCT revealed the lesion in the first case to be a periapical granuloma, due to its large size in all the three dimensions, it was decided to treat it surgically. The rationale was that according to the literature, endodontic surgery done for large lesions has a more favourable and predictable treatment outcome, and the periapical healing is faster, compared to root canal treatment alone. Moreover, the true size, extent, and location of the lesion obtained by CBCT help in the treatment planning for surgery and make it a safe procedure.

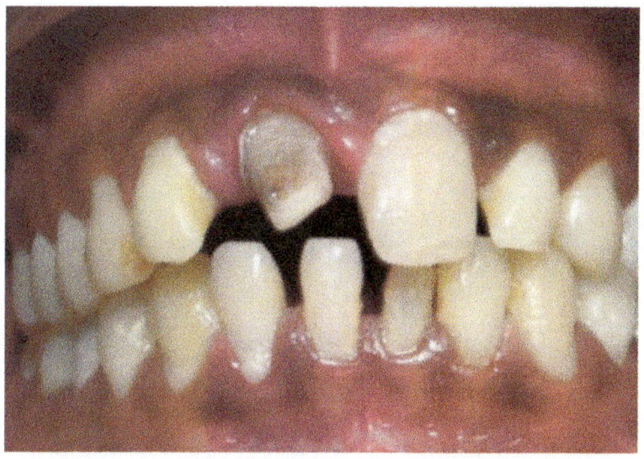

FIGURE 39: Tooth preparation.

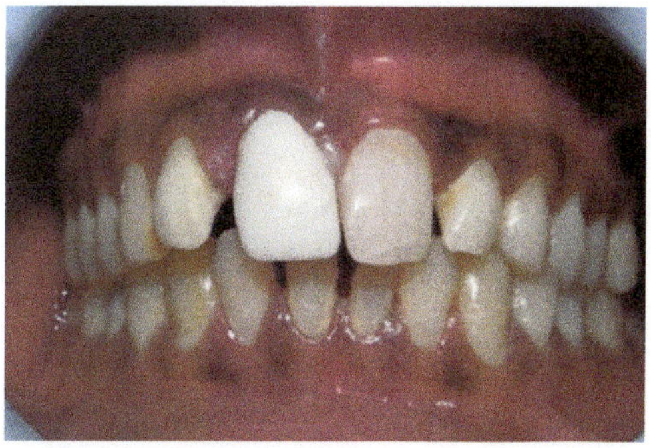

FIGURE 40: Temporisation.

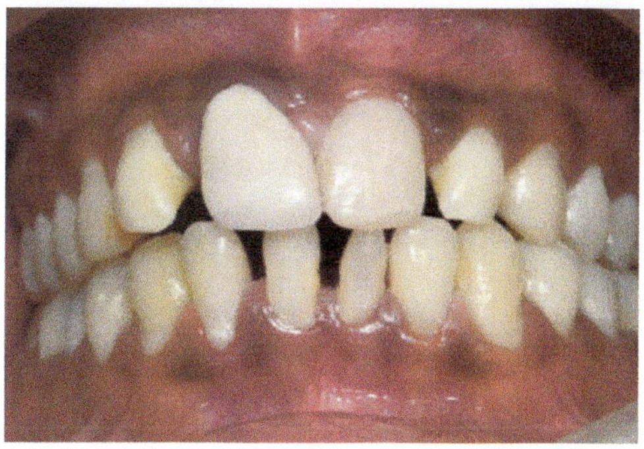

FIGURE 41: PFM crown cementation.

Following endodontic treatment and surgery of a periapical lesion, to be able to determine if the procedure is successful or not, healing of lesions is followed up by radiographic imaging. This can be done by observing changes in the periapical radiolucencies. Healing assessment using conventional and newer three-dimensional imaging includes, but is not limited to, periapical osseous lesions, status after endodontic surgery, and hard tissue deposition in regeneration procedures. Due to a low predictive value of periapical radiographs to distinguish between periapical disease and health, future assessment of endodontic treatment efficacy may include 3D imaging from small field-of-view CBCT units [14]. In a study, the diagnosis using CBCT revealed a lower healed and healing rate for root canal treatment than IOPA radiographs, particularly in roots of molars at the end of one year [15].

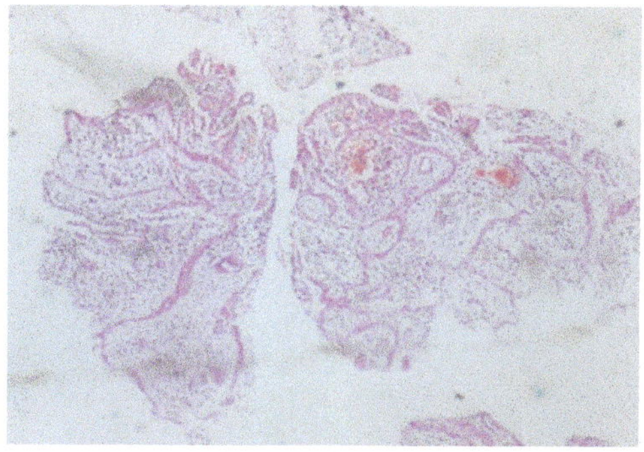

FIGURE 42: Histopathology report: radicular cyst.

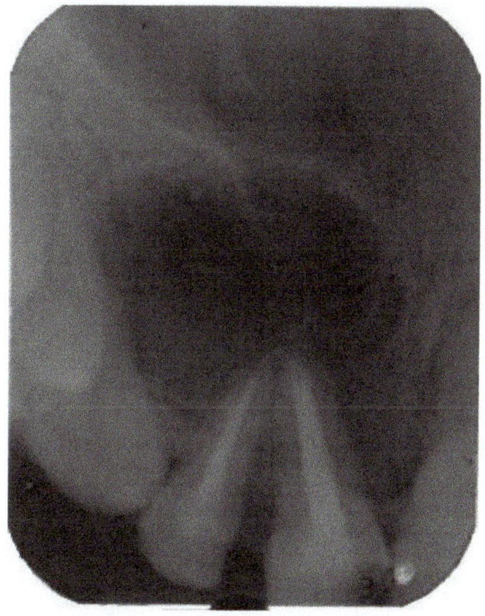

FIGURE 43: 1-month followup IOPA radiograph.

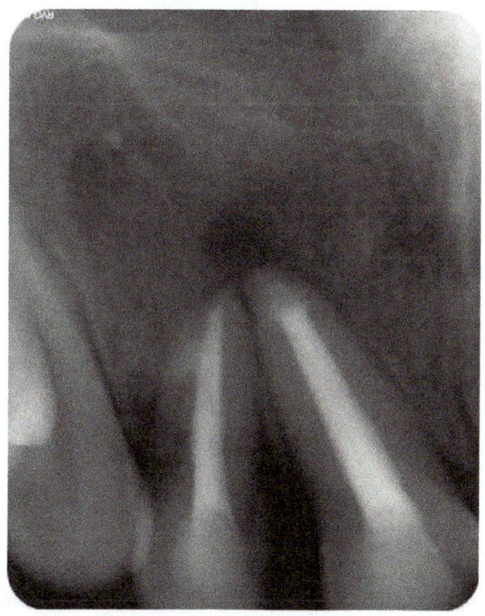

FIGURE 44: 6-month followup IOPA radiograph.

The use of CBCT is advocated in cases where the benefits of this investigation outweigh any potential risks to the patient, such as radiation exposure. Another limitation of

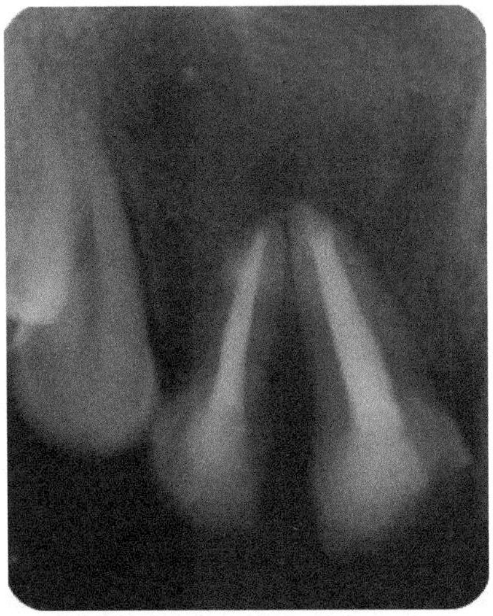

Figure 45: 12-month follow-up IOPA radiograph.

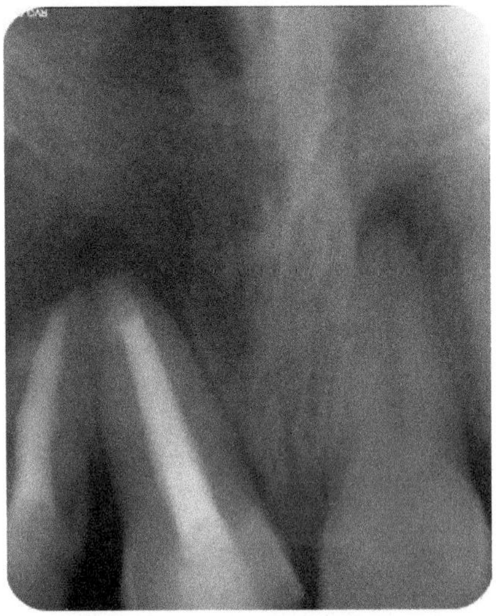

Figure 46: 18-month followup IOPA radiograph.

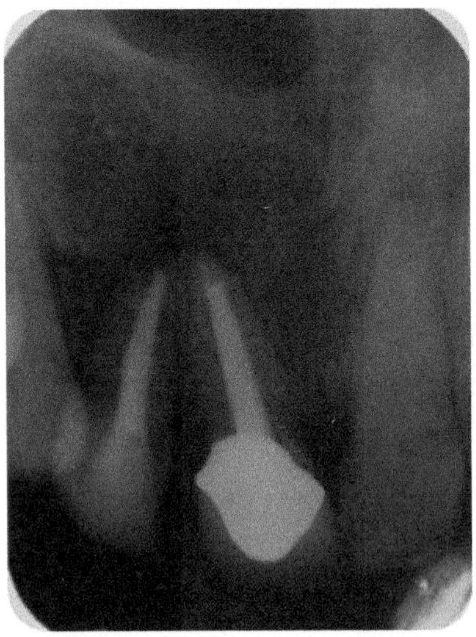

Figure 47: 24-month followup IOPA radiograph.

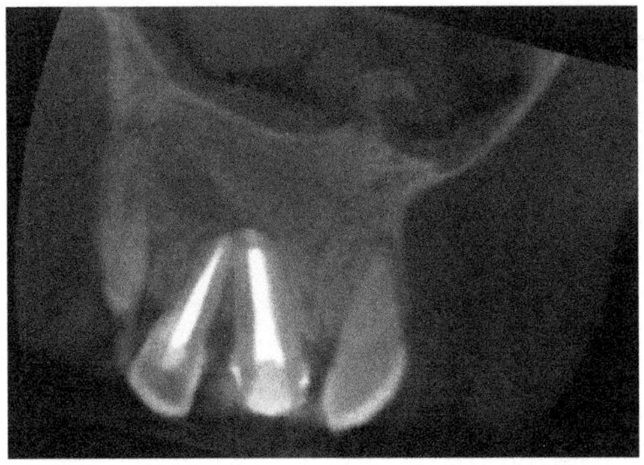

Figure 48: 1-year followup CBCT image in coronal plane.

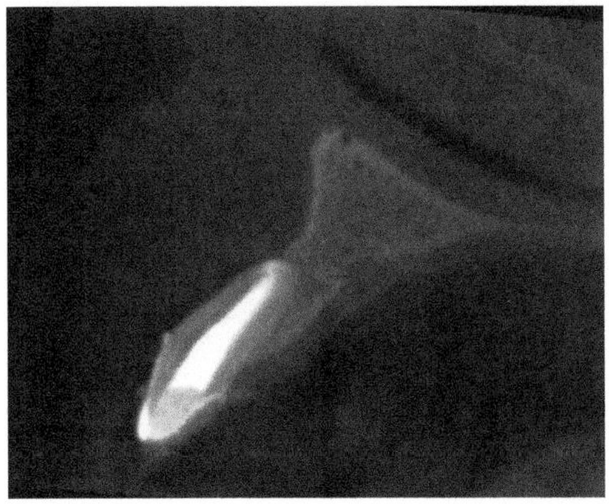

Figure 49: 1-year followup CBCT image in sagittal plane.

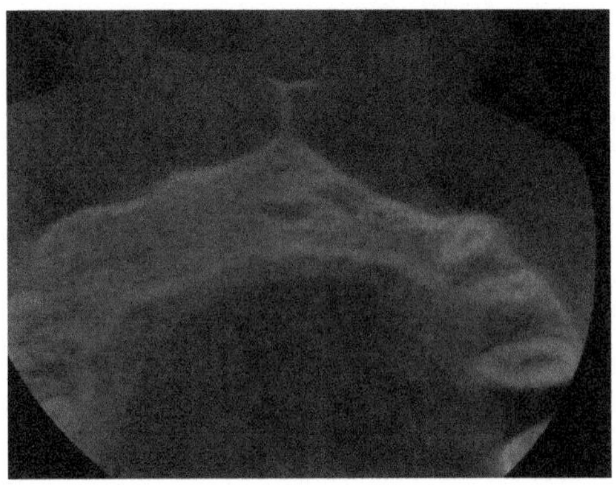

Figure 50: 1-year followup CBCT image in axial plane showing establishment of the buccal and lingual cortical plates.

CBCT is that an endodontic expert is required to analyze the whole lesion manually to search for cystic cavity; thus it is time consuming and prone to human error. Future improvements in CBCT technology may include systems with even more favorable diagnostic yields, lower radiation exposure, and reduced price. For now, CBCT imaging can be seen as a highly useful and, in some situations, an indispensable part of the modern dental imaging armamentarium.

4. Conclusion

This case report revealed that CBCT scan may provide a better, more accurate, and faster method to differentially diagnose a solid from a fluid-filled large periapical lesion or cavity as compared to conventional IOPA radiographs. CBCT also influences the treatment planning and management of such large lesions and is useful for long-term assessment of the outcome of endodontic surgery.

Conflict of Interests

The authors deny any conflict of interests related to this study.

Acknowledgments

The authors acknowledge the contribution of the Department of Oral Pathology (DAPMRV Dental College) with the histopathological diagnosis of the periapical lesions. The authors also acknowledge the expertise of Dr. A. R. Vinod Kumar, MDS (Oral and Maxillofacial Radiology), with the interpretation of the CBCT images.

References

[1] C. Estrela, M. R. Bueno, C. R. Leles, B. Azevedo, and J. R. Azevedo, "Accuracy of cone beam computed tomography and panoramic and periapical radiography for detection of apical periodontitis," *Journal of Endodontics*, vol. 34, no. 3, pp. 273–279, 2008.

[2] F. W. G. de Paula-Silva, M. S. Júnior, M. R. Leonardo, A. Consolaro, and L. A. B. da Silva, "Cone-beam computerized tomographic, radiographic, and histologic evaluation of periapical repair in dogs' post-endodontic treatment," *Oral Surgery, Oral Medicine, Oral Pathology, Oral Radiology and Endodontology*, vol. 108, no. 5, pp. 796–805, 2009.

[3] J. H. S. Simon, R. Enciso, J. M. Malfaz, R. Roges, M. Bailey-Perry, and A. Patel, "Differential diagnosis of large periapical lesions using cone-beam computed tomography measurements and biopsy," *Journal of Endodontics*, vol. 32, no. 9, pp. 833–837, 2006.

[4] A. Balasundaram, P. Shah, M. M. Hoen et al., "Comparison of cone-beam computed tomography and periapical radiography in predicting treatment decision for periapical lesions: a clinical study," *International Journal of Dentistry*, vol. 2012, Article ID 920815, 8 pages, 2012.

[5] S. Patel, A. Dawood, T. Pitt Ford, and E. Whaites, "The potential applications of cone beam computed tomography in the management of endodontic problems," *International Endodontic Journal*, vol. 40, no. 10, pp. 818–830, 2007.

[6] K. M. T. Low, K. Dula, W. Bürgin, and T. von Arx, "Comparison of periapical radiography and limited cone-beam tomography in posterior maxillary teeth referred for apical surgery," *Journal of Endodontics*, vol. 34, no. 5, pp. 557–562, 2008.

[7] Y. H. Liang, G. Li, P. R. Wesselink, and M. K. Wu, "Endodontic outcome predictors identified with periapical radiographs and cone-beam computed tomography scans," *Journal of Endodontics*, vol. 37, no. 3, pp. 326–331, 2011.

[8] D. A. Tyndall and S. Rathore, "Cone-beam CT diagnostic applications: caries, periodontal bone assessment, and endodontic applications," *Dental Clinics of North America*, vol. 52, no. 4, pp. 825–841, 2008.

[9] T. Yoshioka, I. Kikuchi, C. G. Adorno, and H. Suda, "Periapical bone defects of root filled teeth with persistent lesions evaluated by cone-beam computed tomography," *International Endodontic Journal*, vol. 44, no. 3, pp. 245–252, 2011.

[10] S. Patel, A. Dawood, F. Mannocci, R. Wilson, and T. Pitt Ford, "Detection of periapical bone defects in human jaws using cone beam computed tomography and intraoral radiography," *International Endodontic Journal*, vol. 42, no. 6, pp. 507–515, 2009.

[11] F. W. G. D. Paula-Silva, M. K. Wu, M. R. Leonardo, L. A. Bezerra da Silva, and P. R. Wesselink, "Accuracy of periapical radiography and cone-beam computed tomography scans in diagnosing apical periodontitis using histopathological findings as a gold standard," *Journal of Endodontics*, vol. 35, no. 7, pp. 1009–1012, 2009.

[12] P. A. Rosenberg, J. Frisbie, J. Lee et al., "Evaluation of pathologists (histopathology) and radiologists (cone beam computed tomography) differentiating radicular cysts from granulomas," *Journal of Endodontics*, vol. 36, no. 3, pp. 423–428, 2010.

[13] S. Kaya, I. Yavuz, I. Uysal, and Z. Akkus, "Measuring bone density in healing periapical lesions by using cone beam computed tomography: a clinical investigation," *Journal of Endodontics*, vol. 38, no. 1, pp. 28–31, 2012.

[14] C. I. Peters and O. A. Peters, "Cone beam computed tomography and other imaging techniques in the determination of periapical healing," *Endodontic Topics*, vol. 26, pp. 57–75, 2012.

[15] S. Patel, R. Wilson, A. Dawood, F. Foschi, and F. Mannocci, "The detection of periapical pathosis using digital periapical radiography and cone beam computed tomography. Part 2: a 1-year post-treatment follow-up," *International Endodontic Journal*, vol. 45, no. 8, pp. 711–723, 2012.

9

Restoration of Strip Crown with a Resin-Bonded Composite Cement in Early Childhood Caries

Mi-ae Jeong,[1] Ah-hyeon Kim,[2] Youn-soo Shim,[3] and So-youn An[4]

[1] *Department of Dental Hygiene, Kangwon National University, Samcheok, Republic of Korea*
[2] *Department of Preventive Dentistry and Public Oral Health, Research Center for Orofacial Hard Tissue Regeneration, College of Dentistry, Yonsei University, Seoul, Republic of Korea*
[3] *Department of Dental Hygiene, Cheongju University, Cheongju, Republic of Korea*
[4] *Pediatric Dentistry, College of Dentistry, Wonkwang University, Sanbon 435-040, Republic of Korea*

Correspondence should be addressed to So-youn An; 9543sue@hanmail.net

Academic Editors: G. Gómez-Moreno, C. Kitamura, and C. Ledesma-Montes

Background. Early childhood caries is a widely prevalent disease throughout the world. It is necessary to treat this condition in early childhood; however, child behavior management may be particularly challenging during treatment. To overcome this challenge, we used Carigel to remove caries and RelyX Unicem resin cement for strip crown restoration. It not only has the desired aesthetic effect but is also more effective for primary teeth, which are used for a shorter period than permanent teeth are. *Case Presentation.* We report a case of three pediatric patients with early childhood caries, in whom caries was removed by using Carigel to avoid the risk of pulpal exposure associated with high-speed handpieces. Subsequently, aesthetic restoration was performed using strip crown with RelyX Unicem self-adhesive resin cement. *Conclusion.* RelyX Unicem has the following advantages: (1) not requiring have any special skills for the dentist for performing the procedure, (2) decreased occurrence of bubbles during injection of the cement, and (3) overall short duration of the procedure. Thus, it is appropriate for the treatment of pediatric patients whose behavior is difficult to manage. However, further studies are required in order to establish the use of RelyX Unicem as a stable restorative material in early childhood caries.

1. Introduction

Early childhood caries (ECC) commonly affects the maxillary anterior teeth and is characterized by the presence of caries, that is, one or more missing, decayed, or filled tooth surfaces on any primary tooth of children aged less than 71 months [1]. ECC can lead to loss of primary teeth. From the perspective of the health of permanent teeth, proper diet, and aesthetic appreciation, the importance of primary teeth cannot be ignored [2]. In addition, with the loss of primary teeth, children lose the ability to pronounce fricative and sibilant sounds, causing them to develop an inaccurate language pattern. Furthermore, ECC, when left untreated, results in the development of abscesses, pain, and malocclusion. As per national oral health investigation (2010), caries experience rate of primary tooth was 61.4% and average number of decayed teeth was 2.2 in Korean population. The high incidence of ECC also hinders education as it results in nonattendance in school. Moreover, the treatment costs involved becomes a great burden in a country promoting public health care [3]. Therefore, early discovery, diagnosis, and treatment of ECC are necessary.

A painless treatment of dental caries is important in the case of pediatric patients visiting a dentist for the first time. A high-speed handpiece is conventionally used to treat dental caries. This surgical method can prevent unwanted elimination of sound teeth; however, it involves the possibility of damaging the pulp, which may be exposed due to the generation of excessive heat [1, 4].

A new method for treating dental caries that involves no drill, running water, or electricity was presented at the headquarters of the World Health Organization on World Health Day in 1994. This new approach, termed "Atraumatic Restorative Treatment," involves manual cleaning of

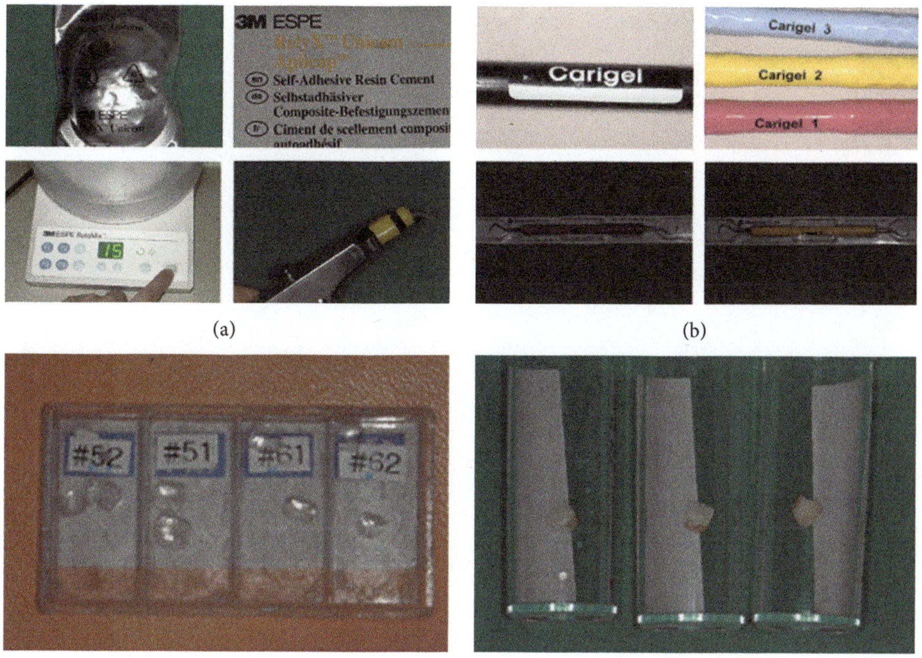

(a) (b) (c) (d)

FIGURE 1: (a) RelyX Unicem. (b) Carigel. (c) Strip crown. (d) Primary tooth restored with RelyX Unicem. The patient used restoration until primary tooth is replaced by permanent tooth.

the dental cavities with hand instruments and restoration of the cavities with an adhesive fluoride-releasing material [5]. In addition, chemomechanical techniques using rotary instruments are an alternative method to conventional caries removal techniques.

In the 1970s, Habib et al. [6] and Kronman et al. [7] studied the effect of a nonspecific proteolytic agent, sodium hypochlorite (NaOCl), on carious dentine. Unfortunately, NaOCl not only dissolved necrotic organic material but also affected sound dentine [8]. Further work led to the development of a new chemomechanical agent Carigel (Foryoudent, Busan, Korea., Figure 1(b)). It consists of a 2-component gel, supplied in 2 different syringes. The first syringe contains glutamic acid, leucine, lysine, sodium chloride, erythrosin, carboxymethylcellulose, water, and sodium hydroxide and has a pH value of 11. The second syringe contains 0.5% NaOCl and alanine aminotransferase.

Full coronal restoration of carious primary incisors is indicated in the following cases: (1) caries is present on multiple surfaces; (2) the incisal edge is involved; (3) extensive cervical decalcification is present; (4) pulpal therapy is indicated; (5) caries may be minor, but oral hygiene is very poor (high-risk patients); (6) the child's disruptive behavior makes placing Class II restorations difficult [9].

The restorative method generally used to treat ECC involves an open-faced stainless steel crown. When the aesthetic demand is high, restoration with a strip crown (3M ESPE, USA., Figure 1(c)) is restrictively performed. With respect to restoration, patients now seem to emphasize on improved aesthetics rather than function, especially in the case of anterior teeth. Using an open-faced stainless steel crown improves the aesthetics more than the stainless steel crown [10]. However, in Korea, the procedure that uses open-faced stainless steel crown has been used for a longer time than the strip crown because the handmade open-faced stainless steel crown is preferred over the commercial open-faced stainless steel crown (e.g., Nusmile, Chang crown). Usually anterior stainless steel crown (e.g., Unitek crowns-stainless steel primary anterior, 3M ESPE, USA, Kids crowns, SHINHUNG company, Korea) are used and they are cemented to the primary anterior tooth. After the cement is hardened, which could take several minutes, the labial surface of anterior stainless steel crown is cut exposing the tooth surface, following which resin is bonded to the tooth surface. However, the cement needs to be hardened before the resin is applied to smooth out the irregular surfaces. Metal is exposed to the marginal region. Thus, in several cases, it is difficult to satisfy patients and guardians who have high aesthetic demands [11].

Composite resin was conventionally used as the restorative material for celluloid strip crown in ECC. Composite resin was first developed by Bowen in the 1960s to strengthen epoxy resin as a filler; since then, several advancements have been made to enhance its physical properties such as its resistance to abrasion, polymerization shrinkage, and bonding strength of dentin. In addition, it is being used extensively to restore anterior teeth for improved aesthetics and to restore posterior teeth without applying too much pressure. However, composite resin is sensitive to the individual skills of a dentist and the process involved is considerably long;

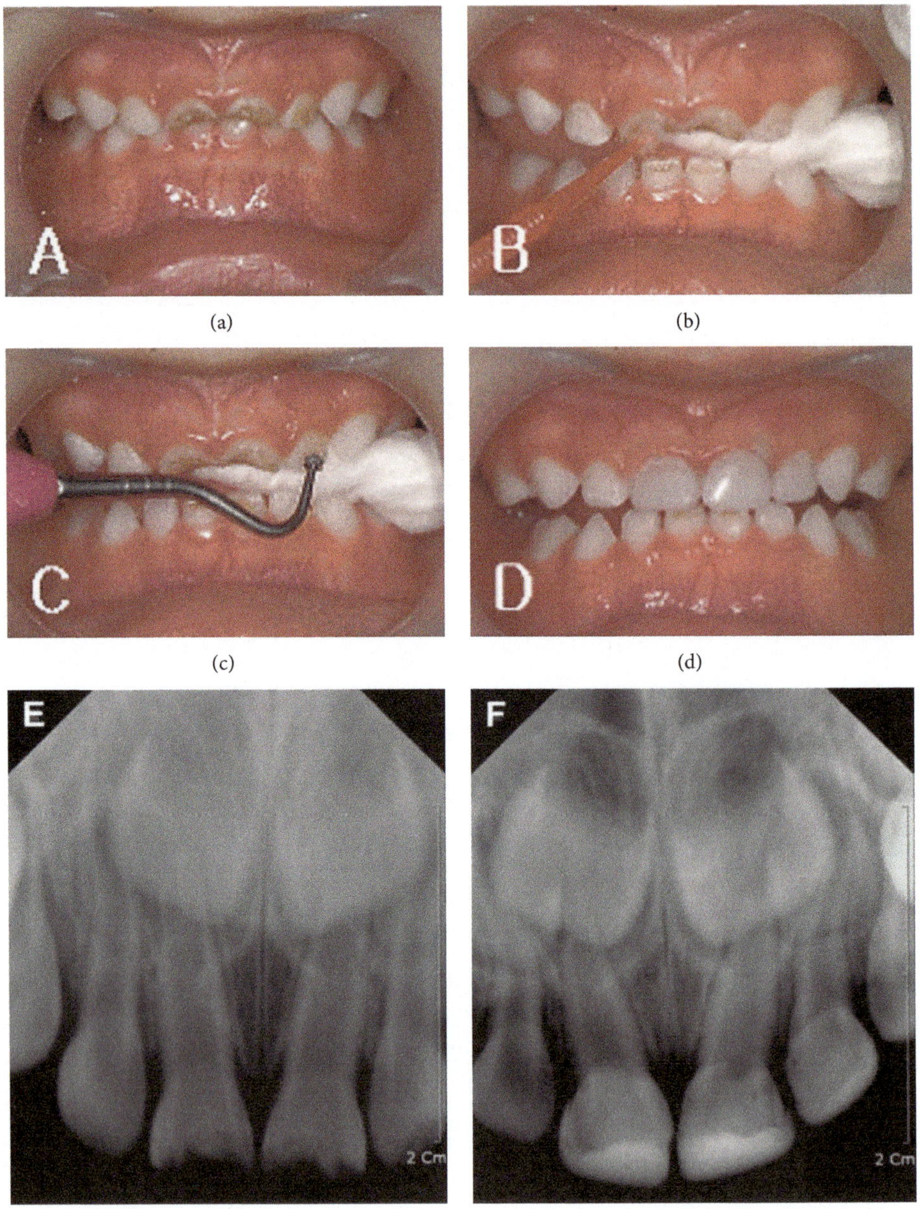

(a) (b) (c) (d) (e) (f)

FIGURE 2: (a) Oral status of the patient before treatment, (b) application of Carigel, (c) removal of dental caries, (d) restoration with RelyX Unicem, (e) radiograph of the patient before treatment, and (f) radiograph of the patient treatment after 8 month.

therefore, it is not convenient for use in pediatric patients, where behavioral management is relatively difficult compared to adults.

Here, we report a case of three pediatric patients with early childhood caries, in whom caries was removed by using Carigel; restoration was performed using a resin-bonded composite cement RelyX Unicem (3M ESPE Dental Products, 2 USA, Figure 1(a)).

2. Case Presentation 1

In February 2010, an 18-month-old Korean girl presented with ECC at the Wonkwang University Dental Hospital (Figure 2(a)). She harbored a fear for dental treatment and was treated using Carigel (FORYOUDENT, Busan, Korea) to avoid the risk of pulp exposure when using a high-speed hand-piece.

According to the manufacturer's instructions, the 2 syringes in which the gel is supplied were maintained at room temperature for approximately 1 hour before treatment [4]. Carigel was applied to the affected area by using a microbrush (Figure 2(b)). After 30 seconds, the gel was absorbed by using hand instrument 1, exclusively designed for Carigel. Caries was removed by using dedicated hand instruments 2 and #3. The process of applying the gel and removing caries by using hand instruments was repeated twice (Figure 2(c)).

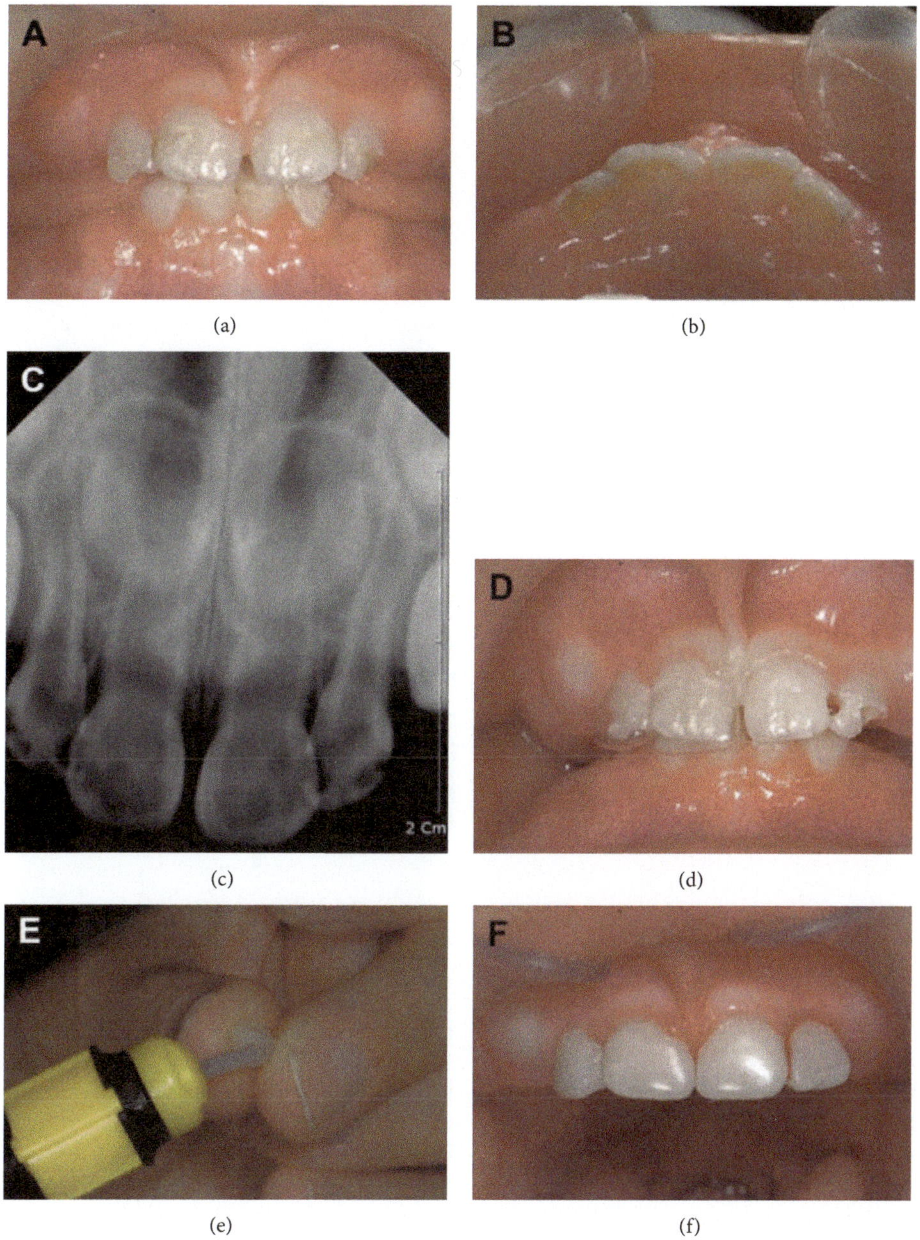

FIGURE 3: (a) Oral status of the patient before treatment (labial surface), (b) oral status of the patient before treatment (lingual surface), (c) radiograph of the patient before treatment, (d) mounting of strip crown on patient's tooth, (e) filling strip crown with RelyX Unicem, and (f) restoration with RelyX Unicem.

After the process of removing caries was completed, a 3-way syringe was used to wash the area to prevent the removed caries residue and gel from remaining on the tooth surfaces. A celluloid crown (3M ESPE, USA) was selected according to the size of the affected tooth after washing, and its shape was modified by clamping after cutting it to the appropriate length. The RelyX Unicem (3M ESPE, USA) was mixed with an automixer and then injected into the crown form followed by an expert surgeon applying the crown form to the affected tooth, which was then removed after photopolymerization (Figure 1(d)).

3. Case Presentation 2

In August 2009, a 16-month-old Korean girl presented with ECC at the Wonkwang University Dental Hospital (Figures 3(a) and 3(b)). Caries did not invade the pulp, but was very close to the pulp (Figure 3(b)). She was treated using Carigel (Foryoudent, Busan, Korea) to avoid the risk of pulp exposure while using a high-speed hand-piece. After the process of removing caries was completed, a 3-way syringe was used to wash the area to prevent the removed caries residue and gel from remaining on the surface of the tooth.

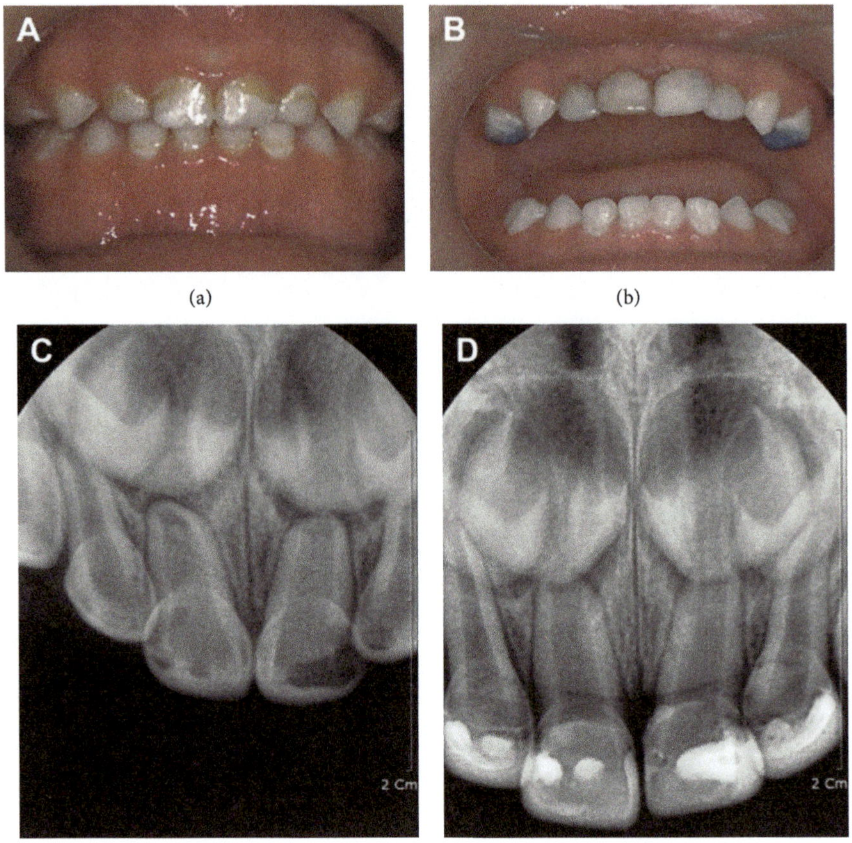

(a) (b) (c) (d)

FIGURE 4: (a) Oral status of the patient before treatment and (b) restoration with RelyX Unicem. In order to avoid anterior teeth biting, 54 and 64 teeth were restored with blue resin. (c) Radiograph of the patient before treatment and (d) radiograph of the patient after treatment.

A celluloid crown (3M ESPE, USA) was selected according to the size of the affected tooth after washing, and its shape was modified by clamping after cutting it to the appropriate length (Figure 3(d)). RelyX Unicem (3M ESPE, USA) was mixed with an automixer and then injected into the crown form (Figure 3(e)) followed by application of the crown form to the affected tooth, which was then removed after photopolymerization (Figure 3(f)).

4. Case Presentation 3

In May 2013, a 22-month-old Korean girl presented with ECC at the Wonkwang University Dental Hospital (Figures 4(a) and 4(c)). She was treated using Carigel (Foryoudent, Busan, Korea) to avoid the risk of pulp exposure while using a high-speed hand-piece. She was treated using Carigel and RelyX Unicem (3M ESPE, USA) in the same way as case 2. In order to avoid anterior teeth biting, 54 and 64 teeth were restored with blue resin (Figure 4(b)).

To meet the rising aesthetic needs, resin-bonded composite strip crowns are the preferred choice of many clinicians, mainly because of the superior aesthetics and the ease of repair in the event that the crown chips or fractures [12]. Restoration of the primary incisors with single bond and Z100 using strip crowns (all by 3M ESPE Dental Products, Seefeld, Germany) is popularly performed in some countries. At our hospital, we also generally used the packable resin Z100 (P shade) as the restorative material for filling the strip crown. In this case, the strip crown could be selected and RelyX Unicem (3M ESPE Dental Products, USA) was used instead of Z100. RelyX Unicem is a unique resin cement. The flexural strength of RelyX Unicem is 63 MPa, which is lower than that of Z100, a packable resin, whose flexural strength is 160 MPa. However, considering that restored primary teeth are used for a shorter period than permanent teeth, RelyX Unicem has the following merits: (1) the dentists performing the procedure do not require any special skills, (2) it facilitates decreased occurrence of bubbles during injection of the material, and (3) it involves a relatively shorter time. Therefore, it is more appropriate for the treatment of caries in pediatric patients, in whom behavioral management may be difficult.

Here, we have reported one such case in which RelyX Unicem was used for the restoration in ECC. We applied this method to a number of children. The majority of patients used restoration until restored deciduous tooth was replaced by permanent tooth (Figure 1(d)). However, to stably use RelyX Unicem as a generally accepted restorative material for primary teeth in pediatric patients with ECC, it is important to compare its physical properties such as microstrength and polymerization shrinkage to those of other restorative materials, which have been traditionally used in laboratories. Further studies must be performed to evaluate the long-term prognosis of ECC treated with Carigel and strip crowns using RelyX Unicem.

Consent

Informed consent was obtained from the guardians of all the three patients.

Conflict of Interests

The authors of this paper state that they do not have any direct financial relation with the commercial identity mentioned in their paper and there is no conflict of interests to declare.

References

[1] American Academy of Pediatric Dentistry, "Definition of early childhood caries," http://www.aapd.org/media/policies.asp.

[2] W. Low, S. Tan, and S. Schwartz, "The effect of severe caries on the quality of life in young children," *Pediatric Dentistry*, vol. 21, no. 6, pp. 325–326, 1999.

[3] S. L. M. Kumarihamy, L. D. Subasinghe, P. Jayasekara, S. M. Kularatna, and P. D. Palipana, "The prevalence of early childhood caries in 1-2 yrs olds in a semi-urban area of Sri Lanka," *BMC Research Notes*, vol. 4, article 336, 2011.

[4] B. Azrak, A. Callaway, A. Grundheber, E. Stender, and B. Willershausen, "Comparison of the efficacy of chemomechanical caries removal (Carisolv) with that of conventional excavation in reducing the cariogenic flora," *International Journal of Paediatric Dentistry*, vol. 14, no. 3, pp. 182–191, 2004.

[5] D. Barmes, "Foreword for proceedings of the IADR symposium minimal intervention techniques for dental caries," *Journal of Public Health Dentistry*, vol. 56, no. 3, p. 131, 1996.

[6] C. M. Habib, J. Kronman, and M. Goldman, "A chemical evaluation of collagen and hydroxyproline after treatment with GK-101 (N chloroglycine)," *Pharmacology and Therapeutics in Dentistry*, vol. 2, no. 3-4, pp. 209–215, 1975.

[7] J. H. Kronman, M. Goldman, C. M. Habib, and L. Mengel, "Electron microscopic evaluation of altered collagen structure induced by N-monochloroglycine (GK-101)," *Journal of Dental Research*, vol. 56, no. 12, pp. 1539–1545, 1977.

[8] R. E. Hand, M. L. Smith, and J. W. Harrison, "Analysis of the effect of dilution on the necrotic tissue dissolution property of sodium hypochlorite," *Journal of Endodontics*, vol. 4, no. 2, pp. 60–64, 1978.

[9] W. F. Waggoner, "Restorative dentistry for the primary dentition," in *Pediatric Dentistry: Infancy through Adolescence*, J. R. Pinkham, Ed., W. B. Saunders, Philadelphia, Pa, USA, 2nd edition, 1994.

[10] M. L. Helpin, "The open-face steel crown restoration in children," *ASDC Journal of Dentistry for Children*, vol. 50, no. 1, pp. 34–38, 1983.

[11] C. R. Hartmann, "The open-face stainless steel crown: an esthetic technique," *ASDC Journal of Dentistry for Children*, vol. 50, no. 1, pp. 31–33, 1983.

[12] D. Ram and A. B. Fuks, "Clinical performance of resin-bonded composite strip crowns in primary incisors: A retrospective study," *International Journal of Paediatric Dentistry*, vol. 16, no. 1, pp. 49–54, 2006.

10

Dual Lesions: A Diagnostic Dilemma

M. P. V. Prabhat,[1] Prasannasrinivas Deshpande,[1] Sarat Gummadapu,[1] Suresh Babburi,[2] Raja Lakshmi Chintamaneni,[1] and Bhavana Sujanamulk[1]

[1] *Department of Oral Medicine and Radiology, Dr. Sudha and Nageswara Rao Siddhartha Institute of Dental Sciences, Chinnaoutpalli, Krishna District, Gannavaram, Andhra Pradesh 521286, India*
[2] *Department of Oral Pathology, Dr. Sudha and Nageswara Rao Siddhartha Institute of Dental Sciences, Chinnaoutpalli, Krishna District, Gannavaram, Andhra Pradesh 521286, India*

Correspondence should be addressed to Prasannasrinivas Deshpande; drprasanna_deshpande@yahoo.com

Academic Editors: R. S. Brown and G. Spagnuolo

Glandular odontogenic cyst (GOC) is a rare aggressive developmental cyst of the jaw. It most commonly occurs in middle-aged people with mandible anterior region being the most affected site. This lesion can present as a unilocular or multilocular radiolucency and has high recurrence rate. The histopathologic features of the GOC are complex and often coincide with the features of dentigerous cyst, radicular cyst, and low-grade central mucoepidermoid carcinoma (CMEC). At times, the microscopic features are so similar to central low-grade mucoepidermoid carcinoma that it becomes highly impossible to distinguish the two entities even with various advanced investigations. The reported case represents one such diagnostic dilemma occurring in the maxilla which is a rare site, and the lesion/s appeared as two distinct entities, that is, GOC and CMEC on either aspects of the same side of maxilla clinically, yet showing continuity on advanced imaging and demonstrating histopathological perplexity.

1. Introduction

In 1987, Padayachee and Van Wyk [1] gave the first description of this kind of cyst and later the term "Glandular Odontogenic Cyst" was introduced in 1988 by Gardner et al. [2]. It is also known as "mucoepidermoid cyst" and "sialo-odontogenic cyst." Clinically it has a slight predilection for men and occurs mostly in middle-aged persons. Most of the reported cases have occurred in the anterior mandible. Radiographically, they are usually multilocular cystic lesions, although unilocular lesions have been reported. They are aggressive lesions and often reach large dimensions. Nevertheless, none of the clinical or radiographic features of GOC are pathognomonic [3].

The histologic features of GOC have been described in detail by several authors [1, 2, 4, 5]. Various histologic features overlap with other entities such as dentigerous cyst, mucous metaplasia in odontogenic cyst, radicular cyst, low-grade central mucoepidermoid carcinoma, and botryoid cyst. The number of typical features necessary for the diagnosis of GOC remains unclear, and there are no specific stains that distinguish GOC from similar lesions [4, 5].

Central mucoepidermoid carcinoma is an extremely rare tumor, representing about 2 to 4% of all mucoepidermoid carcinomas. They are histologically low-grade cancers, usually affecting the mandible as uni- or multilocular radiographic lesions [6].

An article with extensive study on histopathologic features and variants of GOC states that GOC and CMEC may possibly be related, but definitive evidence is still awaited [5].

2. Case Report

A 19-year-old young male reported with swelling in the left side of face since six months. It was insidious in onset with no history of preceding tooth ache or trauma. Swelling was gradually increasing to attain the present size and was associated with mild occasional pain. There were no symptoms of paraesthesia, diplopia, and sinus involvement. His past medical, dental, and personal histories were noncontributory. Extra-oral swelling on left mid-third region measuring about 5 × 4 cms was noted (Figure 1). The overlying surface appeared stretched with no secondary changes. Intraorally,

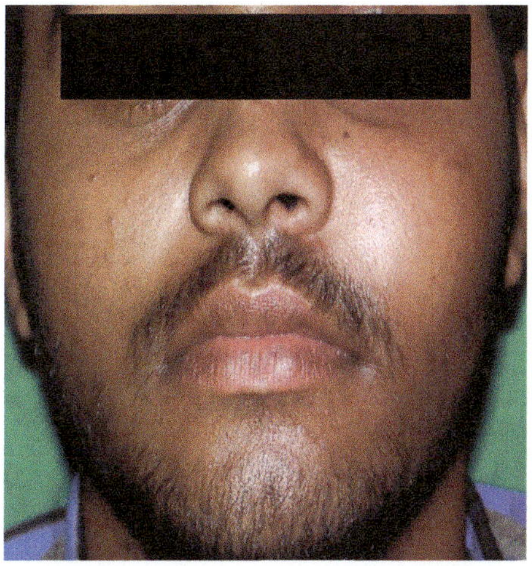

Figure 1: Profile picture showing swelling over the left middle third of face.

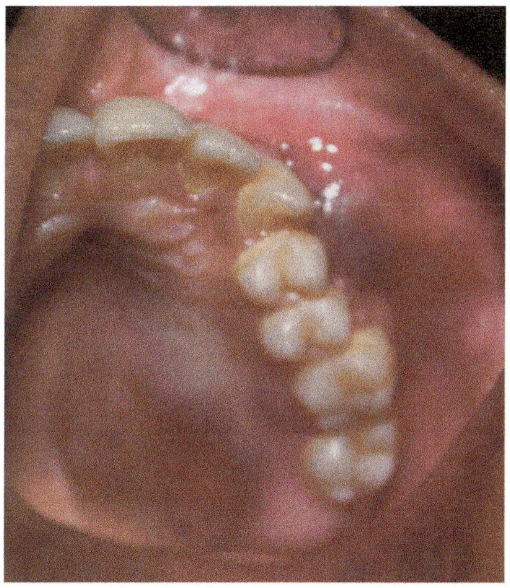

Figure 2: Intraoral swelling over left maxilla.

swelling had obliterated the buccal vestibule from 23 to 25 regions which had a bluish hue and was nontender, soft, and fluctuant with areas of decortications. Palatally a well-defined swelling was seen on left posterior hard palate approximately of 3 × 3.5 cms. Surface had areas of erythema and ulceration. On palpation it was mildly tender due to superficial ulceration and firm in consistency. Grade I mobility was noted with maxillary left premolars (Figure 2).

The history and clinical examination led to an impression of low-grade central salivary gland lesion, namely, mucoepidermoid carcinoma and adenoid cystic carcinoma. Differentials included other odontogenic cysts and tumors, namely, unicystic ameloblastoma, keratocystic odontogenic tumor, and glandular odontogenic cyst.

Orthopantomograph showed multilocular radiolucency over the left maxillary alveolus region as well as large diffuse radiopaque haziness involving the left maxillary sinus region extending posteriorly and causing erosion and obliteration of pterygomaxillary fissure. On CT evaluation an expansile lesion measuring 7 × 4 × 3 cms was observed on left maxilla causing expansion of buccal cortex and deviation of left lateral wall of the nose. The lesion had pushed the lower border of sinus superiorly causing near complete compression of sinus. Inferiorly destruction of the bone was noted in alveolus and palate which was multilocular in pattern. The soft tissue density was seen extending approximately 2 × 1.5 cms into the oral cavity with bone resorption whereas cortical expansion with areas of decortications was seen on buccal aspect. In anterior sections the palatal and buccal lesions appeared as two distinct entities with intact bone in between the two lesions whereas the sections of the posterior aspect of maxilla showed advanced bony destruction with continuity of the buccal and palatal lesions (Figure 3).

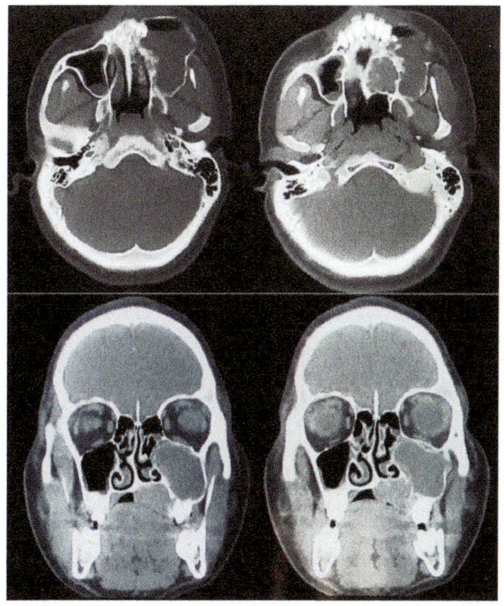

Figure 3: Axial and coronal CT views showing large osteolytic lesion/s involving left maxilla with continuity of buccal and palatal lesions.

Aspiration from buccal lesion yielded brownish color viscous fluid and blood from palatal lesion.

Similarly biopsy was performed individually at both sites. Haematoxylin and eosin staining of buccal lesion showed cystic lining with ciliated pseudostratified squamous epithelium. Goblet cells with multiple microcysts were also noted. The connective tissue stroma was seen with mild inflammatory cells, all of which lead to a diagnosis of glandular odontogenic cyst (Figures 4 and 5). The lesion over the palate showed no evidence of cystic lining but, in contrast, showed presence of infiltrating islands of epithelium comprising mucous cells, epidermoid cells, and intermediate cells. Clear cells in some islands whereas cystic areas in some islands were noted with foci of inflammatory cell infiltrates in the connective tissue leading to a diagnosis of mucoepidermoid carcinoma (Figures 6 and 7).

No clear transition zone of carcinomatous change was noticeable in all the deeper fields examined on excisional biopsy. Mucicarmine staining showed glandular cystic lining with mucicarmine positive mucus cells (Figures 8 and 9)

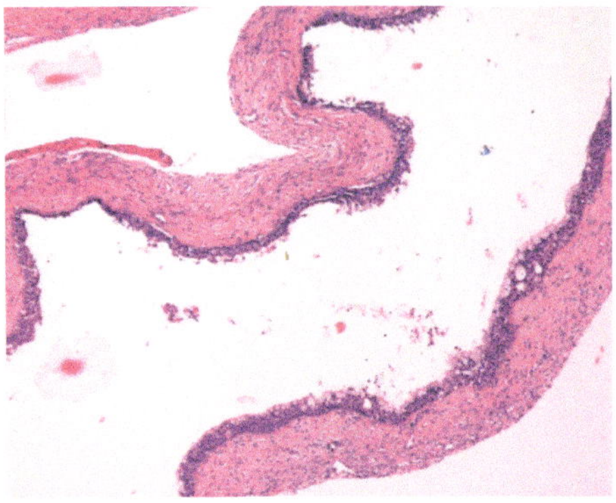

FIGURE 4: Cystic lining with connective tissue stroma (H&E 20x).

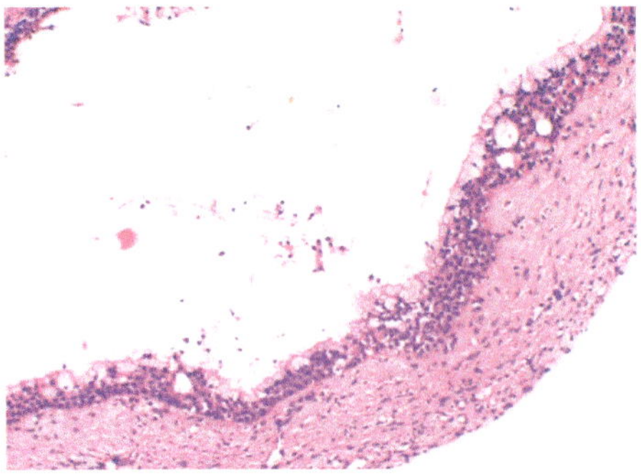

FIGURE 5: Pseudostratified squamous epithelium with multiple microcysts (H&E 20x).

and palatal lesion showing mucicarmine positive mucus cells, clear cells, and intermediate cells with mild mucicarmine positive mucous pooling (Figures 10 and 11).

The patient rejected the further investigations which were advised due to monetary constraints.

A conservative approach in the management was followed considering the age of the patient. Complete enucleation with extensive curettage was carried out, and patient was recalled every 3 months. No signs of recurrence are seen after eight months of follow-up.

3. Discussion

The clinical features in the present case report present a diagnostic dilemma whether to consider it as a single lesion which presents with various clinical features or as two distinct lesions coexisting on the same side of maxilla. Mucoepidermoid carcinoma arising in maxilla was considered as it presents with solid and cystic variant. However a cyst on buccal aspect with a tumor on palate or a sinonasal pathology was also suspected.

Primary central MEC has been reported in the first to seventh decades; however, cases occurring in the fourth and fifth decades are most common. It has slight predilection for posterior mandible and often seen in females. MEC usually presents as a painless swelling. Pain, paraesthesia, numbness, and tooth mobility are usually occasional and late findings. Radiographically they may appear as unilocular or multilocular with or without cortical plate disruption [7]. Based on their clinical behavior they are classified as high- and low-grade MEC, and the present case was a low grade variant.

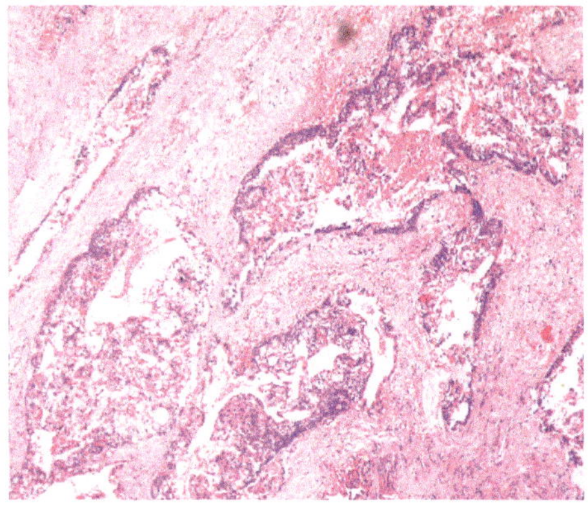

FIGURE 6: Islands of epithelium comprising mucous cells, epidermoid cells, and intermediate cells (H&E 20x).

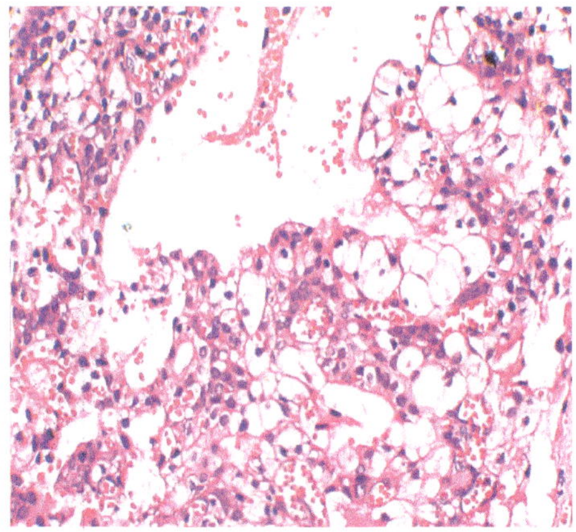

FIGURE 7: Mucous cells, epidermoid cells, and clear cells (H&E 40x).

GOCs are relatively uncommon cysts first reported in 1987. Ever since then, they have remained as interesting controversial favorites for the researchers all over the world. The lesion was initially referred to as a "sialo-odontogenic cyst" and believed to have salivary gland origin, but due to lack of evidence the term "glandular odontogenic cyst" was later adopted by the World Health Organization in 1992 [8].

In the near past, numerous case reports and short series have been reported on GOCs. Therefore, the GOC, although rare, is now a relatively well-known entity. Nevertheless there are no definitive or pathognomonic clinical, radiographic, or histopathological features which aid in diagnosis.

In our case on correlating all the clinical, radiographic, and histopathological findings there were bizarre and overlapping features of GOC and CMEC. Clinically, on buccal aspect, presence of cystic swelling and blood on aspiration was noted in contrast to firm swelling and brownish color viscous fluid on palatal aspect. Radiographic findings revealed buccal cortical expansion with areas of decortications suggestive of cystic lesion whereas palatal lesion showed bony

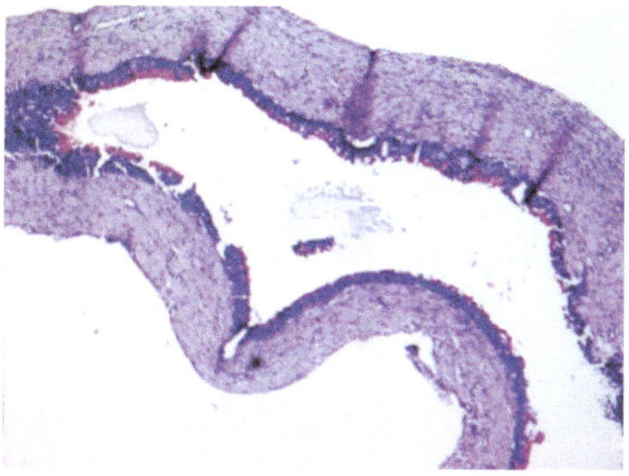

FIGURE 8: Photomicrograph of the lesion showing glandular cystic lining with mucicarmine positive mucus cells (H&E, 10x).

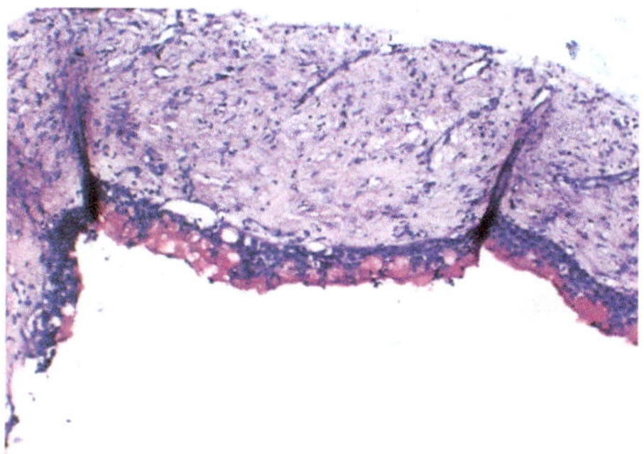

FIGURE 9: High power photomicrograph of the lesion showing glandular cystic lining with mucicarmine positive mucus cells (H&E, 20x).

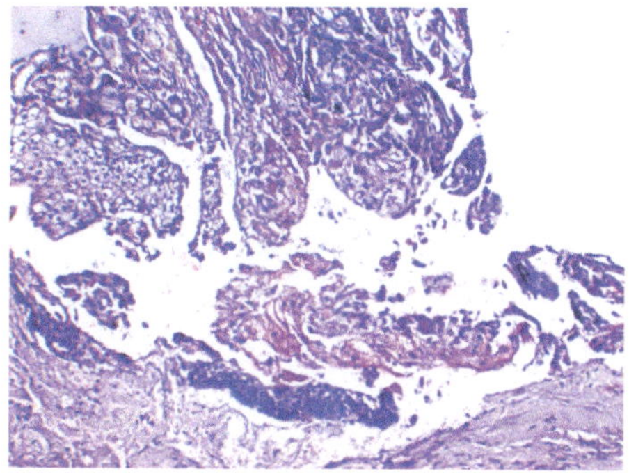

FIGURE 10: Photomicrograph of the lesion showing mucus cells (mucicarmine positive), clear cells, and intermediate cells (H&E, 10x).

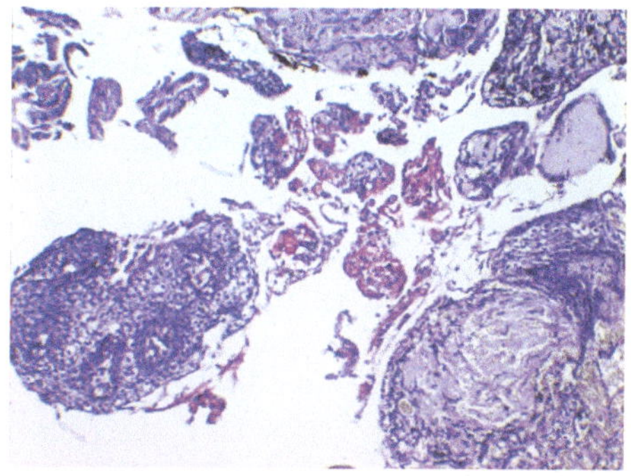

FIGURE 11: Photomicrograph of the lesion showing mucus cells (mucicarmine positive), clear cells, and intermediate cells (H&E, 10x).

resorption with soft tissue infiltrate supporting the clinical findings of tumor. However detailed radiographic evaluation showed continuity in both aspects further enhancing the diagnostic predicament.

A well-known fact of GOC is that it mimics various pathologies occurring in the jaws. In our case, the presence of cystic lining with ciliated pseudostratified squamous epithelium, goblet cells, multiple microcysts, and mucicarmine positive mucous cells in the buccal lesion suggested GOC while palatal lesion showed infiltrating islands of epithelium comprising mucous cells, epidermoid cells and intermediate cells along with clear cells, mucicarmine positive mucus cells with mucous pooling providing a diagnosis of MEC. Overlapping feature on deeper field examinations with no clear field of transition further complicated the diagnosis. A recent article in 2011 analysing 46 cases of GOC with special emphasis on microscopic criteria for diagnosis concludes that at this point of time no enough information is available to determine whether GOC and CMEC share a histopathological spectrum or whether MEC-like changes in GOCs are associated with malignant behaviour [5].

Immunohistochemistry may aid to a smaller extent in differentiating GOC and CMEC. Assessment of the cytokeratin (CK) profile of central MEC and GOC overlaps to a greater extent, but expression of CKs 18 and 19 could be useful in their differential diagnosis [9].

4. Conclusion

Oral cavity may rarely house controversial coexisting lesions which may challenge the diagnosis and acumen of clinician. A specialized oral physician should be aware of such pathologies and work towards solving the mystery as the exact diagnosis is necessary to render proper management. The present case highlights one such diagnostic dilemma which was attempted to be solved with the available resources.

Acknowledgment

The authors would like to thank Dr. R. Subramanyam, Prof, and Head of Department of Oral pathology, for all the help and support rendered.

References

[1] A. Padayachee and C. W. Van Wyk, "Two cystic lesions with features of both the botryoid odontogenic cyst and the central mucoepidermoid tumour: sialo-odontogenic cyst?" *Journal of Oral Pathology*, vol. 16, no. 10, pp. 499–504, 1987.

[2] D. G. Gardner, H. P. Kessler, R. Morency, and D. L. Schaffner, "The glandular odontogenic cyst: an apparent entity," *Journal of Oral Pathology*, vol. 17, no. 8, pp. 359–366, 1988.

[3] S. O. Machado De Sousa, N. T. Cabezas, P. T. De Oliveira, and V. C. De Araújo, "Glandular odontogenic cyst: report of a case with cytokeratin expression," *Oral Surgery, Oral Medicine, Oral Pathology, Oral Radiology, and Endodontics*, vol. 83, no. 4, pp. 478–483, 1997.

[4] X.-N. Qin, J.-R. Li, X.-M. Chen, and X. Long, "The glandular odontogenic cyst: clinicopathologic features and treatment of 14 cases," *Journal of Oral and Maxillofacial Surgery*, vol. 63, no. 5, pp. 694–699, 2005.

[5] C. B. Fowler, R. B. Brannon, H. P. Kessler, J. T. Castle, and M. A. Kahn, "Glandular odontogenic cyst: analysis of 46 cases with special emphasis on microscopic criteria for diagnosis," *Head and Neck Pathology*, vol. 5, no. 4, pp. 364–375, 2011.

[6] A. Munde, R. Karle, R. Metgud, and B. M. Rudgi, "Central mucoepidermoid carcinoma of the mandible," *Indian Journal of Dental Research*, vol. 21, no. 4, pp. 609–610, 2010.

[7] D. L. Raut and S. A. Khedkar, "Primary intraosseous mucoepidermoid carcinoma of the maxilla: a case report and review of literature," *Dentomaxillofacial Radiology*, vol. 38, no. 3, pp. 163–168, 2009.

[8] K. Hussain, H. D. Edmondson, and R. M. Browne, "Glandular odontogenic cysts. Diagnosis and treatment," *Oral Surgery, Oral Medicine, Oral Pathology, Oral Radiology and*, vol. 79, no. 5, pp. 593–602, 1995.

[9] F. R. Pires, S.-Y. Chen, D. E. Da Cruz Perez, O. P. De Almeida, and L. P. Kowalski, "Cytokeratin expression in central mucoepidermoid carcinoma and glandular odontogenic cyst," *Oral Oncology*, vol. 40, no. 5, pp. 545–551, 2004.

11

Use of Zirconia to Restore Severely Worn Dentition

Manish Agrawal,[1] Banashree Sankeshwari,[1] and Channaveer V. Pattanshetti[2]

[1] *Department of Prosthodontics and Crown and Bridge, Bharati Vidyapeeth Dental College and Hospital, Sangli 416 416, India*
[2] *Department of Oral and Maxillofacial Surgery, Bharati Vidyapeeth Dental College and Hospital, Sangli 416 416, India*

Correspondence should be addressed to Manish Agrawal, dragroman@hotmail.com

Academic Editors: Y.-K. Chen and T. Lombardi

The management of tooth wear has been a subject of increasing interest from both preventive and restorative points of view. Severe tooth wear is frequently multifactorial and variable. Successful management is a subject of interest in dentistry. A critical aspect is to determine the occlusal vertical dimension (OVD) and a systematic approach that can lead to a predictable and favorable treatment prognosis. Management of patients with worn dentition is complex and difficult. Accurate clinical and radiographic examinations, a diagnostic wax-up, and determining OVD are crucial. This paper describes the full-mouth rehabilitation of a 47-year-old bruxer with a severely worn dentition.

1. Introduction

Restoration of the severely worn dentition is one of the most challenging procedures in dentistry. In order to successfully restore and maintain the teeth, one must gain insight into how the teeth arrived at this state of destruction. Tooth wear can result from abrasion, attrition, and erosion [1–5].

While all occlusions wear to some degree over the lifetime of the patient, normal physiological wear usually does not require correction [6]. Severe or excessive wear refers to tooth destruction that requires restorative intervention. Severe attritional wear can result from occlusal prematurities that prevent functional or parafunctional movements of the jaw.

Evaluation and diagnosis should account for the patient's diet, history of eating, and/or gastric disorders, along with the present state of the occlusion. Emphasis must be placed on the evaluation of occlusal prematurities preventing condylar seating into the centric relation position [6]. Behavioural factors that may contribute to parafunctional habits and/or nocturnal bruxism are also important to understand and manage in order to successfully restore and maintain a healthier dentition [7]. Once a complete understanding of the etiology of the dentition's present state is appreciated, a treatment plan can be formulated, taking into account the number of teeth to be treated, condylar position, space availability, the vertical dimension of occlusion (VDO), and the choice of restorative material [8].

Full-mouth rehabilitation is the combination of all the different dental specialties under one treatment plan, covering all different dental aspects under one umbrella. Dentistry is a quickly evolving field. New treatments are being created while the old ones are being perfected. Smile makeovers are becoming more common with dental veneers and/or metal-less porcelain crowns. New materials are constantly improving the dental procedures, enhancing the patients comfort. In summation, we could say that full mouth rehabilitation is the combination of dental occlusion, dental balance, and functionality, with dental esthetics.

This paper describes the stages in restoration of severely worn dentition due to bruxism. The steps in treatment of these patients include a comprehensive examination, diagnostic mounting and diagnostic wax-up, careful planning and sequencing of various steps, discussion with the patient about the different treatment alternatives, and careful execution of the treatment plan.

2. Case Report

A 47-year-old male patient reported with the chief complaint of chronic sensitivity with anterior and posterior teeth.

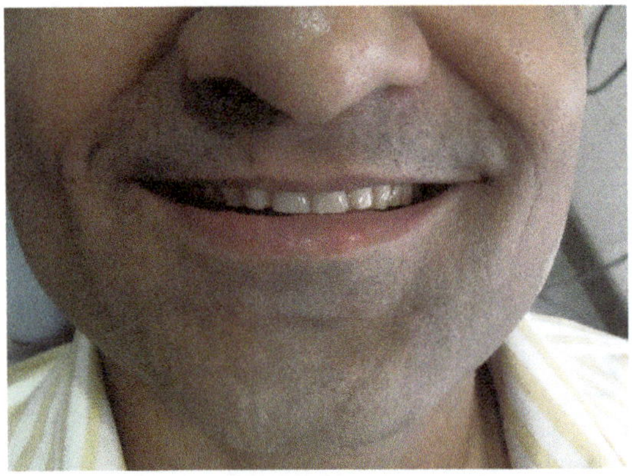

Figure 1: Preoperative extraoral view.

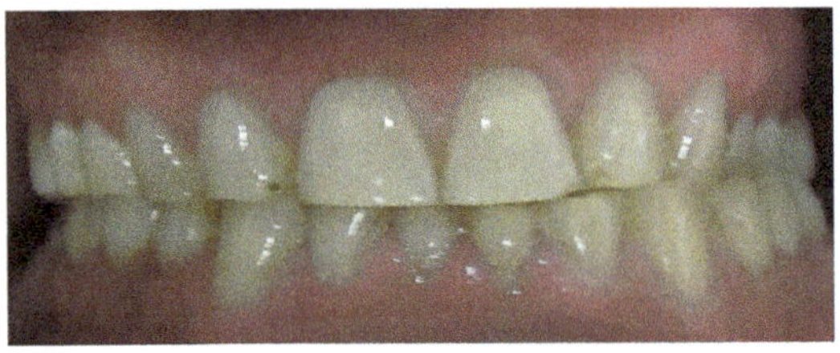

Figure 2: Preoperative intraoral view.

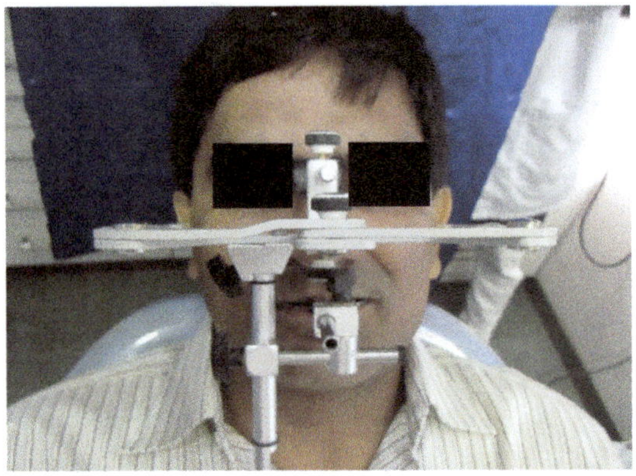

Figure 3: Facebow transfer.

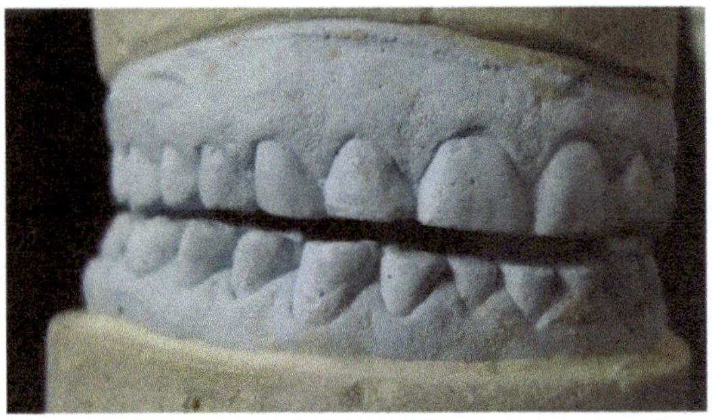

Figure 4: Restoration of vertical dimension on articulator.

Clinical examination revealed severely worn anterior and posterior teeth (Figures 1 and 2). On evaluation and diagnosis, patient's behavioural history related to stress which may have led to parafunctional habits. Endodontic and periodontal status was good except for mandibular left and right central and lateral incisors which needed endodontic treatment. Evaluation of the TMJs was unremarkable, with normal jaw opening and range of motion. No joint sounds, signs or symptoms of instability were evident. Joint loading in centric relation was performed utilizing bimanual manipulation.

Clinical investigation like phonetics—the S sound altered to F due to increased space, signs of wear, interocclusal distance was increased due to wear than normal (2–4 mm), facial appearance showed wrinkles, and drooping commissures at the corner of the mouth indicated loss of vertical dimension.

The findings were explained to the patient, and treatment options were presented. The treatment goals were to restore the lost occlusal vertical dimension (OVD) to correct the occlusal plane, to restore function, and to restore the esthetics of the patient's dentition.

Impressions for study casts were made with irreversible hydrocolloid (Zelgan 2002, Dentsply) material along with a centric relation occlusal record. The patient's casts were mounted on a semiadjustable articulator (Bio-art model A7, Brazil) using facebow record and the centric relation record (Figure 3). The new VDO was set by 3-4 mm increase in incisal guidance pin of the articulator (Figure 4). Occlusal splint was fabricated with the new VD and was designed to offer bilateral contacts of posterior teeth in centric relation (Figure 5). The anterior guidance disoccluded the posterior teeth except in centric relation. The adaptation of the patient to increased VD was evaluated during 6-week period. No muscle tenderness or discomfort in TMJ was noted.

Diagnostic wax-up was performed at the restored VD (Figure 6). It was then followed by prosthetic phase.

Replacing the anteriors and harmonizing the anterior guidance forms the first step in treatment. The mandibular anteriors were prepared to receive all ceramic crowns, gingival displacement was done. Impressions were made with single-step putty-wash technique using addition silicone material (Aquasil, Dentsply, Germany) and casts poured using type IV dental stone (Kalrock, Kalabhai, India). The anterior guidance was established using anterior plane and esthetics as guide. Provisional restorations were fabricated for the mandibular anteriors with autopolymerizing resin using the putty index and were reshaped in the mouth to achieve ideal contour and cemented using eugenol free temporary luting cement (Rely X Temp NE, 3 M ESPE, Germany).

The anterior replacement was followed by management of the posteriors. A putty index was fabricated for the wax-up in each quadrant which served not only as a guide for the tooth preparation in each quadrant but also in the fabrication of provisional restoration.

The posterior quadrants were prepared for full-coverage metal ceramic crowns. Mandibular posteriors were prepared followed by the maxillary posteriors. Gingival displacement

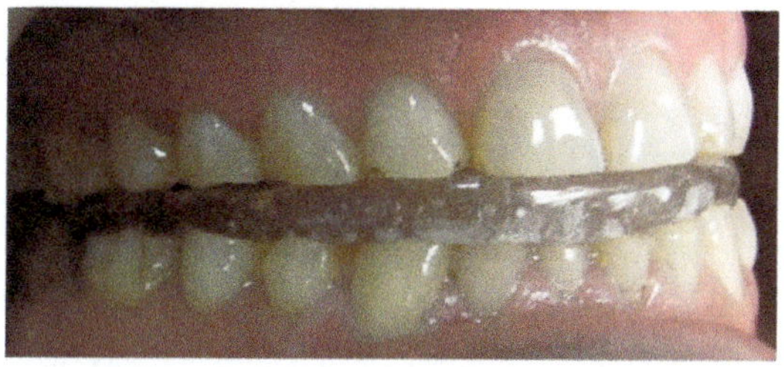

FIGURE 5: Occlusal splint in place.

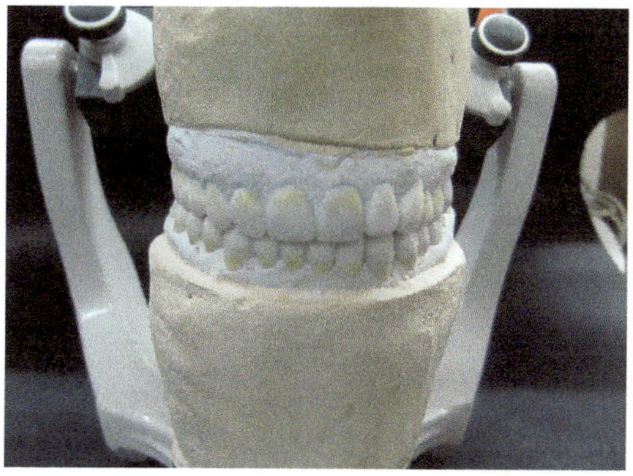

FIGURE 6: Diagnostic wax-up.

was done and impression was made with single-step putty-wash technique using additional silicone material. The working casts were articulated using facebow transfer and interocclusal centric record at previously determined vertical dimension. The provisional restorations were fabricated using putty index by the indirect technique, it was finished and corrected for occlusal interferences and luted with eugenol free temporary luting cement (Figure 7).

Patient's adaptation was monitored for a period of 6 weeks. The patient was assessed for adequate esthetics and functional harmony.

Once the occlusal adjustments, speech and esthetics seemed satisfactory, an occlusal bite record was taken. Definitive impressions were made with additional polyvinyl siloxane (Aquasil, Dentsply, Germany). Casts were mounted on the articulator with facebow transfer and the occlusal bite record in centric and eccentric relations. The final restorations were fabricated and cemented with FugiCEM cement (Figure 8). The scheme of occlusion given to the patient was mutually protected occlusion.

Patient was evaluated for 24 hrs and 48 hrs and necessary occlusal corrections were done. The patient was instructed oral hygiene maintenance and was advised six monthly check-up. A protective splint was fabricated to prevent further damage to the restorations.

3. Discussion

The etiology of occlusal wear for our patient is not fully understood; however, it can be hypothesized that the patient had history of stress which may have led to parafunctional

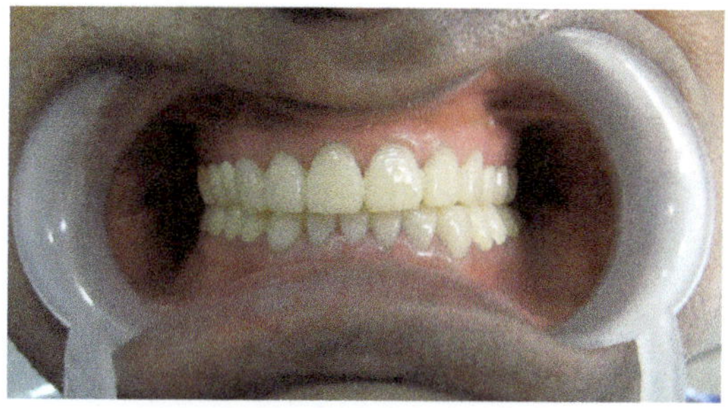

FIGURE 7: Provisional restorations were placed.

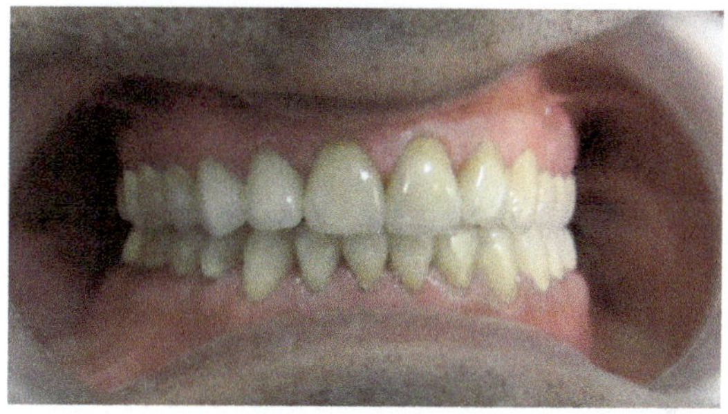

FIGURE 8: Definitive restoration.

occlusal habit and started grinding his anterior teeth. Once the anterior teeth got shorter, the patient lost anterior guidance and developed posterior interferences. The posterior interferences in lateral excursions can activate the masseter and temporalis muscles, enabling the patient to generate more forces to grind his teeth more aggressively [9]. A mutually protected occlusal scheme was used to prevent the destruction of the new prostheses.

Mutually protected articulation is described as "an occlusal scheme in which the posterior teeth prevent excessive contact of the anterior teeth in maximum intercuspation, and the anterior teeth disengage the posterior teeth in all mandibular excursive movements." Studies have shown that in lateral excursive movements [10], the anterior teeth can best receive and dissipate the forces [11] and posterior contacts in excursions appear to provide unfavorable forces to the masticatory system because of the amount and direction of the applied forces [12, 13]. In addition to the use of the mutually protected occlusal scheme, an occlusal splint was fabricated for night wear, and the patient was instructed and trained to keep his teeth apart when not actively chewing.

Zirconia ceramic crowns were selected for the patient's treatment to ensure adequate strength on upper and lower anterior teeth. The primary advantage of a zirconia restoration is esthetic benefit as it is translucent and tooth-colored. A metal-free ceramic crown can transmit a great amount of incident light through to a ceramic core where light is scattered in a natural fashion [14]. Thus, the appearance of definitive restorations may be very close to that of a natural tooth.

Many factors influence the choice of all-ceramic systems for abraded upper incisors. Strength, fit, and esthetics are traditionally considered in the selection of material for full-coverage restorations. Anterior crowns can be fixed to the tooth by traditional cements or resin cements. Traditional cements occupy the space between the restoration and the tooth surfaces but do not provide adhesion between them. Resin cements provide adhesion to both surfaces and can act to transfer force from the restoration to the underlying tooth and strengthen all-ceramic restorations [15].

A protective splint with a medium thermoplastic sheet was fabricated and given to the patient to prevent further tooth damage due to bruxism.

4. Conclusion

Full mouth rehabilitation is a treatment modality which not only focuses on the esthetics and functional aspect of the dentition but also improves upon the health of the whole stomatognathic system. A detailed diagnosis and treatment planning is necessary to achieve predictable success.

References

[1] M. Addy and R. P. Shellis, "Interaction between attrition, abrasion and erosion in tooth wear," *Monographs in Oral Science*, vol. 20, pp. 17–31, 2006.

[2] N. Beyth, E. Sharon, M. Lipovetsky, and A. Smidt, "Wear and different restorative materials—a review," *Refuat Hapeh Vehashinayim*, vol. 24, no. 3, pp. 6–14, 2006.

[3] J. O. Grippo, M. Simring, and S. Schreiner, "Attrition, abrasion, corrosion and abfraction revisited: a new perspective on tooth surface lesions," *Journal of the American Dental Association*, vol. 135, no. 8, pp. 1109–1118, 2004.

[4] R. G. Verrett, "Analyzing the etiology of an extremely worn dentition," *Journal of Prosthodontics*, vol. 10, no. 4, pp. 224–233, 2001.

[5] L. A. Litonjua, S. Andreana, P. J. Bush, and R. E. Cohen, "Tooth wear: ttrition, erosion, and abrasion," *Quintessence International*, vol. 34, no. 6, pp. 435–446, 2003.

[6] P. E. Dawson, *Functional Occlusion: From TMJ To Smile Design*, Mosby, St. Louis, Mo, USA, 2006.

[7] P. Neff, "Trauma from occlusion. Restorative concerns," *Dental Clinics of North America*, vol. 39, no. 2, pp. 335–354, 1995.

[8] B. L. Dahl, G. E. Carlsson, and A. Ekfeldt, "Occlusal wear of teeth and restorative materials. A review of classification, etiology, mechanisms of wear, and some aspects of restorative procedures," *Acta Odontologica Scandinavica*, vol. 51, no. 5, pp. 299–311, 1993.

[9] E. H. Williamson and D. O. Lundquist, "Anterior guidance: its effect on electromyographic activity of the temporal and masseter muscles," *The Journal of Prosthetic Dentistry*, vol. 49, no. 6, pp. 816–823, 1983.

[10] "The glossary of prosthodontic terms," *Journal of Prosthetic Dentistry*, vol. 94, no. 8, pp. 10–92, 2005.

[11] J. P. Standlee, A. A. Caputo, and J. P. Ralph, "Stress transfer to the mandible during anterior guidance and group function eccentric movements," *The Journal of Prosthetic Dentistry*, vol. 41, no. 1, pp. 35–39, 1979.

[12] S. P. Ramfjord, "Dysfunctional temporomandibular joint and muscle pain," *The Journal of Prosthetic Dentistry*, vol. 11, no. 2, pp. 353–374, 1961.

[13] A. Manns, R. Miralles, J. Valdivia, and R. Bull, "Influence of variation in anteroposterior occlusal contacts on electromyographic activity," *The Journal of Prosthetic Dentistry*, vol. 61, no. 5, pp. 617–623, 1989.

[14] S. O. Koutayas and M. Kern, "All-ceramic posts and cores: the state of the art," *Quintessence International*, vol. 30, no. 6, pp. 383–392, 1999.

[15] K. W. Hsu and Y. F. Shen, "Esthetic restoration of infra-occluded retained primary mandibular incisors with all-ceramic crowns in adult dentition," *Chang Gung Medical Journal*, vol. 27, no. 12, pp. 911–917, 2004.

12

Management and Followup of Complicated Crown Fractures in Young Patients Treated with Partial Pulpotomy

Francisco Ojeda-Gutierrez,[1] Brenda Martinez-Marquez,[1] Soraya Arteaga-Larios,[1] M. Socorro Ruiz-Rodriguez,[2] and Amaury Pozos-Guillen[2]

[1] *General Dentistry Department, Facultad de Estomatología, Universidad Autónoma de San Luis Potosí, 2 Dr. Manuel Nava, Zona Universitaria, 78290 San Luis Potosí, SLP, Mexico*

[2] *Pediatric Dentistry Posgraduate Program, Facultad de Estomatología, Universidad Autónoma de San Luis Potosí, 2 Dr. Manuel Nava, Zona Universitaria, 78290 San Luis Potosí, SLP, Mexico*

Correspondence should be addressed to Amaury Pozos-Guillen; apozos@uaslp.mx

Academic Editors: H. C. Gungor and G. Schierano

Two cases of young patients with traumatized permanent teeth having complicated crown fractures are reported. Endodontic management included partial pulpotomy by the Cvek technique; restorative management included resin restoration and reattachment of the teeth fragments. Treatments were considered successful in all cases according to the following criteria: absence of clinical symptoms, absence of X-ray signs of pathology, and presence of pulpal vitality 6 to 25 months after treatment.

1. Introduction

Trauma to the facial area represents a public health problem involving children and adolescents; it generally involves the teeth and their supporting structures. The most frequent causes are falls, traffic accidents, domestic violence, fights, and sports. Most dental injuries occur during the first 2 decades of life, especially between 2 and 3 years and between 8 and 12 years of age, occurring more often in boys than in girls [1–3]. Dental fractures frequently involve only the enamel, or enamel and dentin, without affecting the pulp [4]. Occasionally, however, the pulp is also involved [5–7]. Due to their position, the teeth most frequently affected by dental traumatism are the maxillary incisors: 80% centrals and 16% laterals [8]. Several diagnostic criteria have been used to classify traumatic dental injuries. Ellis and Davery [9], proposed a classification based on a numerical system (I to VIII) and described the extent, using terms like "simple fracture" and "complicated fracture"; this classification considers X-ray examinations and vitality tests.

Treatment of crown fractures with exposed pulp in permanent young teeth depends on the degree of pulp exposure, time between accident and examination, effect of the traumatism, and the stage of root development. Treatment options of crown fractures with pulpal exposure are direct pulp capping, partial pulpotomy, pulpectomy, or extraction. For young patients in whom the exposed pulp maintains its vitality, pulpotomy is the best endodontic treatment option in order to maintain pulpal functions [10–13]. A partial pulpotomy, known as the Cvek technique, is indicated for teeth having the following characteristics: small pulp exposure, treated within 14 days of trauma, caries-free, open apex or thin dentinal walls, and vital and asymptomatic pulp. This technique involves amputation of the pulp 2 mm apical to the affected pulp tissue, but it is not recommended for those cases in which the pulp exposure is extensive or where there has been a 2-week lapse between trauma and treatment [14]. The aim of the present report is to describe the management and followup of 2 cases of dental trauma with complicated crown

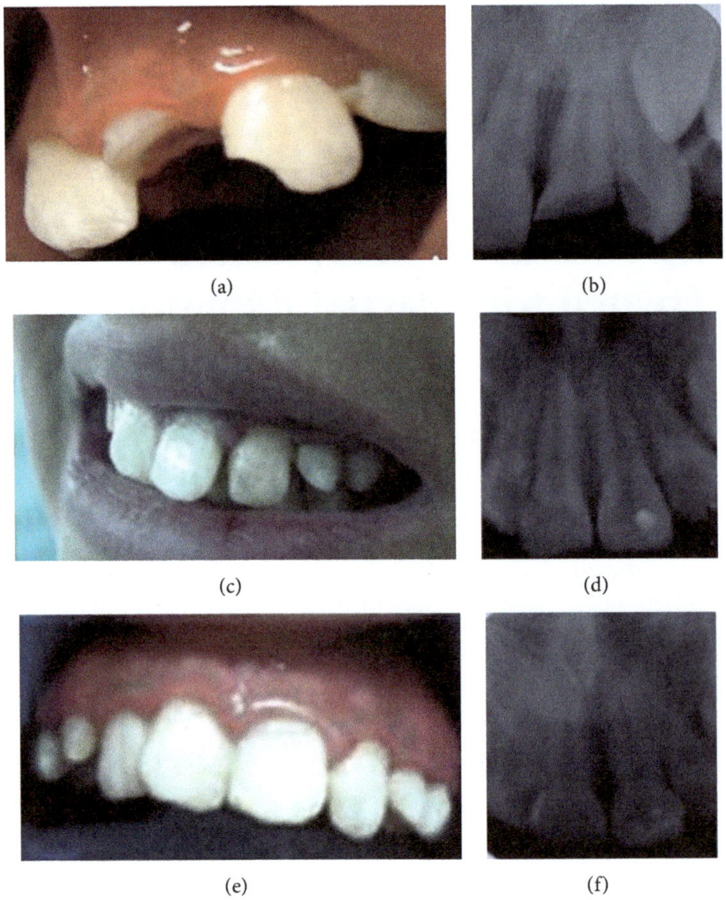

Figure 1: (a) Initial clinical image of patient 4 h after trauma with complicated crown fracture in maxillary left central incisor, with ulcerated and exposed pulp, and enamel crown fracture in left lateral incisor. (b) Initial radiograph showing loss of dental structure, complete root development, closed apices, normal periodontal ligament, and absence of root or alveolar bone fractures. (c) Resin reconstruction and reattachment of tooth fragments after treatment. (d) Posttreatment radiograph showing indirect pulp capping with resin reconstruction in the maxillary left lateral incisor and pulpotomy with reattachment of the dental fragments in the left central incisor. (e-f) Clinical and radiographic examinations 6 months after trauma. Patient showed no periodontal or periapical pathology, nor pulpal signs or symptoms.

fractures who were treated by partial pulpotomy using the Cvek technique.

2. Case Presentation

2.1. Case 1. An 11-year-old boy was referred to our clinic because of crown fractures of the maxillary left central and lateral incisors, presenting to the clinic 4 hours after the trauma. According to his medical history, the patient exhibited neither systemic disease nor relevant problems. Extraorally, there was no apparent trauma to the soft tissues. Intraoral clinical examination revealed a complicated crown fracture of the maxillary left central incisor (class III, Ellis's classification), with ulcerated and exposed pulp, and extensive crown fracture with noticeable dentinal involvement. There was no pulp exposure of the left lateral incisor (class II, Ellis's classification) (Figure 1(a)). For both teeth, periapical radiographic examination showed complete root development, closed apices, no periapical injury, and no alveolar bone fractures (Figure 1(b)). Endodontic treatment included pulpal protection with glass ionomer and for the left lateral incisor, reconstruction with hybrid resin, and partial pulpotomy using the Cvek technique with reattaching of the same teeth fragments for the central incisor. The treatment plan was accepted.

A local anesthetic was administered and the affected teeth were isolated with a rubber dam. For indirect pulp protection in the lateral incisor, a layer of glass ionomer (Vitrebond; 3 M ESPE, St Paul, MN, USA) was applied. Then the tooth was acid-etched using 37% orthophosphoric acid for 30 s, and the acid was eliminated by rinsing with distilled water and drying; dental adhesive (Prime and Bond NT, Dentsply Caulk, Milford, DE, USA) was applied according to the manufacturer's instructions. A hybrid resin (Z-250, 3 M ESPE) was applied using the incremental technique. Each increment was light cured for 40 s. For the partial pulpotomy of the central incisor, a number. 330 tungsten round bur (with continuous saline rinsing) was used to amputate the pulp close to the exposure site to a depth of 2 mm. The blood was noted to be light red, and hemostasis was evident in

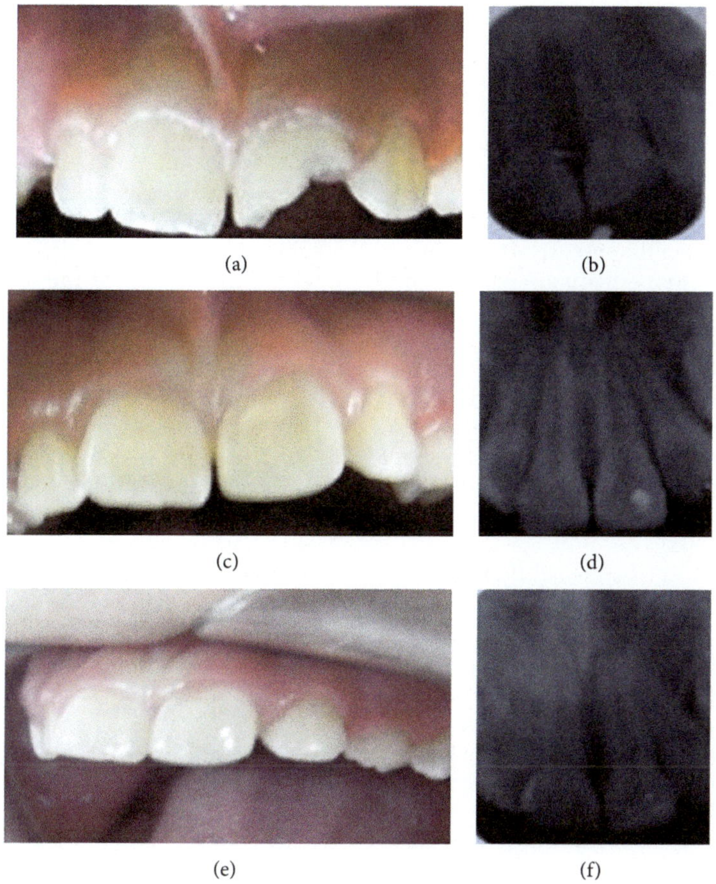

FIGURE 2: (a) Initial clinical image of patient 17 hours after trauma with complicated crown fracture in the maxillary left central incisor. (b) Initial radiograph showing loss of dental structure, complete root development, closed apices, and absence of root or alveolar bone fractures. (c) Resin reconstruction after treatment. (d) Posttreatment radiograph showing partial pulpotomy with resin reconstruction. (e-f) Clinical and radiographic images 25 months after treatment. Patient's teeth were found to be vital; no pain to percussion or palpation, with functional restorations.

2 min. A dressing of calcium hydroxide ($Ca[OH]_2$) paste (Viarden, Mexico City, DF, Mexico) was placed, followed by a coat of glass ionomer (Vitrebond), and photopolymerized for 40 s. The teeth fragments were reattached using a modified Simonsen's technique [7]. Clinical and radiographic examinations were made after treatment (Figures 1(c)-1(d)). Followup appointments took place 1 week, 1 month, and 3 months after treatment, with no pulpal signs or symptoms found. Six months after the trauma, the teeth were found to be vital without periodontal or periapical pathology and the restorations were functional and aesthetically acceptable (Figures 1(e)-1(f)).

2.2. Case 2. A 9-year-old girl was seen in our clinic with trauma to her maxillary left incisor area, received 17 hours previously. Intraoral examination revealed a complicated crown fracture of the left central incisor (class III, Ellis's classification), with ulcerated pulp (Figure 2(a)). Periapical radiographic examination showed completed root formation, closed apices, no periapical injury, and no alveolar bone or radicular dental fractures (Figure 2(b)). Pulp management included partial pulpotomy with the Cvek technique and reconstruction with hybrid resin of both involved teeth. Endodontic and restorative treatments were realized as in the previously reported case 1 (Figures 2(c)-2(d)). Followup appointments were made periodically. At 25 months' followup, the teeth were found to be vital, without periodontal or periapical pathology (Figures 2(e)-2(f)).

3. Discussion

Reports have shown that 25% of school-aged children will experience some kind of dental trauma [15]. Among the child and teenage population, the possibility of suffering orofacial trauma is high and actually is considered a dental public health problem [16]. Crown fractures with pulp exposure represent 18% to 20% of traumatic injuries involving the teeth, the majority being in young permanent teeth [6]. Complicated crown fractures are defined as fractures involving enamel and dentin with pulp exposure. These injuries produce changes in the exposed pulp tissues, and a biological and functional restoration represents an important clinical challenge. In these cases, inflammation or contamination is generally present.

For traumatized teeth with complicated crown fractures in young patients, treatment options include direct pulp capping, partial pulpotomy, cervical pulpotomy, pulpectomy, or extraction, depending on the time between the trauma and treatment of the patient, degree of root development, and size of the pulp exposure. Pulp exposure caused by dental trauma has a better prognosis because of the absence of microorganisms associated with caries. The objective is always to preserve pulp vitality. Pulp capping is recommended for small exposures (1 mm) that have occurred not more than a few hours previously [17]. Partial pulpotomy may be the preferred treatment in cases of extensive pulpal exposure when pulpal vitality and the time elapsed between trauma and treatment allow for this option. A pulpotomy is indicated for those patients wherein the pulpitis has not progressed beyond the coronal pulp, bleeding after amputation is not excessive, and the blood has a normal color [14, 18].

Recently Andreasen et al. [19] estimated that 2 out of 3 children suffer a traumatic dental injury before adulthood and established that the problem of trauma in children is not reflected by the active participation of pediatric dentists in acute treatment, followup, or research on this topic.

Partial pulpotomy has a high success rate in cases with complicated crown fractures in young teeth with pulp exposure [20–24]; however, a long-term followup is necessary to establish this success rate. Cvek reported high success rates in cases of complicated crown fractures treated by partial pulpotomy (96%) having a followup of between 14 and 60 months and 30 hours between trauma and treatment [14]. Partial pulpotomy has the advantage of preserving the cell-rich coronal pulp tissue, which possesses better healing potential and can maintain the physiologic deposition of dentin [20]. Various materials have been proposed as medicaments for pulpotomies such as mineral trioxide aggregate (MTA) and enamel matrix derivative (EMD) [25–27]. MTA's effects on amputated pulpal tissue suggest that the material preserves the pulp tissue and promotes the regeneration of hard tissues [28]. EMD, because of its amelogenin and amelin protein-rich fraction, has the potential to induce a process that seems to imitate normal dentinogenesis; it clearly influences the odontoblasts and endothelial cells of the pulp capillaries to create a hard, calcified barrier over the pulp exposure [27, 29, 30]. However; due to its action, $Ca(OH)_2$ continues to be the material of choice for pulpotomy [6, 7, 23, 24, 31]. This agent prevents bacterial activity and stimulates dentin bridge formation. Its high pH and low water solubility are responsible for its antimicrobial activity and ability to induce hard tissue formation.

The followup for determining the success of treatment is based on clinical and radiographic evaluations. During followup of the 2 cases reported at different periods (6–25 months), no tooth sensitivity or pain was registered; also, no symptoms or radiographic defects were present. Clinical and radiographic examination showed no periodontal or periapical pathology, and the restorations were functionally acceptable and aesthetically gratifying. In the present cases, we decided to use a partial pulpotomy on the affected teeth. For this decision we considered the size of the exposure, interval between the accident and treatment, age of the patient, and maturity of the roots. During followups, we evaluated the vitality of the pulp. The potential for the pulp to recover its vitality depends on several factors such as the state of the pulpal tissue before the trauma, previous inflammation, infection associated with the caries, and the treatment [17, 32–34]. The patients showed no periodontal or periapical pathology, pulpal signs or symptoms, mobility, color changes, edema, fistula, calcification of the root canal, or alterations in the apical region. Another clinical criterion of success is the capacity of the pulp to recover its vitality [35, 36]. The teeth treated in the 2 reported cases were found to be vital, having the formation of dentinal bridges and continuous root development. The treatments substantiated the effectiveness of this pulp procedure, within a postoperative observation time of 6 to 25 months.

Partial pulpotomy represents an excellent alternative for the treatment of traumatized vital teeth. On the basis of these reports, we recommend the partial pulpotomy using the Cvek technique for traumatized teeth with complicated crown fractures.

Acknowledgment

This work was supported partially by PIFI 2012.

References

[1] American Academy of Pediatric Dentistry Council on Clinical Affairs, "Guidelines on management of acute dental trauma," *Pediatric Dentistry*, vol. 30, no. 7, supplement, pp. 175–183, 2009.

[2] P. C. S. Filho, P. S. Quagliatto, P. C. Simamoto Jr., and C. J. Soares, "Dental trauma: restorative procedures using composite resin and mouthguards for prevention," *Journal of Contemporary Dental Practice*, vol. 8, no. 6, pp. 89–95, 2007.

[3] C. M. Forsberg and G. Tedestam, "Etiological and predisposing factors related to traumatic injuries to permanent teeth," *Swedish Dental Journal*, vol. 17, no. 5, pp. 183–190, 1993.

[4] K. Arapostathis, A. Arhakis, and S. Kalfas, "A modified technique on the reattachment of permanent tooth fragments following dental trauma. Case report," *Journal of Clinical Pediatric Dentistry*, vol. 30, no. 1, pp. 29–34, 2005.

[5] G. Cavalleri and N. Zerman, "Traumatic crown fractures in permanent incisors with immature roots: a follow-up study," *Endodontics & Dental Traumatology*, vol. 11, no. 6, pp. 294–296, 1995.

[6] L. P. De Blanco, "Treatment of crown fractures with pulp exposure," *Oral Surgery, Oral Medicine, Oral Pathology, Oral Radiology, and Endodontics*, vol. 82, no. 5, pp. 564–568, 1996.

[7] F. Ojeda-Gutierrez, B. Martinez-Marquez, R. Rosales-Ibanez, and A. J. Pozos-Guillen, "Reattachment of anterior teeth fragments using a modified Simonsen's technique after dental trauma: report of a case," *Dental Traumatology*, vol. 27, no. 1, pp. 81–85, 2011.

[8] J. O. Andreasen, "Etiology and pathogenesis of traumatic dental injuries: a clinical study of 1,298 cases," *Scandinavian Journal of Dental Research*, vol. 78, no. 4, pp. 329–342, 1970.

[9] R. G. Ellis and K. Davery, *The Classification and Treatment of Injuries to the Teeth of Children*, Year Book, Chicago, Ill, USA, 5th edition, 1970.

[10] J. D. McIntyre and W. F. Vann Jr., "Two case reports of complicated permanent crown fractures treated with partial pulpotomies," *Pediatric Dentistry*, vol. 31, no. 2, pp. 117–122, 2009.

[11] K. C. Huth, E. Paschos, N. Hajek-Al-Khatar et al., "Effectiveness of 4 pulpotomy techniques—randomized controlled trial," *Journal of Dental Research*, vol. 84, no. 12, pp. 1144–1148, 2005.

[12] I. Epelman, P. E. Murray, F. Garcia-Godoy, S. Kuttler, and K. N. Namerow, "A practitioner survey of opinions toward regenerative endodontics," *Journal of Endodontics*, vol. 35, no. 9, pp. 1204–1210, 2009.

[13] F. Garcia-Godoy and P. E. Murray, "Recommendations for using regenerative endodontic procedures in permanent immature traumatized teeth," *Dental Traumatology*, vol. 28, no. 1, pp. 33–41, 2012.

[14] M. Cvek, "A clinical report on partial pulpotomy and capping with calcium hydroxide in permanent incisors with complicated crown fracture," *Journal of Endodontics*, vol. 4, no. 8, pp. 232–237, 1978.

[15] P. Krasner and H. J. Rankow, "New philosophy for the treatment of avulsed teeth," *Oral Surgery, Oral Medicine, Oral Pathology and Endodontics*, vol. 79, no. 5, pp. 616–623, 1995.

[16] M. A. Tapias, R. Jiménez-García, F. Lamas, and A. A. Gil, "Prevalence of traumatic crown fractures to permanent incisors in a childhood population: Móstoles, Spain," *Dental Traumatology*, vol. 19, no. 3, pp. 119–122, 2003.

[17] W. H. Liebenberg, "Direct pulp capping considerations during tooth fragment reattachment: a case report," *The Journal of the Dental Association of South Africa*, vol. 48, no. 1, pp. 28–32, 1993.

[18] E. A. V. Maia, L. N. Baratieri, M. A. C. De Andrada, S. Monteiro Jr., and E. M. De Araújo Jr., "Tooth fragment reattachment: fundamentals of the technique and two case reports," *Quintessence International*, vol. 34, no. 2, pp. 99–107, 2003.

[19] J. O. Andreasen, E. Lauridsen, and J. Daugaard-Jensen, "Dental traumatology: an orphan in pediatric dentistry?" *Pediatric Dentistry*, vol. 31, no. 2, pp. 153–156, 2009.

[20] C. D. Fong and M. J. Davis, "Partial pulpotomy for immature permanent teeth, its present and fixture," *Pediatric Dentistry*, vol. 24, no. 1, pp. 29–32, 2002.

[21] A. B. Fuks, A. Cosack, H. Klein, and E. Eidelman, "Partial pulpotomy as a treatment alternative for exposed pulps in crown-fractured permanent incisors," *Endodontics & Dental Traumatology*, vol. 3, no. 3, pp. 100–102, 1987.

[22] R. A. Souza, S. C. N. Gomes, J. D. C. P. Dantas, Y. T. Silva-Sousa, and J. D. Pécora, "Importance of the diagnosis in the pulpotomy of immature permanent teeth," *Brazilian Dental Journal*, vol. 18, no. 3, pp. 244–247, 2007.

[23] D. R. S. Nadia, E. Bresciani, C. E. Francischone, E. B. Franco, and J. C. Pereira, "Partial pulpotomy and tooth reconstruction of a crown-fractured permanent incisor: a case report," *Quintessence International*, vol. 34, no. 10, pp. 740–747, 2003.

[24] I. S. Sonmez and H. Sonmez, "Long-term follow-up of a complicated crown fracture treated by partial pulpotomy," *International Endodontic Journal*, vol. 40, no. 5, pp. 398–403, 2007.

[25] M. Torabinejad and N. Chivian, "Clinical applications of mineral trioxide aggregate," *Journal of Endodontics*, vol. 25, no. 3, pp. 197–205, 1999.

[26] T. Kiatwateeratana, S. Kintarak, S. Piwat, O. Chankanka, S. Kamaolmatyakul, and A. Thearmontree, "Partial pulpotomy on caries-free teeth using enamel matrix derivative or calcium hydroxide: a randomized controlled trial," *International Endodontic Journal*, vol. 42, no. 7, pp. 584–592, 2009.

[27] H. Olsson, J. R. Davies, K. E. Holst, U. Schröder, and K. Petersson, "Dental pulp capping: effect of emdogain gel on experimentally exposed human pulps," *International Endodontic Journal*, vol. 38, no. 3, pp. 186–194, 2005.

[28] R. S. Schwartz, M. Mauger, D. J. Clement, and W. A. Walker III, "Mineral trioxide aggregate: a new material for endodontics," *Journal of the American Dental Association*, vol. 130, no. 7, pp. 967–975, 1999.

[29] N. T. Ishizaki, K. Matsumoto, Y. Kimura, X. Wang, and A. Yamashita, "Histopathological study of dental pulp tissue capped with enamel matrix derivative," *Journal of Endodontics*, vol. 29, no. 3, pp. 176–179, 2003.

[30] A. Garrocho-Rangel, H. Flores, D. Silva-Herzog, F. Hernandez-Sierra, P. Mandeville, and A. J. Pozos-Guillen, "Efficacy of EMD versus calcium hydroxide in direct pulp capping of primary molars: a randomized controlled clinical trial," *Oral Surgery, Oral Medicine, Oral Pathology, Oral Radiology and Endodontology*, vol. 107, no. 5, pp. 733–738, 2009.

[31] A. H. B. Schuurs, R. J. M. Gruythuysen, and P. R. Wesselink, "Pulp capping with adhesive resin-based composite vs. calcium hydroxide: a review," *Dental Traumatology*, vol. 16, no. 6, pp. 240–250, 2000.

[32] F. M. Andreasen, J. G. Norén, J. O. Andreasen, S. Engelhardtsen, and U. Lindh-Strömberg, "Long-term survival of fragment bonding in the treatment of fractured crowns: a multicenter clinical study," *Quintessence International*, vol. 26, no. 10, pp. 669–681, 1995.

[33] P. E. Murray, I. About, P. J. Lumley, G. Smith, J. C. Franquin, and A. J. Smith, "Postoperative pulpal and repair responses," *Journal of the American Dental Association*, vol. 131, no. 3, pp. 321–329, 2000.

[34] D. Tziafas, A. J. Smith, and H. Lesot, "Designing new treatment strategies in vital pulp therapy," *Journal of Dentistry*, vol. 28, no. 2, pp. 77–92, 2000.

[35] I. Jacobsen and B. U. Zachrisson, "Repair of characteristics of root fractures in permanent anterior teeth," *Scandinavian Journal of Dental Research*, vol. 83, no. 6, pp. 355–364, 1975.

[36] L. Feely, I. C. Mackie, and T. Macfarlane, "An investigation of root-fractured permanent incisor teeth in children," *Dental Traumatology*, vol. 19, no. 1, pp. 52–54, 2003.

13

Neuroleptic Malignant Syndrome in a Patient with Tongue Cancer

Osamu Baba,[1] Kenji Yamagata,[1] Yasushi Tomidokoro,[2] Akira Tamaoka,[2] Hiroyuki Itoh,[1] Toru Yanagawa,[1] Kojiro Onizawa,[1] and Hiroki Bukawa[1]

[1] *Department of Oral and Maxillofacial Surgery, Faculty of Medicine, University of Tsukuba, 1-1-1 Tennodai, Ibaraki, Tsukuba City 305-8575, Japan*
[2] *Department of Clinical Pathophysiology of the Neurological Disorders, Faculty of Medicine, University of Tsukuba, Japan*

Correspondence should be addressed to Kenji Yamagata; y-kenji@md.tsukuba.ac.jp

Academic Editors: C. Landes and A. Milosevic

Background. Neuroleptic malignant syndrome (NMS) is a rare but life-threatening complication of neuroleptic drugs, which are used widely in head and neck cancer (HANC) patients who develop delirium. *Methods and Results.* Postoperative delirium in a 39-year-old man with tongue cancer was treated with haloperidol and chlorpromazine. Three days after the first administration of antipsychotics, the patient exhibited elevated body temperature, autonomic and extrapyramidal symptoms, and impaired consciousness. A definitive diagnosis was made using the research diagnostic criteria for NMS in the DSM-IV, and the antipsychotics were immediately discontinued. The patient was given dantrolene and bromocriptine to treat the NMS. The patient's hyperthermia, elevated creatinin kinase (CK), and muscle rigidity improved gradually, with all symptoms of NMS resolving completely by 13 days after the diagnosis. *Conclusions.* HANC surgeons must be alert for early signs of NMS and use antipsychotics conservatively to avoid NMS and its potentially fatal outcome.

1. Introduction

Neuroleptic malignant syndrome (NMS) is a rare but life-threatening disorder caused by an adverse reaction to neuroleptic (antipsychotic) drugs and characterized by hyperthermia, severe muscle rigidity, and changes in autonomic and mental status [1]. Most cases of clinical NMS have been reported by psychiatrists; however, NMS can occur in any setting in which psychotropic drugs are administered. In nonpsychiatric cases treated with neuroleptics, NMS can be difficult to diagnose, particularly because the symptoms are consistent with other, more expected, disorders. However, early diagnosis is extremely important to reduce the risk of death. The frequency of the syndrome ranges from 0.07 to 2.2% in patients treated with neuroleptic drugs, and the mortality is 10 to 30% [2, 3]. Although the frequency of NMS among patients taking neuroleptics has decreased, it remains a significant source of morbidity and mortality in this patient group [4]. To our knowledge, a few reports have been published about NMS in patients with head and neck cancer (HANC) [5, 6]. We report a rare case of NMS that occurred postoperatively in a tongue cancer patient whose surgery consisted of hemiglossectomy, neck dissection, and immediate reconstruction.

2. Case Report

A 39-year-old man came to the Department of Oral and Maxillofacial Surgery, University of Tsukuba Hospital, complaining of a painful mass of the tongue border. His medical, social, and family histories were unremarkable. The diagnosis was tongue cancer (T2N1M0). He received induction chemotherapy of oral fluoropyrimidine, S-1 at 120 mg/day for 2 weeks. After the induction chemotherapy, hemiglossectomy, modified radical neck dissection, and immediate reconstruction with a free forearm flap were performed under general anesthesia, without any complications. The patient was sedated with intravenously administered propofol and dexmedetomidine hydrochloride. Anesthesia was induced and maintained with sevoflurane, propofol, and

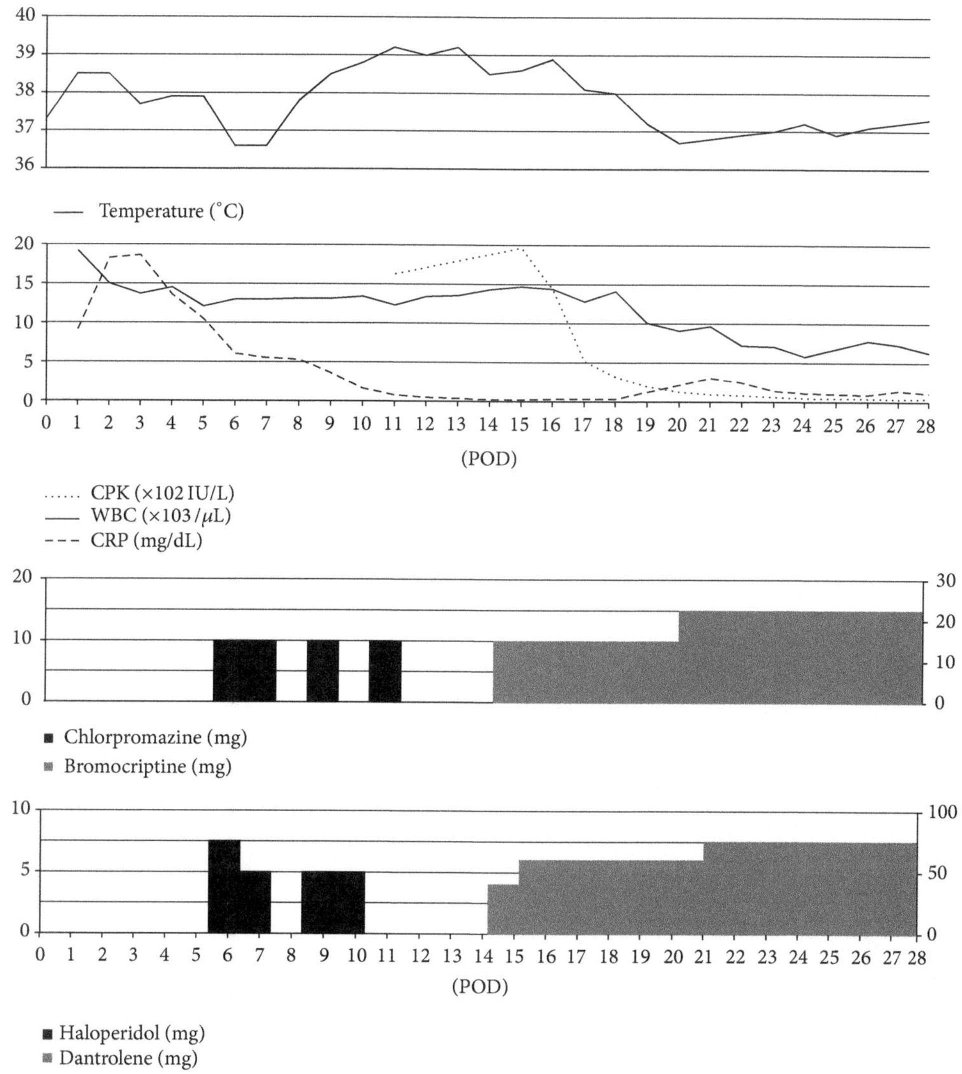

Figure 1: Clinical course of NMS. POD: postoperative days. On POD 15, treatment of NMS began.

dexmedetomidine hydrochloride. The operative time was 10 hours, and the blood loss was 420 mL.

The patient's postoperative clinical course is shown in Figure 1. He was sedated with propofol and dexmedetomidine hydrochloride to prevent postoperative thrombosis in the microvascular anastomosis. On postoperative day 6, the patient became severely agitated, and postoperative delirium was diagnosed. To treat the delirium, 5–10 mg of haloperidol and 10 mg of chlorpromazine were administered intravenously for 5 days. Three days after the first administration of the antipsychotic drugs, the patient's body temperature (BT) rose to over 38.5°C, and severe diaphoresis was observed. Drug-induced fever or infectious disease was suspected, and the antibacterial agent was changed from cefozopran to ciprofloxacin; however, the patient's BT continued to rise.

On the ninth day after the first use of antipsychotic drugs, the patient's hyperthermia continued, and it was accompanied by changes in consciousness level, difficulty closing the mouth, dysphagia, tremor, muscle rigidity, diaphoresis, tachycardia, and elevated blood pressure (Figure 2). The patient's conscious level was confusing. His blood pressure was 143/77 mmHg. Laboratory data on that day showed an elevated white blood cell count (WBC, 14.7 × $10^3/\mu$L), elevated creatinin kinase (CK, 1964 U/l), and a detectable C-reactive protein (CRP) value (0.17 mg/dL). There was a significant discrepancy between the WBC and CRP. Bacterial cultures of the blood and urine were negative. Chest X-ray and brain computed tomography revealed no abnormalities. The patient was referred to the Department of Neurology, where a definitive diagnosis of NMS was made according to the diagnostic research criteria of the DSM-IV [7]. The antipsychotic medications were immediately discontinued.

To treat the NMS, 40 mg of dantrolene was given intravenously, and 15 mg of bromocriptine was delivered by nasogastric tube, 15 days after the first administration of antipsychotics. By the next day, the patient's extrapyramidal and autonomic dysfunction began to improve, and the laboratory data began to return to the normal range. The patient's BT

Table 1: DSM-IV diagnostic criteria of neuroleptic malignant syndrome [7].

(A) The development of severe muscle rigidity and elevated temperature associated with the use of neuroleptic medication
(B) Two (or more) of the following:
(1) diaphoresis
(2) dysphagia
(3) tremor
(4) incontinence
(5) changes in level of consciousness ranging from confusion to coma
(6) mutism
(7) tachycardia
(8) elevated or labile blood pressure
(9) leukocytosis
(10) laboratory evidence of muscle injury (e.g., elevated CPK)
(C) The symptoms in criteria A and B are not due to another substance (e.g., phencyclidine) or a neurological or other general medical conditions (e.g., viral encephalitis)
(D) The symptoms in criteria A and B are not better accounted for a mental disorder (e.g., mood disorder with catatonic features)

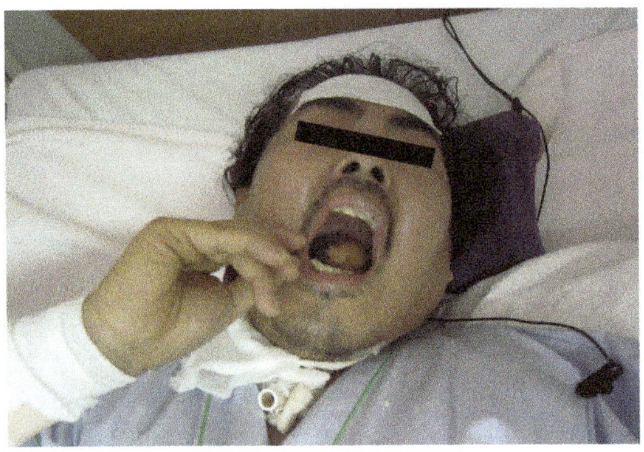

Figure 2: Case patient exhibiting NMS symptoms. Hyperthermia, significant extrapyramidal symptoms, various autonomic symptoms, and impaired consciousness were observed.

resolved to under 37°C, and the CK level decreased to the normal range within 6 days of beginning treatment for the NMS. The patient's muscle rigidity improved gradually, and the symptoms of NMS had completely resolved by 13 days after the date of NMS diagnosis.

3. Discussion

Although the exact pathophysiologic mechanisms of NMS are uncertain, an acute reduction in brain dopamine activity is thought to have a primary role [4, 8–10]. NMS is probably caused by a complex interaction between the neuroleptic medication and host susceptibilities. Familial cluster of NMS and presence of a specific allele of the dopamine D2 receptor gene were reported [11, 12]. Two hypotheses have been proposed to explain the syndrome: (a) the neuroleptic medications cause a blockade of central dopamine receptors, and (b) the neuroleptic medications interact with skeletal muscle defects. In the first hypothesis, dopaminergic receptor blockade by neuroleptics may interfere with central thermoregulation. Heat is produced in response to stimulation by serotonin in the hypothalamus, and dopamine inhibits this process. A dopaminergic blockade would, therefore, reduce the inhibition of the serotonin-induced temperature increase, thus, leading to the hyperthermia seen in NMS [13, 14]. Interference with nigrostriatal dopamine pathways may lead to muscle rigidity and tremor. The second hypothesis posits that NMS shares its pathophysiology with that of malignant hyperthermia [2]. As in patients with malignant hyperthermia, an *in vitro* investigation of tissue samples from NMS patients revealed multiple defects in skeletal muscle, most of which were associated with increased calcium released from the sarcoplasmic reticulum [15].

Major symptoms of NMS include hyperthermia, tachycardia, diaphoresis, muscle rigidity, tremor, mutism, and altered consciousness. Several nonspecific laboratory abnormalities, including elevated CK and leukocytosis, are also seen [10]. The diagnostic criteria of Caroff and Mann [10] and Levenson [16] are considered valid for a definitive diagnosis. However, the above symptoms are for full-blown NMS and are rarely seen early in the disease; therefore, NMS is difficult to diagnose, especially in its early stages. Research criteria from the DSM-IV have been used for the diagnosis of NMS (Table 1) [7]. In the present case, the patient's condition met criterion A and 8 of 10 items of criterion B in the DSM-IV criteria. There were no other identifiable substances, neurologic/medical etiologies, or psychiatric disorders that might better explain the patient's symptoms (criteria C and D). Recently, a novel diagnostic criterion for NMS is published by an international multispecialty consensus group in 2011 for validation [17].

Most neuroleptic medications including "atypical" antipsychotic drugs, carry some risk of causing NMS. Among the typical neuroleptics, haloperidol is the most common associated with NMS, and chlorpromazine, fluphenazine, and levomepromazine are all associated with NMS onset [14]. NMS most often occurs with the initiation of neuroleptics or an increase in dosage, but it is rarely seen after the sudden discontinuation of drug therapy [18].

NMS can be particularly difficult to diagnose, in part because symptoms develop over 24 to 72 hours and can last from 1 to 44 days (about 10 days on average) [19]. Furthermore, there is no typical sequence of symptoms, whereas extrapyramidal symptoms usually occur before autonomic ones. Although mental status change can be an initial symptom of the disorder [20], it is difficult to distinguish from postoperative delirium. In the current patient's case, NMS occurred 3 days after initiation of 2 neuroleptics, haloperidol, and chlorpromazine and lasted through the subsequent 5 days during which these drugs continued to be used. This timing agrees with previous reports [18, 19]. However, it should be mentioned that NMS can occur even after a single dose or after use of for many years [21].

Psychiatric conditions such as catatonia and agitation have been substantiated in case-control studies [22]. In addition, several clinical, systemic, and metabolic factors including undernutrition, dehydration, preexisting abnormalities of the central nervous system, pharmacological and treatment variables, acute medical illness such as surgery, and a history of NMS may be risk factors for NMS, in combination with neuroleptic use [4]. In the case of dehydration, hyperthermia is exacerbated by decreased blood volume, which induces peripheral vasoconstriction and impairs heat dissipation. Other risk factors for NMS may include stress, humidity, and the concomitant use of lithium, anticholinergic agents, or some antidepressants [23]. Nearly 80% of NMS patients have been reported to be undernutrition and dehydration prior to the onset of the disease [8]. The current patient had an increased risk for NMS because of postoperative stress from his prolonged period of admission to intensive care units, dehydration from high fever (over 38.0°C), and postoperative undernutrition, because the patient did not take any oral nutrition before the administration of neuroleptics.

NMS, a life-threatening neurological emergency, requires the immediate discontinuation of neuroleptic medications and the institution of supportive medical therapy, including body fluid volume resuscitation and general cooling [24]. Serial monitoring for hyperthermia, cardiovascular collapse, acute myoglobin-induced renal failure, respiratory failure, and aspiration pneumonia is critical [4, 9, 10]. Dantrolene, a muscle relaxant that is specifically indicated for anesthetic-induced malignant hyperthermia, is also frequently used to treat NMS [4]. Several dopaminergic agents, including bromocriptine and amantadine, have been reported to reverse parkinsonism in NMS [25, 26], reduce time to recovery, and halve mortality rates when used alone or in combination with other treatments [4]. In our case, rapid reversal of the hyperthermia and rigidity were observed within 5 days of starting treatment with dantrolene and bromocriptine. One clinical group reported that benzodiazepines and electric convulsive therapy are effective for treating NMS [4]. At present, it is difficult to compare specific treatments for NMS, because it is rare and unpredictable in its onset and progression, all of which prevent systematic investigations of treatment efficacy.

To our knowledge, only two NMS cases with HANC with the base of the tongue and the soft palate as the primary site have been reported previously [5, 6]. There are some possible explanations for the low incidence of NMS in HANC patients, in comparison with psychiatry and neurology patients. In addition to HANC surgeons not being familiar with NMS, NMS is difficult to diagnose because its symptoms are similar to those of cancer itself and sometimes to other postoperative complications like delirium. Moreover, the occurrence rate of delirium was reported to be 26.3% in patients with major HANC surgery [27]. Neuroleptic medications are widely used in clinical oncology to manage postoperative delirium. We recommend that HANC surgeons bear the possibility of NMS in mind.

In conclusion, although NMS is a rare complication in HANC patients, surgeons must be aware of the clinical features of NMS to detect its early signs and initiate prompt therapy. Furthermore, HANC surgeons should use antipsychotic drugs conservatively and with careful supervision to avoid NMS and its potential lethality.

References

[1] S. N. Caroff, "The neuroleptic malignant syndrome," *Journal of Clinical Psychiatry*, vol. 41, no. 3, pp. 79–83, 1980.

[2] P. Adnet, P. Lestavel, and R. Krivosic-Horber, "Neuroleptic malignant syndrome," *British Journal of Anaesthesia*, vol. 85, no. 1, pp. 129–135, 2000.

[3] S. Stübner, E. Rustenbeck, R. Grohmann et al., "Severe and uncommon involuntary movement disorders due to psychotropic drugs," *Pharmacopsychiatry*, vol. 37, supplement 1, pp. S54–S64, 2004.

[4] J. R. Strawn, P. E. Keck Jr., and S. N. Caroff, "Neuroleptic malignant syndrome," *The American Journal of Psychiatry*, vol. 164, no. 6, pp. 870–876, 2007.

[5] K. Tanaka, T. Akechi, M. Yamazaki, R. Hayashi, Y. Nishiwaki, and Y. Uchitomi, "Neuroleptic malignant syndrome during haloperidol treatment in a cancer patient: a case report," *Support Care Cancer*, vol. 6, no. 6, pp. 536–538, 1998.

[6] Y. Zohar, Y. P. Talmi, R. Sabo, Y. Finkelstein, and A. Korzets, "Neuroleptic malignant syndrome during perphenazine treatment in a patient with head and neck cancer: a case report," *Otolaryngology*, vol. 106, no. 2, pp. 206–208, 1992.

[7] A. P. Association, "Diagnostic and statistical manual of mental disorders: DSM-IV," in *Neuroleptic Malignant Syndrome*, The American Psychiatric Association, Washington, DC, USA, 4th edition, 1994.

[8] K. Nishijima, *Neuroleptic Malignant Syndrome and Related Disoders*, 1st edition, 2010.

[9] B. H. Guze and L. R. Baxter Jr., "Neuroleptic malignant syndrome," *The New England Journal of Medicine*, vol. 313, no. 3, pp. 163–166, 1985.

[10] S. N. Caroff and S. C. Mann, "Neuroleptic malignant syndrome," *Medical Clinics of North America*, vol. 77, no. 1, pp. 185–202, 1993.

[11] K. Otani, M. Horiuchi, T. Kondo, S. Kaneko, and Y. Fukushima, "Is the predisposition to neuroleptic malignant syndrome genetically transmitted?" *British Journal of Psychiatry*, vol. 158, pp. 850–853, 1991.

[12] K. Mihara, T. Kondo, A. Suzuki et al., "Relationship between functional dopamine D2 and D3 receptors gene polymorphisms and neuroleptic malignant syndrome," *The American Journal of Medical Genetics*, vol. 117, no. 1, pp. 57–60, 2003.

[13] R. D. Myers, "Neurochemistry of thermoregulation: two negatives make a positive," *Brain Research Bulletin*, vol. 50, no. 5-6, pp. 453–454, 1999.

[14] G. J. Chandran, J. R. Mikler, and D. L. Keegan, "Neuroleptic malignant syndrome: case report and discussion," *CMAJ*, vol. 169, no. 5, pp. 439–442, 2003.

[15] G. Tollefson, "A case of neuroleptic malignant syndrome: in vitro muscle comparison with malignant hyperthermia," *Journal of Clinical Psychopharmacology*, vol. 2, no. 4, pp. 266–270, 1982.

[16] J. L. Levenson, "Neuroleptic malignant syndrome," *The American Journal of Psychiatry*, vol. 142, no. 10, pp. 1137–1145, 1985.

[17] R. J. Gurrera, S. N. Caroff, A. Cohen et al., "An international consensus study of neuroleptic malignant syndrome diagnostic criteria using the Delphi method," *Journal of Clinical Psychiatry*, vol. 72, no. 9, pp. 1222–1228, 2011.

[18] A. Shalev and H. Munitz, "The neuroleptic malignant syndrome: agent and host interaction," *Acta Psychiatrica Scandinavica*, vol. 73, no. 4, pp. 337–347, 1986.

[19] D. Sierra-Biddle, A. Herran, S. Diez-Aja et al., "Neuroleptic malignant syndrome and olanzapine," *Journal of Clinical Psychopharmacology*, vol. 20, no. 6, pp. 704–705, 2000.

[20] V. R. Velamoor, R. M. G. Norman, S. N. Caroff, S. C. Mann, K. A. Sullivan, and R. E. Antelo, "Progression of symptoms in neuroleptic malignant syndrome," *Journal of Nervous and Mental Disease*, vol. 182, no. 3, pp. 168–173, 1994.

[21] H. G. Pope Jr., H. G. Aizley, P. E. Keck Jr., and S. L. McElroy, "Neuroleptic malignant syndrome: long-term follow-up of 20 cases," *Journal of Clinical Psychiatry*, vol. 52, no. 5, pp. 208–212, 1991.

[22] D. Berardi, M. Amore, P. E. Keck Jr., M. Troia, and M. Dell'Atti, "Clinical and pharmacologic risk factors for neuroleptic malignant syndrome: a case-control study," *Biological Psychiatry*, vol. 44, no. 8, pp. 748–754, 1998.

[23] W. S. Bond, "Detection and management of the neuroleptic malignant syndrome," *Clinical Pharmacy*, vol. 3, no. 3, pp. 302–307, 1984.

[24] J. M. Davis, S. N. Caroff, and S. C. Mann, "Treatment of neuroleptic malignant syndrome," *Psychiatric Annals*, vol. 30, no. 5, pp. 325–331, 2000.

[25] P. Sakkas, J. M. Davis, P. G. Janicak, and Z. Wang, "Drug treatment of the neuroleptic malignant syndrome," *Psychopharmacology Bulletin*, vol. 27, no. 3, pp. 381–384, 1991.

[26] M. R. Rosenberg and M. Green, "Neuroleptic malignant syndrome: review of response to therapy," *Archives of Internal Medicine*, vol. 149, no. 9, pp. 1927–1931, 1989.

[27] K. Yamagata, K. Onizawa, H. Yusa, T. Wakatsuki, T. Yanagawa, and H. Yoshida, "Risk factors for postoperative delirium in patients undergoing head and neck cancer surgery," *International Journal of Oral and Maxillofacial Surgery*, vol. 34, no. 1, pp. 33–36, 2005.

14

Endodontic Management of a Maxillary First Molar with Two Palatal Canals and a Single Buccal Canal

Leila Atash biz Yeganeh, Mamak Adel, Reza Vahedi, and Maryam Tofangchiha

Department of Endodontics, School of Dentistry, Qazvin University of Medical Sciences, Qazvin, Iran

Correspondence should be addressed to Leila Atash biz Yeganeh, yeganehdds@gmail.com

Academic Editors: R. S. Brown and M. W. Roberts

Thorough knowledge of root canal morphology is essential for the endodontic therapy. There are rare variations in canal number and configuration in maxillary molars, which could affect treatment outcome. This paper presents the endodontic management of a maxillary first molar with two palatal canals in one root (Vertucci type IV) and a single buccal canal. In this paper cone-beam computed tomography was made to asses this morphology. This paper is intended to reinforce clinician's awareness of the rare morphology of root canals.

1. Introduction

A thorough knowledge of root canal morphology is an important aspect of root canal treatment. Failures to detect aberrant root canals and to identify extra roots are one of the main causes for failure in the endodontic therapy [1]. Human molars demonstrate relatively high anatomic variations and abnormalities with respect to number of roots and root canals. The literature delineates wide variations in root canal morphology of maxillary first molars. Cleghorn et al. (2006) conducted a comprehensive review of the root and root canal morphology of the human permanent maxillary first molar [2]. Limited number of cases with 2 palatal roots/canals (Table 1) and cases with fused buccal roots have been reported [2, 3]. The frequency of a maxillary first molar with two roots or two palatal canals is very low, 3.9 and 1% respectively [2]. A brief review of recent case reports of extra palatalcanals in maxillary first molars is presented in Table 1.

Baratto-Filho et al. (2009) assessed internal morphology of maxillary first molars by 3 different methods [4]. They found that second palatal canal prevalence in *ex vivo* assessment, 2.05%, in clinical assessment, 0.65%, and by cone-beam computed tomography, 4.55%.

Some of the previous case reports were based on the radiographic examinations of the teeth. Since the radiographic image is a shadow and it is a 2-dimensional image, the best applicative method for precise clarification of the root canal morphology of a tooth is cone-beam computed tomography (CBCT) [5], however it may not to be practical in all clinical situations. This technique offers significant advances in anatomical reconstruction of teeth before and after instrumentation and obturation.

This case report describes nonsurgical therapy of an unusual permanent maxillary first molar with 3 canals: 2 separate palatal canals and one buccal canal, a morphology that has not been reported in published articles that we found in our search. The root canal anatomy was confirmed with the help of spiral CT.

2. Case Report

A 36-year-old male patient referred to the Department of Endodontics of Qazvin University of Dentistry, Iran for implementation of root canal treatment of right maxillary first molar (tooth no. 3), due to carious exposure of the pulp, with a chief complaint of "cavity in the maxillary right first molar but without any history of pain." His medical history was not contributory. Clinically the tooth had a deep carious lesion on the mesiocclusal surface. The tooth was not tender to percussion. There was no mobility and periodontal probing was within normal limits. Pulp vitality testing

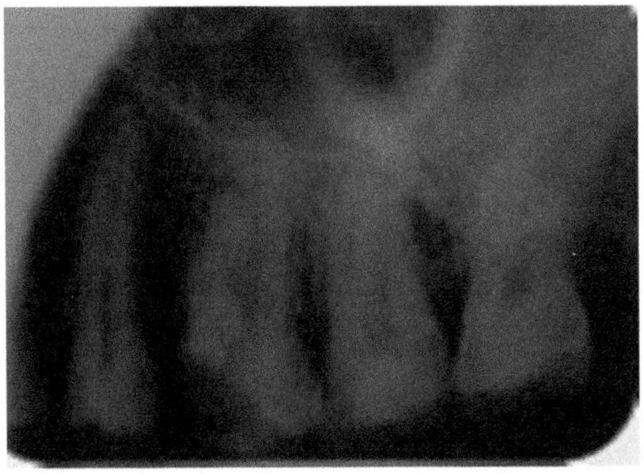

Figure 1: Preoperative radiograph.

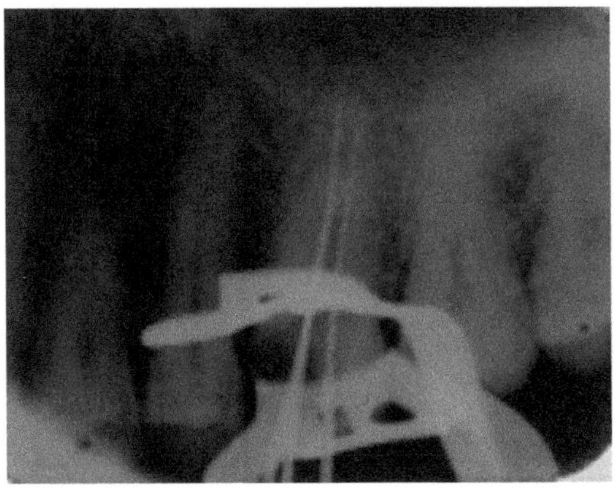

Figure 2: Length-determination radiograph.

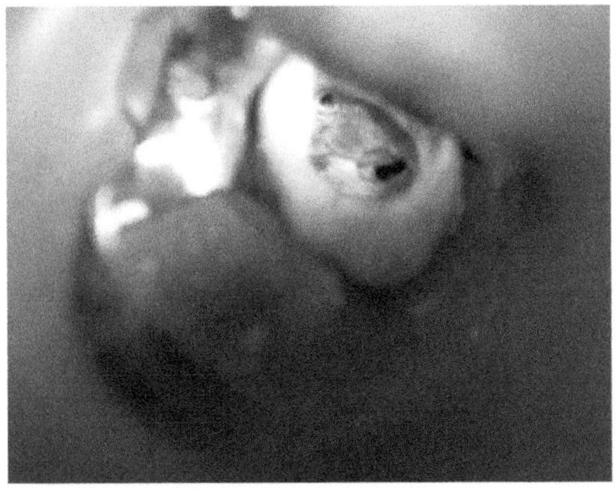

Figure 3: Pulp chamber floor after root canal preparation.

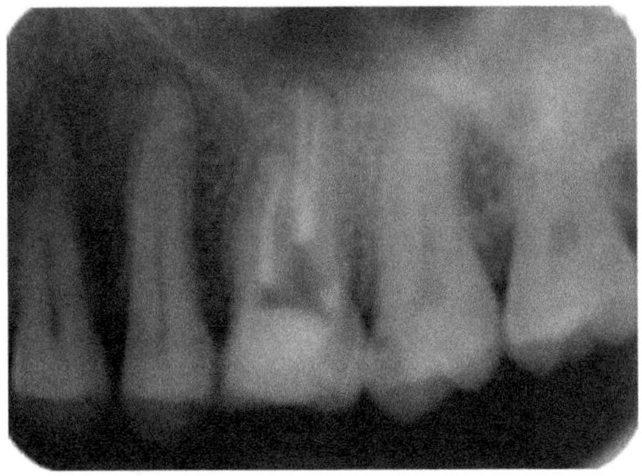

Figure 4: Postoperative radiograph.

Table 1: Review of case reports of two palatal canals in one palatal root in maxillary first molar.

Investigators	Study type	Key information
Johal 2001 [6]	Clinical RCT	2MB, 1DB, 2P
Holderrieth and Gernhardt 2009 [7]	Clinical RCT	2 cases: 2MB, 1DB, 2P
Aggarwal et al. 2009 [8]	Spiral CT	1MB, 1DB, 2P
Deepalakshmi et al. 2009 [1]	Spiral CT	2MB, 1DB, 2P

MB: mesiobuccal, DB: distobuccal, P: palatal.

of the involved teeth with cold (DENRONIC, Aeronova GmbH & Co. KG, Germany) and electric pulp stimulation (Parkel Electronics Division, Farmingdale, NY, USA) were negative, indicative of pulp necrosis. The initial periapical radiograph revealed widening of the apical periodontium and was indicative of an unusual complex root canal anatomy (Figure 1). These findings led to a provisional diagnosis of pulp necrosis with chronic apical periodontitis of the right maxillary first molar, necessitating endodontic therapy.

The patient received local anesthesia of 2% lidocaine with 1 : 80000 epinephrine (Persocaine-E, Darou Pakhsh, Iran). After removing caries of the tooth, a conventional endodontic access opening was made. Rubber dam was placed. Clinical examination with a DG-16 endodontic explorer (Hu-Friedy, Chicago, IL, USA) revealed 3 distinct orifices: two palatals with one large buccal orifice. The conventional triangular access was modified to a trapezoidal shape to improve access to the palatal canals and extended to explore the likely second buccal canal. Surprisingly, clinical and radiographic evaluations confirmed the presence of only one buccal root canal.

After scouting the canals with no.10 and no.15 K-files (Mani INC, Tochigi, Japan), coronal flaring with Protaper Universal Shaping file Sx and S1 (Dentsply, Maillefer, Switzerland) was done. Working lengths were estimated by means of an apex locator (Root ZX, J. Morita Mfg Corp, Kyoto, Japan) and confirmed with a perapical radiograph (Figure 2). The canals were initially instrumented to a size no.15 K-file (Mani INC, Tochigi, Japan), under copious irrigation with 2.5% sodium hypochlorite. Biomechanical preparation was performed using the crown-down technique with Protaper Universal Rotary NiTi files (Dentsply, Maillefer, Switzerland). Figure 3 shows the photograph of the chamber floor after instrumentation. Final irrigation was done with 20 mililiter 2.5% sodium hypochlorite followed by 20 milliliter normal saline irrigation. The canals were dried with paper points and obturated using cold lateral compaction of gutta-percha (GAPADENT Co. LTD, China) and AH 26 sealer (Dentsply Tulsa). The access was

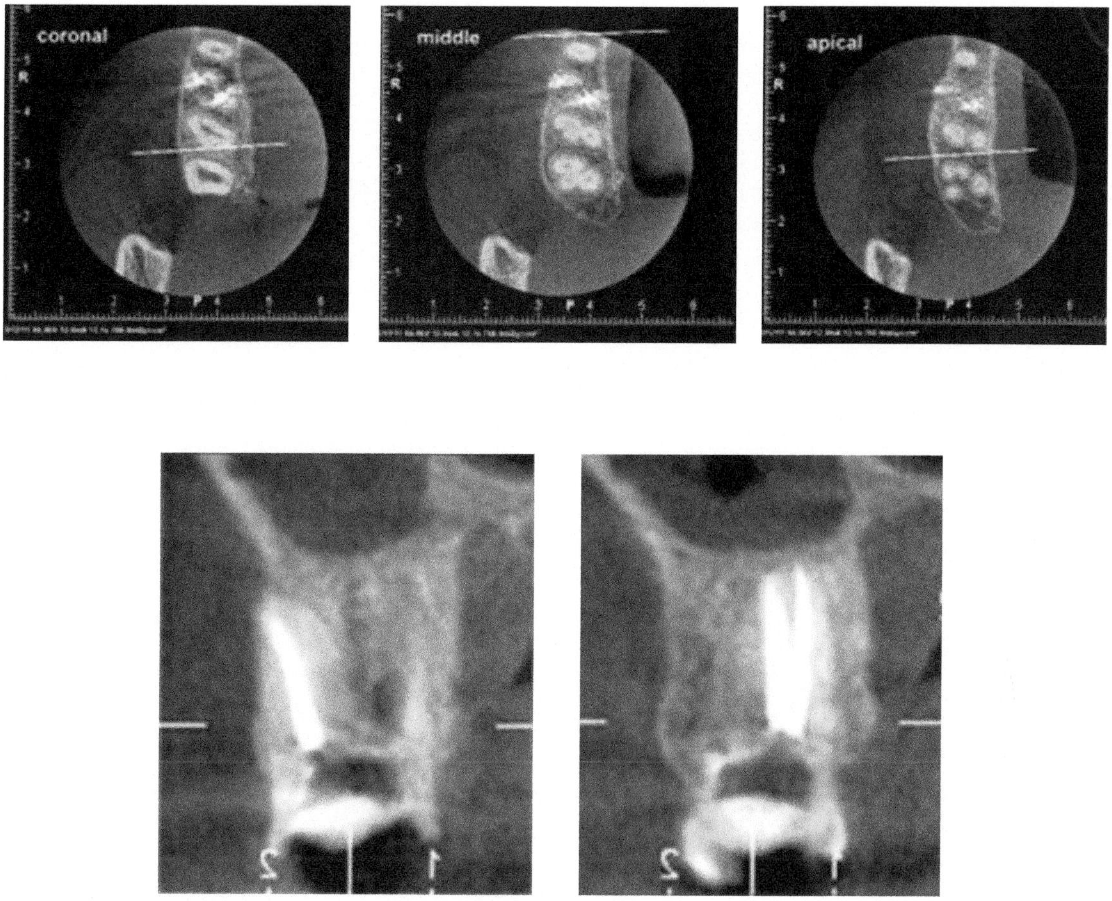

Figure 5: CBCT evaluation.

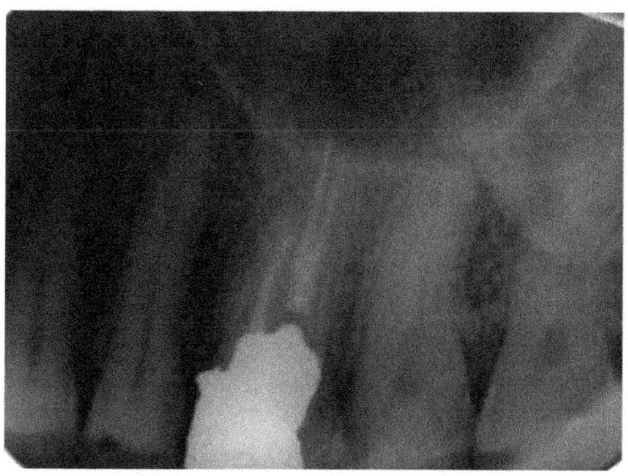

Figure 6: 12 months follow up.

temporarily restored with Cavit (ESPE, Seefeld, Japan). A final radiograph (Figure 4) was taken and the patient was referred to take a cone-beam computed tomography (CBCT) scan for approving this rare and unusual root canal anatomy of the tooth and other possible anomalies.

CBCT revealed the presence of 2 roots including one palatal root with 2 canals; each with a distinct root canal having separate orifices and separate exits and a large buccal root canal (Figure 5). The CBCT data confirmed our clinical and radiographic understanding of canal configuration.

Patient was recalled 12 months later. The tooth was clinically and radiographically asymptomatic (Figure 6).

3. Discussion

The present paper describes the nonsurgical endodontic management of an unusual maxillary first molar with two roots. This case is considerable because of having two palatal canals in a palatal root and one buccal canal in a buccal root. Cleghorn et al. (2006) conducted a comprehensive review of the root and root canal morphology of the maxillary first molar [2]. A thorough literature search in PubMed site was done by the author revealed that the present case is apparently the first reported case of endodontic management of a maxillary first molar with two roots (two palatal canals in one root and a single buccal root canal) that was reported.

The 2-rooted type of the maxillary first molar is rarely reported. Its incidence in the literature is 3.9% [2]. The fusion of the two buccal roots has the prevalence of 0.4% in maxillary first molars [9]. Fava (2001) reported a case of maxillary first molar with two roots; two canals in the buccal root (Vertucci type IV) and one palatal root canal [9].

Nevertheless, presence of only one buccal root with one canal is extremely rare [3, 9]. Gopikrishna et al. (2008) presented the endodontic management of a maxillary first molar with a single-fused buccal root with two canals and 2 palatal roots [3]. After confirmation of this unusual morphology by spiral computerized tomography, incidentally they mentioned that the other maxillary first molar in their reported patient had also a similar morphology, but it had only one buccal canal in its single buccal root.

Incidence of two palatal canals in maxillary first molars is also low (1%). There are some case-reports have been described two palatal canals in one palatal root in maxillary first molars as presented 4 in Table 1. Holderrieth and Gernhardt [7] and Aggarwal et al. [8] reported cases having two palatal canals in a single palatal root representing Vertucci type IV was wrong canal configuration as seen in the presented case.

Radiographs produce only a 2-dimensional image, resulting in superimposition and distortion. Since, it cannot be useful in cases with complex root canal anatomy, it is crucial to use all of the armamentaria to diagnose and treat the entire root canal system [10]. According to previous studies [1, 2, 4, 8] where computerized tomography (CT) was used for definitive diagnosis of morphologic abnormalities in the root canal anatomy, CBCT of the involved tooth was conducted in the present case.

4. Conclusion

The present case was the endodontic management of a maxillary first molar with two palatal canals in one root and one buccal root canal. Although the incidence of a second palatal canal and even a single buccal root canal is not high, it is important to take these abnormalities into consideration during root canal therapy of maxillary molars in order to prevent accidents and ensure successful long-term outcome. We also accentuate the role of CBCT as an objective analytical tool to ascertain root canal morphology in unusual cases.

References

[1] M. Deepalakshmi, R. Miglani, R. Indira, and S. Ramachandran, "Spiral CT diagnosis and endodontic management of an anatomically variant palatal root with two canals in a maxillary first molar," *Indian Journal of Dental Research*, vol. 21, no. 3, pp. 443–445, 2010.

[2] B. M. Cleghorn, W. H. Christie, and C. C. S. Dong, "Root and root canal morphology of the human permanent maxillary first molar: a literature review," *Journal of Endodontics*, vol. 32, no. 9, pp. 813–821, 2006.

[3] V. Gopikrishna, J. Reuben, and D. Kandaswamy, "Endodontic management of a maxillary first molar with two palatal roots and a single fused buccal root diagnosed with spiral computed tomography—a case report," *Oral Surgery, Oral Medicine, Oral Pathology, Oral Radiology and Endodontology*, vol. 105, no. 4, pp. e74–e78, 2008.

[4] F. Baratto Filho, S. Zaitter, G. A. Haragushiku, E. A. de Campos, A. Abuabara, and G. M. Correr, "Analysis of the internal anatomy of maxillary first molars by using different methods," *Journal of Endodontics*, vol. 35, no. 3, pp. 337–342, 2009.

[5] J. Michetti, D. Maret, J. P. Mallet, and F. Diemer, "Validation of cone beam computed tomography as a tool to explore root canal anatomy," *Journal of Endodontics*, vol. 36, no. 7, pp. 1187–1190, 2010.

[6] S. Johal, "Unusual maxillary first molar with 2 palatal canals within a single root: a case report," *Journal of the Canadian Dental Association*, vol. 67, no. 4, pp. 211–214, 2001.

[7] S. Holderrieth and C. R. Gernhardt, "Maxillary molars with morphologic variations of the palatal root canals: a report of four cases," *Journal of Endodontics*, vol. 35, no. 7, pp. 1060–1065, 2009.

[8] V. Aggarwal, M. Singla, A. Logani, and N. Shah, "Endodontic management of a maxillary first molar with two palatal canals with the aid of spiral computed tomography: a case report," *Journal of Endodontics*, vol. 35, no. 1, pp. 137–139, 2009.

[9] L. R. G. Fava, "Root canal treatment in an unusual maxillary first molar: a case report," *International Endodontic Journal*, vol. 34, no. 8, pp. 649–653, 2001.

[10] F. J. Vertucci, "Root canal morphology and its relationship to endodontic procedures," *Endodontic Topics*, vol. 10, no. 1, pp. 3–29, 2005.

15

An Unusual Case Report of Erupted Odontoma

Dhaval Mehta, Nilesh Raval, Sneha Udhani, Viral Parekh, and Chintan Modi

Department of Oral Medicine and Radiology, Karnavati School of Dentistry, 907/A Uvarsad, Gandhinagar, Gujarat 382422, India

Correspondence should be addressed to Dhaval Mehta; drdhaval80@gmail.com

Academic Editors: K. Seymour and P. I. Varela-Centelles

Odontomas are the most common of the odontogenic tumors of the jaws, which are benign, slow growing, and nonaggressive. They are usually asymptomatic and found in routine dental radiographic examination. Odontomas are usually associated with tooth eruption disturbances. Eruption of odontoma in oral cavity is rare entity. Here we report a case of an unusual erupted compound odontoma.

1. Introduction

Odontomas are hamartomas composed of various dental tissues, that is, enamel, dentin, cementum, and sometimes pulp. They are slow-growing, benign tumours. Paul Broca was the first to coin the term "odontoma" in 1867. The World Health Organisation (WHO) defines odontomas as two types: complex odontomas, a malformation in which all dental tissues are present, but arranged in a more or less disorderly pattern; and compound odontomas, a malformation in which all of the dental tissues are represented in a pattern that is more orderly than that of the complex type [1]. The erupted odontomas are the ones which are present coronal to an erupting or impacted tooth or superficially in bone and may have enabled its eruption into the oral cavity [2]. Odontomas erupting into the oral cavity are extremely uncommon, with the first case being reported in English literature in 1980 by Rumel et al. A literature review by Litonjua et al. in 2003 recorded only 14 cases in English literature from 1980 to 2003 [2, 3]. To date, 20 cases of erupted odontomas are reported in the literature; out of these 11 cases are complex odontoma and 9 erupted odontomas are associated with impacted teeth [4].

Here we present a rare case of erupted odontome in maxillary anterior region.

2. Case Report

A 15-year old female patient came with complain of presence of a small hard mass in upper front tooth region and its undesirable appearance was a concern. She had no complaint of pain or any other previous infection.

Patient was fit and well medically. Intraoral examination revealed a small whitish oval tooth like structure present in maxillary anterior region. It is placed superiorly and labially in attached gingival in relation to crown of right maxillary central incisor region (Figure 1). It was hard, nontender, and grade II mobile. Neither expansion of any cortical plates (Figure 2) nor any pus discharge present.

Intraoral periapical radiograph revealed a well-defined radiopaque mass similar to density of dental tissues. It was placed apical to crown of right maxillary central incisor and in interdental bone between maxillary right central and lateral incisors suggesting erupted compound odontoma. Removal of odontoma was done and sent for histopathological report.

Histopathological examination confirmed the specimen to be compound odontoma consisting of organized mass of enamel, dentine, and pulp tissue resembling the structure of tooth (Figure 3).

3. Discussion

Odontoma is the most common odontogenic tumor in maxilla. Compound odontoma most commonly found in the upper incisors and canines areas, followed by the antero- and posteroinferior regions. Complex odontomas are commonly found in the areas of the second and third lower molars. An increased prevalence of these tumors is observed in children and adolescents. These lesions are normally diagnosed by

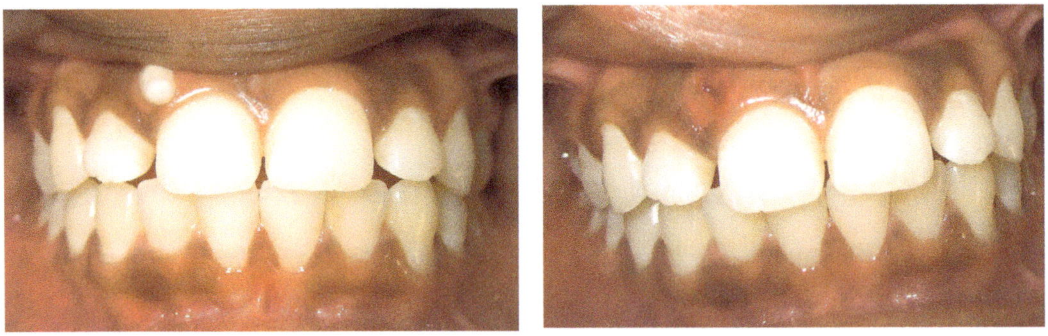

Preoperative (a)

postoperative (b)

FIGURE 1: Compound odontoma in right upper maxillary central incisor region (preoperative and postoperative).

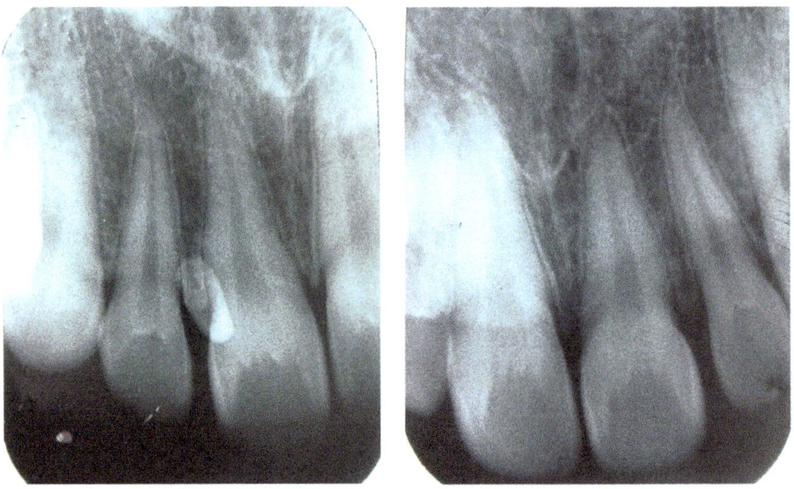

Preoperative (a)

postoperative (b)

FIGURE 2: IOPA showing tooth-like radiopaque structure in right upper maxillary central incisor region suggestive of erupted compound odontoma (preoperative and postoperative).

routine radiological features in the second and third decades of life [5].

Hitchin suggested that odontomas are inherited through a mutant gene or interference, possibly postnatal, with genetic control of tooth development. In humans, there is a tendency for the lamina between the tooth germs to disintegrate into clumps of cells. The persistence of a portion of lamina may be an important factor in the etiology of complex or compound odontomas and either of these may occur instead of a tooth [6].

Odontomas have been associated with trauma during primary dentition, as well as with inflammatory and infectious processes, hereditary anomalies (Gardner syndrome and Hermann syndrome), and odontoblastic hyperactivity, and alterations in the genetic components are responsible for controlling dental development [2].

Usually odontomas are asymptomatic. Clinical indicators of odontoma may include retention of deciduous teeth, noneruption of permanent teeth, pain, expansion of cortical bone, and tooth displacement. Pain and swelling are the most common symptoms when odontomas erupt, followed by malocclusion. Some odontomas appear at very young age and others at old age [3].

Although the odontomas erupting in the oral cavity are controversial, the reason is attributed to the eruptive forces of the apparently impacted teeth, and in cases of absence of teeth, the reasons could possibly be the resorption of alveolar ridge exposing the odontoma, sequestration of overlying bone, alveolar bone remodeling in young adults, or reactive growth of the capsule surrounding odontoma in elderly patients [2, 3].

The mechanism of odontoma eruption appears to be different from tooth eruption because of the lack of periodontal ligament and root in odontoma. Therefore the force required to move the odontoma is not linked to the contractility of the fibroblasts, as in the case for teeth. Although there

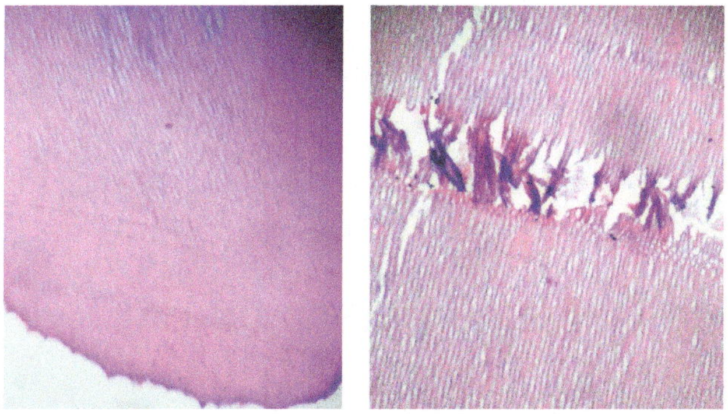

Histopathologic photo

FIGURE 3: Decalcified section showing organized mass of enamel, dentine, and pulp tissue.

is no root formation in odontoma, its increasing size may lead to the sequestration of the overlying bone and, hence, occlusal movement or eruption. An increase in the size of the odontoma over time produces a force sufficient to cause bone resorption [4].

The odontoma presents as a well-defined radiopacity situated in bone, but with a density that is greater than bone and equal to or greater than that of a tooth. It contains foci of variable density. A radiolucent halo, typically surrounded by a thin sclerotic line, surrounds the radiopacity. The radiolucent zone is the connective tissue capsule of a normal tooth follicle. The thin sclerotic line resembles the corticated border seen in a normal tooth crypt. The developmental stages can be identified based on radiologic features and the degree of calcification of the lesion at the time of diagnosis [7]. The first stage is characterized by radiolucency due to the absence of dental tissue calcification, the second or intermediate stage shows partial calcification, and the third or classically radiopaque stage exhibits predominant tissue calcification with the surrounding radiolucent halo described above [8].

Removal of the lesion and enveloping soft tissue with curettage to prevent cystic degeneration is treatment of choice. In case of impacted tooth with compound odontoma, surgical removal of odontoma with orthodontic eruption of impacted tooth is indicated.

4. Conclusion

A rare case of erupted compound odontoma that was about to be exfoliated has been reported. Odontomas rarely erupt into the mouth and tend to be associated with impacted teeth. Despite their benign nature, however, their eruption into the oral cavity can give rise to pain, inflammation, and infection and different clinical appearance.

Conflict of Interests

The authors declare that they have no conflict of interests.

References

[1] H. P. Philipsen, P. A. Reichart, and F. Prætorius, "Mixed odontogenic tumours and odontomas. Considerations on interrelationship. Review of the literature and presentation of 134 new cases of odontomas," *European Journal of Cancer Part B*, vol. 33, no. 2, pp. 86–99, 1997.

[2] C. C. Ragalli, J. L. Ferreria, and F. Blasco, "Large erupting complex odontoma," *International Journal of Oral and Maxillofacial Surgery*, vol. 29, no. 5, pp. 373–374, 2000.

[3] M. Vengal, H. Arora, S. Ghosh, and K. M. Pai, "Large erupting complex odontoma: a case report," *Journal of the Canadian Dental Association*, vol. 73, no. 2, pp. 169–172, 2007.

[4] G. Serra-Serra, L. Berini-Aytés, and C. Gay-Escoda, "Erupted odontomas: a report of three cases and review of the literature," *Medicina Oral, Patologia Oral y Cirugia Bucal*, vol. 14, no. 6, pp. E299–E303, 2009.

[5] S. D. Budnick, "Compound and complex odontomas," *Oral Surgery Oral Medicine and Oral Pathology*, vol. 42, no. 4, pp. 501–506, 1976.

[6] A. D. Hitchin, "The aetiology of the calcified composite odontomes," *British Dental Journal*, vol. 130, no. 11, pp. 475–482, 1971.

[7] L. Junquera, J. C. De Vicente, P. Roig, S. Olay, and O. Rodríguez-Recio, "Intraosseus odontoma erupted into the oral cavity: an unusual pathology," *Medicina Oral, Patologia Oral y Cirugia Bucal*, vol. 10, no. 3, pp. 248–251, 2005.

[8] J. L. Guinta and M. A. Kaplan, "Peripheral soft tissue odontomas," *Oral Surgery, Oral Medicine, Oral Pathology*, vol. 69, no. 3, pp. 406–411, 1990.

16

Multiple Pulp Stones in Primary and Developing Permanent Dentition: A Report of 4 Cases

Mohita Marwaha, Radhika Chopra, Payal Chaudhuri, Atul Gupta, and Jayna Sachdev

Department of Pedodontics & Preventive Dentistry, SGT Dental College, Hospital & Research Institute, Budhera 123505, India

Correspondence should be addressed to Mohita Marwaha, dr.mohitamalhotra@gmail.com

Academic Editors: Y.-K. Chen and M. Machado

Pulp stones are foci of calcification or discrete calcifications in the dental pulp. They are frequently found on bitewing and periapical radiographs, but their occurrence in entire dentition is unusual. We are reporting four cases in which the occurrence of pulp stones ranged from their presence in just primary teeth (Cases 1 and 2) to involvement of young permanent teeth also (Case 3) and even unerupted permanent teeth (Case 4). In all the cases, dental, medical, and family histories as well as the findings from the clinical examination of the patient were not contributory. Histopathological report revealed true denticle. Metabolic evaluation of patients through liver function test, kidney function test, and blood investigation did not show any metabolic disorders. Patients were also evaluated for any systemic, syndromic, or genetic involvement, but this was also noncontributing. Therefore, it is suggested that these unusual cases may be of idiopathic origin.

1. Introduction

Pulp calcifications occurring throughout dentition are uncommon and are usually associated with systemic or genetic diseases such as dentine dysplasia, and dentinogenesis imperfecta [1]. Free pulp stones are found coronally within the pulp tissue and are most commonly seen on radiographs [2]. Pulp stones extending to the entire primary dentition are also infrequent. The purpose of this paper is to present four cases: first with pulp stones in all primary molars with taurodontism, second with pulp calcifications in all primary molars, third with pulp stones in all the primary molars, mandibular permanent central incisors, and first molars, and fourth, with pulp stones in all primary molars, permanent first molars and also in developing unerupted permanent mandibular second molars, permanent mandibular canines, and first premolars. The present case report depicts presence of pulp stones, without any metabolic disturbances and syndrome, which may be suggestive of its idiopathic origin.

Case 1. A 6-year-old girl reported to the clinic with the chief complaint of decayed left posterior teeth since the last three months. Her family/medical history was noncontributory. Intraoral examination revealed several decayed teeth including all the primary molars. So, an OPG was advised which showed taurodontism and pulp stones in all primary molars (Figure 1). Pulpectomy was performed in primary maxillary and mandibular left second molars, and the pulp stones removed from the chamber (Figure 2) were sent for histopathological examination and were found to be true denticle. Primary mandibular right second molar was extracted followed by band and loop space maintainer. The rest of the decayed teeth were restored with glass ionomers cement.

Case 2. A 12-year-old male patient reported to clinic with chief complaint of malaligned teeth in lower front region. Intraoral examination revealed retained primary mandibular incisors. The Panoramic radiograph revealed pulp stones in all primary molars (Figure 3). So, planned treatment was extraction of retained primary mandibular incisors followed by fixed orthodontic therapy. As there was no carious involvement of primary molars, they were left untreated.

Case 3. A 10-year-old male patient reported with the chief complaint of decayed right posterior teeth for 2 months. The family and medical history was noncontributory. Intraoral

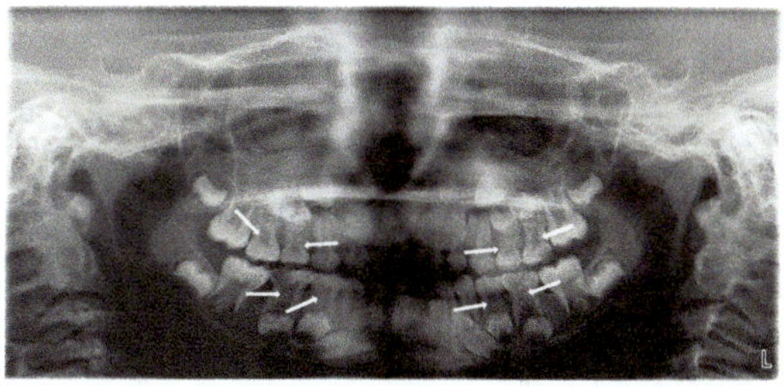

Figure 1: OPG revealing pulp stones and taurodontism in all primary molars (Case 1).

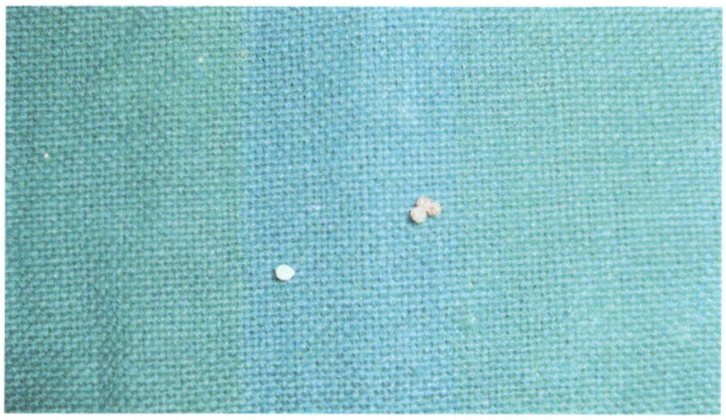

Figure 2: Pulp Stones.

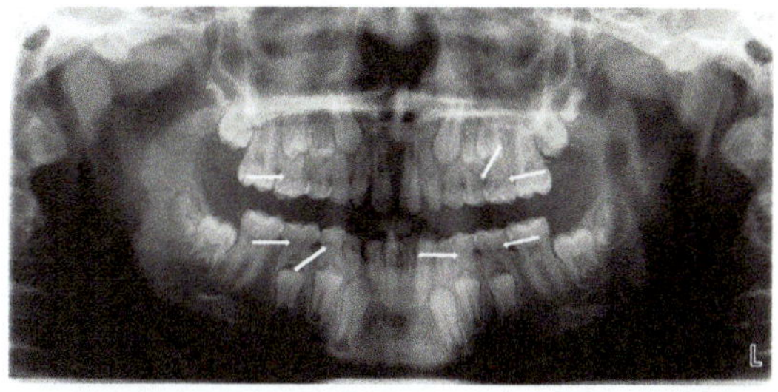

Figure 3: OPG revealing pulp stones in all primary molars (Case 2).

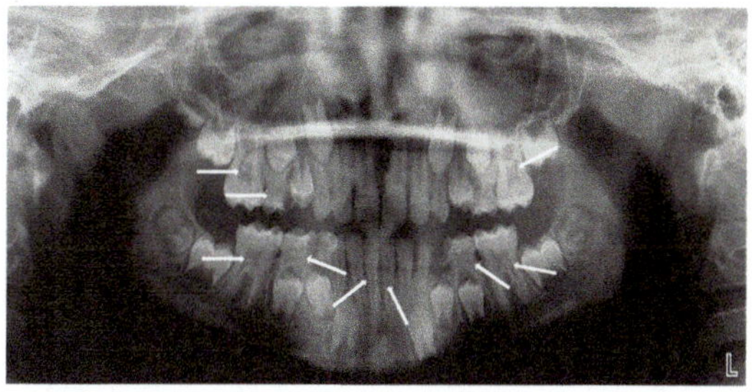

Figure 4: OPG revealing pulp stones in all second deciduous molars, first permanent molars, and mandibular central incisors.

examination revealed deep carious lesions in many teeth. The Panoramic radiograph revealed pulp stones in all second primary molars, permanent first molars, and mandibular central incisors (Figure 4). So, planned treatment was glass ionomer restorations in all decayed teeth; indirect pulp capping was performed in primary maxillary right second molar and extraction of primary mandibular right and left first molars; the remaining asymptomatic teeth were left untreated.

Case 4. An 11-year-old male patient reported with the chief complaint of decayed left posterior teeth for 1 month. Intraoral examination revealed carious lesions in many teeth. The Panoramic radiograph revealed pulp stones in all primary molars and permanent first molars. Also calcifications were observed in developing unerupted permanent mandibular second molars, permanent mandibular canines, and first premolars (Figure 5). So, planned treatment was restorations in all decayed teeth and extraction of primary mandibular right first molar followed by lingual arch.

2. Discussion

Pulp stones are foci of calcification or discrete calcifications in the dental pulp. They may exist freely within the pulpal tissue or embedded/attached to dentine [3]. Stones may occur as a single mass or as several small radio-opacities within pulp chambers or may exist into root canals [4]. A single tooth may have from 1 to 12 stones or even more, with sizes varying from minute particles to large masses [3]. They occur in all tooth types but occur most commonly in molars [2].

Pulp stones can be structurally classified based on location [5]. Structurally, they can be true and false pulp stones. True stones are made up of dentine and lined by odontoblasts, whereas false pulp stones are formed from degenerating cells of the pulp that are mineralized. A third type, "diffuse" or "amorphous" pulp stones, is more irregular in shape [6]. Based on the location, they can be embedded, adherent, and free [5]. Embedded stones are found most frequently in the apical portion of the root, and they are more attached to dentine as compared to adherent stones. Adherent stones are attached to the wall of pulp space, but they are not fully enclosed by dentine. Both adherent and embedded pulp stones can interfere with root canal treatment if they cause occlusion of the canals.

Free pulp stones are found coronally within the pulp tissue and are the most commonly seen on radiographs. They are very common and vary in size from 50 um in diameter to several millimetres where they may occlude the entire pulp chamber [7]. Pulp stones vary in size, ranging from microscopic particles to larger masses that almost obliterate the pulp chamber with only the large masses being radiographically apparent. In all our cases, radiograph examination revealed large pulp stones located in the pulp chamber.

Sayegh and Reed [7] reported that the incidence of calcification in carious teeth from children and young adults (10–34 years old) was nearly 5 times greater than that in noncarious teeth. This supports the theory that pulp calcification is, under normal condition, a physiological process. Under pathological conditions (like caries), the process may speed up. The influence of caries on pulp stone formation may actually be related to properties of dentine such as the number and dimensions of tubules, and

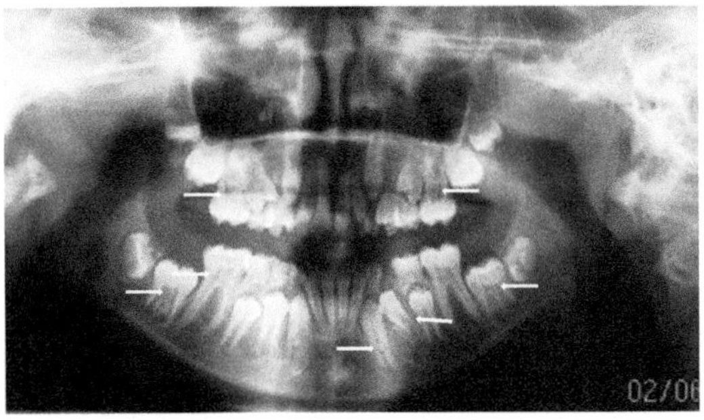

Figure 5: OPG revealing pulp stones in all primary molars and almost in all permanent teeth.

the progression rate, and activity of the disease. These would influence the rate of bacterial toxin penetration. In our cases, although many of the teeth were carious, noncarious teeth and even unerupted teeth had pulp stones suggesting idiopathic aetiology rather than pathological one.

Kumar et al. [8] conducted a study in 120 primary maxillary and mandibular extracted teeth, evaluated them radiographically, and concluded 25% of second molars presented evidence of pulp calcifications and approximately 3% of central incisors were calcified. The low occurrence of pulp calcifications in primary teeth supported the view that the occurrence of pulp calcification increases with age. However, Arys et al. [4] found that age did not have any influence on the occurrence of pulp calcifications. Their study consisted of 42 primary molars with less than one-third of their root resorbed. Forty-two healthy children of both sexes were selected, aged between 5 and 13 yrs. The teeth were examined by microradiography and light microscopy, and results revealed that pulp stones were present in 78% of the molars, with 95% of the material showing some form of pulp calcification. There was lower incidence of pulp stones in treated and carious molars.

Pulp calcification also occurs as sequelae to trauma to the primary dentition [9]. In cases with repeated traumatic injuries, the chances of pulp calcification are doubled compared to single trauma. It is a common finding associated with the healing process following traumatic injuries. Prevalence of pulp calcification in injured primary teeth that were diagnosed by radiographs varied from 6.1% to 35.9%.

Yaacob and Hamid [10] reported that free or attached pulp stones were the most common type of calcification. They selected 120 teeth of children aged between 3 and 11 yrs, examined them histologically, and reported 6.7% of prevalence of pulp stones.

In Cases 1 and 2, pulp stones were noticed along with taurodontism in primary molars. The term taurodontism was first introduced by Sir Arthur Keith in 1913 [11]. The taurodontic teeth are identified by elongated pulp chambers and apical displacement of bifurcation or trifurcation of the roots. Etiology of taurodontism is diverse commonly attributed to the failure of invagination of the epithelial root sheath sufficiently early to form the cynodont. Autosomal transmission of the trait has also been observed. Taurodontism can occur alone limited to one or more teeth or it can be associated with various syndromes like Down's syndrome, Klinefelter's syndrome, and so forth [12, 13]. Taurodontism may be unilateral or bilateral and affects permanent teeth more frequently than primary teeth. Taurodontism may be classified as mild, moderate, and severe (hypo, meso, and hyper, resp.) based on the degree of apical displacement of the pulpal floor [14, 15].

So far, only 2 cases have been reported by Kosinski et al. [14] of pulp stones associated with taurodontism. They demonstrated short, conical, and misshapen roots with pulp stones in the pulp chamber of taurodontic teeth. Mandibular molars are found to be affected more than maxillary molars [16]. The similar findings were recorded in Case 1. As a taurodont shows wide variation in size and shape of pulp chamber with varying degrees of obliteration and canal configuration, root canal therapy becomes a challenge. In Case 4, calcifications were also observed in unerupted developing permanent teeth and till date to the best of our knowledge no case has been reported of the same findings.

In our present cases, the pulp stones were found in young patients, which is contrary to the general concept of pulp stone formation usually seen in older age group or in association with certain syndrome. In our cases, no correlation could be established between pulp stones and any genetic, systemic, or metabolic findings. However, the same findings were reported by Siskos and Georgopoulou [17], Bahetwar and Pandey [18], and Donta et al. [19]. Thus, it may be suggested that these stones were of idiopathic origin. Further studies are required to evaluate the exact mechanism and aetiology of pulp calcification which would be able to clarify the fact that generalized pulp calcification is not merely an age-changed phenomenon attributed for this condition.

References

[1] S. Parekh, A. Kyriazidou, A. Bloch-Zupan, and G. Roberts, "Multiple pulp stones and shortened roots of unknown etiology," *Oral Surgery, Oral Medicine, Oral Pathology, Oral Radiology and Endodontology*, vol. 101, no. 6, pp. e139–e142, 2006.

[2] S. C. White and M. J. Pharoah, *Oral Radiology Principles & Interpretation*, Mosby, St. Louis, Mo, USA, 4th edition, 2000.

[3] G. Bevelander and P. L. Johnson, "Histogenesis and histochemistry of pulpal calcification," *Journal of Dental Research*, vol. 35, no. 5, pp. 714–722, 1956.

[4] A. Arys, C. Philippart, and N. Dourov, "Microradiography and light microscopy of mineralization in the pulp of undemineralized human primary molars," *Journal of Oral Pathology and Medicine*, vol. 22, no. 2, pp. 49–53, 1993.

[5] S. Seltzer and I. B. Bender, *The Dental Pulp*, J.B.Lippincott, Philadelphia, Pa, USA, 3rd edition, 1984.

[6] I. A. Mjor and J. J. Pindborg, *Histology of the Human Tooth*, Munksgaard, Copenhagen, 1st edition, 1973.

[7] F. S. Sayegh and A. J. Reed, "Calcification in the dental pulp," *Oral Surgery, Oral Medicine, Oral Pathology*, vol. 25, no. 6, pp. 873–882, 1968.

[8] S. Kumar, S. Chandra, and J. N. Jaiswal, "Pulp calcifications in primary teeth," *Journal of Endodontics*, vol. 16, no. 5, pp. 218–220, 1990.

[9] A. C. Mello-Moura, G. A. Bonini, C. G. Zardetto, C. R. Rodrigues, and M. T. Wanderley, "Pulp calcification in traumatized primary teeth: prevalence & associated factors," *Journal of Clinical Pediatric Dentistry*, vol. 35, no. 4, pp. 383–387, 2011.

[10] H. B. Yaacob and J. A. Hamid, "Pulpal calcifications in primary teeth: a light microscope study," *The Journal of Pedodontics*, vol. 10, no. 3, pp. 254–264, 1986.

[11] A. Keith, "Problems relating to the teeth of the earlier form of prehistoric man," in *Proceedings of the Royal Society of Medicine*, vol. 6, pp. 103–124, 1913.

[12] A. Genc, F. Namdar, K. Goker, and M. Atasu, "Taurodontism in association with supernumerary teeth," *Journal of Clinical Pediatric Dentistry*, vol. 23, no. 2, pp. 151–154, 1999.

[13] R. Gedik and M. Çimen, "Multiple taurodontism: report of case," *Journal of Dentistry for Children*, vol. 67, no. 3, pp. 216–217, 2000.

[14] R. W. Kosinski, Y. Chaiyawat, and L. Rosenberg, "Localized deficient root development associated with taurodontism: case report," *Pediatric Dentistry*, vol. 21, no. 3, pp. 213–215, 1999.

[15] P. W. Goz and S. C. White, *Oral Radiology (Principle and Interpretation)*, Mosby, St.Louis, Mo, USA, 3rd edition, 1994.

[16] D. S. MacDonald-Jankowski and T. T. L. Li, "Taurodontism in a young adult Chinese population," *Dentomaxillofacial Radiology*, vol. 22, no. 3, pp. 140–144, 1993.

[17] G. J. Siskos and M. Georgopoulou, "Unusual case of general pulp calcification (pulp stones) in a young Greek girl," *Endodontics & Dental Traumatology*, vol. 6, no. 6, pp. 282–284, 1990.

[18] S. K. Bahetwar and R. K. Pandey, "An unusual case report of generalized pulp stones in young permanent dentition," *Contemporary Clinical Dentistry*, vol. 1, no. 4, pp. 281–283, 2010.

[19] C. Donta, K. Kavvadia, P. Panopoulos, and S. Douzgou, "Generalized pulp stones: report of a case with 6-year follow-up," *International Endodontic Journal*, vol. 44, no. 10, pp. 976–982, 2011.

17

A Clinical Report of Nonsyndromic Concomitant Hypo-Hyperdontia

Siddarth Gupta[1] and Hashmat Popat[2]

[1] *School of Dentistry, Cardiff University, Heath Park, Cardiff CF14 4XY, UK*
[2] *Applied Clinical Research and Public Health, School of Dentistry, Cardiff University, Heath Park, Cardiff CF14 4XY, UK*

Correspondence should be addressed to Hashmat Popat; popath@cardiff.ac.uk

Academic Editors: W. L. Adeyemo, R. Crespi, M. De Bruyne, and K. Thongprasom

Although hypodontia and supernumerary teeth are often considered as mutually exclusive conditions, this case report presents an unusual case of hypodontia and a supernumerary tooth occurring simultaneously. An adolescent male was referred to the local hospital department regarding upper arch crowding. Plain film radiographs confirmed the congenital absence of both lower lateral incisors in addition to an unerupted conical supernumerary tooth in the maxillary midline. This condition has been called hypo-hyperdontia and in this paper, we discuss the clinical findings and treatment planning considerations in relation to the limited number of previously reported cases. The case report raises awareness of concomitant hypo-hyperdontia and serves to highlight that concomitant anomalies should be excluded when hypodontia or supernumerary teeth are diagnosed.

1. Introduction

Hypodontia and supernumerary teeth are often considered as two extremes of the same type of dental anomaly. They most commonly occur as mutually exclusive conditions, and each represents its own challenge in terms of treatment planning. On very rare occasions, hypodontia and supernumerary teeth can coexist with the condition termed "concomitant hypodontia and hyperdontia" [1], "oligopleiodontia" [2], or "hypo-hyperdontia" [3]. More recently, the term concomitant hypo-hyperdontia (CHH) has been used. Being an anomaly of extremes, CHH has been associated with conditions such as Ellis-van Creveld syndrome [4], Marfan syndrome [5], and Downs syndrome [6]. Nonsyndromic CHH is very rare with one epidemiological study finding an incidence of 0.3% in an orthodontic population [7]. It is therefore likely that the true incidence in the general population is significantly lower. The aim of this case report is to present a rare finding of CHH in a nonsyndromic adolescent who was referred as part of a routine orthodontic referral. The clinical presentation in relation to previously reported cases is discussed to raise awareness of the condition.

2. Case Report

An 11-year-old, white male was referred to the Department of Child Dental Health, at the local University Dental Hospital for an orthodontic opinion from his general dental practitioner. The medical, dental, and social histories were unremarkable.

2.1. Extraoral Assessment. The patient presented with a class I skeletal relationship with an average Frankfort-mandibular planes angle and lower facial height proportion. There was no significant asymmetry in the transverse plane. The lips were competent, and the nasolabial angle was slightly reduced. An assessment of the temporomandibular joint was unremarkable.

2.2. Intraoral Assessment. In occlusion the patient had a mild class II division 2 incisor relationship in the mixed dentition, with an overjet of 2 mm and an increased, complete to tooth overbite (Figure 1). The upper dental centreline was coincident with the facial midline while the lower dental centreline was displaced 3 mm to the left of the upper.

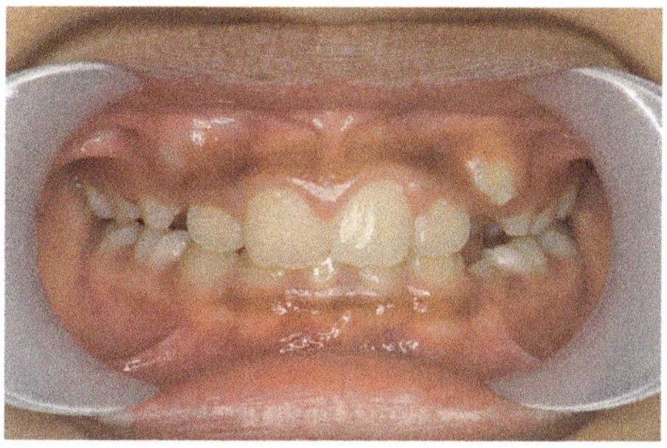

FIGURE 1: Anterior occlusal photograph of dentition.

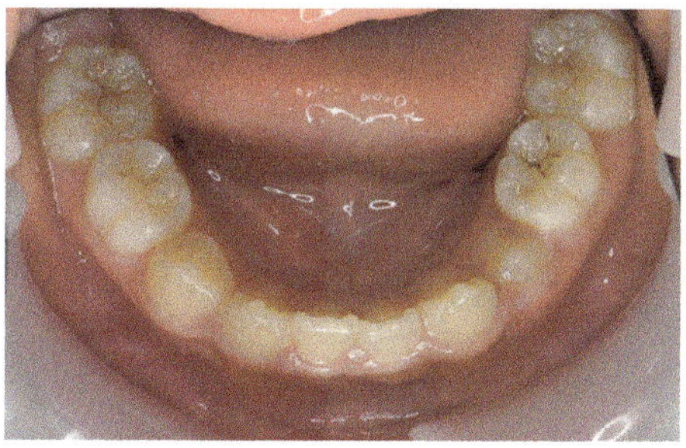

FIGURE 2: Lower occlusal photograph of dentition showing clinical absent lower lateral incisors.

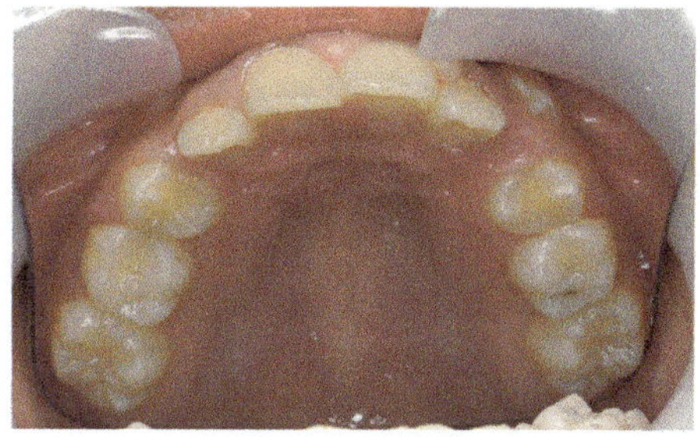

FIGURE 3: Upper occlusal photograph showing crowded permanent canines.

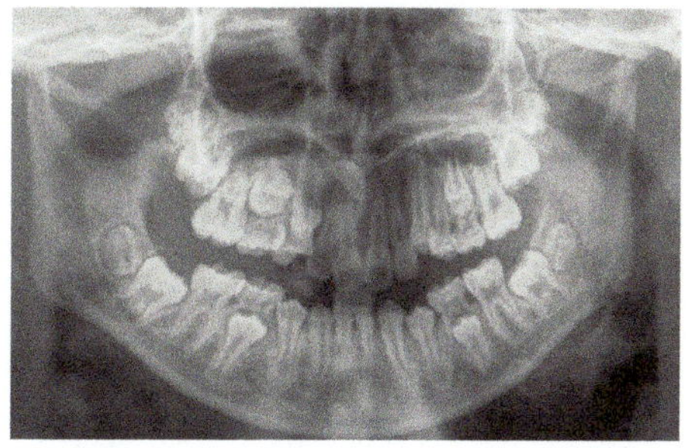

FIGURE 4: Dental pantomogram confirming congenitally absence of lower lateral incisors and upper midline supernumerary.

The lower arch was essentially well aligned; however, both lower permanent lateral incisors were clinically absent (Figure 2).

The upper arch was severely crowded with a lack of space for both upper permanent canines (Figure 3).

The patient's oral hygiene was fair with small amounts of plaque being present in the cervical margins of the posterior dentition. There was occlusal fissure caries present in the lower first permanent molars.

2.3. Radiographic Assessment. A dental pantomogram (Figure 4) revealed the presence of all permanent teeth excluding LL2 and LR2. In addition, an inverted conical supernumerary was found in the maxillary midline close to the root apices of the UR1 and UR2. There was no obvious root resorption of the UR1 and UR2, and all other root lengths appeared normal for the patient's chronological age. Molar stacking was evident in both upper quadrants.

2.4. Treatment Plan. The clinical and radiographic findings were explained to the patient and parents. Oral hygiene instruction, diet advice, and tooth brushing instruction were given. Bite-wing radiographs followed by preventive resin restorations were planned for all four first permanent molars.

Given the reasonable lower arch alignment and aesthetics despite congenitally absent lower lateral incisors, the lower arch was to be treated on a nonextraction basis. Removal of the maxillary first premolars was requested to allow spontaneous eruption of the maxillary permanent canines. There was a discussion with regard to the proximity of the upper midline supernumerary and the roots of the upper incisors. If fixed appliance therapy was to be considered, then the supernumerary would most likely require removal. As the patient and parents were apprehensive regarding a general anaesthetic, the decision was made to review the interarch relationships in a 6-month time and confirm active treatment or accept the malocclusion with regular monitoring of the upper incisor roots and supernumerary.

3. Discussion

The authors have presented a case of CHH in a nonsyndromic patient. The incidence of such a condition in the general population is unknown but is likely to be very rare given the incidence in an orthodontic population has been documented as low as 0.3% [7]. The aetiology of CHH is unclear underlying the complex mechanisms causing hypodontia and supernumerary teeth. The aetiological factors associated with hypodontia include physical disruption of the lamina dura, abnormalities of the dental epithelium, and underlying neural crest derived mesenchyme failing to induce tooth germ production [20]. There is a strong genetic basis with *MSX1*, *TGFA*, and *PAX9* mutations isolated for tooth agenesis [21]. More recently, WNT10A has been isolated and shown to improve the diagnostic yield of DNA testing in isolated nonsyndromic hypodontia [22]. The aetiology of supernumerary teeth includes the phylogenetic theory, the dichotomy theory, and the presence of an overactive lamina dura [23]. Despite a strong genetic basis behind both hypodontia and supernumerary teeth, a study looking at nine patients with CHH found that none of the family members also suffered from CHH [24]. From the current limited literature, CHH

Table 1: Presentation of nonsyndromic CHH in published case reports in English language literature over the last 20 years.

Author	Year	Gender	Age	Hypodontia		Supernumeraries	
				Maxilla	Mandible	Maxilla	Mandible
Hewson et al. [8]	1995	Male	9		LR5	Central incisor	
Zhu et al. [9]	1996	Male	14	UR2, UL2			UL6 region
Scheiner and Sampson [10]	1997	Female	8		LL5, LR5	2 mesiodens	
Segura and Jiménez-Rubio [11]	1998	Male	13	UL2		Mesiodens	
Matsumoto et al. [12]	2001	Female	8	UL5	LL2	UL2	
Sharma [13]	2001	Female	12	UL3		Six supernumeraries	
Oliveira et al. [14]	2002	Female	9		LL5, LR5	Mesiodens	
	2002	Male	8	Gemination		2 mesiodens	
El-Bahannasawy and Fung [15]	2004	Female	4	URC		URD, UR5	
Patchett et al. [16]	2006	Male	9		LL5, LR5	Mesiodens	
Anthonappa et al. [17]	2008	Female	12		LL1, LR1	UL3	
		Male	9	UR5	LL5	UL1	
		Male	11		LL2	UR5	
		Male	5		LLA, LRA, LR2	Mesiodens	
		Male	7		LL1, LR1	2 mesiodens	
		Female	5		LLB, LL2	Mesiodens	
		Male	6		LL5, LR5	Mesiodens	
Varela et al. [7]	2009	Female	Not given		LL5	LR2	
		Male	Not given		LL5, LR5	Mesiodens	
		Male	Not given		LL5	UR2	
		Male	Not given		LL5, LR5		LL2
		Male	Not given	UL2		Mesiodens	
		Female	Not given	UL2		ULB	
		Female	Not given	UL2		URB, UR2	
Marya et al. [18]	2012	Male	20		LL1, LR1		Mesiodens
Nirmala et al. [19]	2013	Female	13	UR3, UL3		Mesiodens	

LL: lower left, LR: lower right, UL: upper left, UR: upper right.

seems to be a result of disturbances to neural crest migration, proliferation, and differentiation when tooth germ formation is initiated [17]. In addition, there is evidence to suggest a model of tooth size and shape discrepancies between hypodontia and supernumerary patients. The more severe the hypodontia, the smaller the mesiodistal width of the teeth formed. Conversely, patients with supernumerary teeth tend to have significantly larger maxillary central and lateral incisors than controls [25].

Whilst hypodontia is more common amongst females and supernumerary amongst males, CHH has been reported to affect both genders equally [25].

Table 1 summarises the phenotypic presentation of non-syndromic cases of CHH reported in the literature over the last 20 years. Two cases of CHH have been reported in the primary dentition, although this is believed to be extremely rare [15]. Abnormalities of the primary dentition are almost certainly likely to be translated to the permanent dentition. The majority of other cases of CHH have presented with missing upper lateral incisors and/or missing lower second premolars. This correlates with teeth most commonly absent in isolated hypodontia [20]. In a similar manner, the most common supernumerary present in CHH appears to be a mesiodens, which mirrors the common presentation of an isolated supernumerary tooth [23].

One case of CHH has reported that a mesiodens was found in conjunction with a missing maxillary lateral incisor [11]. The aetiology of this occurrence of CHH has been speculated as a transposition. However, as the majority of reported cases of CHH are in opposing arches, this theory is unlikely.

Fortunately in the case presented here, the diagnosis of CHH does not seem to have impacted significantly on the treatment plan. Although the supernumerary present was a classic feature of an additional tooth to the normal series, the pattern of hypodontia was not typical. Isolated incidences of congenitally absent mandibular incisors are believed to be in the region of 0.08–0.23% [20], and therefore the presentation is likely to be quite rare.

The body of knowledge on CHH is steadily growing. Literature reviews and case series have helped to recognise a condition which was once thought of as two opposite entities.

4. Conclusion

This case report highlights a routine orthodontic referral presenting with simultaneous occurrence of hypodontia and a supernumerary tooth. Practitioners should be aware that hypodontia and supernumerary teeth may not be mutually exclusive in their presentation.

References

[1] G. E. Camilleri, "Concomitant hypodontia and hyperodontia. Case report," *British Dental Journal*, vol. 123, no. 7, pp. 338–339, 1967.

[2] P. Nathanail, "Letter to the editor," *British Dental Journal*, vol. 129, p. 309, 1970.

[3] A. C. Gibson, "Concomitant hypo-hyperodontia," *British Journal of Orthodontics*, vol. 6, no. 2, pp. 101–105, 1979.

[4] F. N. Hattab, O. M. Yassin, and I. S. Sasa, "Oral manifestations of Ellis-van Creveld syndrome: report of two siblings with unusual dental anomalies," *Journal of Clinical Pediatric Dentistry*, vol. 22, no. 2, pp. 159–165, 1998.

[5] S. K. Mallineni, J. Jayaraman, C. K. Yiu, and N. M. King, "Concomitant occurrence of hypohyperdontia in a patient with Marfan syndrome: a review of the literature and report of a case," *Journal of Investigative and Clinical Dentistry*, vol. 3, pp. 253–257, 2012.

[6] A. G. Acerbi, C. de Freitas, and M. H. de Magalhães, "Prevalence of numeric anomalies in the permanent dentition of patients with Down syndrome," *Special Care in Dentistry*, vol. 21, no. 2, pp. 75–78, 2001.

[7] M. Varela, P. Arrieta, and C. Ventureira, "Non-syndromic concomitant hypodontia and supernumerary teeth in an orthodontic population," *European Journal of Orthodontics*, vol. 31, no. 6, pp. 632–637, 2009.

[8] A. Hewson, J. McCue, P. Kavanagh, and T. McNamara, "Supernumerary central incisor: orthodontic management," *Journal of the Irish Dental Association*, vol. 41, no. 2, pp. 34–35, 1995.

[9] J. F. Zhu, R. Crevoisier, and R. J. Henry, "Congenitally missing permanent lateral incisors in conjunction with a supernumerary tooth: case report," *Pediatric Dentistry*, vol. 18, no. 1, pp. 64–66, 1996.

[10] M. A. Scheiner and W. J. Sampson, "Supernumerary teeth: a review of the literature and four case reports," *Australian Dental Journal*, vol. 42, no. 3, pp. 160–165, 1997.

[11] J. J. Segura and A. Jiménez-Rubio, "Concomitant hypohyperdontia: simultaneous occurrence of a mesiodens and agenesis of a maxillary lateral incisor," *Oral Surgery, Oral Medicine, Oral Pathology, Oral Radiology, and Endodontics*, vol. 86, no. 4, pp. 473–475, 1998.

[12] M. Matsumoto, Y. Nakagawa, S. Sobue, and T. Ooshima, "Simultaneous presence of a congenitally missing premolar and supernumerary incisor in the same jaw: report of case," *Journal of Dentistry for Children*, vol. 68, no. 1, pp. 63–66, 2001.

[13] A. Sharma, "A rare non-syndrome case of concomitant multiple supernumerary teeth and partial anodontia," *Journal of Clinical Pediatric Dentistry*, vol. 25, no. 2, pp. 167–169, 2001.

[14] L. M. Oliveira, L. G. Primo, R. Barcelos, M. B. Portela, and E. P. D. S. Bastos, "Radiographic diagnosis of supernumerary teeth: report of six unusual cases," *ASDC Journal of Dentistry for Children*, vol. 69, no. 2, pp. 175–125, 2002.

[15] E. El-Bahannasawy and D. E. Fung, "Missing C, supplemental D and supplemental premolar all in one quadrant: a case report," *International Journal of Paediatric Dentistry*, vol. 14, no. 6, pp. 461–464, 2004.

[16] C. I. Patchett, A. E. Sargison, and B. O. I. Cole, "Management of a patient exhibiting concomitant supernumerary teeth and hypodontial," *International Journal of Paediatric Dentistry*, vol. 16, supplement 1, pp. C2–C3, 2006.

[17] R. P. Anthonappa, C.-K. Lee, C. K. Y. Yiu, and N. M. King, "Hypohyperdontia: literature review and report of seven cases," *Oral Surgery, Oral Medicine, Oral Pathology, Oral Radiology and Endodontology*, vol. 106, no. 5, pp. e24–e30, 2008.

[18] C. M. Marya, G. Sharma, V. P. Parashar, V. Dahiya, and A. Gupta, "Mandibular midline supernumerary tooth associated with agenesis of permanent central incisors: a diagnostic conundrum," *Stomatologija*, vol. 14, no. 2, pp. 65–68, 2012.

[19] S. Nirmala, S. K. Mallineni, and S. Nuvvula, "Pre-maxillary hypo-hyperdontia: report of a rare case," *Romanian Journal of Morphology and Embryology*, vol. 54, pp. 443–445, 2013.

[20] A. R. Vieira, R. Meira, A. Modesto, and J. C. Murray, "MSX1, PAX9, and TGFA contribute to tooth agenesis in humans," *Journal of Dental Research*, vol. 83, no. 9, pp. 723–727, 2004.

[21] E. Matalova, J. Fleischmannova, P. T. Sharpe, and A. S. Tucker, "Tooth agenesis: from molecular genetics to molecular dentistry," *Journal of Dental Research*, vol. 87, no. 7, pp. 617–623, 2008.

[22] M. van den Boogaard, M. Creton, Y. Bronkhorst et al., "Mutations in WNT10A are present in more than half of isolated hypodontia cases," *Journal of Medical Genetics*, vol. 49, pp. 327–331, 2012.

[23] M. Zadurska, B. Sieminska-Piekarczyk, D. Maciejak, B. Wyszomirska-Zdybel, and J. Kurol, "Concomitant hypodontia and hyperodontia—an analysis of nine patients," *Acta Odontologica Scandinavica*, vol. 70, no. 2, pp. 154–159, 2012.

[24] S. Nuwula, M. Kiranmayi, G. Shilpa, and S. V. S. G. Nirmala, "Hypohyperdontia: agenesis of three third molars and mandibular centrals associated with midline supernumerary tooth in mandible," *Contemporary Clinical Dentistry*, vol. 1, pp. 136–141, 2010.

[25] A. H. Brook, C. Elcock, M. H. Al-Sharood, H. F. McKeown, K. Khalaf, and R. N. Smith, "Further studies of a model for the etiology of anomalies of tooth number and size in humans," *Connective Tissue Research*, vol. 43, no. 2-3, pp. 289–295, 2002.

18

Management of Complex Root Canal Curvature of Bilateral Radix Entomolaris: Three-Dimensional Analysis with Cone Beam Computed Tomography

Muktishree Mahendra,[1] Anand Verma,[2] Sanjeev Tyagi,[1] Santosh Singh,[1] Kapil Malviya,[2] and Ramit Chaddha[2]

[1] *Department of Conservative Dentistry & Endodontics, People's Dental Academy, Bhopal, Madhya Pradesh 462037, India*
[2] *Anand Verma Dental Clinic, C/2-30, Civil Lines, Shamla Hill, Bhopal 462002, India*

Correspondence should be addressed to Muktishree Mahendra; drmuktishree21@gmail.com

Academic Editors: R. Crespi, C. N. Elias, C. Evans, and J. López-López

The meticulous knowledge of anatomic characteristics and their variations is essential for the clinician. Radix entomolaris (RE) is one such anomaly where an extra root is present on the distolingual aspect of the mandibular first molar. 18-year-old patient was referred for the root canal treatment of mandibular right and left first molars. Intraoral periapical radiograph revealed additional periodontal spacing crossing distal root of 36. A CBCT was advised and it confirmed the presence of extra roots both in 36 and 46. CBCT is useful in endodontics as it aids in the identification of essential anatomic structures and determination of radius and angle of root canal curvature which is linked to fracture of the instrument. The classical triangular access cavity was modified to a trapezoidal form to locate the extra canal. All canals were instrumented with controlled memory nickel titanium instruments and obturation was done with single cone technique.

1. Introduction

Success of endodontic therapy depends on the complete cleaning and shaping of the root canal systems, tridimensional obturation, and proper coronary sealing. For that purpose, the knowledge of the morphology of the root canal system as well as its variations is essential. The mandibular first molar is known to display several anatomical variations. The number of roots may also vary in mandibular molars, in which a third additional root, firstly mentioned in the literature by Carabelli [1], is called radix entomolaris. This supernumerary root is located in distolingual position, mainly in the mandibular first molars. When located in the mesiobuccal surface, the anomaly is called radix paramolaris [2]. The frequency of radix entomolaris is less than 5% in Caucasian, African, Eurasian, and Indian populations [3], whereas its bilateral occurrence is less than 2.19% [4]. This extra root is typically smaller and more sharply curved than the distobuccal (DB) root, requiring special attention when root canal treatment is being considered.

CBCT is a noninvasive technique to determine the occurrence of distolingual root and reveals the true nature of macrostructure three-dimensionally and its curvature and angulation [5]. CBCT shows the exact position of distolingual root and hence it helps in tracking the curvature and prevents iatrogenic event that might occur in relation to canal curvature like instrument separation, perforation, ledge formation, and so forth.

2. Case Presentation

18-year-old male patient reported to the dental office with the chief complaint of swelling in lower left back region for last two days as well as pain in lower right back region. The pain was aggravated on taking cold and hot food items and on mastication. The clinical examination revealed the carious

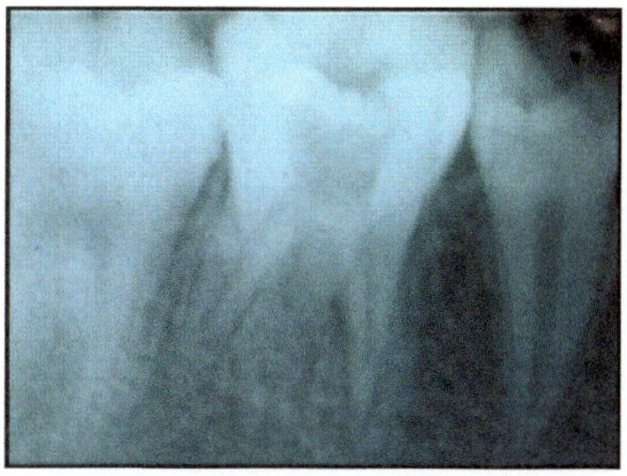

FIGURE 1: Preoperative IOPA of 36.

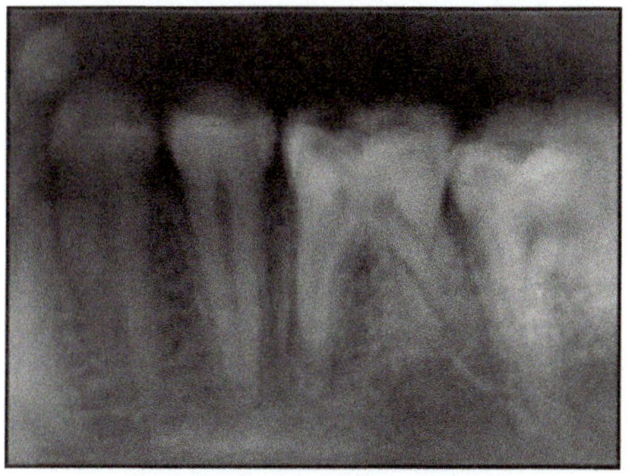

FIGURE 2: Preoperative IOPA of 46.

right and left mandibular first molars. His medical history was noncontributory.

Intraoral periapical radiograph of 36 (Figure 1) revealed deep carious lesion involving the pulp with periapical radiolucency at the root apices and presence of an extra root in 36. On close inspection of radiograph of 46 (Figure 2), an impression of double periodontal ligament space on distal side leads to the suspicion of additional root entity with 46. Based on clinical and radiographic examination, diagnosis of acute apical abscess with 36 and symptomatic irreversible pulpitis with acute apical periodontitis of 46 was established.

A cone beam computerized tomography was advised to confirm the diagnosis of distolingual root. CBCT was done and determined the exact position, angle, and curvature of distolingual root of the permanent mandibular first molars. The morphology of teeth was obtained in oblique (Figure 3), sagittal (Figure 4), axial (Figure 5), curve slicing (Figure 6), and coronal section (Figure 7).

After adequate anaesthesia and isolation with rubber dam, access cavity was prepared using endoaccess kit in the mandibular left first molar. The cavity design was slightly modified by extending more distolingually using ultrasonic tips for exploring extra distal canal orifice. CBCT imaging had shown the severe curvature from the middle third to the apical third in the distolingual root; therefore, the canals were negotiated with pathfinder files. These files create glide path with .02 rotary Ni-Ti instruments till the working length and they glide through the canal and pasts the curvature smoothly. Instrumentation was completed with .04 tapered number 35 Ni-Ti rotary instruments in a crown down fashion till the working length. All the canals were irrigated with 2.5% sodium hypochlorite and 17% EDTA. Calcium Hydroxide was placed into the canals as intracanal medicament. After two weeks, the tooth was asymptomatic and final irrigation was done with ultrasonic passive irrigation for 1 min. Canals were dried with paper point and obturation was done using gutta-percha points and endoflas sealer. Later, the access cavity was sealed with composite.

After completion of 36, endodontic treatment of the mandibular right first molar was initiated. After creating the glide path, biomechanical preparation was using controlled memory NiTi instruments. The canals were irrigated with 2.5% NaOCl and normal saline. Calcium hydroxide was used as intracanal medicament and access opening was sealed with Zinc oxide-eugenol cement. One week later, the tooth was asymptomatic, the canals were dried with paper point, obturation was completed, and access cavity was sealed with composite. Patient was recalled after 1 month and tooth preparation for porcelain fused to metal crown (Figure 8) was done and cemented subsequently.

3. Discussion

The success of endodontic therapy depends on the root canal morphology to some extent, so the clinician should have a thorough understanding of normal anatomy as well as its unusual anatomical configurations. The root canals of the mandibular permanent first molars have several typical anatomical features and anomalies. The presence of four canals is relatively frequent [6], but the presence of two distal roots is uncommon and bilateral presence of three rooted mandibular molar is a rare case. This additional third root, first mentioned in the literature by Carabelli [1] (1844), is called the radix entomolaris (RE), located distolingually in the mandibular molars, mainly the first molars.

The coronal third of distolingual root of RE is fixed partially and completely to the distal root. Based on buccolingual orientation, De Moor et al. [7] have classified RE into three types. Type I refers to straight root or canal. Type II refers to an initially curved entrance which continues as a straight root/root canal. Type III refers to an initial curve in the coronal third of the root canal and a second curve beginning in the middle and continuing to the apical third. In this case, distolingual root of 36 is classified as Type III because severe canal curvature is present in middle third till the apical end. Distolingual root of RE is mostly in buccolingual plane as in conventional radiography (two-dimensional); tooth is visualized in mesiodistal plane only. CBCT [8] is a three-dimensional imaging overcoming these major limitations by visualization of the third dimension and ascertaining the exact location and anatomy of RE.

The location of distolingual canal orifice has an implication for access cavity preparation. The orifice of RE is located far distally from the main distal canal. Hence, the modification of the classical triangular access cavity to a trapezoidal form is required to locate the additional canal orifice and establish the straight line access. The interorifice

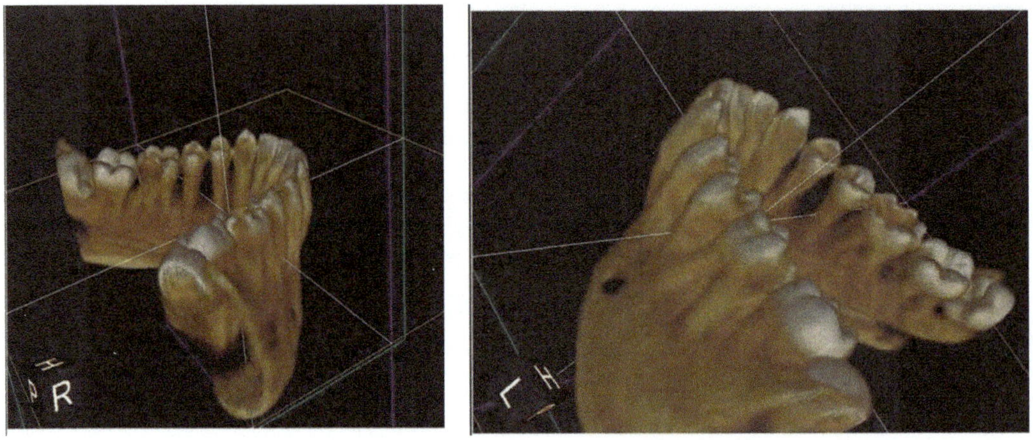

(a) (b)

FIGURE 3: Oblique slicing showing root canal curvature of distolingual root of 36 and 46.

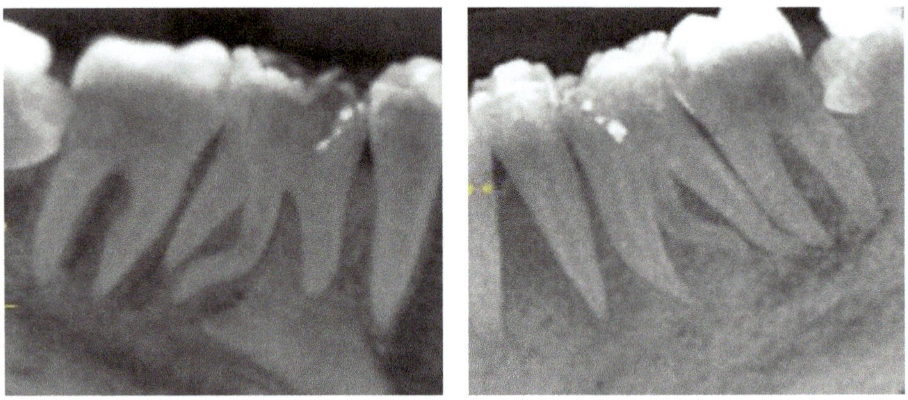

(a) (b)

FIGURE 4: Sagittal view of 36 and 46 showing root canal curvature of distolingual root.

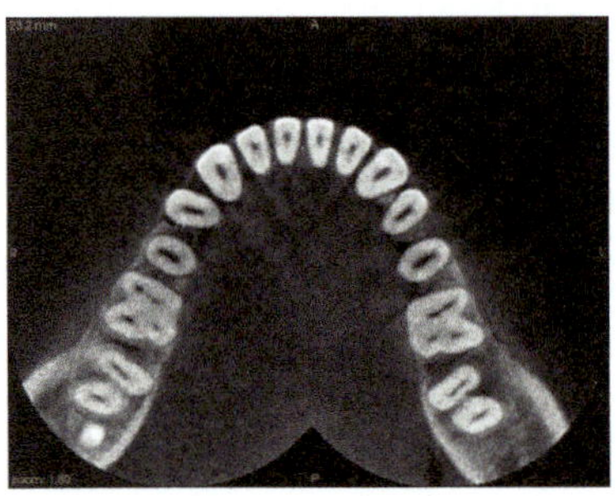

FIGURE 5: Axial views allow the relationship between the additional root and other roots to be assessed.

distance between extra distolingual canal and remaining canals can be measured with CBCT, serving as a useful guideline to locate and treat RE [5, 8]. The axial sectioning of CBCT allows for the exact visualization of distolingual orifice in relation to other canals. Ultrasonic tips help in careful removal of dentin and thus prevent weakening of tooth structure [9].

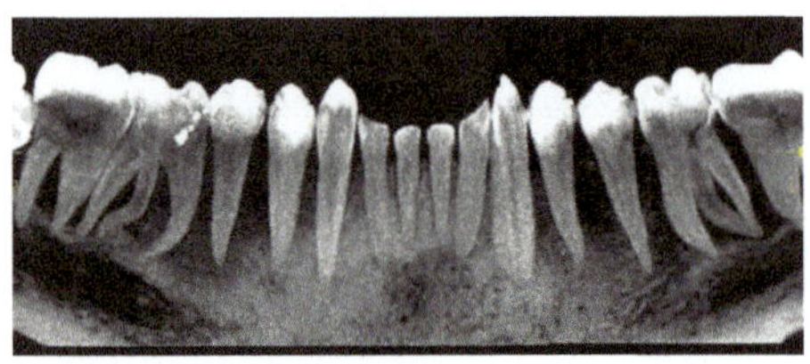

FIGURE 6: Curved slicing section showing 36 and 46.

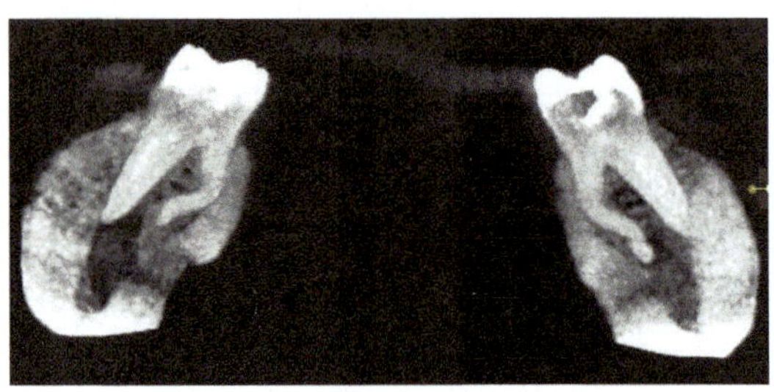

FIGURE 7: Coronal section showing 36 and 46.

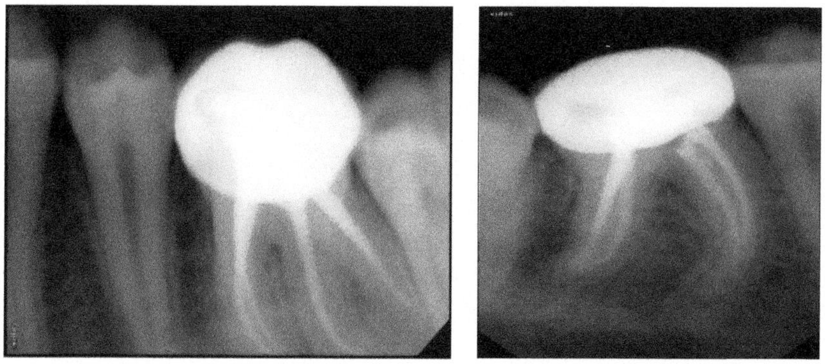

(a) (b)

FIGURE 8: Postoperative IOPA of 36 and 46.

The determination of root canal curvature is a key procedure for endodontic planning. Knowledge of root curvature radius allows for selection of NiTi rotary files and accurate planning of root canal instrumentation. NiTi rotary files undergoe hundreds of cycles of alternating compression and flexure when placed in curved canal. Radius of curvature is the most important factor influencing the cyclic fatigue. The more severe the angle of curvature with small radius of curvature, the greater the cyclic fatigue and thus, lower its life expectancy [10]. Instrument separation increased as radius of curvature decreased. Thus, file design features such as NiTi core diameter, cross-sectional shape, and flute depth should be taken into account while selecting the NiTi rotary instrument for curved canals. In this case, new set of controlled memory flexible NiTi files has been used as they have high resistance to cyclic fatigue and reduce the incidence of instrument separation.

4. Conclusion

Cone beam computed tomography is a practical, noninvasive tool for morphological analysis. It also reduces the radiation dose to which patients are exposed. It helps in accurate diagnosis of the third root and can avoid complications or a "missed canal" during root canal treatment. Failing to realize curvature and radii of canal before treatment can lead to preparation errors—apical zips, perforations, canal blockages, or instrument separation—which can leave the canal unprepared and compromise the outcome of the treatment. Additional aids that help in location of orifices are following law of symmetry and orifice location, DG 16 probe, microopener, sodium hypochlorite "bubble" test, long shank burs, ultrasonic instruments, cbct, and operating microscope.

References

[1] G. Carabelli, *Systematisches Handbuch der Zahnheilkunde*, Braumuller und Seidel, Viena, Austria, 2 edition, 1844.

[2] F. L. Calberson, R. J. De Moor, and C. A. Deroose, "The radix entomolaris and paramolaris: clinical approach in endodontics," *Journal of Endodontics*, vol. 33, no. 1, pp. 58–63, 2007.

[3] M. E. Curzon, "Three-rooted mandibular permanent molars in English Caucasians," *Journal of Dental Research*, vol. 52, no. 1, p. 181, 1973.

[4] C. L. Sabala, F. W. Benenati, and B. R. Neas, "Bilateral root or root canal aberrations in a dental school patient population," *Journal of Endodontics*, vol. 20, no. 1, pp. 38–42, 1994.

[5] T. P. Cotton, T. M. Geisler, D. T. Holden, S. A. Schwartz, and W. G. Schindler, "Endodontic applications of cone-beam volumetric tomography," *Journal of Endodontics*, vol. 33, no. 9, pp. 1121–1132, 2007.

[6] K. Gulabivala, T. H. Aung, A. Alavi, and Y.-L. Ng, "Root and canal morphology of Burmese mandibular molars," *International Endodontic Journal*, vol. 34, no. 5, pp. 359–370, 2001.

[7] R. J. G. De Moor, C. A. J. G. Deroose, and F. L. G. Calberson, "The radix entomolaris in mandibular first molars: an endodontic challenge," *International Endodontic Journal*, vol. 37, no. 11, pp. 789–799, 2004.

[8] M.-G. Tu, H.-L. Huang, S.-S. Hsue et al., "Detection of permanent three-rooted mandibular first molars by cone-beam computed tomography imaging in Taiwanese individuals," *Journal of Endodontics*, vol. 35, no. 4, pp. 503–507, 2009.

[9] G. Plotino, C. H. Pameijer, N. Maria Grande, and F. Somma, "Ultrasonics in endodontics: a review of the literature," *Journal of Endodontics*, vol. 33, no. 2, pp. 81–95, 2007.

[10] J. P. Pruett, D. J. Clement, and D. L. Carnes Jr., "Cyclic fatigue testing of nickel-titanium endodontic instruments," *Journal of endodontics*, vol. 23, no. 2, pp. 77–85, 1997.

Hutchinson-Gilford Progeria Syndrome: A Rare Genetic Disorder

Rajat G. Panigrahi,[1] Antarmayee Panigrahi,[2] Poornima Vijayakumar,[3] Priyadarshini Choudhury,[4] Sanat K. Bhuyan,[1] Ruchi Bhuyan,[5] G. Maragathavalli,[6] and Abhishek Ranjan Pati[1]

[1] *Department of Oral Medicine & Radiology, Institute of Dental Science, Siksha O Anusandhan University, K8 Kalinga Nagar, Bhubaneswar, Odisha 751003, India*
[2] *Department of Pedodontics & Preventive Dentistry, JSS Dental College, JSS University, Sri Shivarathreeshwara Nagara, Mysore, Karnataka 570 015, India*
[3] *Department of Pedodontics & Preventive Dentistry, Tamil Nadu Dr. M. G. R. Medical University, Ragas Dental College & Hospital, No. 191 East Coast Road, Uthandi, Chennai, Tamil Nadu 600096, India*
[4] *Department of Oral Medicine & Radiology, Kalinga Institute of Dental Sciences, KIIT University, Bhubaneswar, Odisha 751024, India*
[5] *Department of Oral Pathology, Institute of Dental Science, Siksha O Anusandhan University, K8 Kalinga Nagar, Bhubaneswar, Odisha 751003, India*
[6] *Department of Oral Medicine & Radiology, Saveetha Dental College, Saveetha University, No. 162 Poonamalee High Road, Vellapanchavadi, Chennai, Tamil Nadu 600077, India*

Correspondence should be addressed to Rajat G. Panigrahi; emaildrrajat@gmail.com

Academic Editors: Y.-K. Chen and M. H. K. Motamedi

Hutchinson-Gilford progeria syndrome (HGPS) is a rare pediatric genetic syndrome with incidence of one per eight million live births. The disorder is characterised by premature aging, generally leading to death at approximately 13.4 years of age. This is a follow-up study of a 9-year-old male with clinical and radiographic features highly suggestive of HGPS and presented here with description of differential diagnosis and dental consideration. This is the first case report of HGPS which showed pectus carinatum structure of chest.

1. Introduction

Hutchinson-Gilford progeria syndrome (HGPS) is an extremely rare but devastating disorder characterised by dwarfism and premature aging [1]. It occurs sporadically with a reported incidence of one in eight millions and male predominance with M : F ratio of 1.5 : 1 and a strong racial susceptibility for Caucasians who represent 97% of patients [2]. The pattern of inheritance is uncertain, though both autosomal dominant and autosomal recessive modes have been proposed [3, 4]. Recent genetic advances have identified LMNA as a causative gene of HGPS. LMNA encodes laminins A and C, which are the main components of intermediate filamentous lamina, function as a structural support, and are essential for DNA replication and mRNA transcription [5]. Though the clinical presentation is typical, conventional radiological and biochemical investigations help in confirming the diagnosis. We present a case of progeria which showed classic physical and radiological changes of HGPS.

2. Case Report

A 12-year-old male reported to the clinic with the chief complaint of decayed teeth in upper and lower anterior teeth region. Past medical history revealed that the first two years of his life were normal followed by failure to gain

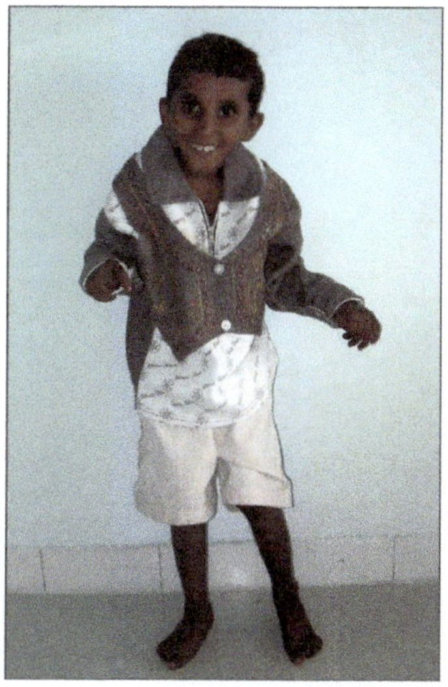

FIGURE 1: It shows a 9-year-old patient standing in an abnormal gait.

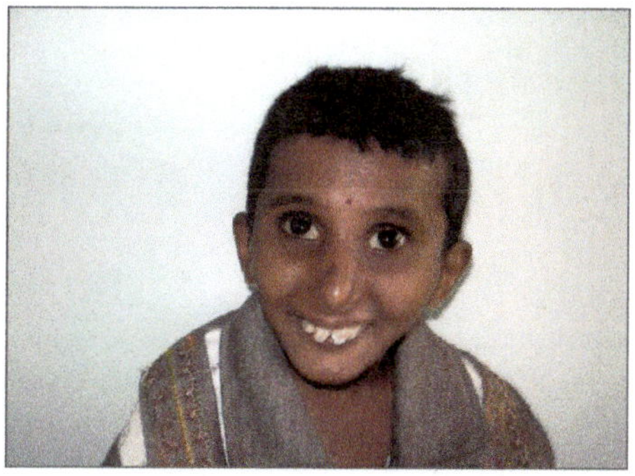

FIGURE 2: It shows the face of the 9-year-old boy showing typical features of progeria.

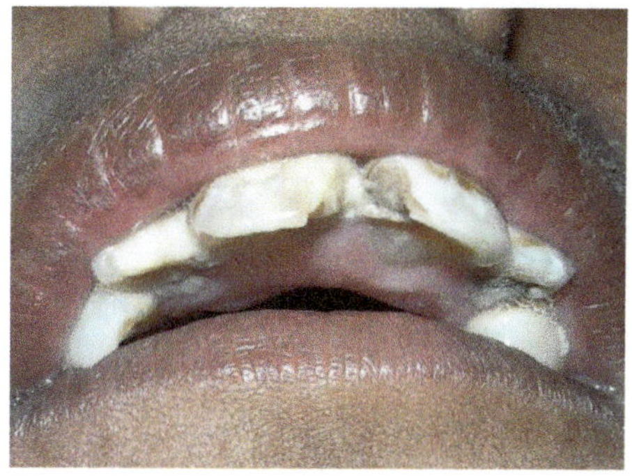

FIGURE 3: It shows the dental condition 2 years back.

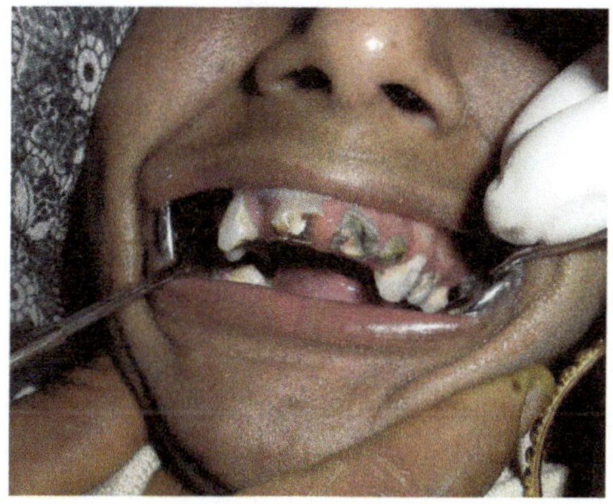

FIGURE 4: It shows the present dental condition.

in both height and weight subsequently followed by loss of hair from scalp and eyebrows. Then he developed stretching of skin and inability to stand or walk properly; however, mental development was normal. Medical history revealed that the patient was undergoing treatment for acute hepatitis (see Figures 1 and 2).

Past dental history revealed that the patient came earlier to the hospital for the treatment of dental caries in the maxillary anterior 2 years back. But no treatment could be done as the patient was uncooperative. This second born child of a nonconsanguineous marriage had an uneventful prenatal history, with an other sibling being normal (see Figures 3 and 4).

No other family members were affected with similar complaints. On general examination, the young patient resembled a "wizened little old person."

He was thin built, poorly nourished, short statured with abnormal gait, thin atrophic skin, loss of subcutaneous fat around the extremities and the skin was coarse, stretched, shiny, and thickened. Chest revealed pectus carinatum structure (see Figures 5 and 6).

Systemic examination revealed that patient had impaired vision, slurring of speech, loss of memory, breathlessness, palpitation, and restricted joint movements with inability to stand or walk.

On extra oral examination, the patient had mild frontal bossing, a beaked nose, protruding eyes, a high pitched voice, and hypoplastic maxilla and mandible with mild mid facial deformity giving "plucked bird appearance." Opening of mouth was restricted (interincisal distance-21 mm) and lateral movements of temporomandibular joint were also restricted.

On intraoral examination, the teeth were of normal size when compared to small size of the jaw, fractured crown irt to 11, root stump irt 12, 15, 16, 21, 22, and dental caries irt 13, 14, 23, 24, 25, 31, 32, 41, 42, 45. High arched palate and partial anodontia were seen.

Based on history and clinical findings, a provisional diagnosis of progeria was made. To confirm the diagnosis, the child was subjected to radiological and biochemical investigations.

Biochemical investigations showed increased serum cholesterol which was 228 mg% and increased urinary excretion of hyaluronic acid.

OPG revealed hypoplastic maxilla, hypoplastic mandible with infantile angle, and multiple missing teeth. The morphology of the condyle appeared to be altered (see Figure 7).

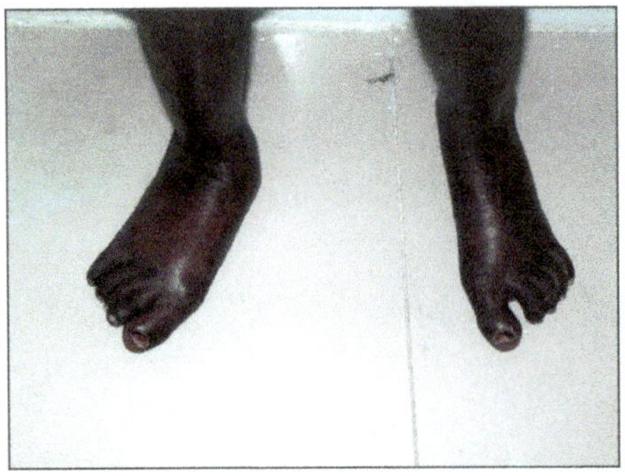

FIGURE 5: It shows the legs of the patient exhibiting shiny and dry skin.

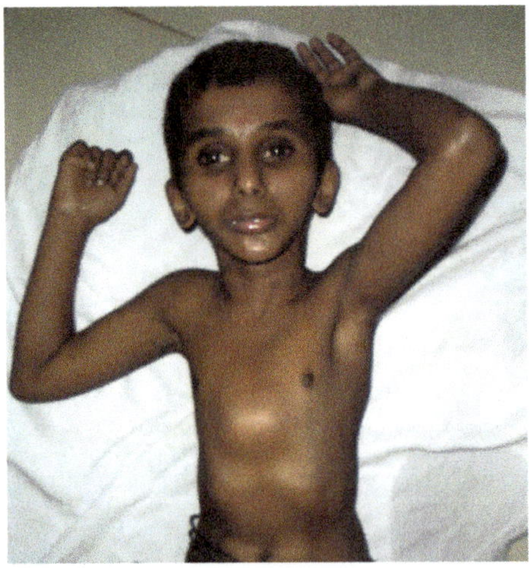

FIGURE 6: It shows the patient being unable to stand and is lying down, and chest showed pectus carinatum structure.

Correlating the history, clinical features, radiographic findings, and laboratory investigations, the findings were consistent with HGP syndrome.

After careful systemic monitoring, extraction of the grossly decayed teeth was planned under antibiotic coverage.

3. Discussion

Progeria is a rare genetic disorder phenotypically characterised by feature of premature aging first described by Hutchinson in 1886 [6]. The term progeria was coined by Gilford in 1904 and is derived from the greek word "gerios" meaning old. DeBusk in 1972 renamed this condition as "Hutchinson-Gilford progeria syndrome" [2]. The rate of ageing in the affected individual is accelerated by seven times that of the normal. The average life span is 13 years (ranging from 7 to 27 years) with occasional survival till the age of 45 years. This is due to various abnormalities of mesodermal tissues and decreased survival time of fibroblasts. De novo mutation of LMNA which encodes for a major constituent of the inner membrane lamina has been reported [5]. Affected children are normal at birth and grow normally until about the end of the first year when both normal growth and weight gain slow down.

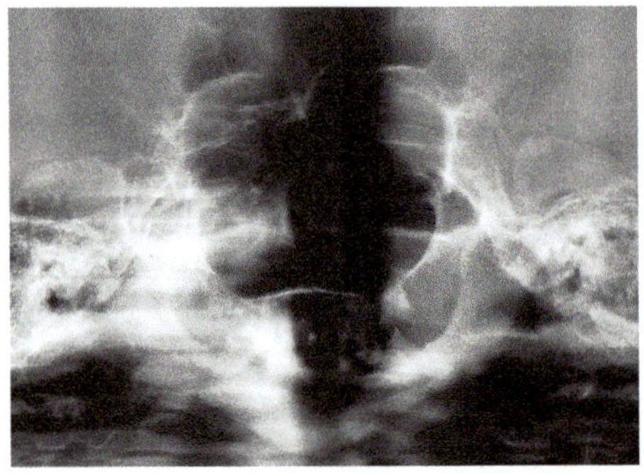

FIGURE 7: It shows the OPG with deformities in the mandible and partial anodontia.

The present case exhibited the typical phenotype of HGPS, showing the initial symptoms in the first year of life, severe growth deficiency, expressive lipodystrophy, loss of hair from scalp and eyebrows along with sclerodermatous changes giving rise to characterstic "Plucked Bird" appearance.

The scalp veins become prominent because of loss of subcutaneous fat and loss of hair. These patients are usually short and thin with an average height of 100 cm and average weight of 12–15 kgs or even less. Delayed dentition and hypodontia are also common [7].

The patient in our case had the classic features which included facial features, alopecia, failure to thrive, poor sexual maturation, and normal intelligence.

Skeletal survey reveals the following radiological features: calvarium is thin and relatively large and the diploic space is absent or very shallow. The face is small with disproportionate small mandible that retains its infantile obtuse angle and short ascending rami. The clavicles are small in caliber and rarefied at birth [8]. This case typically presented with the above mentioned radiographic features confirming the provisional diagnosis.

In progeria, hyperlipidemia is often present with increased low density lipoproteins and increased serum cholesterol level, as seen in our patient. There is also an increase in hyaluronic acid levels that is responsible for sclerodermatous changes and cardiovascular changes.

Death is mainly due to cardiovascular complication like myocardial infarction or congestive cardiac failure. Failure to thrive in patients with progeria may be due to a bioinactive form of growth hormone and lack of vasculogenesis caused by excessive secretion of hyaluronic acid [9].

The differential diagnosis that can be thought of in these cases includes Werner syndrome, acrogeria, Rothmund-Thomson syndrome, and Cockayne syndrome [10].

There is no effective treatment to date. The only available approach towards symptomatic treatment and timely identification and prompt management of complications.

References

[1] R. C. M. Hennekam, "Hutchinson-Gilford progeria syndrome: review of the phenotype," *American Journal of Medical Genetics, Part A*, vol. 140, no. 23, pp. 2603–2624, 2006.

[2] F. L. DeBusk, "The Hutchinson-Gilford progeria syndrome. Report of 4 cases and review of the literature," *The Journal of Pediatrics*, vol. 80, no. 4, pp. 697–724, 1972.

[3] S. Beauregard and B. A. Gilchrest, "Syndromes of premature aging," *Dermatologic Clinics*, vol. 5, no. 1, pp. 109–121, 1987.

[4] M. M. Khalifa, "Hutchinson-Gilford progeria syndrome: report of a Libyan family and evidence of autosomal recessive inheritance," *Clinical Genetics*, vol. 35, no. 2, pp. 125–132, 1989.

[5] D. K. Shumaker, E. R. Kuczmarski, and R. D. Goldman, "The nucleoskeleton: lamins and actin are major players in essential nuclear functions," *Current Opinion in Cell Biology*, vol. 15, no. 3, pp. 358–366, 2003.

[6] W. T. Brown, "Progeria: a human-disease model of accelerated aging," *American Journal of Clinical Nutrition*, vol. 55, no. 6, pp. 1222–1224, 1992.

[7] P. K. Sarkar and R. A. Shinton, "Hutchinson-Guilford progeria syndrome," *Postgraduate Medical Journal*, vol. 77, no. 907, pp. 312–317, 2001.

[8] F. N. Silverman, "Miscellaneous forms of short stature," in *Caffey's Pediatric X-Ray Diagnosis: An Integrated Imaging Approach*, 1993.

[9] M. Zebrower, F. J. Kieras, and W. T. Brown, "Urinary hyaluronic acid elevation in Hutchinson-Gilford Progeria Syndrome," *Mechanisms of Ageing and Development*, vol. 35, no. 1, pp. 39–46, 1986.

[10] A. Ho, S. J. White, and J. E. Rasmussen, "Skeletal abnormalties of acrogeria, a progeroid syndrome," *Skeletal Radiology*, vol. 16, no. 6, pp. 463–468, 1987.

20

Management of Root Fracture: A Novel, Noninvasive Treatment Approach

M. S. Rangareddy,[1] Archana Daga,[1] Y. Vishnu Vardhan,[1] and M. Daneswari[2]

[1] *Panineeya Institute of Dental Sciences, Hyderabad, Andhra Pradesh 500060, India*
[2] *Mamtha Dental College, Khammam, Andhra Pradesh 500060, India*

Correspondence should be addressed to Archana Daga; archanadaga4u@gmail.com

Academic Editors: J. C. de la Macorra and I. El-Hakim

Traumatic injuries to teeth account for approximately 25% of dental conditions where a patient seeks dentist for emergency treatment. Radicular fractures are one such entity which is very challenging to address due to various complications like periodontal communication, increased mobility, and continued pulpal infection leading to necrosis. Radicular fractures in the middle third have long been considered teeth of salvage due to their unfavourable fracture pattern. During the recent years introduction of biomimetic materials has opened the horizon for saving these teeth. In the present case report a novel approach to the management of radicular fractures in the middle third has been presented.

1. Introduction

Traumatic injuries to a tooth range in severity from a simple enamel infraction to a complete exarticulation of tooth also known as avulsion. These injuries account for being the third most common cause for tooth loss where the patient seeks the dentist for emergency treatment [1]. The clinically challenging cases of root fractures due to their complex management involving interdisciplinary/multidisciplinary treatment approach are of particular interest to the clinician [2]. Root fractures are a rare entity where their frequency in permanent teeth is only from 0.5% to 7% and in deciduous teeth is from 2% to 4% [1]. Root fractures occur mainly in the maxillary centrals (68%) and maxillary laterals (27%) mainly due to frontal impact with a rare involvement of only 5% in mandibular incisors [3].

These horizontal fractures are mainly divided on the location of fragment into cervical, middle, and coronal third fractures. Among these entities middle third fractures are relatively more common. Middle third fractures are generally transverse to oblique and may be single or multiple, complete or incomplete [4]. Treatment approach for these fractures is complex involving prognostic considerations like degree of displacement of fracture fragment, patient's age, stage of root growth, mobility of the coronal fragment, and diastasis of the fragments [1].

Endodontic treatment is required in these situations as they lead to pulp necrosis. The various treatment approaches available include either root canal therapy of both fracture fragments [5]; this may be indicated in fracture cases when the segments are not separated and where complete dryness of canal can be obtained. Another treatment approach consists of root canal treatment of the coronal segment only, if this segment shows no mobility [6]. The use of an intraradicular splint in the form of post systems has also been recommended. In the present case reports a novel approach to the management of root fractures is carried out with the use of MTA as intraradicular splint along with aesthetic management with direct and indirect composites.

2. Case 1

An 18-year-old female reported to the Department of Conservative and Endodontics, Panineeya Institute of Dental Sciences, Hyderabad, India, with a chief complaint of broken upper front tooth and mobile upper front tooth for 2 days. On expanding the history, the patient elicited trauma due to road

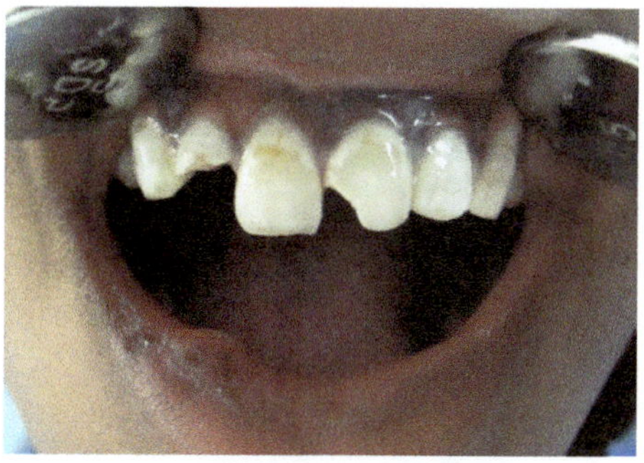

FIGURE 1: Diagnostic photo.

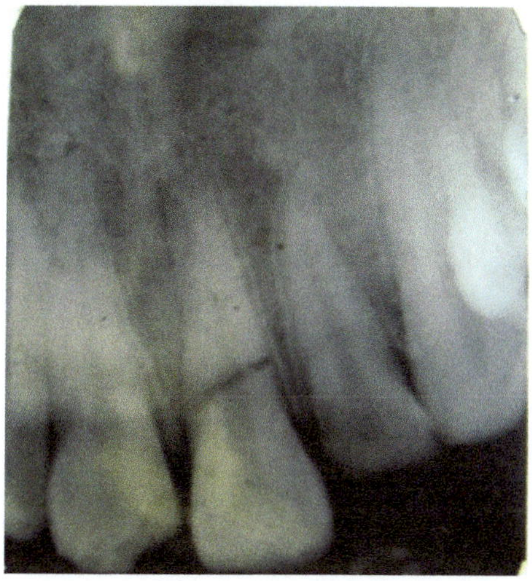

FIGURE 2: Diagnostic radiograph.

traffic accident two days back. Clinical extraoral examination revealed lacerations on the lower lip. Intraoral examination revealed grade II mobility i.r.t 11 and complicated crown fracture i.r.t 12 (Figure 1).

On investigating the intraoral periapical radiograph (Figure 2), a horizontal fracture line was seen i.r.t 11 at the junction of coronal and middle third with minimal displacement of fracture fragments. So the final diagnosis was established as Ellis Class VI fracture i.r.t 11, Ellis Class III fracture i.r.t 12, Ellis Class I fracture i.r.t 21, with moderate dental fluorosis.

Taking into consideration the prognostic factors regarding root fracture i.r.t 11, patient was clearly informed about the various treatment options available either to save the tooth or to send it for extraction. On obtaining the informed consent, a comprehensive treatment plan was devised for the patient which consisted of managing the root fracture i.r.t 11 with MTA as a splint material, post and core rehabilitation for tooth number 12, along with direct and indirect composite restorations.

Initial treatment began with splinting the teeth using orthodontic braided wire and flowable composite as a rigid splint for a period of 6 weeks according to Andreason's protocol (Figure 3).

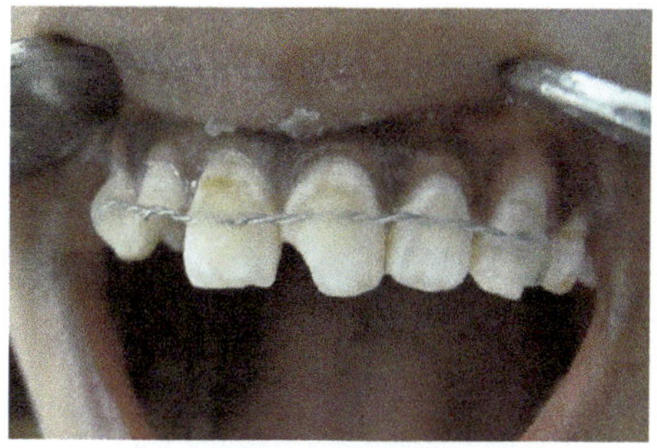

FIGURE 3: Splinting.

Endodontic treatment was initiated i.r.t 11 and 12; after access opening of 12, cleaning and shaping were carried out with hand K-files using step back technique, followed by obturation by using resin sealer (AH Plus; Dentsply; lot number 1209000390, Germany) and lateral condensation method. Later post space preparation was done to receive fibre-post (Quartzix Added Posts; number 2, Landy, Swiss Dental Products Of Distinction) (Figures 4, 5, 6, and 7). The final coronal restoration was planned as indirect composite crown (Adoro Indirect Composite, Ivoclar Vivadent) (Figure 11). For tooth number 11, endodontic treatment was carried out after two weeks confirming pulp necrosis as a result of checking the pulp vitality. After access preparation, number 15 K File was used to negotiate through the fracture fragment (Figure 8). After initial cleaning and shaping using hand files to ensure complete asepsis, two weeks of intracanal calcium hydroxide paste were given (ApexCal, Ivoclar Vivadent). When we could ensure complete dryness of the canal without any bleeding, obturation was carried out with Zinc Oxide Eugenol Sealer (Deepak Enterprises, Mumbai) and lateral condensation of gutta-percha through the complete root. Following this, gutta-percha is carefully removed just below the fracture extension (Figure 9). Later, MTA (Proroot, Dentsply, Germany) is densely packed with hand pluggers (Figure 10) through the fracture fragment and access cavity sealed with flowable composite. Esthetic management for this tooth consisted of a conservative approach of giving indirect composite veneer (Adoro Indirect Composite, Ivoclar Vivadent) (Figure 11).

To address fluorosis, direct composite veneers were given i.r.t 13, 21, 22, and 23 which gave a uniform shade to the patient. Immediate postop evaluation revealed reduction in tooth mobility i.r.t 11 and followup of 6 months did not reveal any periapical changes with the patient remaining asymptomatic (Figure 12).

3. Case 2

A 26-year-old male patient reported to our department with a chief complaint of mobile upper front tooth following a fist injury. On clinical and radiographic examination a diagnosis of Ellis Class VI fracture was established i.r.t 12 (Figures 13 and 14).

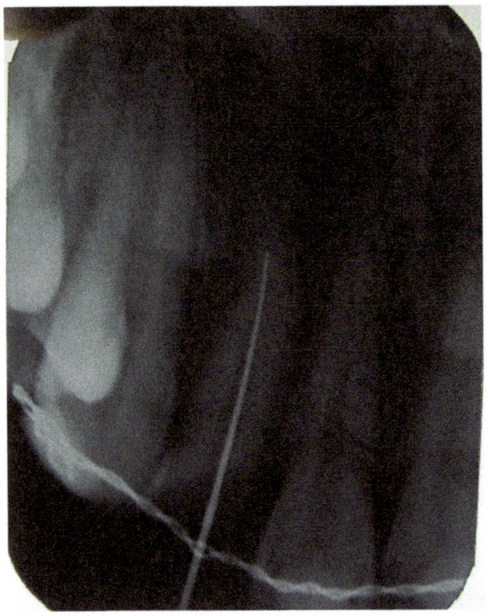

Figure 4: Working length 12.

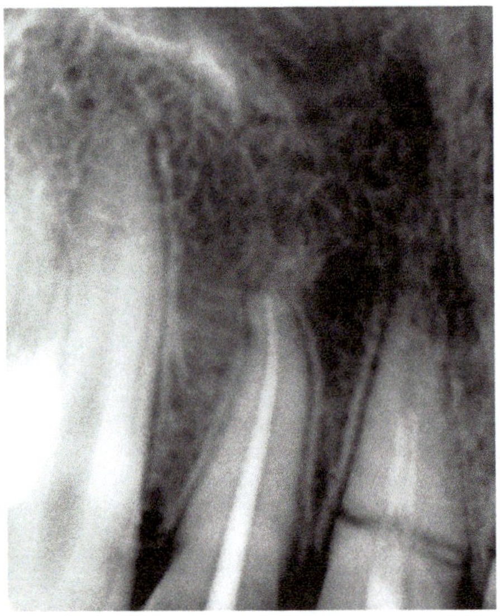

Figure 5: Master cone 12.

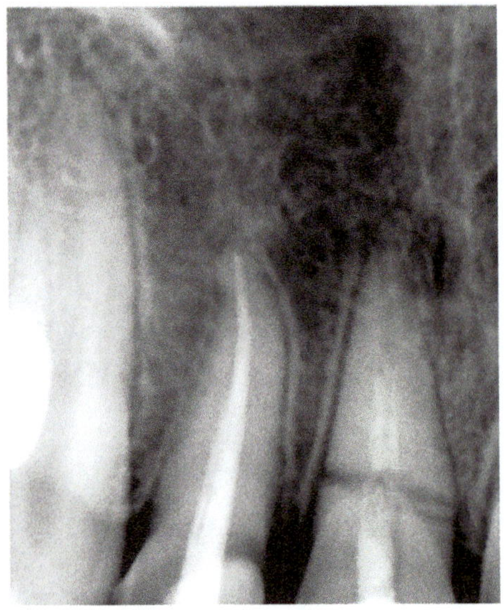

Figure 6: Obturation 12.

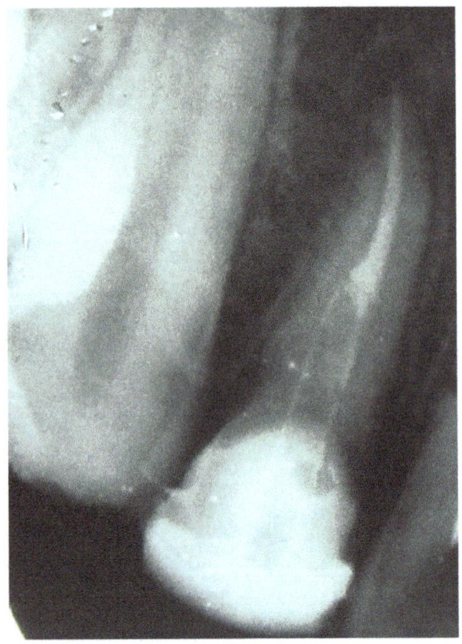

Figure 7: Post and core 12.

The treatment protocol was similar to that of Case 1, where rigid splinting was carried out using orthodontic braided wire and flowable composite for a period of 6 weeks (Figure 15).

Endodontic treatment began two weeks after splinting of teeth, where tooth vitality was checked indicating delayed response, access preparation and pulp extirpation was carried out, and working length was determined (Figure 16). Due to the bayonet configuration of the root, complete instrumentation was done using hand Ni-Ti files by step back technique; following this, complete obturation (Figure 17) was carried out using ZOE sealer and lateral condensation of gutta-percha. And similar intraradicular splinting was carried out like in Case 1 using white MTA (Proroot, Dentsply, Germany) (Figure 18).

Immediate postop evaluation revealed complete resolution of tooth mobility to physiological limits and remaining teeth showed a vital response (Figure 19).

4. Discussion

Management of horizontal middle third root fractures is challenging to an endodontist due to the association of pulpal and periodontal components. Hence the ultimate goal to preserve the natural dentition encourages the possibilities

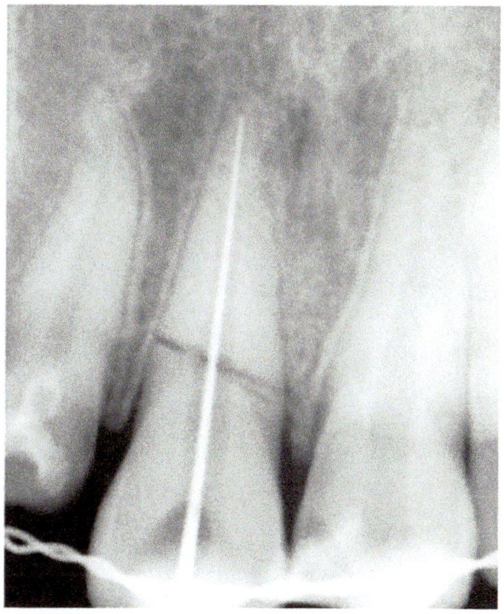

FIGURE 8: Working length 11.

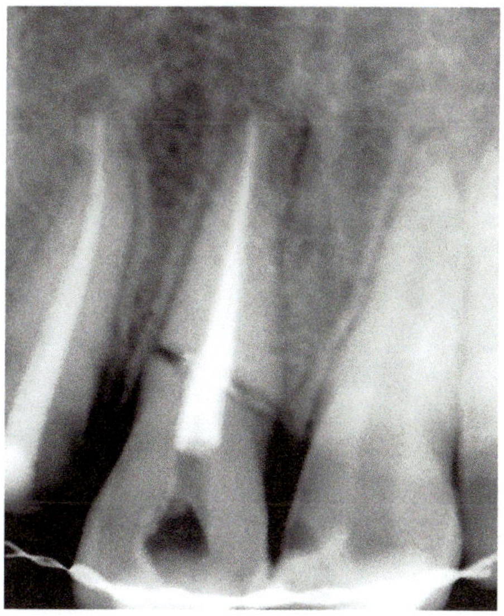

FIGURE 9: Obturation 11.

of new horizons to manage these critical situations. The influence of "preinjury and injury factors" on the healing of intraalveolar root fractures was carried out in a study, whose authors found that the age of the patients, the stage of root growth, mobility of the coronal fragment, dislocation of the coronal fragment, and fragment diastasis exerted the greatest influence on healing at the fracture line and on the occurrence of pulpal necrosis [1]. A recent study by Cvek et al. concluded that 20% of teeth with root fracture lead to pulp necrosis indicating the importance of early endodontic intervention in these patients [7].

In both mentioned cases, the treatment plan was decided based on the level of fracture fragment to the crest of the alveolar bone. As the fragments had the fracture line extending closer to the crest, complete endodontic treatment was

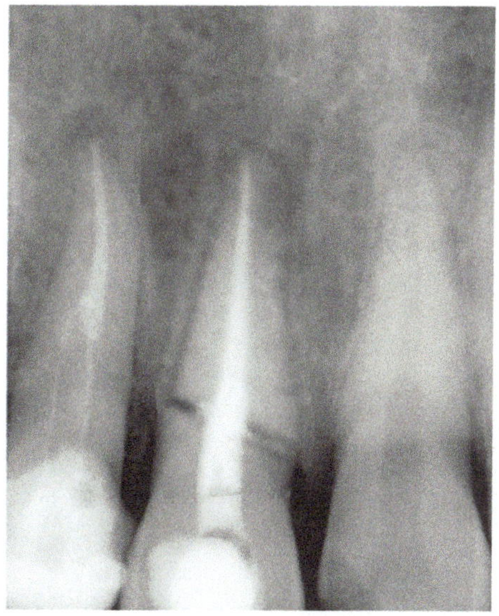

FIGURE 10: MTA placement.

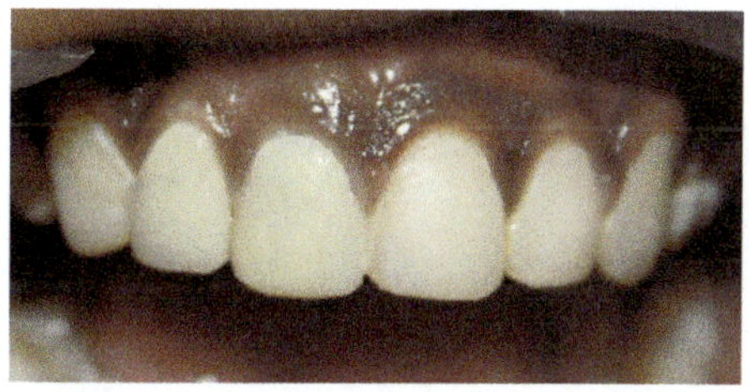

FIGURE 11: Direct and indirect composite restorations.

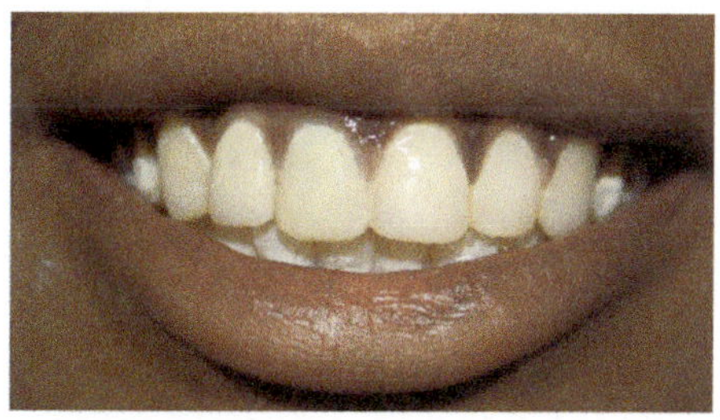

FIGURE 12: Six-month recall.

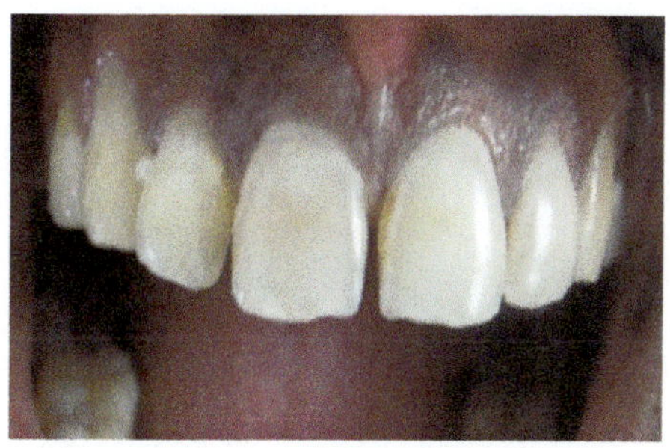

FIGURE 13: Diagnostic picture.

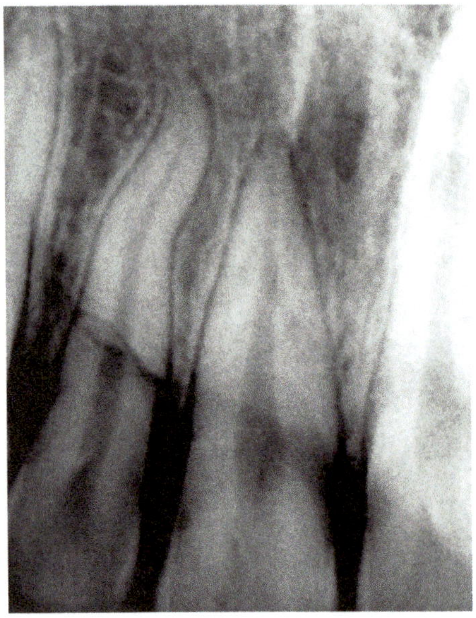

Figure 14: Diagnostic radiograph.

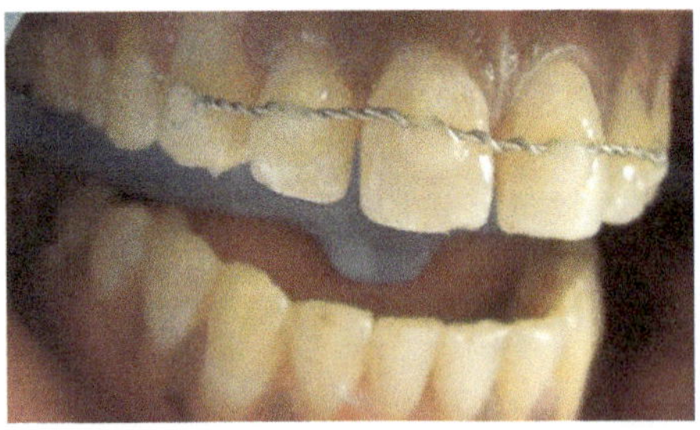

Figure 15: Splinting of teeth.

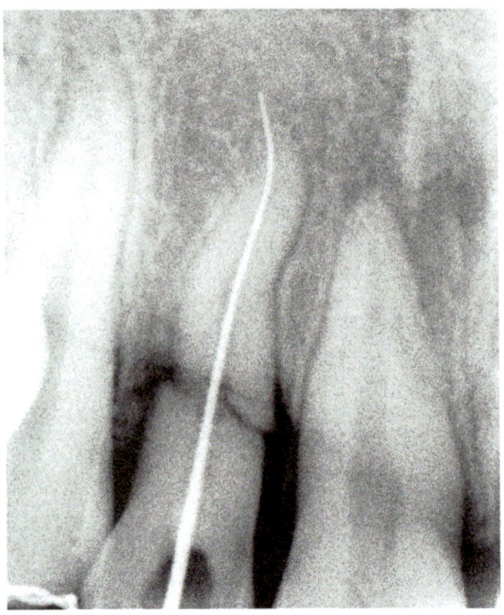

Figure 16: Working length 12.

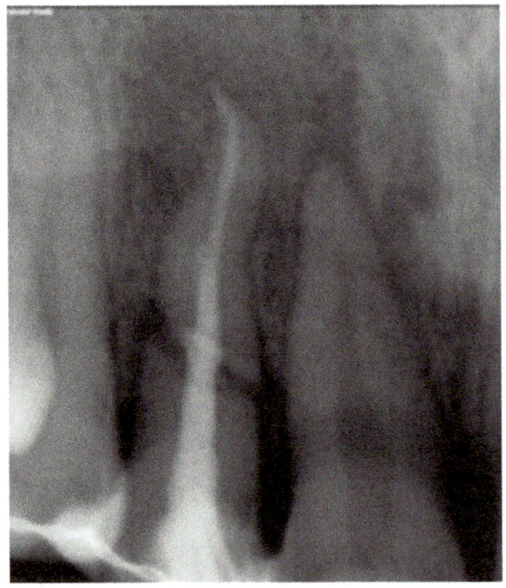

Figure 17: Obturation 12.

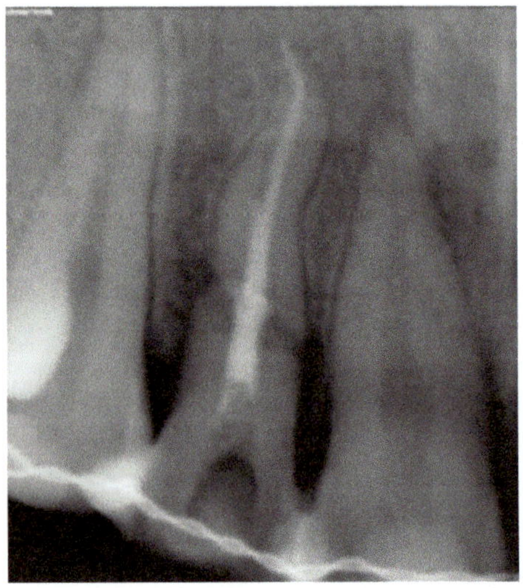

Figure 18: MTA placement.

considered involving both the coronal and apical fragments. Endodontic treatment was carried out as described in the guidelines given by the International Association of Dental Traumatology (IADT) [6]. Nevertheless, vitality was checked two weeks after the trauma and both cases showed delayed response suggestive of pulp necrosis. Cvek et al. reported in their study on the exclusion of the apical fragment due to problems of infection as in case of root fractures [8]. But by doing so there would be a compromise in the crown root ratio of the teeth; hence negotiation and obturation of fracture fragment were also considered. Hand files were used in both cases to preserve maximum intraradicular dentin.

A novel approach of using MTA as a splint material over the fracture fragments was utilised due to its various properties of being osseoinductive, which would result in formation of a hard tissue around the fracture site high pH contributes to its bactericidal effects which creates a sterile environment

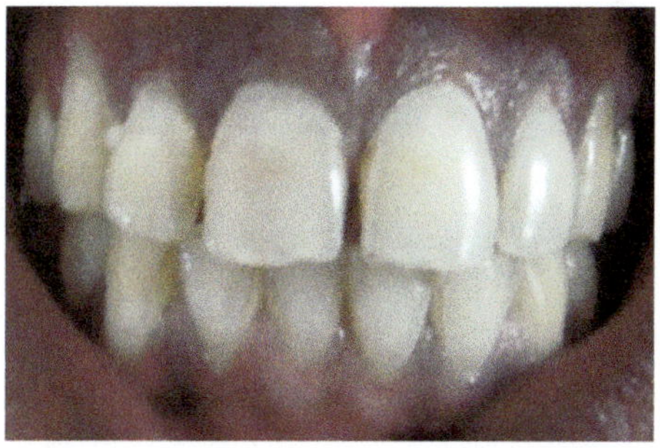

FIGURE 19: Splint removal and followup.

around the fracture site. And it is biocompatible which explains that minor leakage in Case 1 did not contribute to any periodontal changes [9], and it has a hard set stabilization which would contribute to it acting as an intraradicular splint. Furthermore due to its excellent biocompatibility leakage of MTA helps in the healing of periodontal apparatus by forming normal architecture [10].

In Case 1 esthetic rehabilitation was carried out by direct and indirect composites. Indirect composites were used in this case due to their conservation of tooth structure and improved esthetics when compared to direct composites [11].

Short-term followup of both cases have shown promising results of this novel approach. Regular followup along with more clinical trials can confirm this treatment modality for fractured roots.

5. Conclusion

Middle third fractures have long been considered to have a poor prognosis because of lack of understanding the biologic concept of such fracture along with insufficient knowledge to manage these situations.

In recent years introduction and availability of biocompatible materials like MTA have opened the horizons for the clinicians to put forth varied treatment options in the management of mid-root fractures.

Conflict of Interests

The authors declare that there is no conflict of interests regarding the publication of this paper.

References

[1] F. M. Andreasen, J. O. Andreasen, and M. Cvek, "Root fractures," in *Textbook and Color Atlas of Traumatic Injuries to Teeth*, F. M. Andreasen and J. O. Andreasen, Eds., pp. 337–371, Blackwell, Copenhagen, Denmark, 2007.

[2] K. Orhan, A. I. Orhan, and F. T. Oz, "Management of untreated traumatized permanent incisors with crown and root fractures: a case report," *Quintessence International*, vol. 40, no. 8, pp. 647–654, 2009.

[3] M. K. Çalişkan and Y. Pehlivan, "Prognosis of root-fractured permanent incisors," *Endodontics and Dental Traumatology*, vol. 12, no. 3, pp. 129–136, 1996.

[4] D. J. Parekh, R. Sathyanarayanan, and M. T. Manjunath, "Clinical management of mid-root fracture in maxillary central incisors: case reports," *International Journal of Oral Science*, vol. 2, no. 4, pp. 215–221, 2010.

[5] *Ingle's Endodontics-Text Book*, 5th edition.

[6] M. T. Flores, L. Andersson, J. O. Andreasen et al., "Guidelines for the management of traumatic dental injuries. I. Fractures and luxations of permanent teeth," *Dental Traumatology*, vol. 23, no. 2, pp. 66–71, 2007.

[7] M. Cvek, G. Tsilingaridis, and J. O. Andreasen, "Survival of 534 incisors after intra-alveolar root fracture in patients aged 7–17 years," *Dental Traumatology*, vol. 24, no. 4, pp. 379–387, 2008.

[8] M. Cvek, I. Mejàre, and J. O. Andreasen, "Conservative endodontic treatment of teeth fractured in the middle or apical part of the root," *Dental Traumatology*, vol. 20, no. 5, pp. 261–269, 2004.

[9] P. J. C. Mitchell, T. R. Pitt Ford, M. Torabinejad, and F. McDonald, "Osteoblast biocompatibility of mineral trioxide aggregate," *Biomaterials*, vol. 20, no. 2, pp. 167–173, 1999.

[10] C. Main, N. Mirzayan, S. Shabahang, and M. Torabinejad, "Repair of root perforations using mineral trioxide aggregate: a long-term study," *Journal of Endodontics*, vol. 30, no. 2, pp. 80–83, 2004.

[11] M. Thordrup, F. Isidor, and P. Hörsted-Bindslev, "A prospective clinical study of indirect and direct composite and ceramic inlays: ten-year results," *Quintessence International*, vol. 37, no. 2, pp. 139–144, 2006.

21

Orthokeratinized Odontogenic Cyst: A Report of Three Clinical Cases

María del Carmen González Galván,[1] Abel García-García,[2] Eduardo Anitua-Aldecoa,[3] Rafael Martinez-Conde Llamosas,[1] and José Manuel Aguirre-Urizar[1]

[1] *Oral and Maxillofacial Pathology Unit, Dental Clinic Service, Stomatology II Department, UFI 11/25, University of the Basque Country (EHU/EHU), Vizcaya, 48940 Leioa, Spain*
[2] *University of Santiago of Compostela, 15782 Santiago of Compostela, Spain*
[3] *Private Practice, Eduardo Anitua Institute, 01005 Vitoria-Gasteiz, Spain*

Correspondence should be addressed to José Manuel Aguirre-Urizar; josemanuel.aguirre@ehu.es

Academic Editors: A. Epivatianos, A. Markopoulos, and G. Sammartino

The orthokeratinized odontogenic cyst (OOC) is a rare developmental odontogenic cyst that has been considered as a variant of the keratocystic odontogenic tumour (KCOT) until Wright (1981) defined it as a different entity. Surgery is the usual treatment, and recurrence or association with Gorlin-Goltz syndrome has rarely been described. In this report, we presented three cases of this pathology, and we review the principal clinical, histological, radiological, and therapeutic aspects. *Case 1.* A 73-year-old female presents with a slight swelling on the right mandible, associated with an unilocular well-defined radiolucent lesion. *Case 2.* A 27-year-old female presents with a painful mandibular swelling associated with an unilocular radiolucent lesion posterior to the 4.8. *Case 3.* A 61-year-old male was casually detected presents with an unilocular radiolucent lesion distal to the 4.8. *Conclusion.* The OOC is a specific odontogenic clinicopathological entity that should be differentiated from the KCOT as it presents a completely different biological behaviour.

1. Introduction

The orthokeratinized odontogenic cyst (OOC) is a developmental odontogenic cyst relatively rare, arising from the cell rests of the dental lamina [1, 2]. It was first described by Schultz in 1927 [3] as an orthokeratinized variant of the formerly called odontogenic keratocyst, today known as the keratocystic odontogenic tumour. It is not until 1981 that Wright defines this as an independent entity [4].

Since then it has received various designations, such as "orthokeratinized variant of odontogenic keratocyst" or "orthokeratinized cyst of the mandible". It is not until 1998 that Li et al. suggest the term "orthokeratinized odontogenic cyst," which is the most accepted at the present time [2, 5].

The OOC occurs predominantly in males between the third and fourth decades, with a mean age of 33.5 years [2, 5]. The lesion is located mainly in the molar region and posterior mandible [1, 2]. These tumours can reach a large size that causes cortical expansion and presents as a swelling, along with pain, although in most cases it can be detected incidentally during a radiographic examination [1, 2].

Radiographically the cyst appears as a well-circumscribed, unilocular, or multilocular radiolucency that occasionally is associated with an unerupted tooth or with the root without causing resorption [1, 6, 7]. Displacement of neighbouring teeth and of the inferior dental canal has been described [5].

The histopathological analysis confirms the diagnosis which shows a cystic cavity lining composed of a thin and uniform stratified squamous epithelium with a thick granular layer and orthokeratin [1, 8, 9].

A differential diagnostic feature with the keratocystic odontogenic tumour is that no cases of OOC have been associated with nevoid basal cell carcinoma syndrome [8, 10].

Surgical enucleation is the treatment of choice for the OOC, and low recurrence rate has been described between

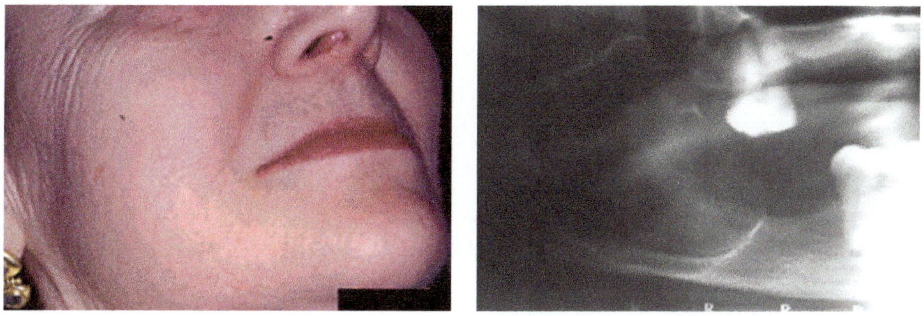

(a) (b)

FIGURE 1: (a) Clinical image. (b) Multilocular radiolucent lesion.

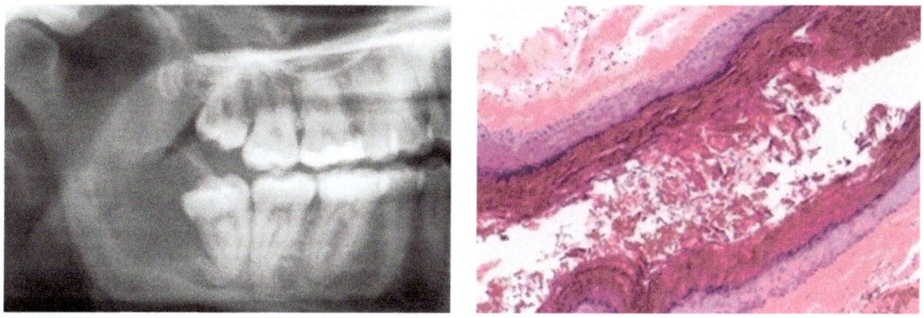

(a) (b)

FIGURE 2: (a) Unilocular radiolucent lesion distal to 4.8. (b) Fibrous connective tissue with a stratified epithelium with orthokeratosis lining.

0 and 2% of cases which is in marked contrast with the 40% recurrence of KCOT [2, 11, 12].

On this paper, we report three clinical cases of the orthokeratinized odontogenic cyst and a review on the main clinicopathological aspects.

2. Clinical Cases

Case 1. A 73-year-old female was referred presenting a slight asymptomatic swelling on the right mandibular angle and ascending ramus of years of evolution (Figure 1(a)). The patient was under treatment with Diclofenac and Piroxicam for arthrosis symptoms and reported no toxic habits.

Radiographically, the lesion appeared as a well-defined multilocular radiolucency on the right posterior mandible and ascending ramus (Figure 1(b)). The computed tomography showed an expansive multilocular and well-defined radiolucency. A fine needle aspiration cytology (FNAC) was performed, and a pearly-white creamy liquid material was obtained. The cytology of the material confirmed the presence of squamous cells.

The complete enucleation of the lesion was performed under general anesthesia, and the material obtained was analyzed for its histopathological figures. Histopathological examination of excised tissue revealed the presence of cystic cavity integrated by dense connective tissue with an inner lining of thin and uniform epithelium with marked granular layer and hyperorthokeratosis. Based on the clinical, radiological, and histological data, a diagnosis of orthokeratinized odontogenic cyst was made. After eleven years of follow-up, no sign of recurrence has been noted.

Case 2. A 27-year-old female presents with a slightly painful swelling in the region of the right inferior third molar of 15 days of evolution, with no other clinical data of interest, nor does she report toxic habits. The orthopantomography shows an unilocular radiolucent lesion, posterior to the 4.8, extending to the ascending ramus (Figure 2(a)). The lesion produced displacement of the molar without causing root resorption. The computed tomography showed the lesion and a slight expansion of the vestibular and lingual walls.

The extraction of the 4.8 and nucleation of the lesion were made under general anaesthesia. In the histopathological analysis, a cystic lesion was recognized with a fibrous connective tissue capsule without inflammation, covered by a stratified epithelium with orthokeratosis and marked granular layer (Figure 2(b)). With the data, the diagnosis of orthokeratinized odontogenic cyst was given.

After the excision of the lesion and the third molar extraction, the pain disappeared.

The outcome was favourable, and after 15 months, no signs of recurrence were recognized.

Case 3. A 61-year-old male who was on a routine dental follow-up presents with a well-defined radiolucent lesion, posterior to the right inferior third molar and extended to the ramus (4.8) on the radiographic exploration (Figure 3(a)). The patient did not show any other signs of interest neither

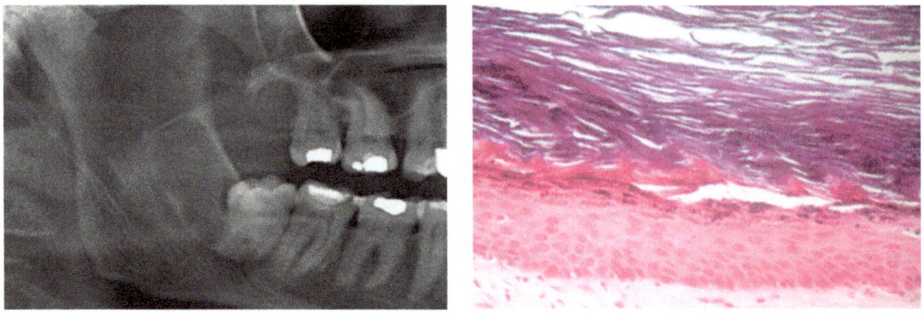

(a) (b)

FIGURE 3: (a) Initial orthopantomography. (b) Fibrous connective tissue with a stratified epithelium with hyperorthokeratosis lining.

toxic habits. The extraction of the 4.8 and enucleation of the lesion were performed under local anaesthesia. On the histopathological analysis, a cystic lesion was recognized with a fibrous connective tissue capsule with no inflammation, covered with a lining of a thin, uniform hyperkeratotic stratified epithelium with marked granular layer.

The cavity was filled with keratin flakes (Figure 3(b)). With this data, the diagnosis of orthokeratinized odontogenic cyst was established.

The outcome was favourable, and after 9 months, no signs of recurrence have been recognized.

3. Discussion

The orthokeratinized odontogenic cyst is an infrequent developmental cyst that occurs most often between the fourth and fifth decades and with a male gender predilection (3, 2 : 1) [1, 2]. Curiously in our cases, two were women and one of them with an advanced age, which we believe to be slow-growing and chronic lesion in an area where extractions were performed without a correct curettage and probably with no previous radiography [1, 5, 11].

As in most cases described previously, our lesions were located in the posterior mandible and extend to the ascending ramus [2, 5, 11]. Swelling is the most frequent symptom and is accompanied on occasions with pain, although in most cases described, the lesion was asymptomatic. The presence of paresthesia, as in Case 2, is a rare sign and is associated with irritative phenomena, such as the infection associated with the impacted third molar [1, 2, 11].

Radiographically, the OOC may appear as a well-defined, unilocular or multilocular, radiolucent solitary lesion associated frequently with impacted teeth, and it on occasions can displace the inferior alveolar nerve. Case 1 presented as a large lesion not associated with teeth. We believe it was slow growing of long evolution. In Cases 2 and 3, the lesions were more typical and related to an impacted molar, located distal to the 4.8 and with no signs of resorption or displacement [2, 7, 11].

Histologically, the OOC shows a cystic cavity lined by a regular stratified squamous epithelium, usually thin and uniform about 4- to 9-cell layers thick. This epithelium presents a defined basal layer that exhibits palisade cuboidal or flat cells, with nuclear hyperchromatism, an intermediate layer of polyhedral cells with eosinophilic cytoplasm, and a thick superficial layer of orthokeratin [1, 2, 8]. This entity must be differentiated from the KCOT that shows a regular epithelium of 5- to 10-cell layers thick with the basal cells lined with an elongated nucleus and the presence of a characteristic superficial corrugated layer of parakeratin [13, 14].

In relation to the immunohistochemical pattern, the OOC does not show activity of the epithelial membrane antigen (EMA) and of the carcinoembrionary antigen (CEA). Moreover, the level of expression of Ki-67 and p53 is lower than on KCOT that suggests a reduced proliferative activity [1, 2, 10]. The reactivity to cytokeratins has showed differences, as OOC stains to cytokeratins 1, 2, and 10 which would suggest a normal differentiation of the epidermis whilst the KCOT reacts to cytokeratins 4, 13, 17, and 19, demonstrating that these are different entities [15].

The differential diagnosis of the OOC includes other radiolucent lesions of the jaws, mainly odontogenic lesions such as dentigerous cyst or paradental cyst [1, 5]. Odontogenic tumours such as ameloblastoma and KCOT should be included. The OOC presents similar radiographic characteristics with the ameloblastoma and the KCOT, such as its tendency to involve the mandibular angle or to appear as a multilocular radiolucency. Unlike these entities, the OOC does not cause root resorption, which is a frequent characteristic on ameloblastomas and KCOT [5].

Conservative surgical removal with complete enucleation of the cystic lesion seems to be the treatment of choice [1, 5, 7].

All our cases were removed with conservative enucleation and have had a periodical follow-up with no recurrence reported to date.

We conclude that the orthokeratinized odontogenic cyst is an independent clinical and pathological entity of the keratocystic odontogenic tumour (KCOT) with a different prognosis. This lesion should be included in differential diagnosis of the radiolucent lesions of the jaws, preferably of the mandibular lesions associated with an impacted tooth.

Acknowledgment

This work was supported by grants from the Department of Education, Universities and Research, Government of the Basque Country (IT-192-07). María del Carmen González Galván is supported by a fellowship from the Itaipu Binacional-Paraguay.

References

[1] T.-J. Li, M. Kitano, X.-M. Chen et al., "Orthokeratinized odontogenic cyst: a clinicopathological and immunocytochemical study of 15 cases," *Histopathology*, vol. 32, no. 3, pp. 242–251, 1998.

[2] Q. Dong, S. Pan, L.-S. Sun, and T.-J. Li, "Orthokeratinized odontogenic cyst A clinicopathologic study of 61 cases," *Archives of Pathology and Laboratory Medicine*, vol. 134, no. 2, pp. 271–275, 2010.

[3] L. Schultz, "Cysts of the maxillae and mandibule," *The Journal of the American Dental Association*, vol. 14, pp. 1395–1402, 1927.

[4] J. M. Wright, "The odontogenic keratocyst: orthokeratinized variant," *Oral Surgery Oral Medicine and Oral Pathology*, vol. 51, no. 6, pp. 609–618, 1981.

[5] D. S. MacDonald-Jankowski and T. K. Li, "Orthokeratinized odontogenic cyst in a Hong Kong community: the clinical and radiological features," *Dentomaxillofacial Radiology*, vol. 39, no. 4, pp. 240–245, 2010.

[6] E. Pérez González, J. López Labady, and M. Villarroel Dorrego, "Quiste odontogénico ortoqueratinizado: una nueva entidad derivada del queratoquiste odontogénico. Revisión de la literatura," *Acta Odontol Venez*, vol. 44, pp. 419–423, 2006.

[7] D. S. MacDonald-Jankowski, "Orthokeratinized odontogenic cyst: a systematic review," *Dentomaxillofacial Radiology*, vol. 39, no. 8, pp. 455–467, 2010.

[8] M. J. A. da Silva, S. O. M. de Sousa, L. Corrêa, A. A. Carvalhosa, and V. C. de Araújo, "Immunohistochemical study of the orthokeratinized odontogenic cyst: a comparison with the odontogenic keratocyst," *Oral Surgery, Oral Medicine, Oral Pathology, Oral Radiology, and Endodontics*, vol. 94, no. 6, pp. 732–737, 2002.

[9] M. Shear, "Odontogenic keratocysts: clinical features," *Oral and Maxillofacial Surgery Clinics of North America*, vol. 15, no. 3, pp. 335–345, 2003.

[10] R. C. K. Jordan, "Histology and ultrastructural features of the odontogenic keratocyst," *Oral and Maxillofacial Surgery Clinics of North America*, vol. 15, no. 3, pp. 325–333, 2003.

[11] T. E. Crowley, G. E. Kaugars, and J. C. Gunsolley, "Odontogenic keratocysts: a clinical and histologic comparison of the parakeratin and orthokeratin variants," *Journal of Oral and Maxillofacial Surgery*, vol. 50, no. 1, pp. 22–26, 1992.

[12] W. Thosaporn, A. Iamaroon, S. Pongsiriwet, and K. H. Ng, "A comparative study of epithelial cell proliferation between the odontogenic keratocyst, orthokeratinized odontogenic cyst, dentigerous cyst, and ameloblastoma," *Oral Diseases*, vol. 10, no. 1, pp. 22–26, 2004.

[13] H. P. Philipsen, "Keratocystic odontogenic tumour," in *Pathology and Genetics of Head and Neck Tumours*, E. L. Barnes, J. W. Eveson, P. Reichart, and D. Sidransky, Eds., World Health Organization Classification of Tumours, pp. 306–307, IARC Press, Lyon, France, 2005.

[14] M. Shear and P. M. Speight, *Cyst of the Oral and Maxillofacial Regions*, Blackwell, Munksgaard, Danmark, 4th edition, 2007.

[15] T. Aragaki, Y. Michi, K.-I. Katsube et al., "Comprehensive keratin profiling reveals different histopathogenesis of keratocystic odontogenic tumor and orthokeratinized odontogenic cyst," *Human Pathology*, vol. 41, no. 12, pp. 1718–1725, 2010.

22

Multiple Supplemental Supernumerary Premolars: Unusual Presentation in a Nonsyndrome Patient

Ashwini Ramakrishna[1] and Kiran B. Rajashekarappa[2]

[1] *Department of Oral Pathology and Microbiology, College of Dental Sciences, Room No. 7, Pavilion Road, Davangere-Karnataka 577004, India*
[2] *Sai Multispecialty Dental Clinic, Vidyanagar Main Road, Davangere, Karnataka 577005, India*

Correspondence should be addressed to Ashwini Ramakrishna; winidoc@rediffmail.com

Academic Editors: A. Celebić and P. Lopez Jornet

Supplementary teeth in the dental arch are a rare occurrence. Though they are mostly reported in association with syndromes they can also present in the absence of systemic pathology. This paper reports a case with multiple supernumerary teeth along with discussion of the frequency, types, complications, and management of such occurrence.

1. Introduction

Extra set of teeth in the dental arch are designated as supernumerary which is a well-known dental phenomenon. This dental anomaly is common to primary and permanent dentitions in which the jaw has more teeth than normal. The term supernumerary frequently encompasses the supplementary teeth which are extra teeth that resemble those of the normal series. This developmental anomaly can occur either in the maxilla or in the mandible and is frequently seen in association with syndromes such as Gardner's syndrome, Cleidocranial dysplasia, Trichorhinophalangeal syndrome, and cleft of the lip and palate. They can also be present in the absence of systemic pathology [1].

Prevalence rate of supernumerary teeth for permanent and primary dentitions is said to be between 0.5%–5.3%, and 0.2%–0.8% respectively [2]. However, the prevalence range depends on the methodology for detection and variation in the population. Supernumerary teeth can be unilateral, bilateral, single, or multiple presenting in either of the jaws. There is an apparent predilection of certain sites for supernumeraries and the most common ones are the maxillary mesiodens, followed by supernumeraries of maxillary molar region and those in mandibular premolar region [3]. The supernumerary premolars are mostly seen in the permanent dentition, the prevalence of which is in between 0.075% and 0.26% and they account for only 10% of all the supernumerary cases [2]. Studies on nonsyndrome multiple supernumerary teeth have found 60.9% of the total sample to occur in the mandible and 44.8% in the mandibular premolar region [4].

Morphologically supernumerary teeth are classified into three types, Tuberculate, Supplemental and Conoid forms. Supplemental, tooth is defined as tooth that may resemble a tooth of the normal series [5]. The presence of multiple supernumerary premolars in the absence of any associated syndromes or systemic conditions is relatively rare. This paper describes multiple unilaterally distributed supplemental type of supernumerary premolars of the mandibular arch.

2. Case Report

A 26-year-old male came to the dental clinic with the chief complaint of pain in the lower left back tooth region. His familial, medical, and dental histories were noncontributory. There was no extra oral deformity in the form of cleft lip or palate and the clavicles were normal. Intraoral examination revealed regular set of permanent dentition along with two completely erupted supernumerary premolars on the left side of the mandibular arch (Figure 1). Both of these teeth presented lingual to the permanent first and second

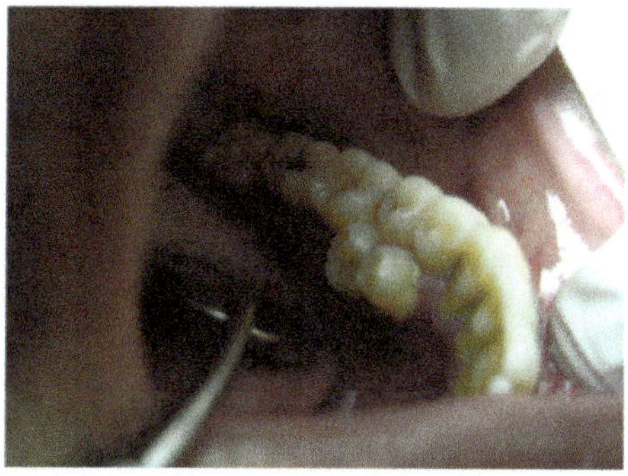

FIGURE 1: Supernumerary premolars presenting lingual to 34, 35.

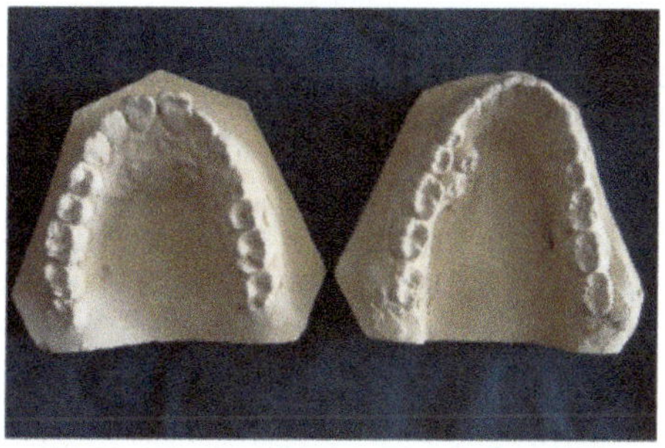

FIGURE 2: Model cast of maxillary and mandibular arch with the pathology.

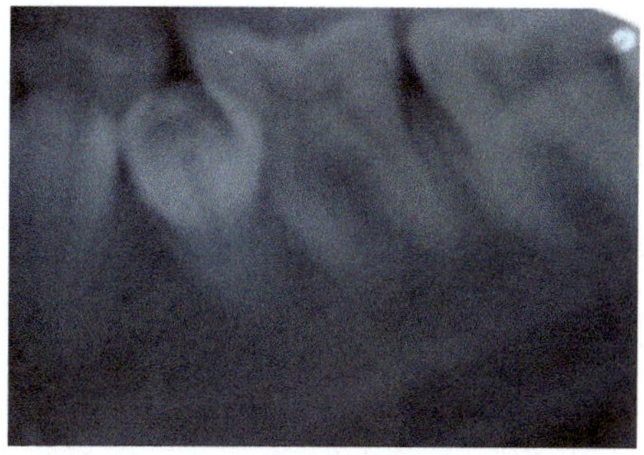

FIGURE 3: Intraoral periapical radiograph of the supernumerary premolars.

premolars and resembled the permanent premolars in morphology and hence were considered as a supplemental type of supernumerary teeth. Generalized plaque and calculus accumulation was present on the teeth along with generalized gingivitis.

Intraoral periapical radiograph (Figure 2) and an orthopantmogram of the patient were taken to evaluate the complete dentition. The radiographs revealed two supernumerary teeth placed lingual to the regular set of mandibular premolars and did not reveal any other impacted or supernumerary teeth or any other pathologies. The supernumerary teeth observed were of normal size and shape with completely formed roots and resembled premolars.

Impressions of upper and lower arches were made and study models were prepared to evaluate the position of the erupted supernumerary teeth and malalignment of the dentition (Figure 3). The patient was informed about the presence of additional number of teeth and was educated about the difficulties associated in maintaining the oral hygiene status and was advised extraction of the same. As family history, medical history, general examination, and extra oral examinations were noncontributory, the diagnosis of nonsyndrome-associated supernumerary was made. Oral hygiene measures were instituted and the follow-up was uneventful.

3. Discussion

The presentation of multiple supernumerary teeth in the absence of association with other systemic diseases or syndromes is rare. The prevalence rates of supernumerary premolars are variedly reported in different studies due to the differences in population, age, ethnicity, and applied radiographic techniques [2]. The most common localization for multiple supernumerary teeth is the premolar region (62.1%) and especially that the lower premolar region is a characteristic location for nonsyndrome multiple supernumerary teeth [6]. And the literature states that supernumerary premolars are more frequent in males than females [2]. A majority of supernumerary premolars are of the supplemental type and develop later than their normal counterparts. Patients with a previous history of supernumerary teeth have a 24% possibility of developing single or multiple supernumerary premolars at a later age [7].

Numerous theories have been proposed for the development of supernumerary teeth. The oldest is the theory of Atavism which proposed the development of supernumerary teeth as related to phylogenetic reversion to extinct primates with three pairs of incisors. However, these theories have been discounted now. Two other popularly accepted theories are the Dichotomy theory, which stated that the splitting of the tooth bud into two equal or different-sized parts results in the formation of two teeth of equal size, or one normal and one dysmorphic tooth, respectively [4], and Dental Lamina Hyperactivity theory, which suggests that supernumeraries are found as a result of local, independent, and conditioned hyperactivity of dental lamina [5]. Since individuals with some other dental anomalies and developmental disorders are the ones who frequently present with the supernumerary teeth, combination of hereditary and environmental factors have also been considered in the etiology [6].

Supernumerary teeth can be classified based on morphology as accessory and supplemental and based on syndrome as syndrome associated and nonsyndrome associated [8]. The prevalence for nonsyndrome multiple supernumerary teeth is less than 1%. The male to female ratio has been reported as 9 : 2 [6]. Supernumerary teeth are associated with Gardner's syndrome, Cleidocranial dysplasia, Fabry-Anderson Syndrome, Ehlers-Danlos Syndrome, Down's syndrome, Crouzon's Disease, Hallermann Streiff Syndrome, and Orodigitofacial Dysostosis.

Supernumeraries may erupt normally or may remain impacted or inverted in the jaw or reach heterotopic position or show abnormal eruptive patterns. Various pathological conditions such as delayed eruption or noneruption, displacement of permanent teeth, resorption or malformation of adjacent roots, and cystic formation may be caused because of these teeth [6]. Their occurrence has also been noted in gingiva, soft palate, nasal cavity, maxillary sinus, sphenomaxillary fissure, ophthalmic conchae, maxillary tuberosity, incisive suture, and between the orbit and the brain [9].

Supernumerary teeth are usually asymptomatic and most cases are an incidental finding during a dental visit. Usually if the teeth are asymptomatic, it can be left in place and kept under observation. Surgical removal should be considered based on the pathological sequelae associated with it. And an orthopantomogram should be advised as a part of routine investigation to rule out the presence of multiple supernumerary teeth. In the premolar area, common complications associated with supernumerary teeth are cyst formation (9%) and damage to neighbouring teeth (13%) [8]. Also reports of compression of the supernumerary premolars on the adjacent teeth and their closeness to the mental and inferior dental nerves may lead to pain [2]. Supernumeraries can be associated with other dental anomalies, such as hypodontia, taurodontism, germination, and macrodontia [6].

The treatment methods and the timing of surgical removal of supernumerary premolars is much debated among clinicians [10]. Formation of supernumerary premolars are often delayed, and these teeth generally develop on the lingual side of the normal premolars. Developing crypts of the supernumeraries in young patients may be masked by the roots of the normal premolars, which makes early detection on routine radiographs difficult [11]. Hence it is imperative to evaluate the patient clinically and radiologically when a single supernumerary is detected to rule out association with syndromes and for its appropriate and timely management. And it is important on our part to educate the patient about the complications which can arise when the patient is reluctant to the therapy.

References

[1] S. Mali, F. R. Karjodkar, S. Sontakke, and K. Sansare, "Supernumerary teeth in non-syndromic patients," *Imaging Science in Dentistry*, vol. 42, no. 1, pp. 41–45, 2012.

[2] G.-Ş. Kaya, G. Yapıcı, M. Ömezli, and E. Dayı, "Non syndromic supernumerary premolars," *Medicina Oral Patologia Oral y Cirugia Bucal*, vol. 16, no. 4, pp. e522–e525, 2011.

[3] K. Parikh and N. C. Soni, "Non-Syndrome multiple supplemental supernumerary teeth," *The Journal of Ahmedabad Dental Collge and Hospital*, vol. 1, no. 2, pp. 43–47, 2010.

[4] A. Shah, D. S. Gill, C. Tredwin, and F. B. Naini, "Diagnosis and management of supernumerary teeth," *Dental Update*, vol. 35, no. 8, pp. 510–520, 2008.

[5] P. Pallavi Pandey, V. Arun Prasad Rao, R. Shetty, N. Venugopal Reddy, and M. Preeti, "Non syndrome associated bilateral supernumerary teeth in the maxillary premolar region," *International Journal of Dental Case Reports*, vol. 2, no. 3, pp. 21–25, 2012.

[6] A. Açikgöz, G. Açikgöz, U. Tunga, and F. Otan, "Characteristics and prevalence of non-syndrome multiple supernumerary teeth: a retrospective study," *Dentomaxillofacial Radiology*, vol. 35, no. 3, pp. 185–190, 2006.

[7] R. Sharma, P. Sharma, P. Kumar, and P. Kumar, "Non-syndromal multiple supernumerary premolars in siblings- a case report," *Indian Journal of Dental Sciences*, vol. 3, no. 4, pp. 78–80, 2012.

[8] N. Kalra, S. Chaudhary, and S. Sanghi, "Non-syndrome multiple supplemental supernumerary teeth," *Journal of Indian Society of Pedodontics and Preventive Dentistry*, vol. 23, no. 1, pp. 46–48, 2005.

[9] S. Chandra Raj, H. Malini Rath, J. Mishra, and A. Kumar Barik, "Multiple non-syndromic hyperdontia—report of an unusual case," *International Journal of Clinical Dental Science*, vol. 2, no. 3, pp. 77–80, 2011.

[10] S. Gupta and M. Goswami, "Asymptomatic nonsyndromic multiple supernumerary premolars," *International Journal of Clinical Paediatric Dentistry*, vol. 5, no. 1, pp. 84–86, 2012.

[11] S.-Y. Cho, "Supernumerary premolars associated with dens evaginatus: report of 2 cases," *Journal of the Canadian Dental Association*, vol. 71, no. 6, pp. 390–393, 2005.

Transmigration of Mandibular Canines

N. Umashree,[1] Avinash Kumar,[2] and Tejavathi Nagaraj[3]

[1] *Department of Oral Medicine and Maxillofacial Radiology, Al-Badar Dental College and Hospital, Gulbarga, Karnataka, India*
[2] *Department of Orthodontics and Dentofacial Orthopedics, Al-Badar Dental College and Hospital, Gulbarga, Karnataka, India*
[3] *Department of Oral Medicine and Maxillofacial Radiology, Sri Rajiv Gandhi College of Dental Sciences and Hospital, Karnataka, India*

Correspondence should be addressed to N. Umashree; dr.umashree@gmail.com

Academic Editors: R. Crespi and Y. Nakagawa

The purpose of this paper is to present the first case of unusual reverse oblique (110 degrees to midsagittal plane) migration of mandibular right canine crossing the jaw midline and piercing the lower border of the mandible at the level of the opposite canine and also to report two more cases of transmigrated mandibular canine and one case of transmigrating mandibular canine. Mandibular canines are "cornerstone" of dental arch; their importance is manifested by their efficiency in masticatory function, stability of dental arch, and aid in maintaining natural facial expression. Early detection of this anomaly can help preserving these canines by orthodontic intervention or by surgical transplantation. This developmental anomaly is properly diagnosed by radiographic evaluation, which is primarily based on the panoramic radiograph. In patients with overretained deciduous canines or missing permanent canines, an intraoral radiograph should be supplemented with panoramic radiograph. This paper discusses the importance of early diagnosis of canine transmigration in treatment planning and reviews the various possible treatment options.

1. Introduction

Migration of teeth is a well-documented ectopia, the mechanism that causes the migration of a tooth is still not clear [1]. An impacted tooth migrates to a location some distance away from the site of its development but usually remains within the same side of the arch [2]. Migration of a tooth across the jaw midline without the influence of any pathological entity is called transmigration [3]. The intraosseous migration of a tooth apparently starts during the early mixed dentition stage and may take place over a period of many years [4].

The incidence of transmigration has increased over the past 50 years with the introduction of dental panoramic tomography. Aydin et al. reported a panoramic radiographic survey of 4500 patients in a Turkish subpopulation, which revealed 14 cases of canine transmigration, out of which six were maxillary and eight mandibular canines, with an incidence of 0.31% [5]. Javid reported a radiographic survey of 1000 students which revealed only 1 case of transmigrated impacted mandibular canine [6]. Aktan and associates reported a panoramic radiographic survey of 5000 patients and observed that transmigration of impacted mandibular canines was greater than the maxillary canines. Women were affected more often than men [7]. Most of the cases reported in the literature were unilateral mandibular canine transmigration [3–6] and a very few were cases of bilateral canine transmigration [8, 9].

The aim of this paper is to report the first unusual case of reverse oblique migration of mandibular right canine crossing the jaw midline and piercing the lower border of the mandible which has never been reported in the literature so far. We also report additional two cases of transmigrated mandibular canine and one case of mandibular canine with a tendency to transmigrate. This paper also discusses the importance of early diagnosis in treatment planning and reviews the various possible treatment options for canine transmigration.

2. Case Reports

Case 1. A 20-year-old male presented with pain in front of the ear while opening and closing the mouth for one year. Intraoral examination revealed permanent maxillary

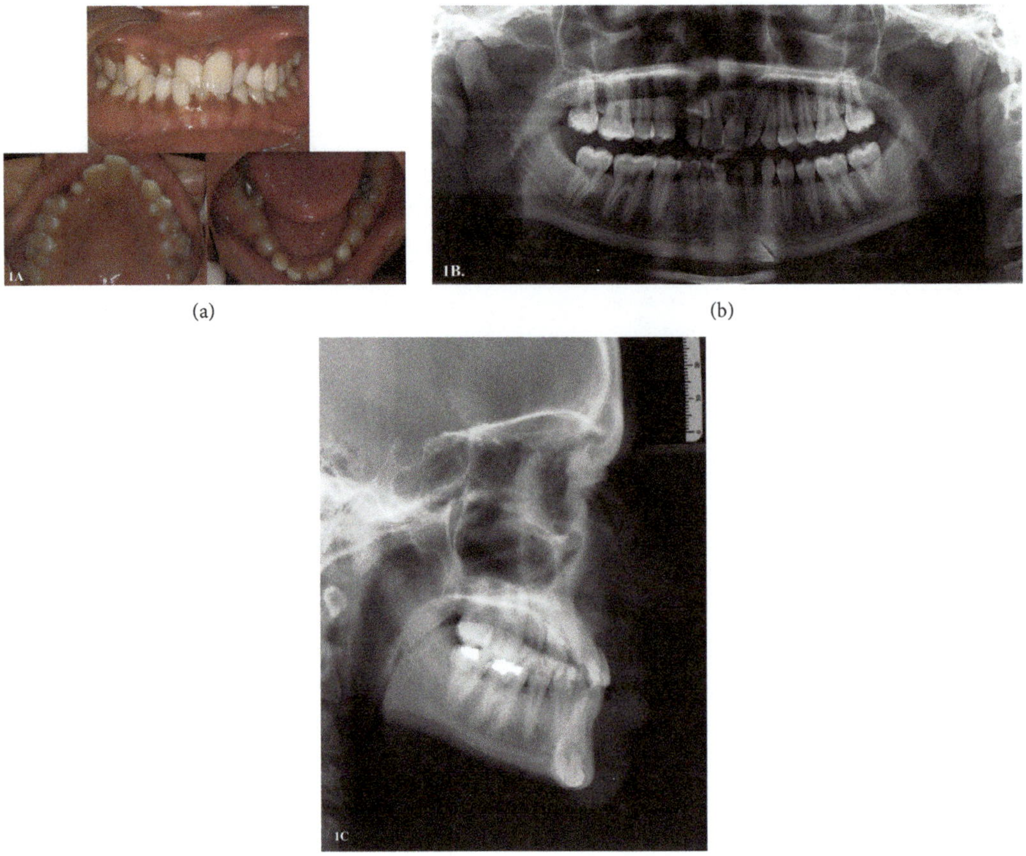

(a) (b) (c)

Figure 1: (a) Intraoral photographs showing clinically missing upper right canine, lower right canine and central incisors, and retained deciduous lower right canine and central incisor. (b) Panoramic radiograph showing impacted upper right canine and a reverse obliquely transmigrated lower right canine with its crown piercing the lower border of mandible at the level of opposite canine. (c) Lateral cephalogram showing obliquely lying lower right canine near the lower border of mandible.

right central and lateral incisor in cross-bite, peg-shaped maxillary lateral incisors, clinically missing permanent maxillary right canine, mandibular central incisors, and right canine, and retained deciduous mandibular right canine and left central incisor. TMJ examination revealed clicking and deviation of the jaw to right side while closing the mouth (Figure 1(a)). A panoramic radiograph was requested, which revealed impacted and ectopically erupting maxillary right canine, congenitally missing lower central incisors and reverse oblique (110° to midsagittal plane) transmigration of mandibular right canine crossing the jaw midline and piercing the lower border of the mandible and causing erosion of the inner (endosteal) cortex at the level of opposite canine. The radiographic position of the tooth was not in accordance with the classification given by Mupparapu [10] for mandibular canine transmigration (Figure 1(b)). The lateral cephalogram revealed obliquely lying permanent mandibular right canine near the lower border of mandible (Figure 1(c)). No pathologic finding was associated with the transmigrated tooth. Surgical removal of the canine was decided. However, the patient declined the surgical intervention as the tooth was asymptomatic. The patient was informed of the consequence of pathologic fracture and was scheduled for periodic radiographic monitoring.

Case 2. A 30-year-old female presented with the chief complaint of pain in upper left molar area. Intraoral examination showed a decayed upper first molar, and tooth simulating a mandibular left canine in the midline; the tooth was rotated and retained deciduous lower left canine. An intraoral periapical radiograph revealed erupted and transmigrated mandibular left canine in midline (Figure 2). The radiographic position of tooth was in accordance with type 5 transmigration pattern classified by Mupparapu [10]. The patient was informed of the condition and orthodontic alignment and reshaping of midline canine tooth with central incisor, and left lateral incisor with canine crown was decided for esthetic and functional reasons.

Case 3. A 15-year-old female patient presented with the chief complaint of protruded upper front teeth. Intraoral examination revealed increased overjet, retained deciduous mandibular right canine, and clinically missing permanent right canine. Panoramic radiograph revealed transmigrated

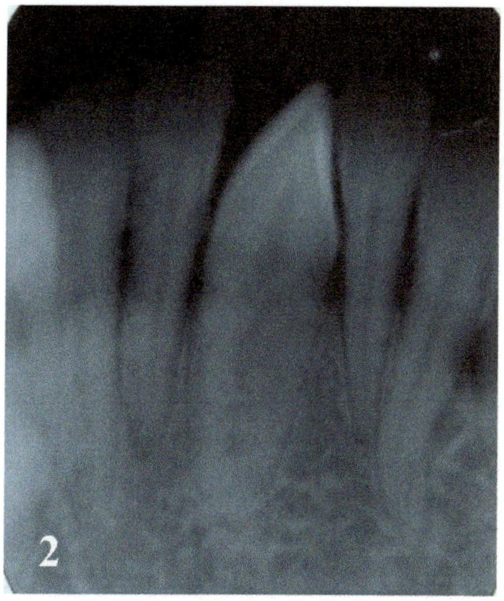

FIGURE 2: Periapical radiograph showing transmigrated and erupted lower left canine in the midline.

permanent right mandibular canine under the apices of the incisors. The radiographic position of tooth was in accordance with type 1 mandibular canine transmigration classified by Mupparapu [10] (Figure 3(a)). There was no pathologic finding associated with the transmigrated tooth. Surgical removal of the canine was done due to its unfavorable position (Figure 3(b)). Extraction of deciduous mandibular right canine and replacement with an endosseous implant and crown was advised.

Case 4. A 12-year-old female patient presented with a complaint of spacing between upper front teeth. Intraoral examination revealed all deciduous canines intact and clinically nonpalpable all permanent canines, retained deciduous lower lateral incisors and clinically missing permanent lower lateral incisors. A Midline diastema was present in the upper arch. Panoramic radiograph revealed congenitally missing lower lateral incisors and an ectopically erupting mandibular right canine excessively tilted mesially (Figure 4). According to Howard's [11] criteria for canine transmigration, the axial inclination of mandibular right canine to midsagittal plane was 45°, and in addition it was associated with congenitally missing lower lateral incisors; hence, there is an increased tendency for the mandibular right canine to transmigrate. Therefore, preventive and interceptive treatment such as an extraction of the deciduous canine, surgical exposure of the ectopically erupting permanent canine followed by orthodontic treatment to pull the canine into the dental arch to its ideal position, was advised.

3. Discussion

Tarsitano et al. defined transmigration as a phenomenon in which an unerupted mandibular canine migrates, crossing the mandibular midline [12]. According to Joshi [3] migration of a tooth across the jaw midline without the influence of any pathological entity is called as transmigration. Javid [6] suggested that transmigration should be considered when half the length of the crown crosses the midline.

In 2002, Mupparapu [10] classified mandibular canine transmigration depending on its path of deviation into five types. Type 1: canine positioned mesioangularly across the midline within the jaw bone, labial or lingual to anterior teeth, and the crown portion of the tooth crossing the midline (45.6%). Type 2: canine horizontally impacted near the inferior border of the mandible below the apices of the incisors (20%). Type 3: canine erupting either mesial or distal to the opposite canine (14%). Type 4: canine horizontally impacted near the inferior border of the mandible below the apices of either premolars or molars on the opposite side (17%). Type 5: canine positioned vertically in the midline (the long axis of the tooth crossing the midline) irrespective of eruption status (1.5%).

In the present study, the radiographic appearance of the transmigrated canine in Case 3 was in accordance with type 1. In Case 2, the radiographic position of the tooth was in accordance with type 5, where the transmigrated mandibular left canine was erupted in the midline. Case 1 was not in accordance with any of the types described previously, as mandibular right canine was in a reverse oblique (110° to midsagittal plane) position, crossing the jaw midline, and piercing the lower border of the mandible at the level of the opposite canine. Hence, Case 1 is the first of its kind being reported in the literature.

Pérez et al. [13] observed patients in the age ranging from 8 to 74 years old, with the mean age being 21.9 ± 13.4 years old. The greatest prevalence of transmigrated canines was found in the age group that ranges from 0 to 20 years, which accounted for 56.7% of the sample. The incidence of transmigrated canines is much higher in females than in males and there is no plausible reason why it occurs more often in women [3, 5, 7, 9, 12, 14].

The frequency of canine transmigration is more in the mandible than maxilla. It may be due to the larger distance between the root apices and lower border of mandible, and as the migratory canine is lodged in the symphyseal area, this area will grow larger to accommodate the migratory canine. Transmigration of maxillary canines is very rare, which may be due to the shorter distance between the roots of maxillary incisors and the floor of the nasal fossa and restriction of the path of tooth movement by the roots of adjacent teeth [14].

The etiology of this rare developmental anomaly is not yet known and there are many contributing factors to its occurrence. Heredity has been suggested as a causative factor. The most commonly accepted explanation is the abnormal displacement of the dental lamina in the embryonic life and noneruption of such canines. Noidine [15] emphasized that even a very small obstacle, such as a small root fragment or an odontoma, would be sufficient to divert a tooth from its normal path of eruption. Ando et al. [16] suggested that agenesis of permanent lateral incisors may result in deviated path of eruption and hence the transmigration. In our first case described previously, transmigrated mandibular canine was associated with congenitally missing central incisors which could be the cause for the transmigration.

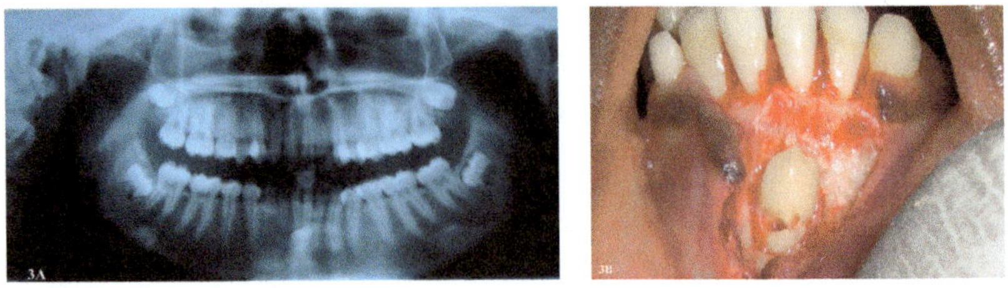

(a) (b)

FIGURE 3: (a) Panoramic radiograph showing transmigrated lower right canine under the apices of the incisors. (b) Surgically exposed transmigrated lower right canine.

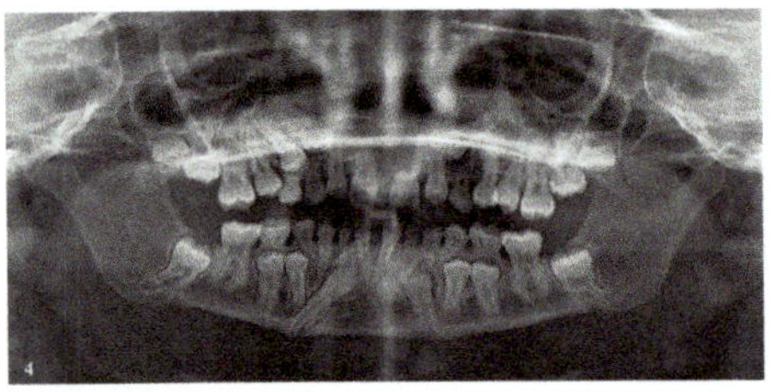

FIGURE 4: Panoramic radiograph showing an ectopically erupting mandibular right canine excessively tilted mesially and agenesis of lower lateral incisors.

Al-Waheidi [17] suggested that transmigrated canines are usually associated with a cystic lesion and that the presence of a cyst at the crown of the canine may facilitate the migration process. Other authors, such as Joshi and Howard, did not report any associated cystic lesions with transmigration. However, the role of cystic lesions in the etiology of transmigration is difficult to determine. A cyst is an expansive lesion and is more likely to displace the tooth in any direction in the path of the least resistance. Among the transmigrated mandibular canine, cases reported here, 2 impacted and 1 erupted, were not found to be associated with any pathology.

3.1. Diagnosis. The presence of transmigration must be suspected in cases where lower permanent canine is clinically absent from the dental arch along with an abnormal retention of lower deciduous canine. The prolonged retention of the deciduous canine is quite often a reliable clue leading to the discovery of its impacted permanent successor. In this present paper retained deciduous canine was present in all four cases supporting the findings by Joshi [3] and Pérez et al. [13] in which 70.8% and 48% of the sample had retained deciduous canines, respectively.

The other clinical factors associated with canine transmigration are agenesis of lateral incisors, proclined lower incisors, and deviated dental midline [16]. When two or more of these characteristics are present and the patient is 10-to-13 year old, the patient should be evaluated radiographically for impaction and transmigration of permanent canine. Clinically, transmigration is usually asymptomatic. Joshi [3] reported that symptoms such as pain or oppression of mandibular nerve owing to the transmigration of canine in their patients were not observed.

It is possible in the routine checkup that the intraoral periapical radiograph may fail to reveal transmigrated canines. These canines may not be visible in periapical radiographs as some lie horizontally below the inferior alveolar canal or migrate toward the midline. This emphasizes the importance of a panoramic radiograph in diagnosis of canine transmigration. In Case 1, transmigration was detected only on panoramic radiograph. Since the advent of panoramic radiography, it has become very easy to detect a migratory tooth.

Howard [11] observed the influence of the axial inclination of impacted canines on its migration. The author observed that those canines with axial inclination between 25° and 30° to the midsagittal plane represent a group of unerupted canines that are displaced but not migrating across the mandibular midline. Those impacted canines that are between 30° and 95° are a group that tends to cross the midline. An overlap appears to exist between 30° and 50°. When this angle exceeds 50°, crossing the midline becomes a rule. Joshi [3] reported the axial inclination to the midsagittal plane of migratory canine ranged from 45° to 95°. However, in our first case the described inclination of transmigrated tooth to midsagittal plane was 110^0 which has not been reported in the literature.

Ando et al. [16] observed transmigration of canine in their patient for 6 years. During this time, the canine moved from its original position to a place near the mental foramen on the opposite side. They also suggested that the greatest amount of movement of transmigratory canine is more rapid before the formation of its root. However, Dhooria et al. [18] observed a fairly rapid movement even after completion of the root formation, about 3 to 4 mm in one of their patients during 1 year. Whereas in our first case, the mandibular right canine is transmigrated in a reverse oblique angulation, piercing the lower border of the mandible. A very thin plate of periosteal cortical bone is left covering the crown of the tooth. The tooth apex is closed and the patient is twenty-year old; if the tooth still has its inherent eruptive force, it may pierce the lower border of the mandible.

3.2. Treatment Options. Treatment considerations for transmigrated tooth depend on the stage of development, distance

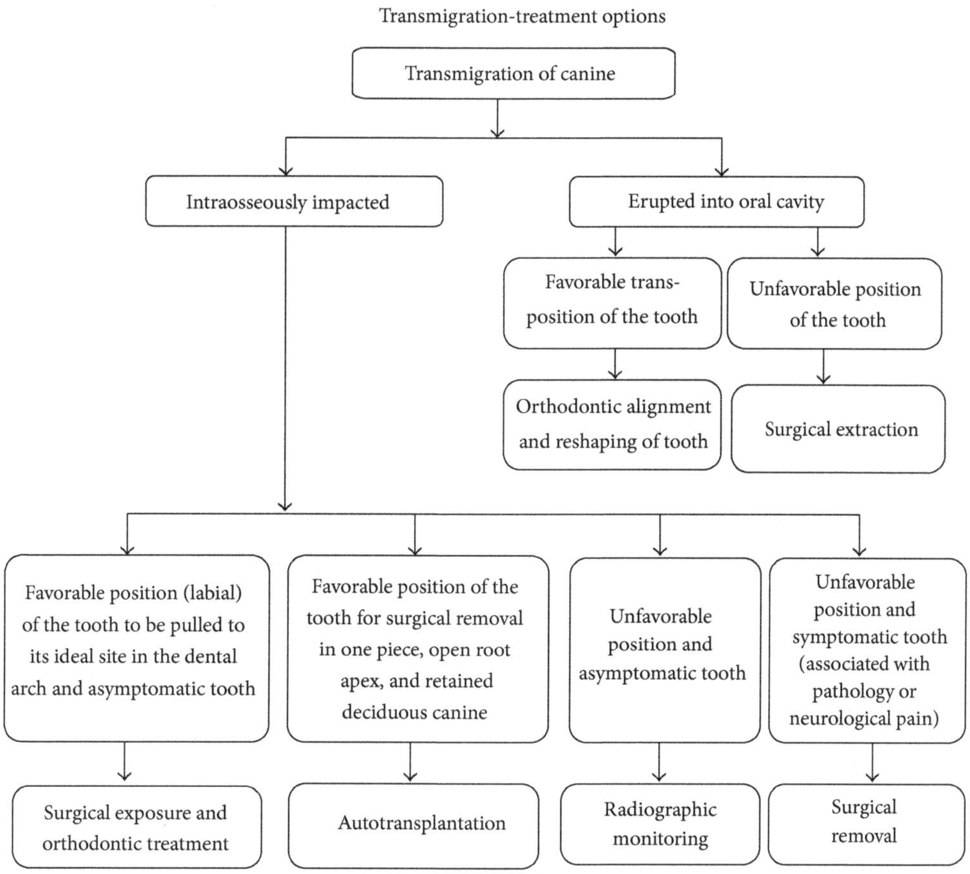

FIGURE 5: Flowchart depicting the various treatment options to aid in decision making for the management of canine transmigration.

of migration, and position and angulation of the tooth when it is diagnosed.

3.2.1. Preventive and Interceptive Treatment. A small root fragment or an odontoma interferes with the normal path of the eruption of the tooth, hence, their removal would facilitate its eruption. Taguchi et al. [19] reported, after removal of the odontoma and surgical exposure an improvement in the position of the associated canines. Vichi and Franchi [20] suggested that an 8-to 9-year-old patient with an excessive mesial inclination of the unerupted mandibular permanent canine should be kept under critical observation with periodical panoramic radiographic examination. If the position of the unerupted mandibular canine is observed to progressively tilt more to the mesial, interceptive measures should be taken. The preventive and interceptive treatment includes extraction of the retained deciduous canine and surgical exposure of the impacted canine followed by orthodontic treatment. This emphasizes the importance of early diagnosis to correct this problem before the tooth migrates too far from its original location.

3.2.2. Surgical Exposure and Orthodontic Treatment. The transmigrated canine, when detected early, can be surgically exposed and moved to its ideal position by using orthodontic forces. Wertz [21] reported the successful correction of three cases using orthodontic treatment, where lower canine was transmigrated labially. Kumar and associates [22] recently reported one case of successful eruption of transmigrated lower left canine after orthodontic traction, which was located with its crown below the apices of the right central incisor. However, if the crown of such a tooth migrates past the opposite incisor area or if the apex is seen to have migrated past the apex of the adjacent lateral incisor, it might be mechanically impossible to bring it into place [2].

Transplantation is another approach to save the transmigrated tooth. If the transmigrated canine is in favorable position for surgical removal in one piece asymptomatically and there is sufficient space with retained deciduous canine, transplantation may be undertaken. Timing of transplant is very important since a primary objective is to obtain maximum root length. The procedure is best performed when the root length of the tooth is between one-half and three-fourths complete for the reestablishment of blood supply. The prognosis is diminished as the root apex nears closure. The length of time from removal to reinsertion should be minimal; ideally, this is a nonstop relocation. Desiccation of the periodontal ligament can cause resorption, ankylosis, and failure [23]. Howard [11] transplanted a transmigrated canine when there was enough space, and retained deciduous canine was present to accommodate the tooth. Slagsvold and Bjercke autotransplanted the premolars with partly formed roots with successful results [24, 25].

Retrograde endodontic treatments have been performed simultaneous to transplantation with varying degrees of success; such treatment introduces a foreign substance into the site, possibly inducing an inflammatory reaction, but it greatly increases the length of the procedure and the time the transplant remains out of the mouth. Further, such manipulation will assuredly traumatize the root surface [23]. It would be more judicious to perform the root canal treatment after the periodontal ligament attachment has readapted if such treatment proves necessary. Verma et al. [26] reported a successful transplantation of transmigrated mandibular right canine (type 2 of Mupparapu) into the prepared socket of retained deciduous canine. After one year of followup they observed good periodontal condition with no gingival recession, but they also noted external root resorption at the distal side of the apex in the panoramic radiograph and axial section of CT scan.

3.2.3. Surgical Removal. Wetz [21] stated that once the canine crown migrated past the adjacent lateral incisor root apex, orthodontically it is impossible to reposition the tooth to its ideal position and in cases where the transmigrated canine is associated with pathology or neurological symptoms, surgical removal is indicated. Bruszt [27] clearly showed that the transmigrated tooth maintains its nervous innervation from the side where the germ is formed. Joshi [3] suggested that it is important to anesthetize the nerve of the side to which the canine belongs, when the extraction is to be attempted under local anesthesia. However, if general anesthesia is to be used, this problem does not arise. He also suggested that the surgical removal of a transmigrated tooth should be done as far as possible through an intraoral approach. Nevertheless, if necessary, an extra oral approach can be used in extreme unusual cases of canine transmigration.

3.2.4. Radiographic Monitoring. Impacted and transmigrated tooth can be left in place if it is symptomless and not associated with any pathology. In these patients, a series of periodic radiographs should be taken to check the status of the transmigrated tooth. A continuous worsening of position or development of cystic lesion and in case of severe root resorption of adjacent teeth, surgical removal is indicated [2].

3.2.5. Transmigrated and Transpositioned Canine. In cases where the transmigrated canine is erupted and transpositioned in the dental arch, the tooth can be orthodontically aligned and recontoured accordingly. Trakyali et al. [28] reported the management of a transmigrated lower right canine, which was erupted between the left central and lateral incisors. The crown was recontoured to simulate a lateral incisor, and an acceptable aesthetic and functional outcome was gained.

A flowchart is provided which summarizes the various treatment options mentioned previously to guide in the decision making for management of canine transmigration (Figure 5).

4. Conclusion

With early radiographic detection and timely interception with surgical and orthodontic treatment, mandibular canines which have an increased tendency towards transmigration can be guided to erupt to its ideal position in the dental arch. However, if transmigration is detected at a later stage, autotransplantation is a better treatment option. Future studies may lead to a better understanding of this complex natured developmental anomaly leading to improvement in diagnosis and treatment.

References

[1] Y. Shapira, G. Borell, M. M. Kuftinec, and O. Nahlieli, "Bringing impacted mandibular second premolars into occlusion," *Journal of the American Dental Association*, vol. 127, no. 7, pp. 1075–1078, 1996.

[2] S. Camilleri and E. Scerri, "Transmigration of mandibular canines—a review of the literature and a report of five cases," *Angle Orthodontist*, vol. 73, no. 6, pp. 753–762, 2003.

[3] M. R. Joshi, "Transmigrant mandibular canines: a record of 28 cases and a retrospective review of the literature," *The Angle Orthodontist*, vol. 71, pp. 12–22, 2001.

[4] S. Peck, "On the phenomenon of intraosseous migration of nonerupting teeth," *American Journal of Orthodontics and Dentofacial Orthopedics*, vol. 113, no. 5, pp. 515–517, 1998.

[5] U. Aydin, H. H. Yilmaz, and D. Yildirim, "Incidence of canine impaction and transmigration in a patient population," *Dentomaxillofacial Radiology*, vol. 33, no. 3, pp. 164–169, 2004.

[6] B. Javid, "Transmigration of impacted mandibular cuspids," *International Journal of Oral Surgery*, vol. 14, no. 6, pp. 547–549, 1985.

[7] A. M. Aktan, S. Kara, F. Akgünlü, and S. Malkoç, "The incidence of canine transmigration and tooth impaction in a Turkish subpopulation," *European Journal of Orthodontics*, vol. 32, pp. 575–581, 2010.

[8] M. R. Joshi, N. R. Daruwala, and H. C. Ahuja, "Bilateral transmigration of mandibular canines," *British Journal of Orthodontics*, vol. 9, no. 1, pp. 57–58, 1982.

[9] M. M. Kuftinec, Y. Shapira, and O. Nahlieli, "A case report. Bilateral transmigration of impacted mandibular canines," *The Journal of the American Dental Association*, vol. 126, no. 7, pp. 1022–1024, 1995.

[10] M. Mupparapu, "Patterns of intra-osseous transmigration and ectopic eruption of mandibular canines: review of literature and report of nine additional cases," *Dentomaxillofacial Radiology*, vol. 31, no. 6, pp. 355–360, 2002.

[11] R. D. Howard, "The anomalous mandibular canine," *British Journal of Orthodontics*, vol. 3, pp. 117–119, 1976.

[12] J. J. Tarsitano, J. W. Wooten, and J. T. Burditt, "Transmigration of nonerupted mandibular canines: report of cases," *The Journal of the American Dental Association*, vol. 82, no. 6, pp. 1395–1397, 1971.

[13] A. M. Pérez, M. I. L. Berrocal, C. B. Dorado, F. F. Cáliz, and J. M. M. González, "Transmigrated canines: review and update," *Journal of Clinical and Experimental Dentistry*, vol. 3, no. 3, pp. e235–e239, 2011.

[14] F. S. Ryan, P. Batra, H. Witherow, and M. Calvert, "Transmigration of a maxillary canine. A case report," *Primary Dental Care*, vol. 12, no. 2, pp. 70–72, 2005.

[15] A. M. Nodine, "Aberrant teeth, their history, causes, and treatment," *Dental Items of Interest*, vol. 65, pp. 440–451, 1943.

[16] S. Ando, K. Aizaea, T. Nakashima, Y. Sanka, K. Shimbo, and K. Kiyokawa, "Transmigration process of impacted mandibular cuspid," *The Journal of Nihon University School of Dentistry*, vol. 6, pp. 66–71, 1964.

[17] E. M. H. Al-Waheidi, "Transmigration of unerupted mandibular canines: a literature review and a report of five cases," *Quintessence International*, vol. 27, no. 1, pp. 27–31, 1996.

[18] H. S. Dhooria, R. S. Sathawane, R. N. Mody, and S. B. Sakarde, "Transmigration of mandibular canines," *Journal of the Indian Dental Association*, vol. 58, no. 9, pp. 348–357, 1986.

[19] Y. Taguchi, J. Kurol, H. Kobayashi, and T. Noda, "Eruption disturbances of mandibular permanent canines in Japanese children," *International Journal of Paediatric Dentistry*, vol. 11, no. 2, pp. 98–102, 2001.

[20] M. Vichi and L. Franchi, "The transmigration of the permanent lower canine," *Minerva Stomatologica*, vol. 40, no. 9, pp. 579–589, 1991.

[21] R. A. Wertz, "Treatment of transmigrated mandibular canines," *American Journal of Orthodontics and Dentofacial Orthopedics*, vol. 106, no. 4, pp. 419–427, 1994.

[22] S. Kumar, A. S. Urala, A. T. Kamath, P. Jayaswal, and A. Valiathan, "Unusual intraosseous transmigration of impacted tooth," *Imaging Science in Dentistry*, vol. 42, pp. 47–54, 2012.

[23] W. M. Northway and S. Konigsberg, "Autogenic tooth transplantation. The 'state of the art'," *American Journal of Orthodontics*, vol. 77, no. 2, pp. 146–162, 1980.

[24] O. Slagsvold and B. Bjercke, "Autotransplantation of premolars with partly formed roots. A radiographic study of root growth," *American Journal of Orthodontics*, vol. 66, no. 4, pp. 355–366, 1974.

[25] O. Slagsvold and B. Bjercke, "Indications for autotransplantation in cases of missing premolars," *American Journal of Orthodontics*, vol. 74, no. 3, pp. 241–257, 1978.

[26] S. L. Verma, V. P. Sharma, and G. P. Singh, "Management of a transmigrated mandibular canine," *Journal of Orthopaedic Science*, vol. 11, no. 1, pp. 23–28, 2012.

[27] P. Bruszt, "Neurological anomaly associated with extreme malposition of a mandibular canine," *Oral Surgery, Oral Medicine, Oral Pathology*, vol. 11, no. 1, pp. 89–90, 1958.

[28] G. Trakyali, S. K. Cildir, and N. Sandalli, "Orthodontic treatment of a transmigrated mandibular canine: a case report," *Australian Orthodontic Journal*, vol. 26, no. 2, pp. 195–200, 2010.

Dentinal Dysplasia Type I: A Case Report with a 6-Year Followup

Sezin Ozer,[1] Bora Ozden,[2] Feyza Otan Ozden,[3] and Kaan Gunduz[4]

[1] *Department of Pediatric Dentistry, Faculty of Dentistry, Ondokuz Mayıs University, Atakum, 55139 Samsun, Turkey*
[2] *Department of Oral and Maxillofacial Surgery, Faculty of Dentistry, Ondokuz Mayıs University, 55139 Samsun, Turkey*
[3] *Department of Periodontology, Faculty of Dentistry, Ondokuz Mayıs University, Kurupelit, 55139 Samsun, Turkey*
[4] *Department of Oral Diagnosis and Radiology, Faculty of Dentistry, Ondokuz Mayıs University, Kurupelit, 55139 Samsun, Turkey*

Correspondence should be addressed to Sezin Ozer; sezinsezgin78@yahoo.com

Academic Editors: I. Anic, P. I. Varela-Centelles, and E. F. Wright

Introduction. Dentin dysplasia is a rare disturbance of dentin formation characterized by normal enamel but atypical dentin formation with abnormal pulpal morphology that is inherited as an autosomal pulpal morphology. *Case Presentation.* A 7-year-old female who had problems in chewing function was referred to Oral and Maxillofacial Surgery Department at the Faculty of Dentistry in Ondokuz Mayıs University. In the radiographic examination, it was determined that some of the unerupted permanent teeth of the patient had short, blunted, and malformed roots with obliterated pulp chambers, although the bone below the teeth showed well-defined margins. This unusual case of generalized short roots presents a case demonstrating both classic and atypical features of dentinal dysplasia type I (DDI) in the mixed and permanent dentitions. *Conclusion.* There are still many issues in the diagnosis and management of patients with dentin dysplasia. Early diagnosis, clinical and radiographic findings, as well as treatment of this condition and the initiation of effective preventive strategies may help prevent or delay loss of dentition.

1. Introduction

Dentin is a mineralized tissue constituting the body of a tooth, serving as a protective covering for the pulp and as a support for overlying enamel and cementum [1]. Dentin dysplasia is an autosomal-dominant trait, affecting either the primary or both the primary and secondary dentitions for approximately one patient in every 100.000 [1, 2]. Dentinal dysplasia (DD) is classified into type I (DDI; radicular dysplasia) and type II (DDII; coronal dysplasia) in order to indicate the parts of the primarily involved teeth which affect both dentitions [2].

DDI is characterized by the presence of primary and permanent teeth with normal morphology of crown, but without rudimentary root development, incomplete or total obliteration of the pulp chamber, and periapical radiolucent areas or cysts [3, 4]. In DDI, teeth eruption is usually normal, but a delayed dental eruption pattern has also been reported [5]. Teeth are more resistant to dental caries, and clinically normal attrition has been found in both dentitions [6]. Because of short roots, DDI may be the extreme mobility and premature exfoliation of teeth, either spontaneously or with minor trauma [1].

Histopathologically, the enamel and the immediately subjacent dentin appear normal. Deeper layers of dentin show atypical tubular patterns with amorphous, atubular areas, and irregular organization. On the pulpal side of the normal appearing mantle of dentin, globular or nodular masses of abnormal dentin are seen. Dysplastic areas have been shown to exhibit tubules which are blocked and shunted from their normal course by numerous denticles [7, 8].

For DDI, treatment aims to remove sources of infection or pain, restore aesthetics, and protect posterior teeth from wear. Treatment varies according the age of the patient, severity of the problem, and presenting complaint [4]. However, the goal of the treatment is to retain the teeth for as long as possible. Because of the shortened roots, the prognosis for prolonged tooth retention is poor. When the teeth were lost prematurely, prosthetic replacement including dentures,

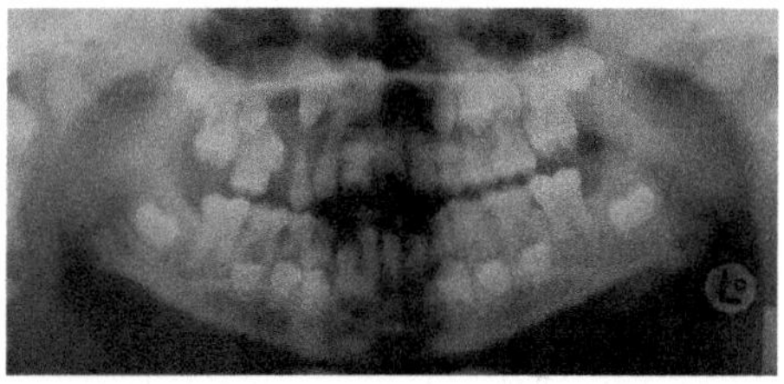

Figure 1: Panoramic radiographic view of the patient at first visit.

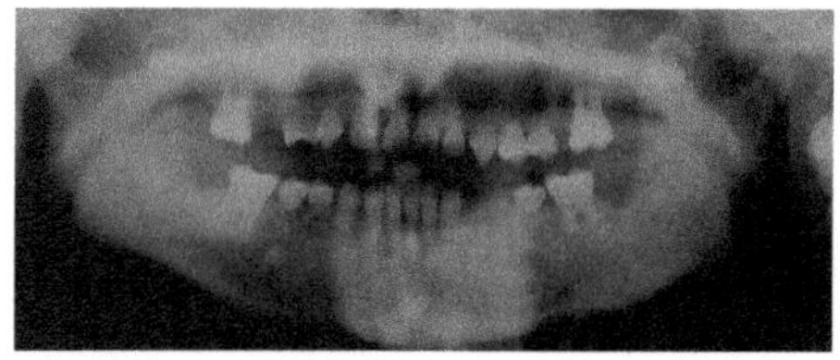

Figure 2: Panoramic radiographic view of the patient at last visit.

overdentures, partial dentures, and/or dental implants may be required [9].

This paper describes a case of DDI in a 7-year-old girl, highlighting the clinical and radiographic variations of the defect and the importance of the preventive care in this anomaly.

2. Case Presentation

A 7-year-old female was referred to the Department of Oral and Maxillofacial Surgery at Ondokuz Mayıs University, Faculty of Dentistry. The patient had some complaints in chewing function. The patient's medical history revealed chronic renal insufficiency and hypertension and received peritoneal dialysis five times a day.

The extraoral examination revealed no abnormality. The intraoral examination revealed that the patients' oral hygiene was poor, and there were plaque deposits present in all quadrants. Only the maxillary left first primary molar had caries. The patient was in the mixed dentition, and the first permanent molars showed abnormal occlusal morphology. And the patient had class 2 malocclusion with anterior open bite.

In the radiographic examination, there was a radiolucent cystic lesion at right maxilla, first permanent molars and incisors were erupted, and the root development was incomplete. The permanent second molars were unerupted and had no root formation, while the other unerupted permanent teeth had short, blunted, and malformed roots with obliterated pulp chambers, and bone below the teeth showed well-defined margins (Figure 1).

Treatment strategy consisted of instructing the patient in oral hygiene and provision of treatment to enhance mastication and improve esthetics. Treatment was initiated with compomer restoration of the maxillary first primary molar. Then, dietary and oral hygiene instructions as well as fluoride supplements were suggested to the patient. The primary teeth had no mobility and infection, so they were not extracted. The possible complications were explained to the patient and her family, and then the patient was followed up. Depending upon clinical and radiographic examinations, the patient was diagnosed with DDI. Family history revealed no such abnormality among other family members.

During the controls, the primary teeth of the patient were physiologically lost. The permanent maxillary right second premolar, the mandibular left first premolar, the mandibular third molars, and the second molars were extracted due to extensive mobility. However, the patients' oral hygiene was good, and the gingiva was healthy.

After six years, the permanent teeth were still in the mouth, and the patients' oral hygiene was still good. Complete obliteration of pulp chambers was noted in both erupted permanent teeth, and also they had no mobility, they were healthy and had no caries (Figure 2).

In this case, because of patient's age, dental implants and the other prosthetic management strategies were not suggested. The patient is still followed up.

3. Discussion

DDI is a genetic defect of dentin formation, although its etiology is still considered a mystery [1]. Wesley et al. proposed that the condition is caused by an abnormal interaction of odontoblasts with ameloblasts leading to abnormal differentiation and/or function of the ectomesenchymal-derived odontoblasts [8, 10]. DDI should be differentiated from DDII, dentinogenesis imperfect, and odontodysplasia [11]. The present case exhibited features of DDI defined in the study, including clinically normal crowns, radiographic obliteration of pulp chambers, rootless teeth, and cystic lesion. Malocclusion is not a specific feature of DDI, but a few cases of malocclusion have been reported in association with this disorder [12]. In this case, class 2 malocclusion with anterior open bite was observed.

DD is usually an autosomal dominant condition [1], and there is a 50% chance that a child born to an affected parent will himself be affected [9]. But, in this patient, there was no familial history of the disease, so she was considered to be the first generation sufferer. Some association has also been reported between dentine dysplasia and osseous chances in addition to sclerotic bone formation [13], but this patient had no signs of other pathologic conditions.

Management of patients with DD has presented dentists with many problems. Extraction has been suggested as a treatment alternative for teeth with pulp necrosis and periapical abscess. Endodontic treatment is contraindicated in teeth with total obliteration of root canals and pulp chambers [12]. Tidwell and Cunningham in 1979 concluded that the results of endodontic treatment might not be successful, but though challenging; they provided an alternative to extraction [6]. Orthodontic treatment is suggested; however, further resorption of the roots, loosening of teeth, and premature exfoliation may occur due to the resistance of the short roots to the orthodontic forces [14]. However, followup and routine conservative treatment is another important choice of treatment [15]. In DDI, because of the shortened roots, early tooth loosing from periodontitis is frequent [9]. For the maintenance of periodontal health of the mobile teeth, oral hygiene must be established and maintained. In this case, followup and routine conservative treatment plan was preferred for the patient, because the teeth had no mobility and the patient's oral hygiene was good. However, because of the early age of the patient, dental implants and the other prosthetic management strategies were not suggested. The patient is still followed up.

4. Conclusion

DDI is an unusual abnormality of dentin which leads premature exfoliation of the primary and permanent teeth. The treatment for children with DDI mainly aims effective preventive care because the early loss of the teeth from periodontitis is frequent. The oral hygiene of the children must be established to have natural teeth as long as possible. The pediatric dentist has an important role in the early diagnosis of this disorder in guiding patient to prolong the retention of affected teeth.

References

[1] J. W. Kim and J. P. Simmer, "Hereditary dentin defects," *Journal of Dental Research*, vol. 86, no. 5, pp. 392–399, 2007.

[2] C. J. Witkop, "Hereditary defects of dentin," *Dental Clinics of North America*, vol. 19, no. 1, pp. 25–45, 1975.

[3] R. A. Depprich, M. A. Ommerborn, J. G. K. Handschel, C. D. Naujoks, U. Meyer, and N. R. Kübler, "Dentin dysplasia type I: a challenge for treatment with dental implants," *Head and Face Medicine*, vol. 3, article 31, 2007.

[4] M. J. Barron, S. T. McDonnell, I. MacKie, and M. J. Dixon, "Hereditary dentine disorders: dentinogenesis imperfecta and dentine dysplasia," *Orphanet Journal of Rare Diseases*, vol. 3, article 31, 2008.

[5] S. M. Scola and P. G. Watts, "Dentinal dysplasia type I. A subclassification," *British Journal of Orthodontics*, vol. 14, no. 3, pp. 175–179, 1987.

[6] E. Tidwell and C. J. Cunningham, "Dentinal dysplasia: endodontic treatment, with case report," *Journal of Endodontics*, vol. 5, no. 12, pp. 372–376, 1979.

[7] E. D. Shields, D. Bixler, and A. M. El-Kafrawy, "A proposed classification for heritable human dentine defects with a description of a new entity," *Archives of Oral Biology*, vol. 18, no. 4, pp. 543–553, 1973.

[8] M. Melnick, L. S. Levin, and J. Brady, "Dentin dysplasia type I: a scanning electron microscopic analysis of the primary dentition," *Oral Surgery Oral Medicine and Oral Pathology*, vol. 50, no. 4, pp. 335–339, 1980.

[9] American Academy on Pediatric Dentistry Council on Clinical Affairs, "Guideline on oral heath care/dental management of heritable dental development anomalies," *Pediatric Dentistry*, vol. 30, no. 7, supplement, pp. 196–201, 2008.

[10] R. K. Wesley, G. P. Wysocki, S. M. Mintz, and J. Jackson, "Dentin dysplasia Type I. Clinical, morphologic, and genetic studies of a case," *Oral Surgery Oral Medicine and Oral Pathology*, vol. 41, no. 4, pp. 516–524, 1976.

[11] L. Özer, H. Karasu, K. Aras, B. Tokman, and E. Ersoy, "Dentin dysplasia type I: report of atypical cases in the permanent and mixed dentitions," *Oral Surgery, Oral Medicine, Oral Pathology, Oral Radiology and Endodontology*, vol. 98, no. 1, pp. 85–90, 2004.

[12] N. E. Steidler, B. G. Radden, and P. C. Reade, "Dentinal dysplasia: a clinicopathological study of eight cases and review of the literature," *British Journal of Oral and Maxillofacial Surgery*, vol. 22, no. 4, pp. 274–286, 1984.

[13] M. E. Morris and R. H. Augsburger, "Dentine dysplasia with sclerotic bone and skeletal anomalies inherited as an autosomal dominant trait. A new syndrome," *Oral Surgery Oral Medicine and Oral Pathology*, vol. 43, no. 2, pp. 267–283, 1977.

[14] C. J. Witkop, "Clinical aspects of dental anomalies," *International Dental Journal*, vol. 26, no. 4, pp. 378–390, 1976.

[15] S. Ravanshad and A. Khayat, "Endodontic therapy on a dentition exhibiting multiple periapical radiolucencies associated with dentinal dysplasia Type 1," *Australian Endodontic Journal*, vol. 32, no. 1, pp. 40–42, 2006.

25

Computer Guided Implantology Accuracy and Complications

Vincenzo Bruno,[1] Mauro Badino,[1] Francesco Riccitiello,[1] Gianrico Spagnuolo,[1] and Massimo Amato[2]

[1] *Department of Neurosciences, Reproductive and Odontostomatological Sciences, University of Naples Federico II, Naples, Italy*
[2] *Medical School, University of Salerno, Salerno, Italy*

Correspondence should be addressed to Gianrico Spagnuolo; gspagnuo@unina.it

Academic Editors: G. Gómez-Moreno and G. Schierano

The computer-based method allows the computerized planning of a surgical implantology procedure, using computed tomography (CT) of the maxillary bones and prosthesis. This procedure, however, is not error-free, unless the operator has been well trained and strictly follows the protocol. A 70-year-old woman whom was edentulous asked for a lower jaw implant-supported prosthesis. A computer-guided surgery was planned with an immediate loading according to the NobelGuide technique. However, prior to surgery, new dentures were constructed to adjust the vertical dimension. An interim screwed metal-resin prosthesis was delivered just after the surgery; however, after only two weeks, it was removed because of a complication. Finally, a screwed implant bridge was delivered. The computer guided surgery is a useful procedure when based on an accurate 3D CT-based image data and an implant planning software which minimizes errors.

1. Introduction

The computer-based technique allows the virtual planning of a surgical implantology procedure by using a CT/CBCT of the maxillary bones and prosthesis [1–3] with an analysis of the jaw in all three dimensions. Therefore, it is possible to plan a precise position of the implant respect to the anatomical structures as well as the prostheses, improving the predictability of implant placement, obtaining a prosthetically driven planning [4]. An accurate surgical guide is generated that is also used by the dental technician to fabricate a definitive cast with the precise position of the implants before the surgery. Therefore, a definitive or interim prosthesis can be constructed prior to the surgical procedure, therefore, obtaining an immediate function.

The NobelGuide (Nobel Biocare AB, Göteborg, Sweden) technique permits the surgical installation of the implants without raising a flap, reducing significantly the operating time and the impact on the patient and patient's morbidity (postoperative pain and swelling) [5]. Several studies [3, 6, 7] reported a cumulative survival rate similar to the conventional surgical procedures, with a few complications.

In the present case report, immediate implant borne prostheses were construct via a computer-assisted implantology and prosthodontics; however, a late surgical complication occurred and in turn CAD/CAM titanium implant bridge was delivered.

2. Case Presentation and Results

A 70-year-old Caucasian woman came into our practice and was in good physical health with no medical risks. She had been wearing two complete dentures (Figure 1) and desired to rehabilitate her edentulous jaws by an implant-retained prosthesis. Two new complete dentures were manufactured to adjust the vertical and horizontal dimensions and to enhance her aesthetic outlook (Figures 2(a), 2(b), 2(c), and 2(d)).

A panoramic radiograph and two spiral computed tomograms (CT) were taken. The first CT was taken of the mandible with the prostheses and a silicon index for the occlusion. The second CT was taken of the denture duplication, using gutta-percha markers (Figure 3). The double scanning system is necessary, because the density of the radiographic mask is similar to that of soft tissues, and

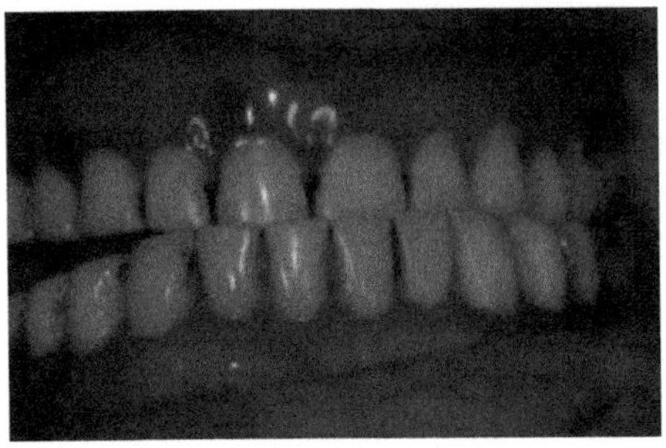

FIGURE 1: Initial dentures worn out with an altered occlusion.

a single scan might not be sufficient to distinguish between the two. After loading the two tomograms into the NobelGuide software (Nobel Biocare, AB), the images were converted and coupled. Then, three-dimensional (3D) planning was performed, which entails positioning the implants in accordance with anatomical structures, such as the mental foramina and mandibular nerve and the prostheses (prosthetic driven planning) (Figure 4).

The surgical template and laboratory products were ordered, allowing the dental technician to produce a definitive cast model with an accurate position for future implants, obtained from the surgical template. Therefore, this model reproduces the jaw bone and dental prosthesis with a space in between representing the gingiva and mucosa. The cast was then mounted on an articulator using the prostheses replica and the bite index. A reinforced interim prosthesis was made through the diagnostic waxing obtained from the previous prostheses.

On the day of surgery, preoperative antibiotics (Amoxicillin 1 g 12 hourly) were given orally 1 day prior to surgery and were continued for another 5 days postoperatively. Local anesthetic was administered, and the surgical template was blocked intraorally using pins (Figure 5), according the position obtained from the casts mounted in articulator. In particular, a surgical bite, to transfer the position, is fabricated from the casts previously mounted in articulator. The gingiva was cut using a circular scalpel, and the osteotomies were performed by following strict protocol [2]. According to the protocol, the osteotomes for the implants were prepared through metallic cylinders which are inserted in the template using a series of drilling sleeves with different diameters that completely coincide with the series of twist drills, taps, and implant holders/mounts. Thus, the drilling is guided and the drill can be moved only along the planned axis avoiding any wobbling. Using this protocol the implant position is precisely transferred from digital position to the mouth.

The first two implants were positioned, but good primary stability was not established. The template was removed, showing that the implants were positioned buccally (Figure 6). The implants were then unscrewed/removed, and the operator made the decision to continue the surgery free hand and open flap. A new osteotomy was performed distally, but this action resulted in being too close to the mandibular foramina (Figure 7); therefore another osteotomy was performed mesially (Figure 8). The other osteotomies were performed, and five implants were placed (Figure 9). Finally, the last denture was adapted to the new implant positions (Figure 10), and the reinforced interim prostheses fabricated could not be delivered.

Two weeks later, the patient called stating that while she made a wide yawn, she heard a noise in the mandible and currently has pain with any movement. A Cone Beam CT was taken, and a hairline fracture was detected (Figures 11(a) and 11(b)). The patient was then referred to a maxillofacial surgeon, who stated that no surgery was required. However, the prostheses needed to be unscrewed, to allow the mandible to rest, and the patient was asked to follow a soft diet for 2 months. Two months later, a CAD/CAM titanium implant bridge was constructed to complete the procedure (Figures 12(a), 12(b), 12(c), 12(d), and 12(e)).

3. Discussion

Van Steenberghe et al., 2005 [2], by using an immediately loaded CAD-CAM manufactured fixed complete dentures computer-designed procedure, reported an implant cumulative survival rate after 5 years of 91.5%. In particular, there was a difference between the nonsmoking group (98.9%) and the smoking group (81.2%), with a mean marginal bone loss of 2.6 mm for the smoking group and 1.2 mm for the nonsmoking group.

Gillot et al., 2010 [7], reported an implant survival rate of 98.1%, and of the 211 implants loaded, four were lost (1.9%). Even so, the prosthetic survival rate was 100%. It is still interesting to note that the most commonly used implant lengths were between 10 and 13 mm; these lengths represent 75% of the overall pool of implants, and in particular, the 13 mm and 15 mm lengths represent the 52.13% [7]. Therefore, a conclusion can be drawn that good results can be obtained with the use of longer implants.

Vasak et al., 2012 [8], presented similar results regarding the implant survival rate (98.8%), adding more details concerning the mean marginal bone level at 1 year (1.44 mm; SD 1.35; $n = 98$) and reporting an increment of all the clinical parameters of the soft tissue conditions.

The flapless surgery, based on keyhole surgery, entails less intense pain and for shorter periods of time [5]. Moreover, this minimal invasive technique reduces surgery time and swelling, compared to conventional treatment [5]. This treatment also reduces the number of appointments and chair time for the patient as well as for the dentist.

However, prosthetic and surgical complications [9] are reported in the literature using the computer-aided implantology. Authors [9] have also stated that it is particularly important to have a "strict adherence" to the protocol, to prevent any complications. Schneider et al. [10] reported early surgical complications such as the lack of primary stability, which has been resolved by the use of wider implants, bone augmentation, or no loading.

D'haese et al. [11], in a literature review, reported that there is a substantial deviation between the implant planned and the one placed. This deviation can vary from a mean angular of 2.71° (range 0.4–8, SD 1.9), with a mean deviation

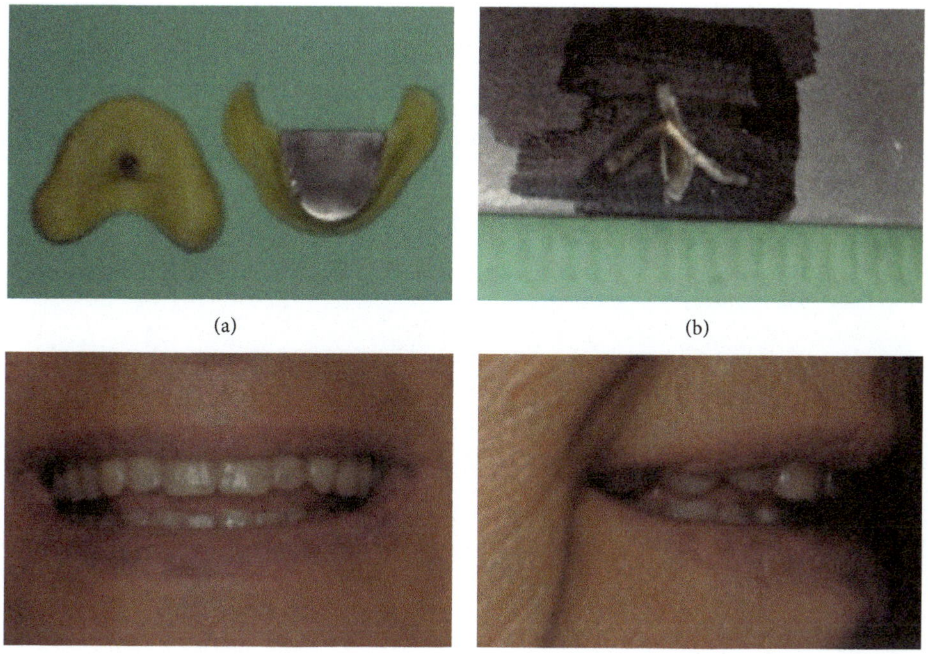

(a) (b) (c) (d)

FIGURE 2: Registration of the gothic arch, according to central bearing point (CBP), to restore the correct interarch relationships ((a), (b)), the new dentures in use ((c), (d)).

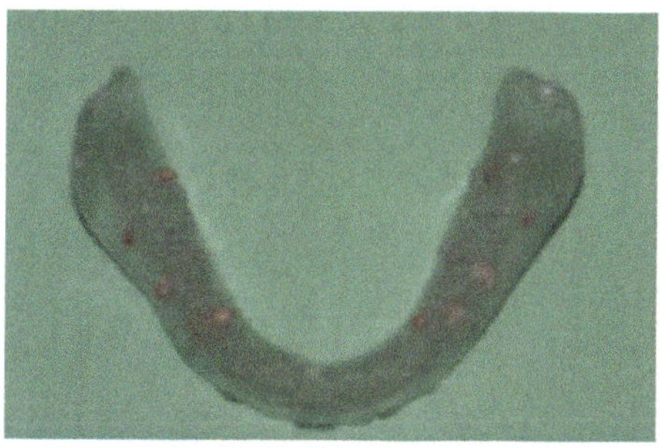

FIGURE 3: The low denture duplicated and with the gutta-percha markers to be used for the CT.

at the apex of 1.0 mm (range 0.2–3.0, SD 0.7) [11], to 7.9° (range 0.7–24.9, SD 4.7), with a mean deviation at the apex of 1.6 mm (range 0–4.2, SD 1.2) [12].

Another point to consider is the deformation of the stereolithographic surgical guide caused by the incorrect setting of the ISO values for the segmentation of the scan denture [13]. Stumpel concluded that the evaluation of the produced surgical guide before the clinical use might be prudent [13]. To avoid this arbitrary setting, Nobel Biocare has introduced the calibration procedure using a unique calibration object. This procedure permits obtaining a calibration of the scan in relation of the object, resulting in a production of surgical templates with a better stability and precision.

We would also like to point out that in this case the protocol was strictly followed and the surgeon was extremely experienced. However, the first two implants showed a poor torque during the last rotation, resulting in a lack of primary stability. The position of the implants did not coincide with the digital position as planned in the software.

The explanation of the complication can be referred to a sum of different errors as reported by Valente et al. [14] and summarized in the following.

The different types of errors which could occur during a CT guided implant surgery and prosthetics are as follows.

(1) Errors during image acquisition and data processing, on average less than 0.5 mm.

(2) Error during surgical template production, typically around 0.1 to 0.2 mm for CAM with stereolithography.

(3) Error during template positioning and movement of the template during the drilling.

(4) Mechanical error caused by the bur-cylinder gap.

(5) In template-assisted surgery, the height of the template necessitates very long burs.

In particular, it is evident that the support area of the denture was extremely reduced, and the surgical guide, with 5 holes, has still less contact with the mucosa.

In this case report, the desire to conclude the treatment with an immediate delivery of the prostheses a superficial valuation of the impact to perform three holes so close in the mandible and the subsequent increase of load during mastication due the implant borne prosthesis. Likewise, the presence of 5 splinted implants reduce the elasticity of the mandible during the opening of the mouth. Moreover,

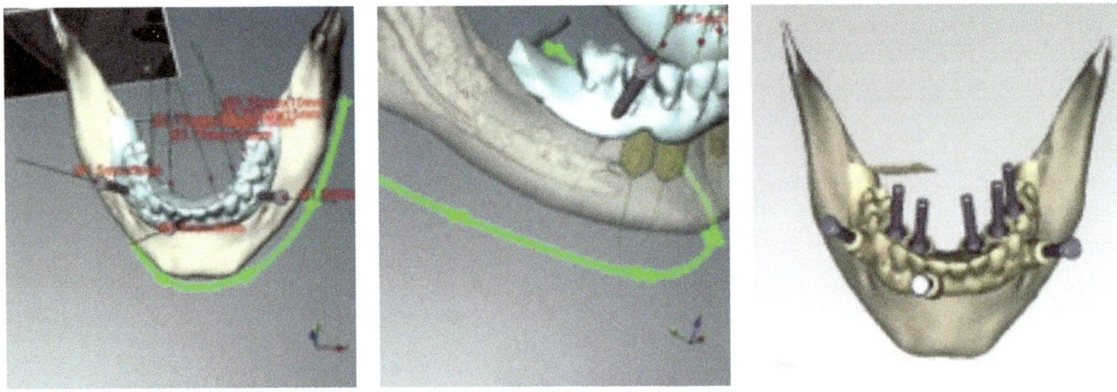

Figure 4: Representative images from the software with the driven prosthetic implants planned.

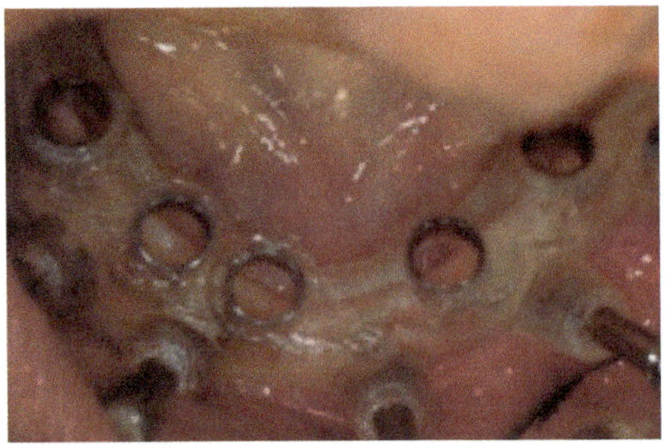

Figure 5: The surgical template in situ.

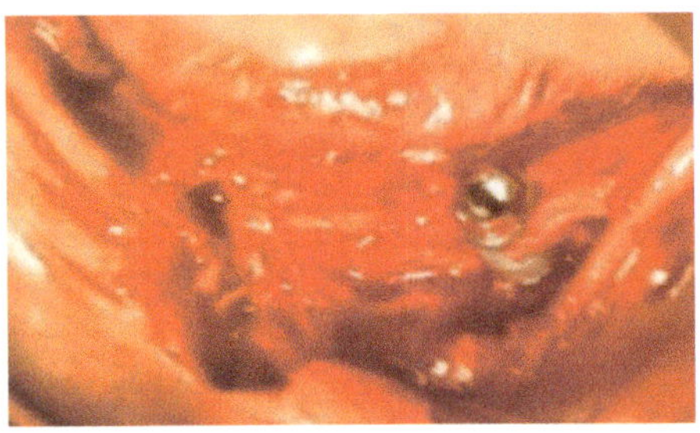

Figure 6: An image, out of focus, with the implants' position too buccal.

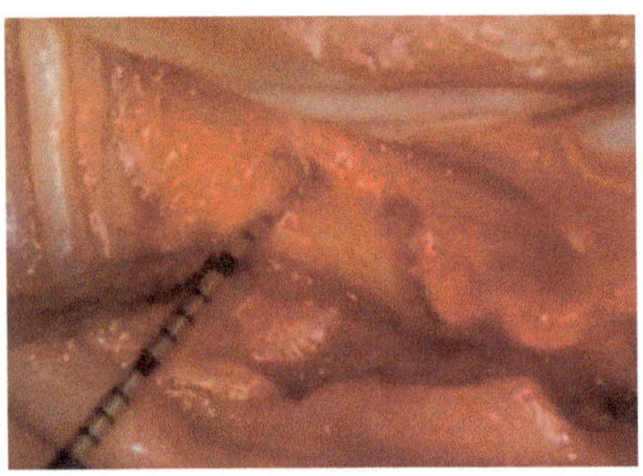

Figure 7: The distal osteotome intimate to the alveolar nerve.

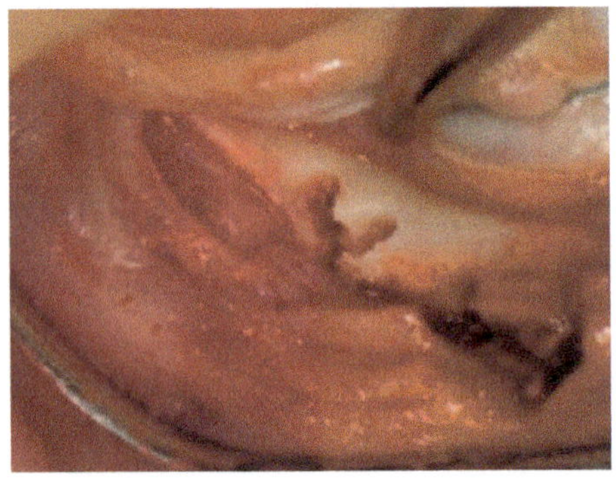

Figure 8: The two osteotomes very close.

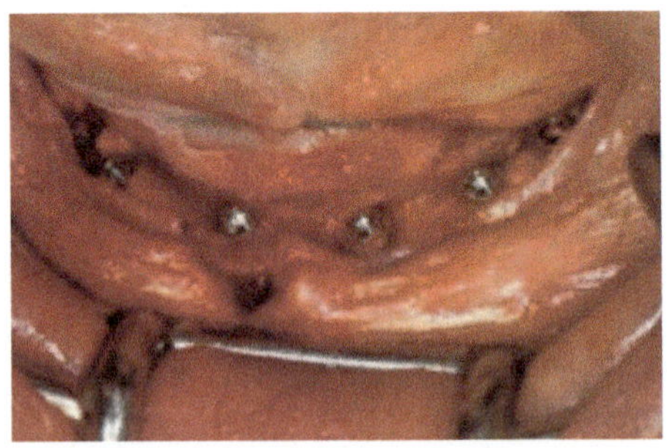

Figure 9: All the five implants placed free hand.

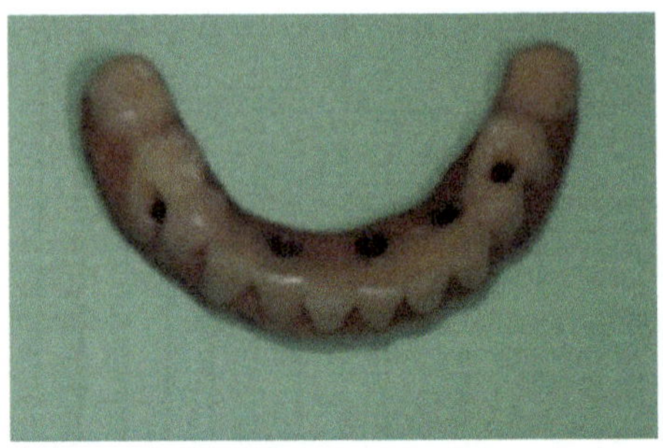

Figure 10: The denture modified to be used as interim implant borne prosthesis.

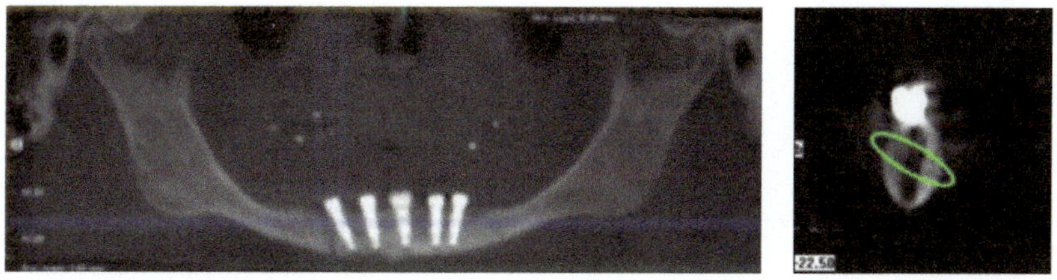

(a) (b)

FIGURE 11: The CBCT (a) and a slice (b) where the hairline fracture is evident.

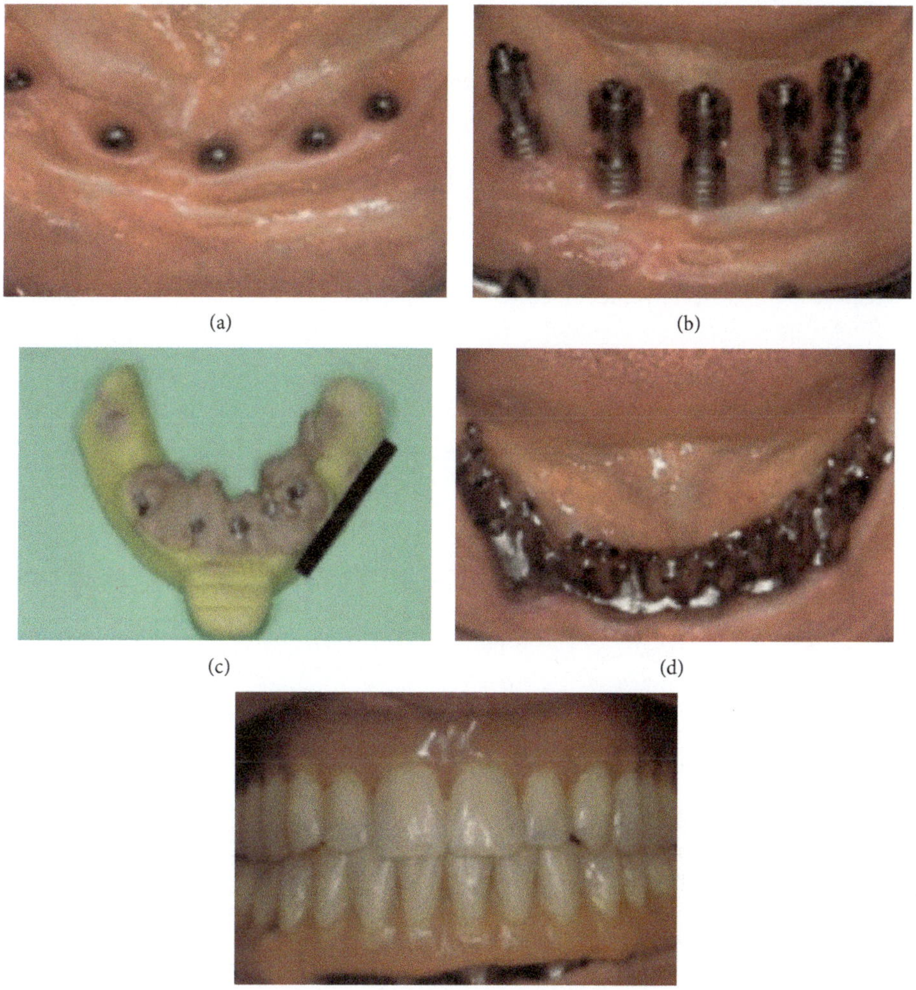

(a) (b) (c) (d) (e)

FIGURE 12: The healed mucosa and the osseointegrated implants (a). The impression abutments where the angulation of the distal right implant is inserted and evident (b). The impression was taken using plaster (c). The try-in of the screwed titanium implant bridge (d). The titanium implant bridge delivered (e).

the splinted implants might cause an increase of stress in the distal bone [15], exactly in the zone of the hairline fracture.

The NobelGuide system is a reliable treatment modality, but not without its complications. Strict adherence to the system protocol is only one key to prevent complications. Likewise, it is important during the planning to respect all maximum deviations as the safety margins [16] recommended by the planning software (Figure 13).

As well as it is important to do the calibration of the scan obtaining the minor deformation of the surgical template. Finally, it is useful a verification of the volumetric congruence of the produced surgical guide and the scan denture [13]. This

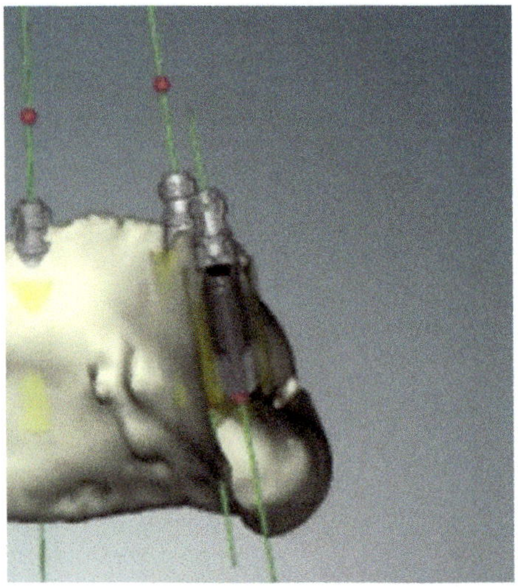

FIGURE 13: The yellow shade representing the safety area.

verification can be attained using a vinyl polyether silicone (VPS) to check the fit of the surgical guide. The thickness of the VPS material indicates space between the guide and the tissue.

Conflict of Interests

The authors declare that they have no conflict of interests.

References

[1] D. van Steenberghe, I. Naert, M. Andersson, I. Brajnovic, J. van Cleynenbreugel, and P. Suetens, "A custom template and definitive prosthesis allowing immediate implant loading in the maxilla: a clinical report," *International Journal of Oral and Maxillofacial Implants*, vol. 17, no. 5, pp. 663–670, 2002.

[2] D. van Steenberghe, R. Glauser, U. Blombäck et al., "A computed tomographic scan-derived customized surgical template and fixed prosthesis for flapless surgery and immediate loading of implants in fully edentulous maxillae: a prospective multicenter study," *Clinical Implant Dentistry and Related Research*, vol. 7, no. 1, pp. 11–20, 2005.

[3] A. M. Sanna, L. Molly, and D. van Steenberghe, "Immediately loaded CAD-CAM manufactured fixed complete dentures using flapless implant placement procedures: a cohort study of consecutive patients," *Journal of Prosthetic Dentistry*, vol. 97, no. 6, pp. 331–339, 2007.

[4] J. Katsoulis, P. Pazera, and R. Mericske-Stern, "Prosthetically driven, computer-guided implant planning for the edentulous maxilla: a model study," *Clinical Implant Dentistry and Related Research*, vol. 11, no. 3, pp. 238–245, 2009.

[5] T. Fortin, J. L. Bosson, M. Isidori, and E. Blanchet, "Effect of flapless surgery on pain experienced in implant placement using an image-guided system," *International Journal of Oral and Maxillofacial Implants*, vol. 21, no. 2, pp. 298–304, 2006.

[6] M. Hultin, K. G. Svensson, and M. Trulsson, "Clinical advantages of computer-guided implant placement: a systematic review," *Clinical Oral Implants Research*, vol. 23, pp. 124–135, 2012.

[7] L. Gillot, R. Noharet, and B. Cannas, "Guided surgery and presurgical prosthesis: preliminary results of 33 fully edentulous maxillae treated in accordance with the nobelguide® protocol," *Clinical Implant Dentistry and Related Research*, vol. 12, no. 1, pp. e104–e113, 2010.

[8] C. Vasak, R. J. Kohal, S. Lettner, D. Rohner, and W. Zechner, "Clinical and radiological evaluation of a template-guided (nobelguide) treatment concept," *Clinical Oral Implants Research*, 2012.

[9] L. T. Yong and P. K. Moy, "Complications of computer-aided-design/computer-aided-machining-guided (NobelGuide) surgical implant placement: an evaluation of early clinical results," *Clinical Implant Dentistry and Related Research*, vol. 10, no. 3, pp. 123–127, 2008.

[10] D. Schneider, P. Marquardt, M. Zwahlen, and R. E. Jung, "A systematic review on the accuracy and the clinical outcome of computer-guided template-based implant dentistry," *Clinical Oral Implants Research*, vol. 20, no. 4, pp. 73–86, 2009.

[11] J. D'haese, T. van de Velde, A. Komiyama, M. Hultin, and H. de Bruyn, "Accuracy and complications using computer-designed stereolithographic surgical guides for oral rehabilitation by means of dental implants: a review of the literature," *Clinical Implant Dentistry and Related Research*, vol. 14, pp. 321–335, 2012.

[12] N. van Assche, D. van Steenberghe, M. Quirynen, and R. Jacobs, "Accuracy assessment of computer-assisted flapless implant placement in partial edentulism," *Journal of Clinical Periodontology*, vol. 37, no. 4, pp. 398–403, 2010.

[13] L. J. Stumpel, "Deformation of stereolithographically produced surgical guides: an observational case series report," *Clinical Implant Dentistry and Related Research*, vol. 14, pp. 442–453, 2012.

[14] F. Valente, G. Schiroli, and A. Sbrenna, "Accuracy of computer-aided oral implant surgery: a clinical and radiographic study," *International Journal of Oral and Maxillofacial Implants*, vol. 24, no. 2, pp. 234–242, 2009.

[15] M. Radnai, B. Erdohelyi, P. I. Szabo, and E. Varga, "Stress in the mandible with splinted dental implants caused by limited flexure on mouth opening: an in vitro study," *International Journal of Experimental Dental Science*, vol. 1, pp. 8–13, 2012.

[16] C. Vasak, G. Watzak, A. Gahleitner, G. Strbac, M. Schemper, and W. Zechner, "Computed tomography-based evaluation of template (NobelGuide)-guided implant positions: a prospective radiological study," *Clinical Oral Implants Research*, vol. 22, no. 10, pp. 1157–1163, 2011.

Multidisciplinary Management of a Fused Tooth

Derya Demircioglu Guler,[1] Emine Sen Tunc,[1] Nursel Arici,[2] and Nilüfer Ozkan[3]

[1] *Department of Pediatric Dentistry, Faculty of Dentistry, Ondokuz Mayis University, Kurupelit, 55139 Samsun, Turkey*
[2] *Department of Orthodontics, Faculty of Dentistry, Ondokuz Mayis University, Kurupelit, 55139 Samsun, Turkey*
[3] *Department of Oral and Maxillofacial Surgery, Faculty of Dentistry, Ondokuz Mayis University, Kurupelit, 55139 Samsun, Turkey*

Correspondence should be addressed to Derya Demircioglu Guler; dt_deryad@hotmail.com

Academic Editors: L. Manuel Junquera Gutierrez and D. Torrés-Lagares

Objective. Fusion is a dental anomaly that arises through the union of two adjacent teeth. The case report presents multidisciplinary management of a fused maxillary anterior tooth. *Case Report.* A 10-year-old boy was referred to the pediatric dental clinic with the chief complaint of a large upper anterior tooth. Intraoral and radiographic examinations indicated fusion between the permanent maxillary right central incisor and a supernumerary tooth. According to the treatment plan, the fused tooth was sectioned, and the mesial portion was removed. The remaining tooth section was restored with composite resin, and the diastema between the central incisors was closed with orthodontic treatment. After an 18-month followup period, the tooth showed no sign of pathosis. *Conclusion.* The technique described here offers a simple and effective method for restoring a fused tooth that reestablishes function, shape, and esthetics.

1. Introduction

Tooth fusion is a rare developmental anomaly that stems from the embryogenic union of two teeth originating from two or more tooth germs [1, 2]. Although the exact etiology of fusion is unclear, pressure or physical force producing close contact between two developing tooth buds has been reported as a possible cause, and trauma, genetic and environmental factors have also been implicated as contributing factors [3–6]. Moreover, fused teeth may form part of syndromes such as achondrodysplasia, chondroectodermal dysplasia, focal dermal hypoplasia, and osteopetrosis [7–11].

The literature suggests fusion has a higher incidence in deciduous dentition (0.5%–2.5%) than in permanent dentition (0.1%–1.0%) [7, 12, 13]. Fused teeth are found predominantly in the anterior region, with incisors and canines the most frequently affected [14, 15]. These anomalies may be bilateral or unilateral [14, 16]. The incidence of fusion does not vary by sex [7, 12]. Fused teeth may occur in both the maxilla and mandible, but they are more frequently present in the mandible [17].

The majority of fused teeth show an anomalous broad crown and two distinct root canals. Clinically, the crowns appear melded together, with a small groove between the mesial and distal parts. Fused teeth may be characterized by one pulp chamber divided into two root canals, two independent endodontic systems, or one common pulp canal [5, 15, 18].

This case report presents the surgical separation and orthodontic treatment of a maxillary central incisor fused with a supernumerary tooth.

2. Case Report

A 10-year-old boy was referred to the paediatric dental clinic with the chief complaint of the unpleasant appearance of a large anterior tooth. His medical history was noncontributory. There was no family history of dental anomalies, and there was no previous trauma to the teeth or jaws. The patient was a single child of a nonconsanguineous marriage.

Intraoral examination revealed a large maxillary right central incisor, with a small groove observed on the labial and palatal aspects of the crown (Figure 1). Response to pulp

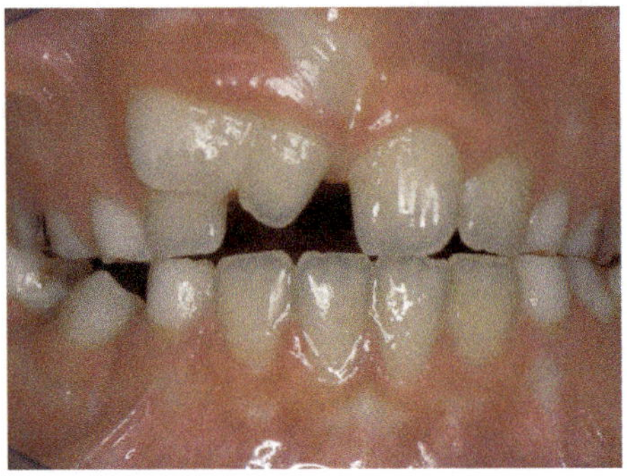

FIGURE 1: Clinical appearance of fused tooth.

testing was normal, no caries were detected, and there was no significant periodontal pocketing. The patient was in mixed dentition and had crowding in the anterior region due to a lack of space. The total number of teeth was normal.

Radiographic examination revealed fusion of the maxillary right permanent central incisor with a supernumerary tooth. According to the radiographs, the fused tooth had two distinct roots, with no connection between the pulp chambers and canals. No periapical radiolucency associated with these teeth was detected (Figures 2(a) and 2(b)).

An orthodontic examination was conducted, and an initial treatment plan was developed that aimed to separate the fused supernumerary tooth and then correct the arch discrepancy with orthodontic treatment. The treatment objectives and alternatives were explained to the patient and his parents who provided their written consent prior to treatment.

The teeth were anaesthetized (Ultracain D-S, Istanbul, Turkey), and buccal and palatal flaps were raised. Some bones were removed below the buccal groove in order to locate the point at which the two roots separated. The crown was sectioned with a diamond bur (Midwest, Dentsply, IL, USA), and the mesial part of the tooth was removed (Figures 3(a) and 3(b)). The root surfaces were examined, and no pulpal association was detected (Figure 3(c)). The remaining distal tooth was restored with composite resin (Gradia Direct, GC Corporation, Tokyo, Japan), and the flaps were sutured (Figure 3(d)). Following surgery, the patient was prescribed chlorhexidine mouthwash (Orasept, Biofarma İlaç San. ve Tic. A.Ş, İstanbul, Turkey). Sutures were removed one week postoperatively.

Fixed orthodontic treatment was then agreed in order to correct the position of the central tooth, and routine orthodontic records (plaster model, photographs, and radiographs) were obtained. Clinical examination and analysis of the records showed the maxillary right central tooth to be infrapositioned. Cephalometric analysis showed the upper and lower jaws to be in normal position in the sagittal plane in relation to the base of the cranium, but the right upper central tooth was found to be protruding slightly due to the fusion. In order to eliminate the malocclusion, a fixed orthodontic appliance was planned using 0.022 inch Gemini MBT metal brackets (3 M Unitek, USA). Following placement of the maxillary incisor brackets, an arch wire (16 Heat Active Nickel-Titanium, 3 M Unitek) was connected to the bracket slots to correct the position of the maxillary right central tooth (Figure 4(a)).

At the fixed appliance adaptation appointment, the patient was instructed on oral hygiene and prohibited foods and was called back for routine orthodontic controls once a month. When the maxillary right central incisor had moved into the correct position in the arch, $0.019'' \times 0.025''$ Heat Active Nickel-Titanium and $0.019'' \times 0.025''$ stainless steel arch wires were attached to correct the midline diastema. At the end of a 13-month followup period, orthodontic treatment using fixed mechanics was found to have achieved adequate positioning of the central teeth. Following fixed orthodontic treatment, a Hawley appliance was constructed for retention (Figure 4(b)).

Once orthodontic treatment had been completed, the maxillary central teeth were reshaped with composite resin (Gradia Direct, GC Corporation, Tokyo, Japan) for aesthetic reasons. Teeth were checked for possible complications once every three months. After an 18-month followup period, the maxillary right central tooth showed no sign of periapical pathosis (Figures 5(a) and 5(b)) and responded positively to electric pulp testing. Followup examinations indicated that treatment had successfully restored both esthetics and function. Probing revealed no periodontal pocketing around the central incisor, and there was good attachment; however, long-term followup is required.

3. Discussion

Fused teeth may lead to serious esthetic problems and malocclusions, especially when supernumerary elements are involved. Owing to the abnormal shape and size of crown(s) and root(s) as well as misalignment, treatment usually requires a multidisciplinary approach to address both endodontic and esthetic issues [9, 19, 20].

Depending on factors such as location of the connecting area, root-development stage, and patient age, treatment of fused teeth may vary [15]. One option involves extraction of the fused tooth after completion of root-canal therapy, removal of the unwanted part, and reimplantation of the tooth into its original site [21, 22]. However, because the root surface of the reimplanted tooth lacks a periodontal membrane, ankylosis may be expected [23]. In the present case, based on the location of the connecting area, the root-development stage, and the patient's age, a more conservative treatment option was selected. Because the fused tooth possessed two separate roots and canals, extraction of the mesial part of the tooth was chosen to solve the esthetic problems and obtain space for alignment. Although endodontic treatment may be necessary even when no pulpal communication is visualized between two fused teeth, in the case presented here, no pulpal exposure was observed following separation, and no endodontic therapy was required. Difficulties in the observation of the surgical area require clinicians to check

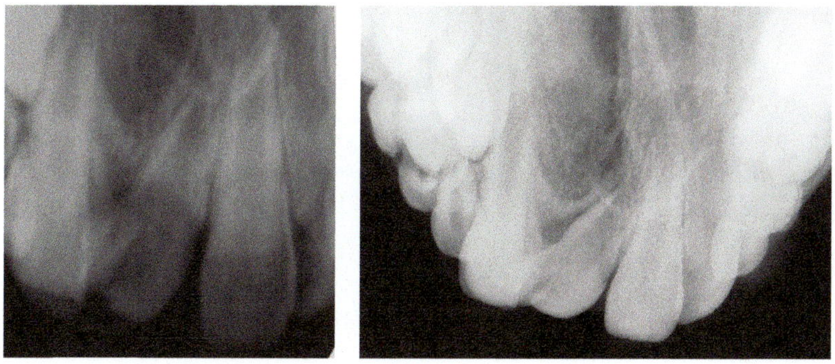

(a) (b)

FIGURE 2: Radiographic appearance of fused tooth.

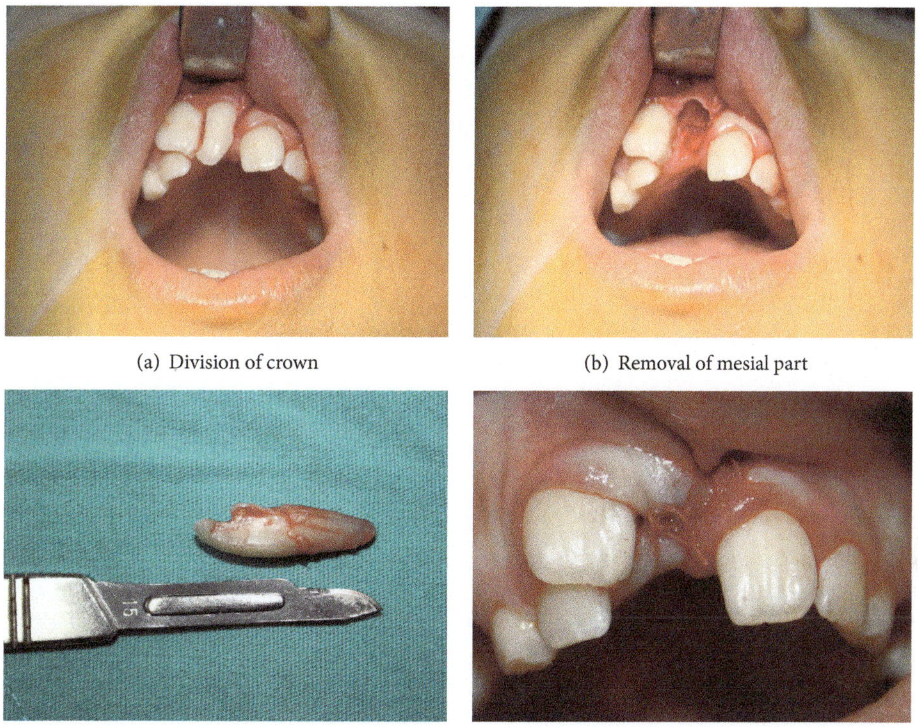

(a) Division of crown

(b) Removal of mesial part

(c) Visualization of any pulpal communication

(d) Suturing of surgical area following operation

FIGURE 3: Surgical procedures.

carefully for any possible pulpal exposure, and detailed radiographic followup examinations are essential for avoiding late-term complications.

In the present case, following hemisection of the crown, the remaining part was restored with traditional composite resin. Some case reports have described postoperative complications such as hypersensitivity, reversible pulpitis, and external root resorption [22]. In this case, no pathological findings were observed radiographically, and the tooth responded positively to electric pulp testing at the one-year recall. Followup indicated that treatment had successfully restored both esthetics and function. No periodontal pocketing was found around the central incisor upon probing, and the attachment was good. Most importantly, the patient was pleased with the esthetic outcome of treatment.

4. Conclusion

Gemination and fusion are frequently responsible for periodontal, endodontic, orthodontic, and esthetic problems. The excellent esthetic and functional results obtained in the case presented here are attributable to scientific knowledge,

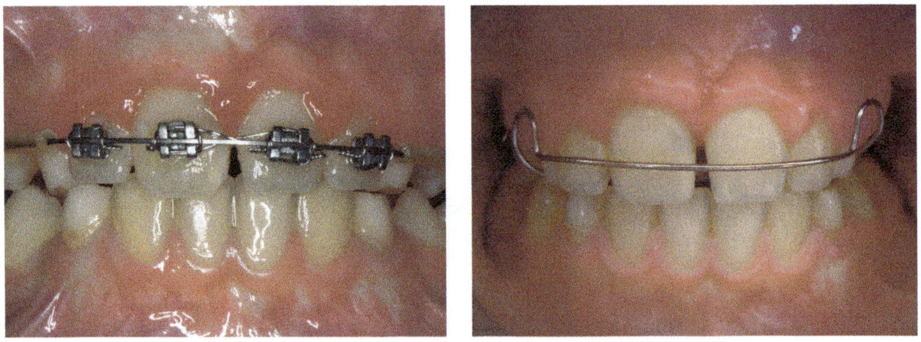

(a) Fixed orthodontic period (b) Hawley appliance

FIGURE 4: Orthodontic therapy.

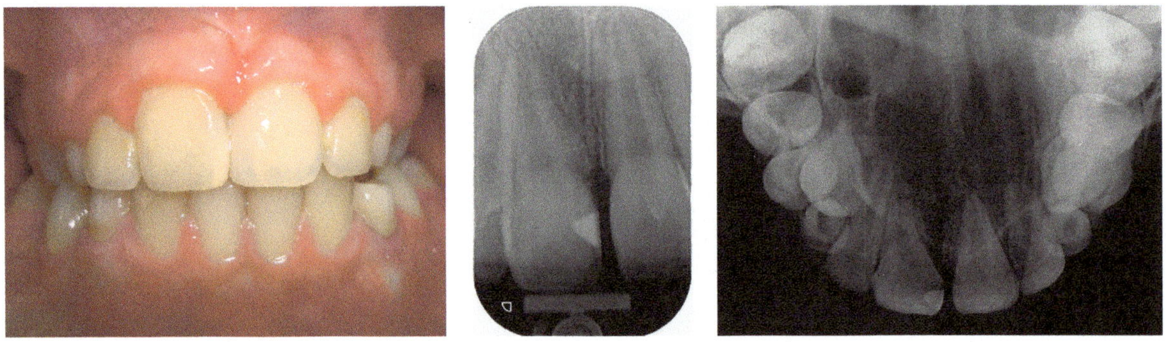

(a) (b) (c)

FIGURE 5: Clinical and radiographic appearance at 18-month followup.

broad experience, and team work, where individual experts in specialized fields contributed to the selection of the most suitable treatment possible.

References

[1] A. Knežević, S. Travan, Z. Tarle, J. Šutalo, B. Janković, and I. Ciglar, "Double tooth," *Collegium Antropologicum*, vol. 26, no. 2, pp. 667–672, 2002.

[2] M. K. Caroll, "Fusion and Gemination in alternate dentitions," *Oral Surgery Oral Medicine and Oral Pathology*, vol. 69, no. 5, p. 655, 1990.

[3] R. J. Lowell and A. L. Solomon, "Fused teeth," *Journal of the American Dental Association*, vol. 68, p. 762, 1964.

[4] W. G. Shafer, M. K. Hine, and B. M. Levy, *A Textbook of Pathology*, WB Saunders, Philadelphia, Pa, USA, 4th edition, 1983.

[5] C. L. Mader, "Fusion of teeth," *The Journal of the American Dental Association*, vol. 98, no. 1, pp. 62–64, 1979.

[6] E. Moody and L. B. Montgomery, "Hereditary tendencies in tooth formation," *The Journal of the American Dental Association*, vol. 21, pp. 1774–1776, 1934.

[7] A. H. B. Schuurs and C. van Loveren, "Double teeth: review of the literature," *Journal of Dentistry for Children*, vol. 67, no. 5, pp. 313–325, 2000.

[8] N. L. Crawford, S. North, and L. E. Davidson, "Double permanent incisor teeth: management of three cases," *Dental update*, vol. 33, no. 10, pp. 608–610, 2006.

[9] T. Cetinbas, S. Halil, M. O. Akcam, S. Sari, and S. Cetiner, "Hemisection of a fused tooth," *Oral Surgery, Oral Medicine, Oral Pathology, Oral Radiology and Endodontology*, vol. 104, no. 4, pp. e120–e124, 2007.

[10] S. Karaçay, U. Gurton, H. Olmez, and G. Koymen, "Multidisciplinary treatment of "winned"

permanent teeth: two case reports," *Journal of Dentistry for Children*, vol. 71, no. 1, pp. 80–86, 2004.

[11] G. Oliván Rosas, J. López Jiménez, M. J. Giménez Prats, and M. Piqueras Hernández, "Considerations and differences in the treatment of a fused tooth," *Medicina Oral*, vol. 9, no. 3, pp. 224–228, 2004.

[12] C. Schulze, "Developmental abnormalities of the teeth and the jaws," in *Thoma's Oral Pathology*, R. J. Gorlin and H. M. Goldman, Eds., pp. 96–183, Mosby, St. Louis, Mo, USA, 6th edition, 1970.

[13] T. D. Blaney, G. R. Hartwell, and R. Bellizzi, "Endodontic management of a fused tooth: a case report," *Journal of Endodontics*, vol. 8, no. 5, pp. 227–230, 1982.

[14] G. M. Delany and L. I. Goldblatt, "Fused teeth: a multidisciplinary approach to treatment," *The Journal of the American Dental Association*, vol. 103, no. 5, pp. 732–734, 1981.

[15] M. Hülsmann, R. Bahr, and U. Grohmann, "Hemisection and vital treatment of a fused tooth—literature review and case

report," *Endodontics and Dental Traumatology*, vol. 13, no. 6, pp. 253–258, 1997.

[16] C. S. Budd, D. E. Reid, J. C. Kulild, and R. N. Weller, "Endodontic treatment of an unusual case of fusion," *Journal of Endodontics*, vol. 18, no. 3, pp. 133–137, 1992.

[17] A. H. Brook and G. B. Winter, "Double teeth. A retrospective study of "geminated" and "fused" teeth in children," *British Dental Journal*, vol. 129, no. 3, pp. 123–130, 1970.

[18] E. S. Reeh and M. ElDeeb, "Root canal morphology of fused mandibular canine and lateral incisor," *Journal of Endodontics*, vol. 15, no. 1, pp. 33–35, 1989.

[19] C. Gadimli and Z. Sari, "Interdisciplinary treatment of a fused lower premolar with supernumerary tooth," *European Journal of Dentistry*, vol. 5, no. 3, pp. 349–353, 2011.

[20] B. Ozden, K. Gunduz, S. Ozer, A. Oz, and F. O. Ozden, "The multidisciplinary management of a fused maxillary central incisor with a talon cusp," *Australian Dental Journal*, vol. 57, no. 1, pp. 98–102, 2012.

[21] T. Demir, U. Ates, B. Cehreli, and Z. C. Cehreli, "Autotransplantation of a supernumerary incisor as a replacement for fused tooth: 24-month follow-up," *Oral Surgery, Oral Medicine, Oral Pathology, Oral Radiology and Endodontology*, vol. 106, no. 4, pp. e1–e6, 2008.

[22] H. Kayalibay, M. Uzamis, and A. Akalin, "The treatment of a fusion between the maxillary central incisor and supernumerary tooth: report of a case," *Journal of Clinical Pediatric Dentistry*, vol. 20, no. 3, pp. 237–240, 1996.

[23] J. O. Andreasen and L. Kristerson, "The effect of limited drying or removal of the periodontal ligament. Periodontal healing after replantation of mature permanent incisors in monkeys," *Acta Odontologica Scandinavica*, vol. 39, no. 1, pp. 1–13, 1980.

27

Sinus Lift and Transantral Approach to Root Fragment Removal

Andrea Enrico Borgonovo,[1] Federica Rizza,[2] Adele Dudaite,[2] Rachele Censi,[3] and Dino Re[2]

[1] *School of Oral Surgery, University of Milan, Via Festa del Perdono 7, 20122 Milano, Italy*
[2] *Department of Oral Rehabilitation, Istituto Stomatologico Italiano, University of Milan, Via Pace 21, 20122 Milano, Italy*
[3] *Department of Periodontology and Implantology III, Istituto Stomatologico Italiano, Via Pace 21, 20122 Milano, Italy*

Correspondence should be addressed to Federica Rizza; rizza.federica@gmail.com

Academic Editors: R. Crespi, E. Mijiritsky, and G. Schierano

The aim of this case report is to present a case of root fragment removal during planned sinus lift procedure. After failed molar tooth extraction, we chose to retrieve the residual root apex with transantral approach not to damage excessively bone volume. Without changing primary implant rehabilitation purpose, the fragment removal procedure was performed prior to implant placement during necessary sinus lift surgery. Higher visibility of surgical field was achieved. The root fragment residual was removed without an additional surgery appointment avoiding postoperative discomfort. The goal is to underline the importance of being able to change planning during intrasurgical complications. It is most appropriate to operate with safe and simple procedures to reduce surgical discomfort for the patient.

1. Introduction

Various treatment modalities are available for replacing a single missing tooth: removable partial denture, fixed partial denture, or dental implant. The choice is influenced by clinical-, dentist- and patient-immanent factors [1], but both dentist and patient increasingly choose to avoid to damage neighbouring teeth and to rehabilitate with endosseous implant [2].

Traditionally, before placing dental implants, the compromised teeth are removed and the extraction sockets are left to heal for 3-4 months [3].

Sometimes complications may happen and it is important to be able to plan again a surgical procedure limiting damage and discomfort for the patient.

The most frequent extraction complication is certainly the root/apex fracture in the alveolus [4]. When it occurs in upper jaw, it is important to manage it to preserve the socket and avoid an oroantral fistula.

Removal of a root through the alveolar opening without the removal of bone from the extraction socket is not always possible and excessive bone removal may result in chronic complications and lack of bone volume for the following implant restoration [5].

In the literature there are some studies about removal of a foreign body from the maxillary sinus [6–9]. These studies suggest to have a clear view of the surgical field and so to use Caldwell-Luc technique that permits the elimination of blind procedures, however, removing a large portion of the anterior maxillary wall. Otherwise, this technique remains invasive and traumatic, with consequent complication rates associated [10], like swelling, infection, orbital hematoma, visual disturbances, infraorbital nerve damage, and oroantral fistula.

In this clinical report, we are presenting a case in which the fragment was not dislocated in the maxillary sinus, but it was retained in the palatal alveolar bone under Schneiderian membrane. The surgeon decided to leave the fragment knowing that it will be removed during the planned sinus lift procedure for endosseous implant rehabilitation.

This decision favourably resulted in a minimal damage for the patient and a reduction of surgical appointment.

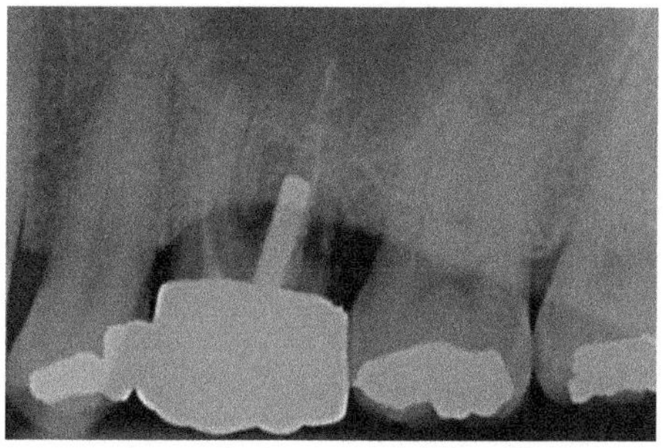

FIGURE 1: Initial X-ray examination.

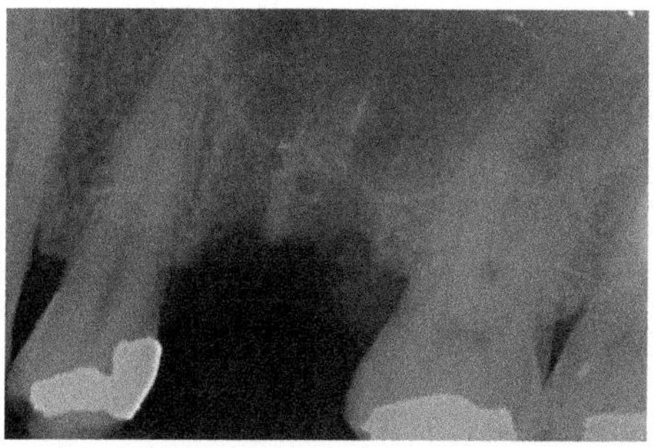

FIGURE 2: X-ray examination after first extraction: residual root and insufficient bony support.

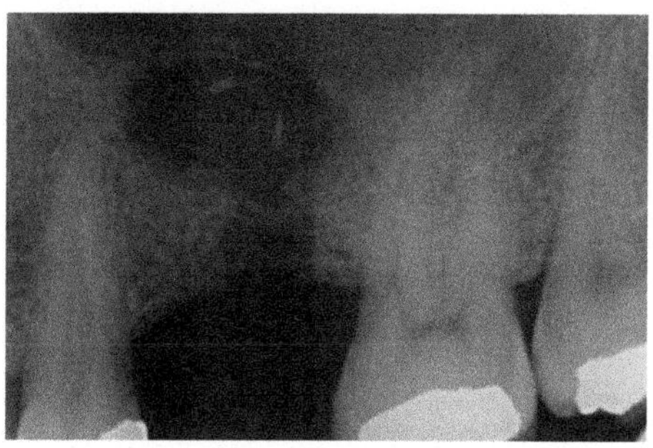

FIGURE 3: Bone lesion occurred trying to retrieve the residual fragment before sinus lift approach.

2. Case Report

A 51-year-old male patient (R.R.), with good general health (ASA 1), nonsmoker, was referred to our department for rehabilitation of the first molar (Figure 1). The tooth was periodontally compromised, with mobility of II degree and furcation interest. It was decided to extract it and in the second phase, after 3-month-healing period, make a single-tooth implant restoration with the bone volume augmentation.

The first attempt to extract this tooth was made by nonexpert oral surgeon and the palatal residual root was left inside (Figure 2).

Also during a second session with a specialist, it was difficult and complicated to remove the entire root, which was fragile and fell apart.

To avoid a higher bone loss and oroantral communication (Figure 3), it was decided to leave the last apical fragment in the alveolus. The primary purpose had not changed, and it was chosen to retrieve the residual root apex during sinus lift procedure, because antrostomy approach would help to remove it with a major visibility of the surgical field.

After the healing period, a further accurate radiographic exam was necessary. As for any other sinus floor elevation case, reformatted computer tomography (CT) scans were required to examine insufficient bony support (Figure 4).

This exam also revealed the palatal position of the residual root apex. Surgery was performed under local block anesthesia (posterior superior alveolar nerve, greater palatine nerve, and buccal infiltration from the canine to the first molar). An intrasulcular and crestal incision was performed and a full-thickness mucoperiostal flap was reflected to expose the maxillary and palatal wall (Figures 5 and 6).

An antrostomy with 5 mm diameter was made approximately from the distal root of first premolar to mesial root of second molar (Figure 7).

The membrane was elevated from the bone and we could see the root fragment adjacent to the sinus floor. The residual was removed without difficulty with hemostatic clamps (Figures 8(a) and 8(b)).

Afterwards, implant was placed using a conventional approach: drills were used to prepare the fixture bed and the implant of 4,3 Ø in diameter and 11,5 mm of length (NobelReplace Select, NobelBiocare, Göteborg, Sweden) was installed protecting elevated sinus membrane. The insertion torque was of 35 N/cm, measured with a manual torque wrench by the operator. Particulate graft material (Geistlich Bio-Oss) was inserted between Schneiderian membrane and sinus floor and also between implant and vestibular tissue to fill the gap (Figure 9(a)).

In the lateral bony windows collagen membrane was installed to reinforce and keep stable graft material (Figure 9(b)).

The wound was closed primarily and detached sutures were positioned.

Pharmacological management was with antibiotic therapy (oral amoxicillin and clavulanic acid 875 mg + 125 mg every 8 hours) and nonsteroidal anti-inflammatory drugs (ibuprofen 600 mg, as needed by the patient).

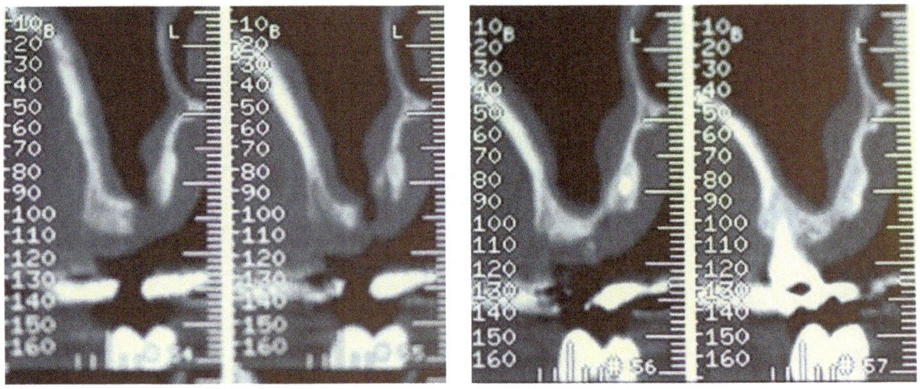

(a) (b)

FIGURE 4: ((a), (b)) Radiographic exams (paraxial images) also revealed not only the residual root apex in the palatal side, but also insufficient bone volume.

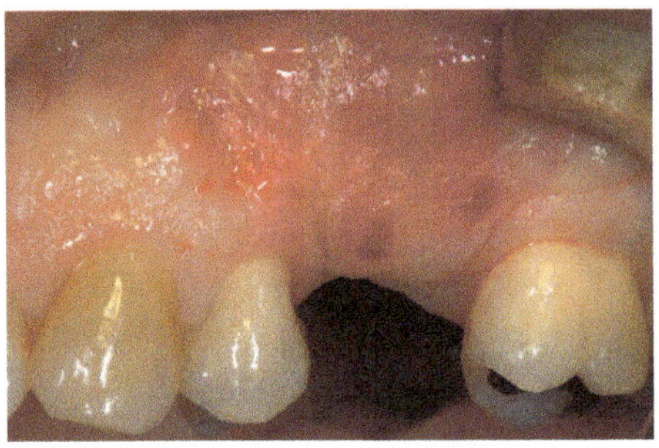

FIGURE 5: Surgical site.

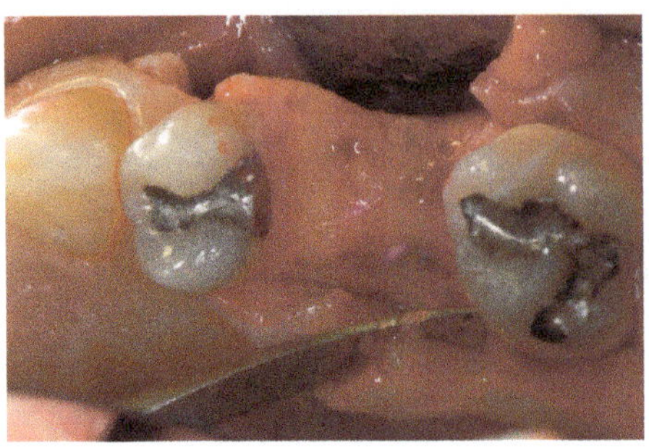

FIGURE 6: Alveolar bone exposed.

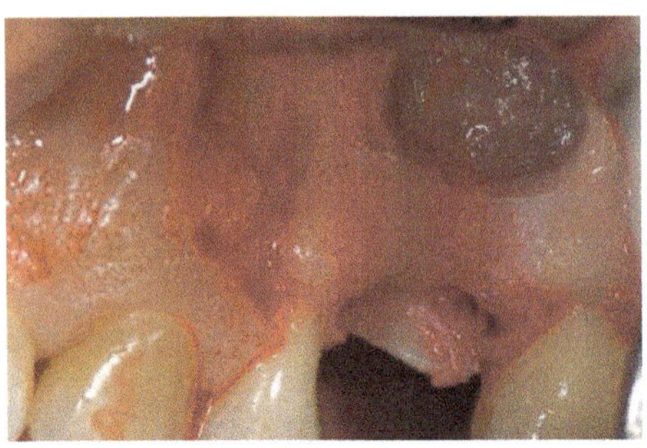

FIGURE 7: Antrostomy on the lateral maxillary wall.

Sutures were removed after fifteen days and no postoperative complications were present. No signs of infection, inflammation, or maxillary sinusitis were detected.

After three-months, the second-stage operation was carried out to expose the fixture and cover screw was placed (Figure 10). Radiograph examination showed (Figure 11) correct osteointegration, displaying good bone filling and the successful fractured apex retrieval (Figure 12).

3. Discussion

Extraction is the most common surgery performed in the dental office. Although most cases are simple, complications can occur.

The fracture of a root is the most frequent complication of exodontia [11]. It occurs accidentally and may cause severe problems as infection, residual cyst, and, in case of displacement of the fragment, an oroantral fistula [12].

In endodontically treated teeth, fracture resistance decreases, and the amount of stress in dental tissues increases in the face of functional forces. These stresses are vertical and oblique forces, which are the basis of masticatory function and increase the possibility of fracture both of crown and root. The restoration types play an important role in the clinical prognosis of these endodontically treated teeth [13]. Many studies have revealed the ideal restorative approaches that increase fracture resistance of remaining dental tissues after endodontic treatment and enables minimal stress transmission [14, 15]. However, when there is a strong patient's interest on preserving a compromised tooth, it must be clearly underlined that endodontically treated teeth are more weak and with a high probability of fracture and possible complications.

In case of the fractured fragment retrieval the visibility of surgical area takes a very important role.

Trying to access the apex with a blind procedure could determinate unjustified aggressive treatment with worse prognosis of alveolus healing influencing bone insufficiency in the area.

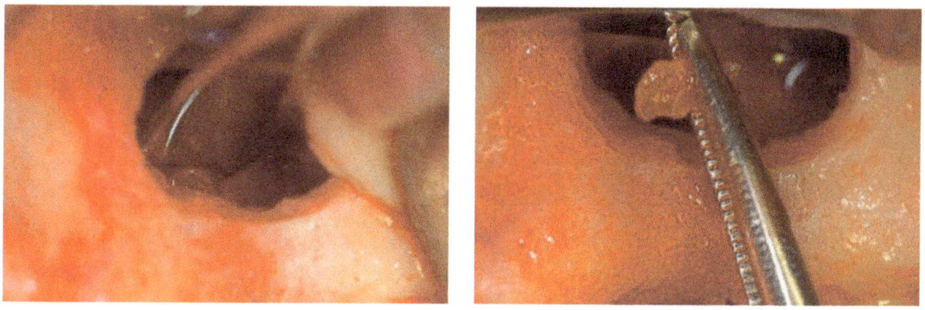

(a) (b)

FIGURE 8: (a), (b): Intra-operative images during retrieval of residual root apex through the antrostomy.

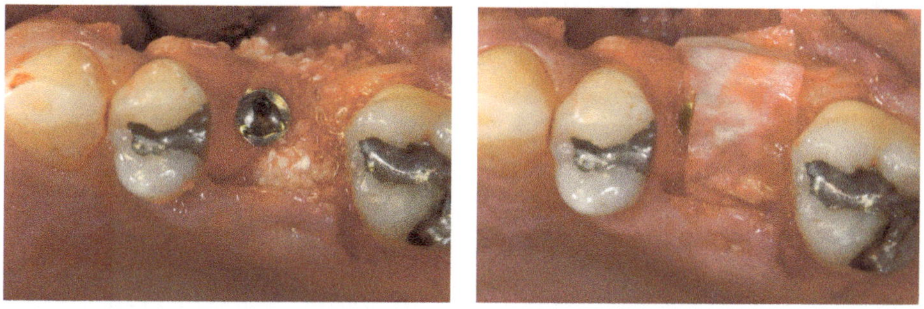

(a) (b)

FIGURE 9: (a) Insertion of graft material; (b) collagen membrane positioned.

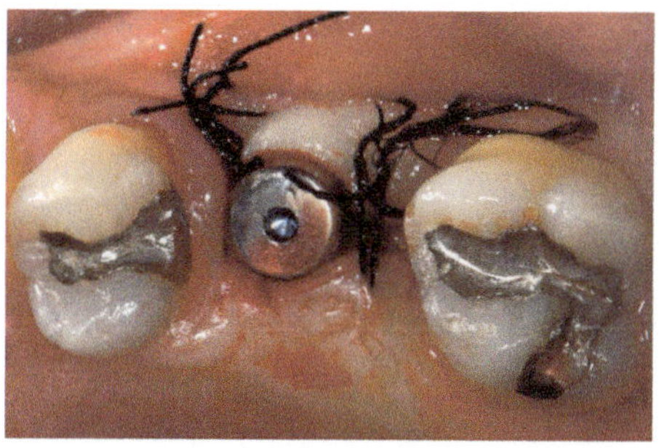

FIGURE 10: Reopening after 3 months.

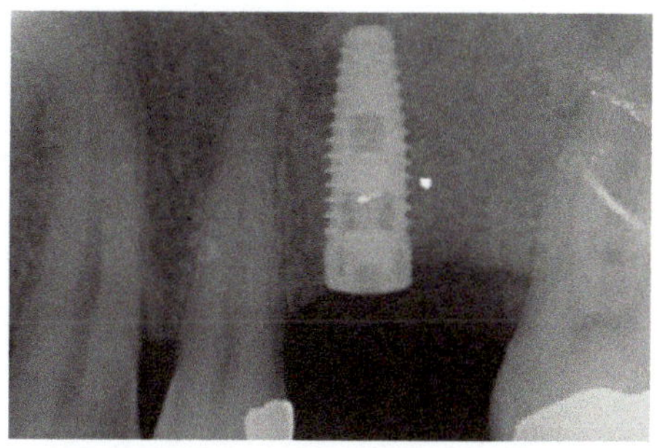

FIGURE 11: X-ray control after 3 months.

Furthermore, the inadequate bone volume of our patient required a surgery to enhance it for implant placement and a higher bone volume loss had to be prevented by all means. It was decided to perform an antrostomy procedure with implant rehabilitation and simultaneous retrieval of the root fragment. The necessity of a sinus lift surgery determines adequate healing time (in our case it was 3 months) to be sure to achieve the correct primary coronal stability.

There are cases present in the literature of foreign bodies displacement into maxillary sinus, because of the increased oral implant migration. If the search is restricted just to fractured root, the results highlight correlation with extraction of maxillary third molars.

Even if a foreign body is a root or an oral implant, the migration of foreign bodies into paranasal sinuses is certainly a severe complication and it needs a proper procedure for its retrieval to avoid chronic infections. Most authors chose Caldwell-Luc technique [16–18]. This approach provides direct access to the sinus but may result in the partial loss of functions of the sinus. For that reason the most frequently used technique is the functional endoscopic sinus surgery (FESS) [19]. This technique is minimally invasive, recreating competent sinus ostial patency, and provides access to drain and clean the cavity exudates.

In case of a foreign body migration into sinus, it is important to emphasize that patients do not always show symptoms. In the literature there are reports of asymptomatic cases [16] and reports of patients with infections, such as acute and chronic sinusitis [16, 20, 21]. But it would be appropriate to remove all foreign bodies present in the maxillary sinus,

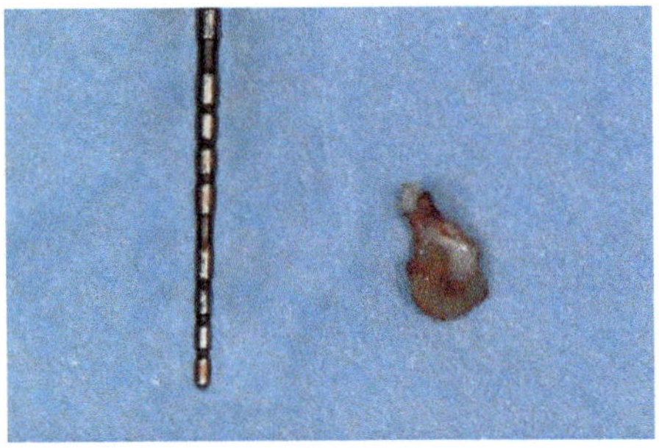

FIGURE 12: Retrieved residual root fragment.

because of the interference with the sinus clearance and the inflammatory response of the sinus membrane.

In our case the fractured root was not in the sinus but still retained by the sinus membrane.

Lifting up the Schneiderian membrane permits to open the surgical area, with a better view and to reach the residual fragment with noninvasive instrument like haemostatic clamps.

With this work, we want to underline the importance of being able to change planning during intrasurgical complications. It is most appropriate to operate with safe and simple procedures to reduce surgical discomfort for the patient.

References

[1] F. A. Al-Quran, R. F. Al-Ghalayini, and B. N. Al-Zu'bi, "Single-tooth replacement: factors affecting different prosthetic treatment modalities," *BMC Oral Health*, vol. 11, no. 1, article 34, 2011.

[2] P. Bouchard, F. Renouard, D. Bourgeois, O. Fromentin, M. H. Jeanneret, and A. Beresniak, "Cost-effectiveness modeling of dental implant vs. bridge," *Clinical Oral Implants Research*, vol. 20, no. 6, pp. 583–587, 2009.

[3] R. Adell, U. Lekholm, B. Rockler, and P. I. Branemark, "A 15-year study of osseointegrated implants in the treatment of the edentulous jaw," *International Journal of Oral Surgery*, vol. 10, no. 6, pp. 387–416, 1981.

[4] G. Venkateshwar, M. Padhye, A. Khosla, and S. Kakkar, "Complications of exodontia: a retrospective study," *Indian Journal of Dental Research*, vol. 22, no. 5, pp. 633–638, 2011.

[5] S. Uckan and D. Buchbinder, "Sinus lift approach for the retrieval of root fragments from the maxillary sinus," *International Journal of Oral and Maxillofacial Surgery*, vol. 32, no. 1, pp. 87–90, 2003.

[6] I.-Y. Huang, C.-M. Chen, and F.-H. Chuang, "Caldwell-Luc procedure for retrieval of displaced root in the maxillary sinus," *Oral Surgery, Oral Medicine, Oral Pathology, Oral Radiology and Endodontology*, vol. 112, no. 6, pp. e59–e63, 2011.

[7] A. Sethi, K. M. Cariappa, and A. Chitra, "Root fragment in the ostium of the maxillary sinus," *British Journal of Oral and Maxillofacial Surgery*, vol. 47, no. 7, pp. 572–573, 2009.

[8] D. Flanagan, "A method to retrieve a displaced dental implant from the maxillary sinus," *The Journal of Oral Implantology*, vol. 35, no. 2, pp. 70–74, 2009.

[9] A. Borgonovo, A. Fabbri, R. Boninsegna, M. Dolci, and R. Censi, "Displacement of a dental implant into the maxillary sinus: case series," *Minerva Stomatologica*, vol. 59, no. 1-2, pp. 45–54, 2010.

[10] J. DeFreitas and F. E. Lucente, "The Caldwell-Luc procedure: institutional review of 670 cases: 1975–1985," *Laryngoscope*, vol. 98, no. 12, pp. 1297–1300, 1988.

[11] G. Venkateshwar, M. Padhye, A. Khosla, and S. Kakkar, "Complications of exodontia: a retrospective study," *Indian Journal of Dental Research*, vol. 22, no. 5, pp. 633–638, 2011.

[12] E. J. Woolley and M. Patel, "Subdural empyema resulting from displacement of a root into the maxillary antrum," *British Dental Journal*, vol. 182, no. 11, pp. 430–432, 1997.

[13] I. Yıkılgan and O. Bala, "How can stress be controlled in endodontically treated teeth? A 3D finite element analysis," *The Scientific World Journal*, vol. 2013, Article ID 426134, 7 pages, 2013.

[14] A. Elayouti, M. I. Serry, J. Geis-Gerstorfer, and C. Löst, "Influence of cusp coverage on the fracture resistance of premolars with endodontic access cavities," *International Endodontic Journal*, vol. 44, no. 6, pp. 543–549, 2011.

[15] M. Hammad, A. Qualtrough, and N. Silikas, "Effect of new obturating materials on vertical root fracture resistance of endodontically treated teeth," *Journal of Endodontics*, vol. 33, no. 6, pp. 732–736, 2007.

[16] G. M. Raghoebar and A. Vissink, "Treatment for an endosseous implant migrated into the maxillary sinus not causing maxillary sinusitis: case report," *International Journal of Oral and Maxillofacial Implants*, vol. 18, no. 5, pp. 745–749, 2003.

[17] P. Galindo, E. Sánchez-Fernández, G. Avila, A. Cutando, and J. E. Fernandez, "Migration of implants into the maxillary sinus: two clinical cases," *International Journal of Oral and Maxillofacial Implants*, vol. 20, no. 2, pp. 291–295, 2005.

[18] S. D. Schaefer, S. Manning, and L. G. Close, "Endoscopic paranasal sinus surgery: indications and considerations," *Laryngoscope*, vol. 99, no. 1, pp. 1–5, 1989.

[19] M. Chiapasco, G. Felisati, A. Maccari, R. Borloni, F. Gatti, and F. di Leo, "The management of complications following displacement of oral implants in the paranasal sinuses: a multicenter clinical report and proposed treatment protocols," *International Journal of Oral and Maxillofacial Surgery*, vol. 38, no. 12, pp. 1273–1278, 2009.

[20] J.-W. Kim, C. H. Lee, T.-K. Kwon, and D. K. Kim, "Endoscopic removal of a dental implant through a middle meatal antrostomy," *British Journal of Oral and Maxillofacial Surgery*, vol. 45, no. 5, pp. 408–409, 2007.

[21] H. G. El Charkawi, A. S. El Askary, and A. Ragab, "Endoscopic removal of an implant from the maxillary sinus: a case report," *Implant Dentistry*, vol. 14, no. 1, pp. 30–35, 2005.

28

Idiopathic Orofacial Granulomatosis with Varied Clinical Presentation

Rathy Ravindran[1] **and Anila Karunakaran**[2]

[1] *Department of Oral and Maxillofacial Pathology, Azeezia College of Dental Science & Research, Diamond Hills, Meeyannoor, Kollam-691537, Kerala State, India*
[2] *Department of Oral and Maxillofacial Pathology, Kannur Dental College, Anjarakandy, Mamba, Kannur-670611, Kerala State, India*

Correspondence should be addressed to Rathy Ravindran; aswathysundaran1@yahoo.co.in

Academic Editors: C. Landes, P. Lopez Jornet, and K. Seymour

Orofacial granulomatosis is a granulomatous disease of orofacial region, which can occur for a variety of reasons. The clinical features are highly variable and sometimes so insidious that signs and symptoms are not frequently severe to cause alarm. The lips are most commonly involved with persistent/recurrent swelling. The medical history is very important as Crohn's disease and sarcoidosis can present oral manifestation. Other causes like mycobacterial infection, foreign body reaction, fungal infection, and allergy were excluded with further investigation to establish diagnosis. Here and we report a case of orofacial granulomatosis with a review of the literature.

1. Introduction

Orofacial granulomatosis (OFG) is a chronic inflammatory disorder characterized by persistent or recurrent soft tissue enlargement, oral ulceration, and a variety of orofacial features. The term orofacial granulomatosis was proposed by Wiesenfield et al. in 1985. Focal granulomas may occur anywhere in the oral mucosa or in the subcutaneous tissue of the skin where they present as localized firm mass that are occasionally multinodular. When diagnosis of noncaseating granuloma is made microscopically, the patient should be evaluated for several systemic diseases such as crohn's disease, sarcoidosis, TB and the local processes (Table 1) that may be responsible for similar oral lesion has to be ruled out. Orofacial granulomatosis is a term which encompasses variety of clinical presentation that upon biopsy reveal presence of nonspecific granulomatosis inflammation. Here we report a case of idiopathic orofacial granuloma and the etiology, diagnostic approach and treatment of orofacial granulomatosis reviewed.

2. Case Report

A 40-year-old male patient reported to our OPD with complaint of swelling of lower lip. The patient gave a history of similar swelling 8 months back which was biopsied at another hospital and the report is unavailable. The medical history was noncontributory. Intraoral examination revealed diffuse swelling of lower lip (Figure 1). On palpation the swelling was nodular with diffuse margin, soft to firm in consistency. A provisional diagnosis of mucocele was made. Routine hematological examination was performed and all were with normal limits. Biopsy of the lip lesion revealed circumscribed aggregates of noncaseating granulomatous inflammation consisting of lymphocyte and epithelioid histiocytes with multinucleated giant cells. The granuloma consists of central aggregates of histiocytes with peripheral rim of inflammatory cells chiefly lymphocytes (Figures 2 and 3). The fibrous connective tissue showed areas of vascularity, multiple granulomas containing lot of giant cells suggestive of granulomatous lesion (Figure 4). Following this, patient

Table 1: Oral granuloma.

Systemic causes	Local causes
Chronic granulomatous disease	Chronic oral infection
Crohn's disease	Foreign material
Sarcoidosis	Allergy
Tuberculosis	

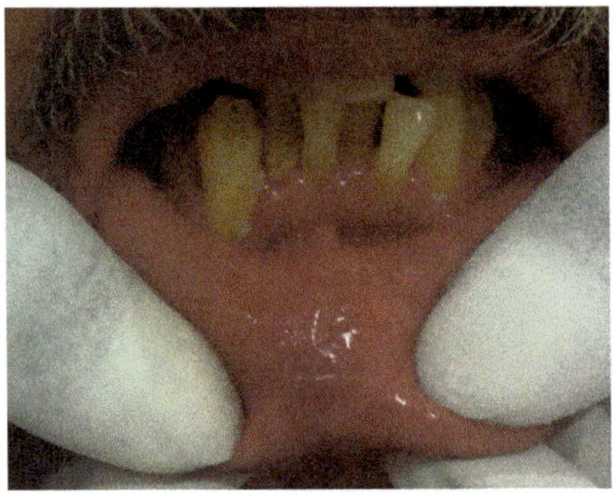

Figure 1: Diffuse swelling of lower lip.

was thoroughly investigated to rule out the list of granulomatous disease. Hematological investigation was performed for RBC count, differential count, platelet count, Hb%, ESR, serum folate, iron, and serum ACE (Angiotensin converting enzyme) levels were found to be within normal limits. The Mantoux test was negative. The chest radiograph did not reveal any pathology. Periodic acid Schiff stain for fungal organism and acid fast bacilli stain for mycobacteria were negative. No foreign material was detected. The patient gave no history of allergy. As the patient had normal hematological value and the medical history was not contributory for intestinal manifestation, further investigation for Crohn's disease was not undertaken.

The above investigation ruled out tuberculosis, sarcoidosis, fungal infection, and Crohn's disease. The diagnosis of idiopathic orofacial granulomatosis was made. The patient reported with recurrent swelling. The patient was treated with biweekly intralesional injection of triamcinolone acetonide with simultaneous topical clobetasol propionate for 4 weeks. On review patient showed improvement. On followup for a period of one year the patient showed no recurrences.

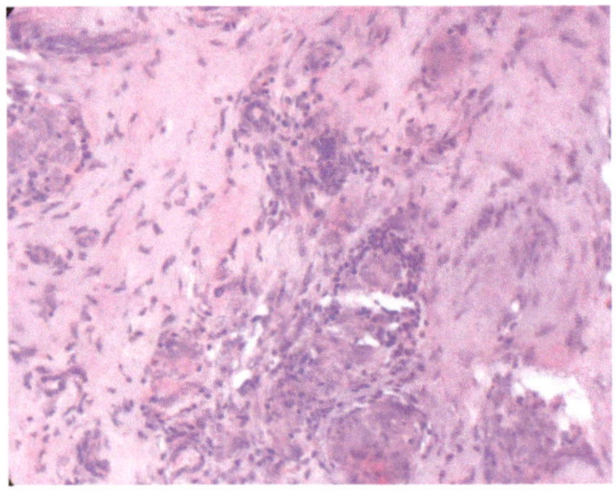

Figure 2: Aggregates of noncaseating granulomas (H&E 10x).

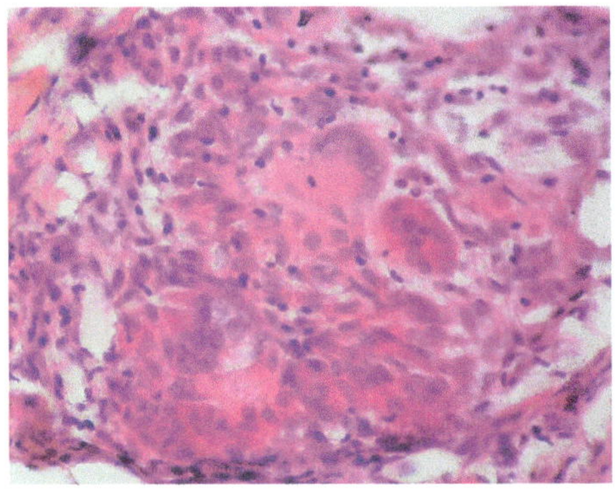

Figure 3: Granuloma showing peripheral lymphocytes, central histiocytes, and giant cell (H&E 40x).

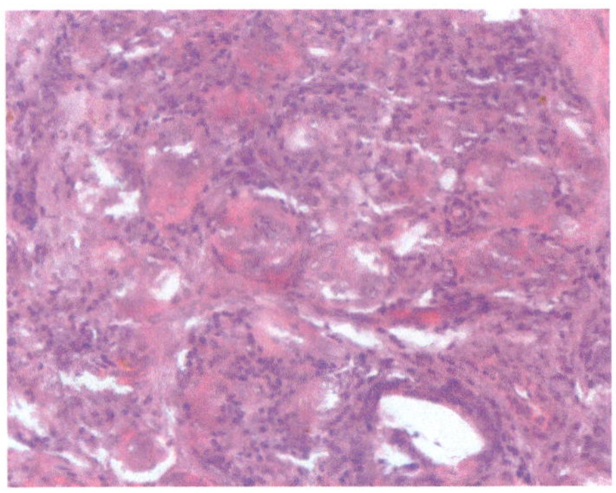

Figure 4: Granuloma with many multinucleated giant cells (H&E 40x).

3. Discussion

The clinical and histopathological features of orofacial granulomatosis can be produced by a variety of underlying causes; this diagnosis is beginning of patient's evaluation [1, 2]. The conditions with granulomatous lesion histologically include Melkersson-Rosenthal syndrome, Crohn's disease, sarcoidosis, TB, hypersensitivity reaction, and angioneurotic edema [3] (Table 2).

In the present case the clinician's provisional diagnosis was mucocele and hence the lesion was submitted for histopathological examination. The clinical presentation of intraoral mucocele in some cases of sarcoidosis which led to its diagnosis has been reported [3].

On histopathological diagnosis of noncaseating granulomatous inflammation, systemic evaluation was undertaken. The hematological evaluation and chest radiograph ruled out sarcoidosis and tuberculosis [4, 5]. Since the patients hematological investigation was within normal limits and did not give history of signs and symptoms of gastrointestinal discomfort further investigation of colonoscopy and biopsy is not required [2, 6]. Investigations were performed to exclude diseases with similar clinical and histopathological feature.

TABLE 2: Differential diagnosis of orofacial granulomatosis.

Disease	Features different to OFG
Crohn's disease	Have illeal and/or rectal disease
Sarcoidosis	Pulmonary, cutaneuos, lacrimal, salivary, neurological, skeletal features
Allergic angioedema	Nonpitting oedema of lips, tongue, pharynx, face. History of atopic disease
Miescher's cheilitis	Labial enlargement, similar histopathology to OFG
Melkerson-Rosenthal syndrome	Labial enlargement, fissuring of tongue, facial nerve palsy variant of OFG
Cheilitis glandularis	Labial enlargement with ulcers. Mild acute and chronic inflammation (without granuloma) within minor salivary glands of lip
Tuberculosis	Rarely lips. Usually contain caseating granuloma

Orofacial granulomatosis is a disease with wide spectrum of clinical presentation. The causative agent in the present case is unknown; hence it is categorized as idiopathic Orofacial granulomatosis.

The exact cause of orofacial granulomatosis is still unknown, although several theories have been suggested including infection, genetic predisposition, and allergy [7]. The etiological agents such as food substances, food additives, dental material microbiological agents have been proposed, but its pathogenesis is uncertain. A delayed type of hypersensitivity reaction appears to play a role, but the antigen inducing immunological reaction varies in individuals. The evidence for role of genetic predisposition to disease is sparse. Tilakaratne et al. propose the term idiopathic orofacial granulomatosis as better term for cases restricted to oral region without any identifiable known granulomatous disease and diagnosis should not be changed until patient develops systemic manifestation of specific granulomatous condition [8]. The various treatment modalities include intralesional injection, topical and systemic steroids, and surgical excision [9].

4. Conclusion

Orofacial granulomatosis can be a distinct clinical disorder or can be an initial presentation of underlying systemic disease such as crohn's disease or sarcoidosis. Hence an early diagnosis of orofacial granulomatosis can identify an underlying disease as cases have been reported which had initial manifestation of orofacial granulomatosis. Hence followup for the patient is advised as a step in prevention of a possible systemic granulomatous disease.

Conflict of Interests

The authors declare that they have no conflict of interests.

References

[1] L. R. Eversole, "Orofacial granulamatosis and other inflammatory lesion," in *Essential of Oral Medicine*, pp. 245–251, BC Decker, 2002.

[2] G. Karthikeyan, M. Arvind, N. D. Jayakumar, and M. Khakar, "Idiopathic Orofacial granulamatosis in a young patient : a rare entity," *Journal of Oral and Maxillofacial Pathology*, vol. 16, no. 3, pp. 432–434, 2012.

[3] B. W. Neville, D. D. Damm, C. M. Allen, and J. E. Bouquot, *Oral and Maxillofacial Pathology*, W.B. Sanders, Philadelphia, Pa, USA, 3rd edition, 2004.

[4] L. Suresh and L. Radfar, "Oral sarcoidosis: a review of literature," *Oral Diseases*, vol. 11, no. 3, pp. 138–145, 2005.

[5] J. Mar Coval and J. Mana, "Specific, (granulomatosis) oral lesions of sarcoidosis: report of two cases," *Medicina Oral Patologia Oral y Cirugia Bucal*, vol. 15, no. 3, pp. e456–e458, 2010.

[6] T. Bogenrieder, G. Rogler, T. Vogt, M. Landthaler, and W. Stolz, "Orofacial granulomatosis as the initial presentation of Crohn's disease in an adolescent," *Dermatology*, vol. 206, no. 3, pp. 273–278, 2003.

[7] T. K. Thomas, R. S. Neelakandan, D. Bhargava, and A. Deshpande, "Orofacial granulomatosis: a clinicopathologic correlation," *Head and Neck Pathology*, vol. 5, no. 2, pp. 133–136, 2011.

[8] W. M. Tilakaratne, J. Freysdottir, and F. Fortune, "Orofacial granulomatosis: Review on aetiology and pathogenesis," *Journal of Oral Pathology and Medicine*, vol. 37, no. 4, pp. 191–195, 2008.

[9] B. Grave, M. McCullough, and D. Wiesenfeld, "Orofacial granulomatosis—a 20-year review," *Oral Diseases*, vol. 15, no. 1, pp. 46–51, 2009.

Intraductal Papilloma: Atypical Presentation

P. Ramaswamy,[1] Tanya Khaitan,[1] A. Anuradha,[2] B. Praveen Kumar,[1] and S. Sudhakar[1]

[1] *Department of Oral Medicine and Radiology, St. Joseph Dental College and Hospital, Duggirala, Eluru, Andhra Pradesh 534003, India*
[2] *Department of Oral and Maxillofacial Pathology, St. Joseph Dental College and Hospital, Duggirala, Eluru, Andhra Pradesh 534003, India*

Correspondence should be addressed to P. Ramaswamy; ramomdr@gmail.com

Academic Editors: L. Junquera and K. Seymour

Ductal papillomas have unique papillary features arising from the salivary gland duct system. They comprise three rare benign adenomas, namely, inverted ductal papilloma, sialadenoma papilliferum, and intraductal papilloma. Intraductal papilloma is an extremely rare benign salivary gland tumor that occurs most commonly in the minor salivary glands. Here, we are presenting a case report of intraductal papilloma in an 18-year-old patient.

1. Introduction

Salivary gland neoplasms are uncommon; only 10–15% of cases are reported in the minor salivary glands [1].

Benign papillary lesions that arise from the ductal system of salivary glands include intraductal papilloma, inverted ductal papilloma, and sialadenoma papilliferum. These ductal papillomas are considered to be relatively rare but generate considerable interest because of their remarkable similarities and variations in clinical and histological appearance [2]. They represent adenomas with unique papillary features, a nonaggressive biologic behavior, and a predilection for the minor salivary glands [3].

Intraductal papilloma is a rare benign lesion showing a characteristic papillary growth of ductal epithelium. It appears as a submucosal small nodule predominantly in lip and buccal mucosa [4]. They tend to occur in the middle-aged and elderly and rarely in children [3]. Here, we are reporting an infrequent case of intraductal papilloma in an 18 year old patient.

2. Case Report

An 18-year-old male patient reported having a complaint of growth in the left half of the lower lip region since 2 months. The patient's history revealed that he had noticed the growth 2 months back which initially started as a small growth and gradually increased over a period of 1 month to attain the present size. There was history of mild and occasional pain associated with the growth. The patient claimed that there was no history of paraesthesia or numbness and no similar lesion elsewhere. The medical, dental, family, and personal histories were noncontributory.

Intraoral examination revealed presence of solitary, well-defined and oval-shaped, nodular exophytic growth (Figure 1) on the left half of the lower labial mucosa measuring approximately 9 × 7 mm in size. Anteroposteriorly, it extends 0.5 cm from the vermilion border of lower lip to 1 cm from the lower vestibular area. Mediolaterally, the growth extends 1.5 cm away from the midline to 1.5 cm in front of the left corner of mouth. The surface over the growth appears whitish in the centre and erythematous in the periphery. On palpation, the growth was sessile, slight tender, and firm in consistency and arose from the underlying soft tissue.

Based on the history, clinical features and the nature of the growth, a provisional diagnosis of irritational fibroma was considered. Differential diagnoses of fibrosed mucocele, peripheral giant cell granuloma, and extragingival pyogenic granuloma were considered. The patient was subjected to complete hematological examination, and all the parameters were within normal limits. The growth was being excised and specimen was sent for histopathological evaluation.

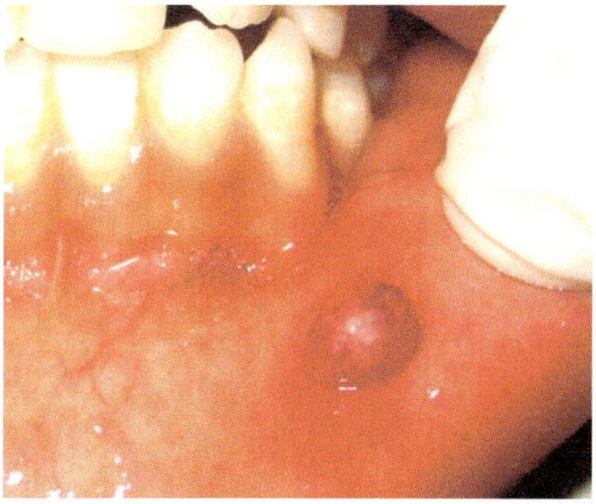

FIGURE 1: Solitary, well-defined and oval-shaped, nodular exophytic growth on the left half of the lower labial mucosa.

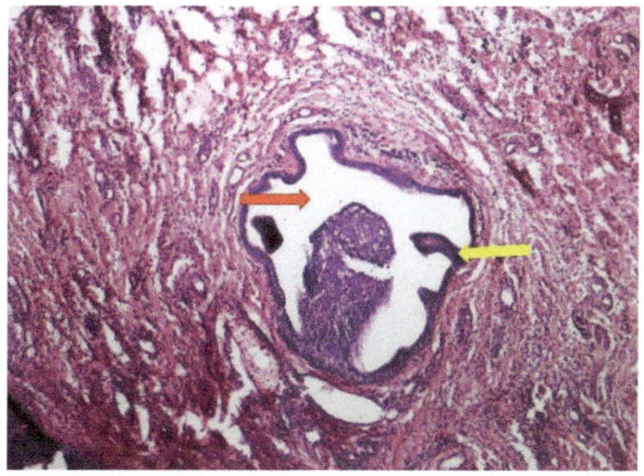

FIGURE 2: Histopathological section of H&E specimen (40x) showing minor salivary gland with atrophy of the acinar cells (red arrow) and with large dilated duct is partly double walled and partly stratified squamous with numerous papillary fronds (yellow arrow) extending into the lumen.

On microscopic examination, the specimen showed stratified squamous epithelium with acanthosis, parakeratosis, and intracellular edema. The underlying connective tissue is delicate with mild chronic inflammatory infiltrate, numerous dilated engorged capillaries, extravasated red blood cells and mast cells. Minor salivary gland with atrophy of the acinar cells, (red arrow) and with large dilated duct is partly double walled and partly stratified squamous with numerous papillary fronds (yellow arrow) extending into the lumen (Figure 2). The papillary fronds are bland with mucous cells. Based on the clinical features and histopathology, final diagnosis of intraductal papilloma was established.

The patient was being followed up after 10, days and healing lesion was found on examination (Figure 3).

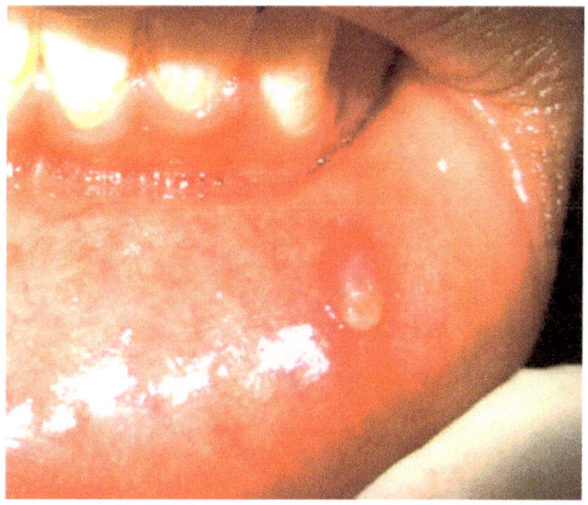

FIGURE 3: Healing areas seen post-operatively after 10 days.

3. Discussion

Intraductal papillomas of the breast are relatively common lesions with an incidence of approximately 2–3% in humans [5]. The exact incidence of intraoral intraductal papilloma is not easy to evaluate in the literature due to the inconsistent terminology as the term "papillary cystadenoma" is often applied instead of the term "intraductal papilloma" [2].

Intraductal papilloma is a luminal papillary proliferation of duct epithelium that arises from a segment of the interlobular or excretory duct and causes unicystic dilatation [3]. This is also known as "simple ductal papilloma" [6].

The pathogenesis of intraductal papilloma is still uncertain. Brannon et al. [2] stated that these lesions originate from the salivary gland duct epithelium, most likely the excretory duct.

These tumors usually present as asymptomatic, well-defined solitary submucosal masses or swellings that vary in size from less than 1–1.5 cm [7]. The lesion often has a reddish color [6]. The ages of patients have ranged from 29 to 77 years, with mean age of 54 years. Gender distribution has remained essentially even [7]. The minor salivary glands are more frequently involved than the major glands. Intraductal papillomas are most commonly found in the lips and buccal mucosa followed by palate and tongue. Of the major glands, the parotid is most frequently involved [3].

In contrast to intraductal papillomas, papillary cystadenomas are morphologically multicystic with numerous small-to-medium-sized cystic spaces. In the papillary cystadenoma, the intraluminal growth is often characterized by multiple papillary projections with a variety of epithelial cell types, but usually the papillary growth occupies the lumen to a limited degree [3]. In inverted ductal papilloma, the character of the proliferating epithelium is predominantly epidermoid, whereas in intraductal papilloma, it is columnar or cuboidal epithelium and/or mucous cells [7].

Microscopically, this papilloma appears to arise in the duct system at a deeper level relative to the mucosal surface. The proliferating epithelium is a characteristic of the ductal epithelium in this location. The cyst wall is lined by a single or double layer of cuboidal and columnar cells. Extending into the lumen are several to numerous papillary fronds that have thin fibrovascular cores which form a complex branching structure that creates an appearance of islands of tumor. These papillary projections are covered by the same cuboidal and columnar ductal epithelia [7].

The blockage of a salivary gland duct can result in ductal ectasia and hyperplasia of the ductal epithelium. This epithelial hyperplasia forms the intraluminal papillary projections, and these changes cause chronic inflammation, fibrosis, and atrophy of adjacent salivary gland lobules [2, 4].

Immunohistochemical studies have supported an origin of these tumors in ductal luminal cells, ductal epithelium, and excretory duct epithelium. Ishikawa et al. [8] showed that the tumor cells facing the lumina were strongly positive for keratin and epithelial membrane antigen (EMA) and partly reactive for lactoferrin and S-100. Hara et al. [9] proved that tumor cells show high reactivity to human cytokeratin M-630 and CAM, moderate reactivity to low molecular weight keratin, and partial reactivity to S-100, amylase, and EMA. These reports proposed the excretory duct epithelium as an origin of the lesion. Nagao et al. [10] affirmed that tumor cells are reactive for cytokeratin (AE1/AE3, CAM5.2), EMA, and S-100 and negative for cytokeratin 14, lactoferrin, and SMA and proposed then origin as ductal luminal cells.

Excision is curative, and these tumors are not known to recur. In fact, if small enough, all types of papillomas of the major salivary glands may be removed in the dental clinic with only local anaesthesia [7].

References

[1] P. Jansisyanont, R. H. Blanchaert Jr., and R. A. Ord, "Intraoral minor salivary gland neoplasm: a single institution experience of 80 cases," *International Journal of Oral and Maxillofacial Surgery*, vol. 31, no. 3, pp. 257–261, 2002.

[2] R. B. Brannon, J. J. Sciubba, and M. Giulani, "Ductal papillomas of salivary gland origin: a report of 19 cases and a review of the literature," *Oral Surgery, Oral Medicine, Oral Pathology, Oral Radiology, and Endodontics*, vol. 92, no. 1, pp. 68–77, 2001.

[3] R. B. Brannon and J. J. Sciubba, "World Health Organization classification of tumours," in *Pathology and Genetics of Head and Neck Tumours*, L. Barns, J. W. Eveson, P. Reichart, and D. Sidransky, Eds., pp. 272–273, IARC, Lyon, France, 2005.

[4] A. Tomonao, M. Kishino, T. Masuda et al., "Intraductal papilloma arising from sublingual minor salivary gland: case report and immunohistochemical study," *Oral Surgery, Oral Medicine, Oral Pathology, Oral Radiology, and Endodontology*, vol. 107, pp. e34–e37, 2009.

[5] K. S. Sahu, P. K. Singh, B. P. Singh et al., "Breast intraductal papilloma," *Jurnalul de Chirurgie (Iași)*, vol. 8, no. 2, 2012.

[6] M. S. Greenburg and M. Gick, *Burket's Oral Medicine Diagnosis and Treatment*, BC Decker, Ontario, Canada, 11th edition, 2003.

[7] G. L. Ellis and P. L. Auclair, "Ductal papillomas," in *Surgical Pathology of the Salivary Glands*, G. L. Ellis, P. L. Auclair, and D. R. Gnepp, Eds., pp. 238–252, Saunders, Philadelphia, Pa, USA, 1991.

[8] T. Ishikawa, S. Imada, and N. Ijuhin, "Intraductal papilloma of the anterior lingual salivary gland. Case report and immunohistochemical study," *International Journal of Oral and Maxillofacial Surgery*, vol. 22, no. 2, pp. 116–117, 1993.

[9] H. Hara, T. Oyama, K. Omori et al., "Fine needle aspiration cytology of an intraductal papilloma originating in a sublingual gland: a case report," *Acta Cytologica*, vol. 43, no. 3, pp. 457–463, 1999.

[10] T. Nagao, I. Sugano, O. Matsuzaki, H. Hara, Y. Kondo, and K. Nagao, "Intraductal papillary tumors of the major salivary glands: case reports of benign and malignant variants," *Archives of Pathology and Laboratory Medicine*, vol. 124, no. 2, pp. 291–295, 2000.

30

Dental Treatments under the General Anesthesia in a Child with Keratitis, Ichthyosis, and Deafness Syndrome

Sera Sımsek Derelioglu, Yücel Yılmaz, and Sultan Keles

Department of Pedodontics, Faculty of Dentistry, Atatürk University, 25240 Erzurum, Turkey

Correspondence should be addressed to Sera Sımsek Derelioglu; simseksera@gmail.com

Academic Editors: A. Milosevic and N. Shah

KID syndrome is a rare genodermatosis characterized by keratitis, ichthyosis, and sensorineural deafness. Although the dermatological, ophthalmologic, and sensorineural defects are emphasized in the literature, oral and dental evaluations are so superficial. In this case report, dental and oral symptoms of a three year and five months old boy with KID syndrome, suffering severe Early Childhood Caries (s-ECC) and dental treatments done under General Anesthesia (GA) were reported.

1. Introduction

Keratitis-ichthyosis-deafness (KID) syndrome is congenital ectodermal disorder without a clear mode of inheritance and is characterized by erythrokeratoderma, sensorineural hearing loss, and vascularizing keratitis [1–5]. KID syndrome is usually associated with less severe keratoderma and a milder hearing problem, but the eye involvement (keratitis) may eventually lead to impaired vision [3]. Keratitis is rather a late finding and may not sometimes be seen [6]. The cause of KID syndrome was identified as a germline missense mutation in the *GJB2* (gap junctionβ-2) gene encoding for connexin-26, which is essential for gap function formation in various tissues [7, 8]. Mutations in the GJB2 gene encoding connexin 26 are detrimental to function of cochlea, palmoplantar epidermis, hair follicles, corneal epithelium, and sweat glands and ducts, causing nonsyndromic sensorineural deafness, palmoplantar keratoderma and hearing impairment, Vohwinkel syndrome, and KID syndrome [8–11].

The first component required for diagnosis is characteristic skin findings which are usually present at birth or in early infancy. The well-demarcated, erythematous, hyperkeratotic plaques with verrucous surface are distributed over face and extremities alternating with smoother areas [3]. Hyperkeratotic plaques over the face give patients an appearance of premature aging [12].

The second one is presence of sensorineural hearing loss. The third component is ophthalmologic defects, which can progress total blindness [13].

Most patients have sparse or absent scalp hair, eyebrows, and eyelashes [3]. Nails may be thickened, deformed, brittle, white, hypoplastic, or normal. In some patients teeth are normally developed, but in others they may be defective and they are likely to develop caries [3, 14–17]. However, oral mucosa, status of the primary teeth and development of permanent teeth of the children with KID syndrome, and treatment approaches for those children have not been investigated so far. Here, we report the dental restorative treatments provided for a three-year and five-month-old boy—with prediagnosed KID syndrome—under general anesthesia in a hospital setting in order to eliminate his infectious teeth and to restore his carious teeth.

2. Case Report

2.1. Medical and Dental Histories. A 3-year and 5-month-old boy was admitted to our dental clinic for treatment of his extensive carious and infectious teeth. His skin was dry with well-demarcated lesions, and there were plaques of mild hyperkeratosis on the knees and elbows. Eyebrows and eyelashes were completely absent. The hair was short, dry, and sparse. He had a cochlear implant because of sensorineural

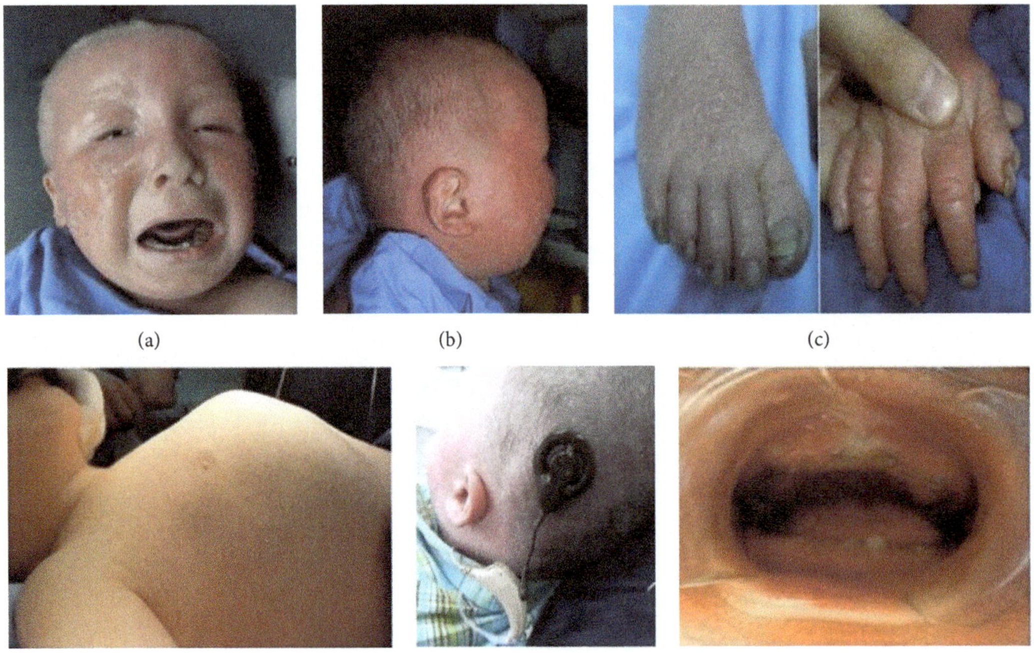

FIGURE 1: (a) Erythematous hyperkeratotic patches over the skin and the eyebrows and eyelashes are sparse in the photograph of this case. (b) Erythematous hyperkeratotic patches over the skin and the eyebrows and eyelashes are sparse in the photograph of this case. (c) View of hand, foot, and nails. (d) Pigeon chest. (e) Cochlear implant. (f) Intraoral view before the treatment.

hearing loss. The patient consulted an ophthalmologist for eye functions. The ophthalmologist did not note any visual problem of the patient. The patient had a history of Atrial Septal Defect (ASD) that continued until 2 years of age and later closed spontaneously. Since the patient had a neurosensory deafness, his ability to speak was less than his peers. However, he was uncooperative, but not mentally retarded. The patient's physical appearance had the typical findings of KID syndrome except for the diagnosis of "pigeon chest (pectus carinatum)," although he had no respiratory problems due to pigeon chest (Figure 1). He can walk by himself without any assistance. None of his family members were physically and medically disabled.

He had not received any dental treatment before. The oral mucosa was unremarkable. Intraoral examination of the child's tongue, lip mucosa, buccal mucosa, hard and soft palate, and sublingual region revealed no pathological findings. Hypoplasia, diffuse or limited opacities, fluorosis, and developmental abnormalities such as dentinogenesis imperfecta and amelogenesis imperfecta were not seen on the enamels or enamel residues. However, teeth 81, 82, 83, 84, 85, 72, 73, and 74 were vital; but with extensive caries. Teeth 51, 53, 52, 54, 55, 61, 63, 64, and 65 were nonvital because of severe caries. Two pediatric dentists diagnosed s-ECC (severe early child caries) by considering family history and dental findings (Figures 1 and 2). From ages 3 to 5, one or more cavitated, missing (due to caries), or filled smooth surfaces in primary maxillary anterior teeth or a decayed, missing, or filled score of ≥4 (age 3), ≥5 (age 4), or ≥6 (age 5) surfaces also constitutes s-ECC [18].

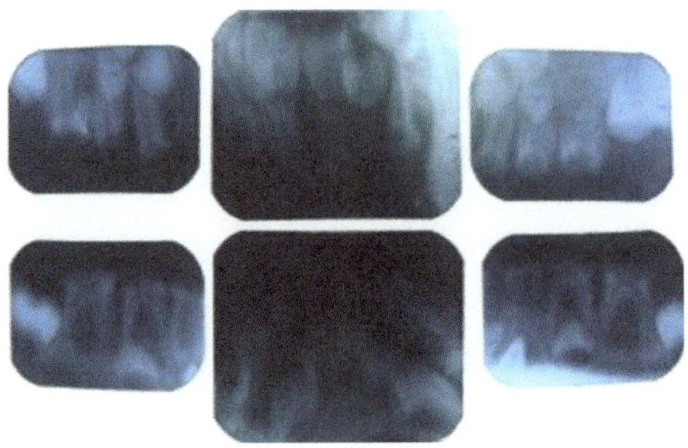

FIGURE 2: Periapical radiographs showing sEEC.

The child declaimed against the dental treatment and his skin was overstretched and sensitive. Also, he came from a rural area. Since the treatment could not be provided in dental office conditions, we discussed and decided that his dental treatment would be best provided under general anesthesia in a hospital setting.

2.2. General Anesthesia. Before each treatment session, he was referred to a cardiologist, a general pediatrician, and a radiologist in order to clear his medical status for general anesthesia. General anesthesia was induced by 2% sevoflurane using a face mask, according to a standard protocol, after an injection of the neuromuscular blocker

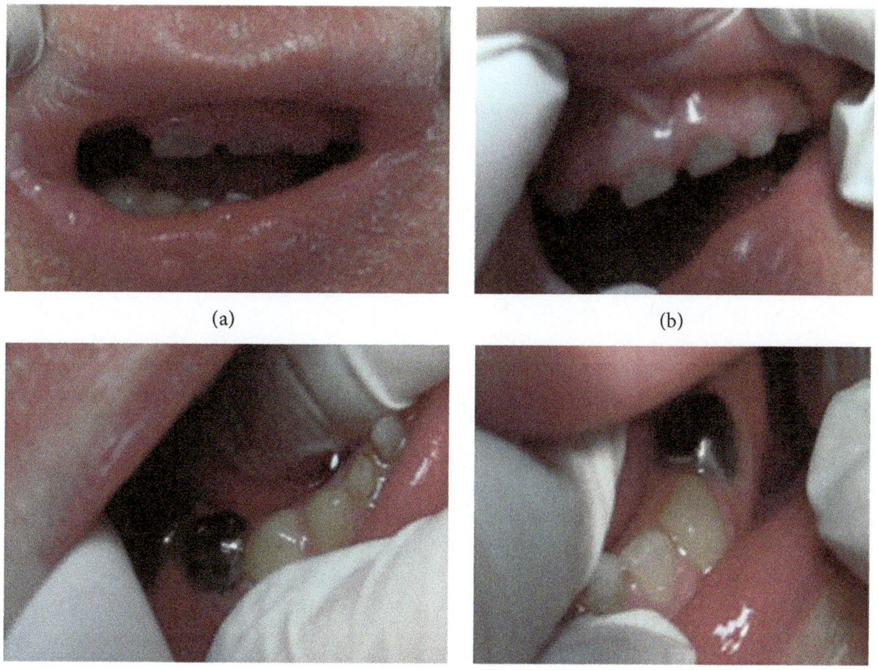

(a) (b) (c) (d)

FIGURE 3: Intraoral view after the dental treatment.

agent, vecuronium. The anesthesia was maintained by intravenously administered propofol. Atropine and neostigmine were administered to reverse the vecuronium-induced muscle relaxation when the dental procedures were completed. The patient was intubated nasotracheally in order to obtain unobstructed surgical access into the patient's mouth, which was kept open using a molt mouth prop. A saliva ejector was used to control oral moisture, and aspiration was prevented by placing moist sterile gauze in the pharyngopalatine area. The local anesthetic agent, articaine with epinephrine, was used when oral surgery and endodontic treatment were required.

2.3. Dental Treatments. The aim of this dental treatment was to restore his aesthetics, speech, and chewing capacity and to eliminate the chronically infected teeth.

The carious lesions of teeth 81, 82, 83, 72, and 73 were removed using round steel burs and the cavities were then prepared using self-etch dentin bonding agent, followed by incremental compomer resin restoration. Sof-Lex discs were used for contouring and polishing of the restored teeth.

The pulp of the three teeth (84, 85, and 74) was removed by a spoon excavator, and bleeding was arrested with gentle pressure from a sterile cotton wool pledget (CWP) moistened with saline. A 20% ferric sulphate solution was applied to pulp stumps for 15 seconds via a CWP. After CWP was removed, zinc oxide-eugenol cement was directly placed over pulp stumps, and then the tooth was restored with high viscosity glass-ionomer cement. The prefabricated stainless steel crowns (SSC) (3M/ESPE, St. Paul, MN, USA) for pulpotomised 84, 85, and 74 teeth were cemented using luting resin-modified glass-ionomer cement.

The root canals of teeth 51, 53, 61, and 63 were filled with a calcium hydroxide + iodoform mixture paste. Then, mixture paste was removed from root canal for a distance of 2 to 3 mm. The coronal part was reconstructed by a strip crown plus compomer.

The local anesthetic agent, articaine with epinephrine, was injected before tooth extraction. The chronically infected six teeth (52, 54, 55, 64, 65, and 75) were extracted and their alveolar sockets were sutured.

After completion of the dental treatments, the patient was transferred to the recovery room, where he recovered uneventfully from the general anesthesia. All dental procedures were completed without any problems, and the entire operation took about 90 minutes. After an oral examination (Figure 3), he was discharged from the hospital the next day.

The restorations were evaluated in terms of color, aesthetics, phonetics, and parent's general satisfaction. Their scores for each evaluation criterion at each follow-up visit were ranged from excellent to good [19].

3. Discussion

The pathology which is first described by Burns in 1915 with congenital keratoderma, keratitis, and deafness findings was named KID syndrome by Skinner et al. in 1981 [1, 2]. In the world literature, nearly 100 with KID syndrome were reported [20]. Our case was identified as KID syndrome by a pediatrician and a dermatologist in 2007. Therefore, we have not signed a genetic test up again, because it would not be ethical.

In our case, there were not only three characteristic symptoms such as ichthyosiform dermatosis, neurosensorial deafness, and but also sparse and absent eyebrow and eyelashes, nail malformations, and ASD as compatible with other case reports. The patient had a normal visual function. A vascularizing keratitis of the corneas, the third major feature of KID syndrome, occurs in about three-fourths patients. The eye symptoms usually occur by early adolescence though at some times these may appear during the fourth decade [6, 21]. The eye lesions of the KID syndrome are expressed later than the other alterations and although they are usually detected in childhood [14, 22–24], they may not evolve with symptom until puberty [25–27]. However, we had also a pigeon chest finding in our case which was not remarked in any other case reports. Pigeon chest is presented in Marfan syndrome [28], Noonan syndrome [29], Osteogenesis Imperfecta [30], Shprintzen-Goldberg syndrome [31], Loeys-Dietz syndrome [32], and Ehler-Danlos syndrome [33]. It has been specified that fatigue and asthma—ranging from mild to moderate levels—due to shortness of breath can be seen in the presence of pigeon chest [34]. In our case, we were not informed about such a symptom during the consultation before general anesthesia.

Our patient received his cochlear implant in 2009 due to hearing disability. His speaking ability was less than his peers and he had just started to make sentences. We decided to treat the child under general anesthesia because of his uncooperative manner that originated from his younger age and his communication problems. In our decision, we also considered the fact that travelling would be a problem for the far living family since the child had a lot of caries and infectious teeth should be treated for a long period of sessions. Additionally, the child's skin was so overstretched that if we chose to treat the patient with medical fixation, we could cause the skin to be cracked.

It has been stated that oral manifestations of KID syndrome might be leukokeratosis, patches of the oral mucosa, and deep fissures of the tongue or dental abnormalities [3, 15]. There were no symptoms related with tongue and mucosa. Those tissues were completely normal. Dental abnormalities in KID syndrome were mentioned in the literature [3]. However, types of the dental abnormalities were not present in the literature. We concluded that the dental situation of our patient was not the result of the KID syndrome. There was no evidence of any hereditary shape, color, or calcification disorders. Our patient was evaluated meticulously by two pediatric dentists. Two pediatric dentists decided by consensus that dental findings of the patient matched with s-ECC score for the ages over four years and his dental infections were aroused from the pulpal infections induced by the growth of the carious lesions. Our case had received no previous dental treatment. Additionally, permanent teeth were evaluated radiographically against the existence of structure and shape deformations. No structural deformation and calcification disorder were observed in permanent tooth germs. Excessive dental tissue loss or missing primary anterior teeth (space) in children may produce speech impediments of which the most familiar type is interdental (frontal) lisp, described as the inability to correctly pronounce the sounds of s, z, sh, zh, ch, and/or j, also known as the sibilant consonants [35, 36]. Children with such developmental phonetic disorders may also learn the erroneous pronunciations of those sibilants permanently and get wrong habitual tongue movements. Missing teeth in children may cause some psychological problems due to aesthetical reasons and mocking and stigmatizing of the other children because of the lips as well. Thus, in our case the nonvital upper and the lower incisors and canines were treated with root canal therapy and consequently restored with mushroom crowns. In this case, mushroom crowns are preferred because they have high clinical performance and gain utmost patient satisfaction.

In our case, the primary molars (52, 54, 55, 64, 65, and 75) which could not be treated due to extensive chronic infection were extracted. Vital teeth with deep dentine caries were restored with SSC following the ferric sulphate pulpotomy. When restorations were evaluated in accordance with Patient Satisfaction Scale (PSS), full parent satisfaction—especially for the anterior restorations, was obtained. Removable partial denture for children for the prematurely lost primary molars was planned at a later date, when the patient grew older and became more cooperative.

Ventura et al. recommended that the duration of day-stay general anesthesia for a patient should be between 40 minutes and 180 minutes [37]. The duration of the dental surgery for our patient was 120 minutes and postoperation stay was two days. So the duration for the two-day stay general anesthesia was fully in compliance with the recommendation.

4. Conclusion

(1) Dental evaluations of children with KID syndrome and also patients' and their families' oral hygiene trainings are important for the prevention of dental problems.

(2) If the children with KID syndrome had so many caries, they would have been treated under general anesthesia due to communicational and dermatological problems.

(3) Supplementary dental treatments should be necessary for the patients with KID syndrome in order for the delayed speech affiliated with their hearing impediments to progress normally and also to help eliminating pronunciation disorders and psychological problems probably arising from the missing teeth.

Conflict of Interests

The authors declare that they have no conflict of interests.

References

[1] B. A. Skinner, M. C. Greist, and A. L. Norins, "The keratitis, ichthyosis, and deafness (KID) syndrome," *Archives of Dermatology*, vol. 117, no. 5, pp. 285–289, 1981.

[2] F. S. Burns, "A case of generalized congenital erythroderma," *Journal of Cutaneous Diseases*, vol. 33, pp. 255–260, 1915.

[3] H. Caceres-Rios, L. Tamayo-Sanchez, C. Duran-Mckinster, M. De La Luz Orozco, and R. Ruiz-Maldonado, "Keratitis,

ichthyosis, and deafness (KID syndrome): review of the literature and proposal of a new terminology," *Pediatric Dermatology*, vol. 13, no. 2, pp. 105–113, 1996.

[4] C.-Y. Yang, Y.-J. Chen, and J.-L. Shen, "Keratitis, ichthyosis and deafness syndrome—a case report and literature review," *Dermatologica Sinica*, vol. 26, no. 3, pp. 151–156, 2008.

[5] G. Ülker, A. Kılıç, M. Gönül, S. Külcü Çakmak, and T. Ünal, "A case with KID Syndrome: keratitis-ichthyosis-deafness," *Turkiye Klinikleri Journal of Dermatology*, vol. 19, no. 2, pp. 104–106, 2009.

[6] E. M. Messmer, K. R. Kenyon, O. Rittinger, A. R. Janecke, and A. Kampik, "Ocular manifestations of keratitis-ichthyosis-deafness (KID) syndrome," *Ophthalmology*, vol. 112, no. 2, pp. e1–e6, 2005.

[7] A. B. Carey, W. A. Burke, and H. M. Park, "Malignant fibrous histiocytoma in keratosis, ichthyosis, and deafness syndrome," *Journal of the American Academy of Dermatology*, vol. 19, no. 6, pp. 1124–1126, 1988.

[8] S. Yotsumoto, T. Hashiguchi, X. Chen et al., "Novel mutations in GJB2 encoding connexin-26 in Japanese patients with keratitis-ichthyosis-deafness syndrome," *British Journal of Dermatology*, vol. 148, no. 4, pp. 649–653, 2003.

[9] L. Miteva, "Keratitis, ichthyosis, and deafness (KID) syndrome," *Pediatric Dermatology*, vol. 19, no. 6, pp. 513–516, 2002.

[10] W. Jurecka, E. Aberer, M. Mainitz, and O. Jurgensen, "Keratitis, ichthyosis, and deafness syndrome with glycogen storage," *Archives of Dermatology*, vol. 121, no. 6, pp. 799–801, 1985.

[11] L.-G. Chia and W.-M. Li, "Clinical and electrophysiological studies in a patient with keratitis, ichthyosis and deafness (KID) syndrome," *Journal of Neurogenetics*, vol. 4, no. 1, pp. 57–64, 1987.

[12] K. Langer, K. Konrad, and K. Wolff, "Keratitis, ichthyosis and deafness (KID)-syndrome: report of three cases and a review of the literature," *British Journal of Dermatology*, vol. 122, no. 5, pp. 689–697, 1990.

[13] S. Sonoda, E. Uchino, K.-H. Sonoda et al., "Two patients with severe corneal disease in KID syndrome," *American Journal of Ophthalmology*, vol. 137, no. 1, pp. 181–183, 2004.

[14] S. M. Elsayed, N. S. Seifeldeen, and H. Bolz, "Connexin 26 (GJB2) mutation in KID syndrome: an Egyptian patient," *The Egyptian Journal of Medical Human Genetics*, vol. 12, pp. 91–93, 2011.

[15] X.-B. Zhang, S.-C. Wei, C.-X. Li et al., "Mutation of GJB2 in a Chinese patient with keratitis-ichthyosis-deafness syndrome and brain malformation," *Clinical and Experimental Dermatology*, vol. 34, no. 3, pp. 309–313, 2009.

[16] S. Criton and J. Vincent, "Keratitis, ichthyosis and deafness (KID) syndrome," *Indian Journal of Dermatology, Venereology and Leprology*, vol. 61, no. 5, pp. 312–313, 1995.

[17] M.-L. Bondeson, A.-M. Nyström, U. Gunnarsson, and A. Vahlquist, "Connexin 26 (GJB2) mutations in two Swedish patients with atypical Vohwinkel (mutilating keratoderma plus deafness) and KID syndrome both extensively treated with acitretin," *Acta Dermato-Venereologica*, vol. 86, no. 6, pp. 503–508, 2006.

[18] American Academy of Pediatric Dentistry Guidelines, "Policy on early childhood caries (ECC): classifications, consequences, and preventive strategies," *Oral Health Policies, and Clinical Guidelines*, pp. 47–49, 2012.

[19] C. Roberts, J. Y. Lee, and J. T. Wright, "Clinical evaluation of and parental satisfaction with resin-faced stainless steel crowns," *Pediatric Dentistry*, vol. 23, no. 1, pp. 28–31, 2001.

[20] M. E. Gonzalez, B. E. Tlougan, H. N. Price, R. Patel, H. Kamino, and J. V. Schaffer, "Keratitis-ichthyosis-deafness (KID) syndrome," *Dermatology Online Journal*, vol. 15, no. 8, article 11, 2009.

[21] A. J. Kanwar, S. Ghosh, S. Handa, G. P. Thami, and S. Kaur, "Keratitis, ichthyosis, deafness (KID) syndrome—the first report from India," *Clinical and Experimental Dermatology*, vol. 18, no. 4, pp. 386–388, 1993.

[22] A. Abdollahi, Z. Hallaji, N. Esmaili et al., "KID syndrome," *Dermatology Online Journal*, vol. 13, no. 4, article 11, 2007.

[23] A. Y. Jan, S. Amin, P. Ratajczak, G. Richard, and V. P. Sybert, "Genetic heterogeneity of KID syndrome: identification of a Cx30 gene (GJB6) mutation in a patient with KID syndrome and congenital atrichia," *Journal of Investigative Dermatology*, vol. 122, no. 5, pp. 1108–1113, 2004.

[24] J. Mazereeuw-Hautier, E. Bitoun, J. Chevrant-Breton et al., "Keratitis-ichthyosis-deafness syndrome: disease expression and spectrum of connexin 26 (GJB2) mutations in 14 patients," *British Journal of Dermatology*, vol. 156, no. 5, pp. 1015–1019, 2007.

[25] K. Tuppurainen, J. Fraki, S. Karjalainen, L. Paljarvi, R. Suhonen, and M. Ryynanen, "The KID-syndrome in Finland. A report of four cases," *Acta Ophthalmologica*, vol. 66, no. 6, pp. 692–698, 1988.

[26] V. Shanker, M. Gupta, and A. Prashar, "Keratitis-ichthyosis-deafness syndrome: a rare congenital disorder," *Indian Dermatol Online Journal*, vol. 3, no. 1, pp. 48–50, 2012.

[27] D. Watanabe, M. Zako, Y. Tamada, and Y. Matsumoto, "A case of keratitis-ichthyosis-deafness (KID) syndrome," *International Journal of Dermatology*, vol. 46, no. 4, pp. 400–402, 2007.

[28] H. C. Dietz, "Marfan syndrome," in *GeneReviews*, R. A. Pagon, T. D. Bird, C. R. Dolan et al., Eds., University of Washington, Seattle, Wash, USA, 1993.

[29] J. E. Allanson and A. E. Robers, "Noonan syndrome," in *GeneReviews*, R. A. Pagon, T. D. Bird, C. R. Dolan et al., Eds., University of Washington, Seattle, Wash, USA, 1993.

[30] A. LoMauro, S. Pochintesta, M. Romei et al., "Rib cage deformities alter respiratory muscle action and chest wall function in patients with severe Osteogenesis Imperfecta," *PLoS ONE*, vol. 7, no. 4, Article ID e35965, 2012.

[31] M. T. Greally, "Shprintzen-goldberg syndrome," in *GeneReviews*, R. A. Pagon, T. D. Bird, C. R. Dolan et al., Eds., University of Washington, Seattle, Wash, USA, 1993.

[32] B. L. Loeys and H. C. Dietz, "Loeys-dietz syndrome," in *GeneReviews*, R. A. Pagon, T. D. Bird, C. R. Dolan et al., Eds., University of Washington, Seattle, Wash, USA, 1993.

[33] Z. H. Zaidi, "Ehlers-Danlos syndrome with congenital herniae and pigeon breast," *British Medical Journal*, vol. 2, no. 5145, pp. 175–176, 1959.

[34] M. de Souza Coelho and P. S. F. de Guimarães, "Pectus carinatum," *Jornal Brasileiro de Pneumologia*, vol. 33, no. 4, pp. 463–474, 2007.

[35] J. S. Rathbone and J. C. Snidecor, "Appraisal of speech defects in dental anomalies with reference to speech improvement," *The Angle Orthodontist*, vol. 29, no. 1, pp. 54–59, 1959.

[36] O. F. Khabour, F. S. Mesmar, F. Al-Tamimi, O. B. Al-Batayneh, and A. I. Owais, "Missense mutation of the EDA gene in a Jordanian family with X-linked hypohidrotic ectodermal dysplasia:

phenotypic appearance and speech problems," *Genetics and Molecular Research*, vol. 9, no. 2, pp. 941–948, 2010.

[37] E. Ventura, E. Levy, M. Friedman, and H. Gat, "General anesthesia for complete oral rehabilitation in children," *ASDC Journal of Dentistry for Children*, vol. 48, no. 1, pp. 33–35, 1981.

31

True Generalized Microdontia and Hypodontia with Spondyloepiphyseal Dysplasia

Anita Singhal,[1] Parul Singhal,[2] Ranjan Gupta,[3] and Kush Dev Jarial[4]

[1] *Department of Oral Pathology and Microbiology, H.P. Government Dental College and Hospital, Shimla, Himachal Pradesh 171001, India*
[2] *Department of Pedodontics and Preventive Dentistry, H.P. Government Dental College and Hospital, Shimla, Himachal Pradesh 171001, India*
[3] *Department of Prosthodontics, H.P. Government Dental College and Hospital, Shimla, Himachal Pradesh 171001, India*
[4] *Department of Pediatrics, Indira Gandhi Medical College & Hospital, Shimla, Himachal Pradesh 171001, India*

Correspondence should be addressed to Anita Singhal; dr.anitathakur@gmail.com

Academic Editors: S. G. Boynes, V. Brailo, L. Gallego, and M. T. Martins

Spondyloepiphyseal dysplasia (SED) is a descriptive term used for group of inherited disorders of bone growth resulting in short stature, skeletal abnormalities, and problems with hearing and vision. SED have three major forms, SED congenital, pseudoachondroplastic SED, and SED tarda. SED tarda is milder than SED congenita. True generalized microdontia is a rare condition in which all the teeth are abnormally small. This is a report of a rare case having SED with generalized microdontia in a 26-year-old patient.

1. Introduction

SED refers to a heterogeneous group of disorders with primary involvement of vertebrae and epiphyseal centers of long bones. Three major types of SED are recognized SED congenital, pseudoachondroplastic SED, and SED tarda. Spondyloepiphyseal dysplasia (SED) was first described in 1966 by Spranger and Wiedemann and is now also known as Wiedemann-Spranger syndrome [1]. SED congenita is inherited as an autosomal dominant condition and is associated with a highly disproportional reduction in growth and severe coxa vara, and the milder tarda form which is an X-linked recessive condition, in which growth in adolescence is defective after normal childhood development. Clinically, SED is characterized by short stature (120 to 140 cm), often significant lordosis, pectus carinatum and may have associated features of myopia, retinal detachment, deafness, cleft lip cleft palate, and muscular hypotonia [2]. The genetic modes for SED tarda are various. Initially heredity was described as X-linked, but in later reports both autosomal dominant and autosomal recessive transmission have been demonstrated. In patients of SED tarda, the development up to 5–10 years of age is usually normal after which mild disproportionate trunk and shortening becomes evident. In some patients, the condition remains unrecognized until adolescent years and may become clinically apparent with hip pain, scoliosis or lordosis. SED is rare with its prevalence being approximately 3-4 per million population [3]. The term microdontia (microdentism, microdontism) is defined as the condition of having abnormally small teeth [4]. In generalized microdontia, the teeth are small, the crowns and roots are short, and normal contact areas between the teeth are frequently missing [5]. Shafer, Hine, and Levy divided microdontia into three types: (1) microdontia involving only a single tooth; (2) relative generalized microdontia due to relatively small teeth in large jaws; and (3) true generalized microdontia, in which all the teeth are smaller than normal [6]. According to these authors, aside from its occurrence in some cases of pituitary dwarfism, true generalized microdontia is exceedingly rare. Literature review of MEDLINE/PubMed base did not show any case of SED with microdontia. Here, we report a rare case of SED associated with true generalized microdontia.

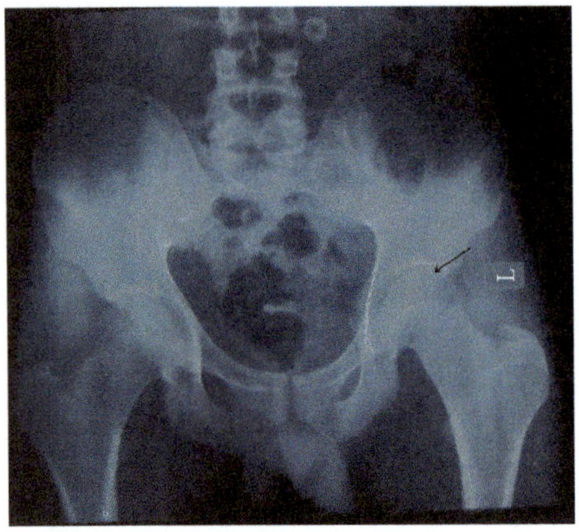

FIGURE 1: Pelvic X-ray showing spina bifida oculta at L5, femoral epiphysis compressed on left sides.

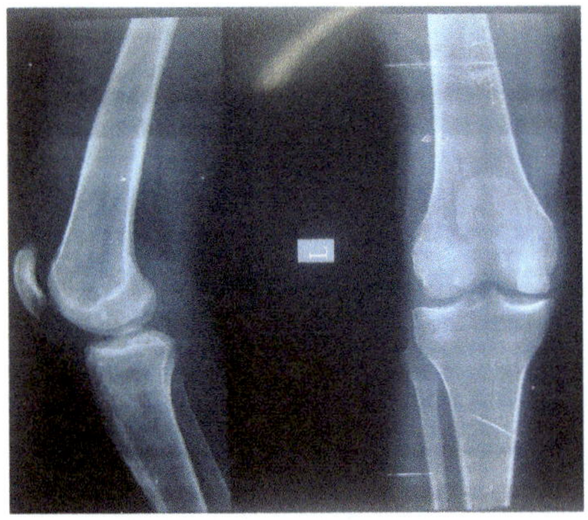

FIGURE 2: X-ray knee joint showing maldeveloped patella with osteoporosis in right side inferior pubic ramus, lower end of femur, and upper end of tibia.

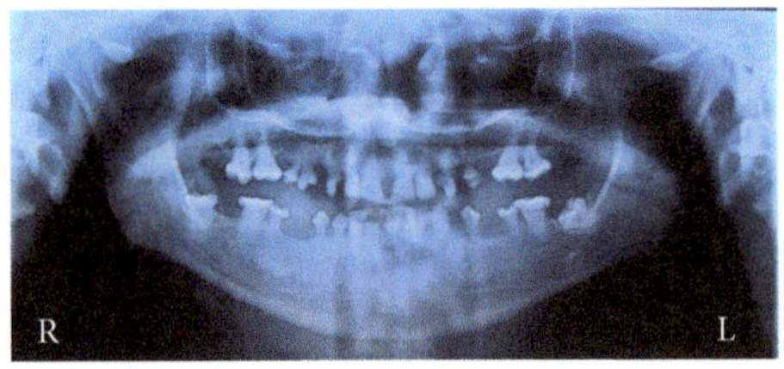

FIGURE 3: OPG shows conical tooth roots floating over alveolar bone with dilacerations.

2. Case Report

A 26-year-old male patient reported with complaint of mobile and missing teeth accompanied with sensitivity to hot and cold since last few months. Patient was not able to eat and chew properly. History of pain in the leg bones while sitting and walking and pain in hand and feet on their movement were present for the last four years. The patient did not complain of pain in any of the joints. Patient also had impaired vision for which he was diagnosed having cataract four years back and was surgically treated for the same then. Patient gave history of hearing deficiency and back pain for past 3 years. On physical examination his height was found to be 65.95 inches with thin stature. Upper segment to lower segment ratio was 0.87, normal being 0.89 to 0.95. this was suggestive of skeletal dysplasia. Hand, wrist, pelvic, and spinal radiographs of the patient were taken. Spinal radiograph revealed loose bodies. Hand wrist radiographs showed normal bone. Pelvic radiographs showed spina bifida oculta at L5 level and femoral epiphysis compressed on left side (Figure 1). Osteoporosis was seen in the inferior pubic ramus right side, lower end of femur, and upper end of tibia. Patella was maldeveloped (Figure 2). DEXA (dual-emission X-ray absorptiometry) scan of the patient was done. DEXA scan score for the patient was between −1 and −2.5. It revealed that patient was osteopenic. Patient was advised calcium supplements and physiotherapy. On oral examination mouth opening was normal. Patient presented with true generalized microdontia. Morphology of the teeth was maintained. Teeth number 23 and 25 were congenitally missing. Caries was present in multiple teeth. Orthopantomogram of the patient showed severe bone loss in relation to all teeth. Teeth number 13, 14, 15, 25, 26, 27, 31, 33, 34, 42, and 44 had dilacerated roots. 37 and 47 were impacted. Teeth appeared small conical floating over alveolar bone. (Figure 3). 44, 34, and 35 were extracted due to extreme mobility and 36 was extracted due to caries. Tooth measurements were made on the diagnostic casts of patient's dentition. Patient was the second of three siblings (2 brothers and one sister); all others did not have any of these findings. There was no family history of similar complaints. Comparison of the patient's tooth measurement was done with anatomic average dental measurements in Tables 1 and 2.

Pedigree and genetic testing showed the condition as autosomal recessive. Based on all the clinical, radiolographical, and genetic findings, final diagnosis of spondyloepiphyseal dysplasia tarda with generalized microdontia was made. Carious teeth were restored with composite restoration and missing teeth were replaced by interim removable partial denture. Physiotherapy is advised to the patient and he is under routine followups.

3. Discussion

Spondyloepiphyseal dysplasias are a spectrum of disorders comprising of SED congenita, pseudoachondroplastic SED, and SED tarda [7]. SED congenita is a specific skeletal dysplasia inherited as autosomal dominant disorder which is evident at birth. Cleft palate is common and over half of the patients have high grade myopia and/or retinal detachment. SED tarda is customarily used for the X-linked recessive disorder; however, autosomal dominant and recessive forms have been described. The most consistent radiologic findings in SED are a dysplastic odontoid process, flattened vertebrae, and small and deformed (femoral) epiphyses (long-bone metaphyseal involvement is variable). In the cervical spine of children with SED congenita, atlantoaxial instability is the most commonly encountered and most dangerous problem,

Table 1: Measurements in millimeters were made on clinical crown of diagnostic casts (right side).

Tooth (right side) (U/L)	Anatomic average crown length of teeth (U/L)	Crown length of patient's teeth (U/L)	Anatomic average mesiodistal width of teeth (U/L)	Mesiodistal width of patient's teeth (U/L)
Central incisor	10.5/9	6.5/5	8.5/5	6/4.5
Lateral incisor	9/9.5	5/4	6.5/55	5/5
Canine	10/11	6/5.5	7.5/7	5/4
First premolar	8.5/8.5	5/—	7/7	5/—
Second molar	8.5/8.5	3.5/—	7/7	3.5/—
First molar	7.5/7.5	4.5/—	10/11	8/—
Second molar	7/7.5	5/—	9/10.5	7.5/—
Third molar	6.5/7	—	8.5/9.5	—

Anatomic averages taken from *Textbook of Dental Anatomy and Physiology, R. C. Wheeler.*

Table 2: Measurements in millimeters were made on clinical crown of diagnostic casts (left side).

Tooth (left side) (U/L)	Anatomic average crown length of teeth (U/L)	Crown length of patient's teeth (U/L)	Anatomic average mesiodistal width of teeth (U/L)	Mesiodistal width of patient's teeth (U/L)
Central incisor	10.5/9	5/5.5	8.5/5	7/4.5
Lateral incisor	9/9.5	5/5.5	6.5/55	6/4
Canine	10/11	5.5/5.5	7.5/7	5/5
First premolar	8.5/8.5	4.5/5	7/7	4.5/5
Second molar	8.5/8.5	—/2	7/7	—/5
First molar	7.5/7.5	4/4	10/11	8/3.5
Second molar	7/7.5	—	9/10.5	6/—
Third molar	6.5/7	—	8.5/9.5	—

Anatomic averages taken from *Textbook of Dental Anatomy and Physiology, R. C. Wheeler.*

found in 30–40%. The major clinical characteristics of SED tarda are pain, stiffness, and limitations to the movements of the lumbar spine and multiple joints combined with a waddling gait as was seen in present case. Progressive symptomatic osteoarthritis of the hips and knees may be seen. Atlantoaxial instability may be present and patients may present with neurologic deficits. Scoliosis or thoracic kyphosis with exaggerated lumbar pain in the back and hips with limitation of motion in these joints are frequent by the teens [2]. Adult height of the patients with SED varies from 52 to 62 inches. In general as a rule, patients with disproportionate stature have some form of skeletal dysplasias, whereas those with relatively normal body proportions have some form of endocrine, nutritional, metabolic, or other nonskeletal defects [8]. Anomaly with ocular, skeletal, craniofacial, dental and somatic developmental defects, termed as Axenfeld-Rieger syndrome (ARS), has been reported [9]. Presentation of the symptoms of the present case were quite different than that of ARS except for the hypodontia and the microdontia. In ARS microdontia is generally found in the bimaxillary anterior region, whereas in our case microdontia was generalized. Besides from its occurrence in some cases of pituitary dwarfism, true generalized microdontia is exceedingly rare [10]. Cleft palate and missing teeth are frequently reported to be associated with SED. True generalized microdontia associated with SED has never been reported in literature. The patient had two missing teeth but no cleft was present. The initiating factor or factors responsible for microdontia remain obscure. Mutation in developmental regularity genes is known to cause variety of dental defects [11]. Both genetic and environmental factors are involved in the complex etiology of microdontia The development of a tooth has been shown to have ectodermal, mesodermal, and neural crest contributions. The variation in size of a particular tooth arises during the period when the form of the tooth is being determined by the enamel organ and the sheath of Hertwig at the bell stage of enamel organ. The determination of the form of the crown is thought to be related to different regions of the oral epithelium or to the ectomesenchyme. Studies have shown that different regions of the oral epithelium rather than the underlying ectomesenchyme are initially responsible for the shape of the crown [12] Bones dating from the middle ages which were excavated at Alborg, Denmark, proved evidence for generalized microdontia resulting from intrauterine growth retardation [13]. There is no cure for spondyloepiphyseal dysplasia, but a great deal can be done to provide support and compensate for disabilities. An ophthalmologist should examine the patient at an early stage. Congenital cataracts should be treated surgically. Recurrent middle ear infections should be treated to prevent hearing impairment. Hip joint defects and arthrosis sometimes require surgical intervention. Spinal defects are treated with a corset brace but may require surgery.

Microdonts having good root length and bone support are given crowns. If microdonts are lost prematurely, they can then be replaced by removable partial dentures. In adults dental implants can be used with normal-sized teeth. We have presented a case of SED with generalized microdontia here and future studies are needed to find the association basis between the symptoms and there prevalence.

References

[1] J. Spranger and H. R. Wiedemann, "Dysplasia spondyloepiphysaria congenita," *Helvetica Paediatrica Acta*, vol. 21, pp. 598–611, 1966.

[2] A. S. Choonia and N. M. Salgar, "Spondylo-epiphyseal dysplasia congenita—a variant," *Bombay Hospital Journal*, vol. 54, no. 1, pp. 125–129, 2012.

[3] R. Wynne-Davies, C. Hall, and B. M. Ansell, "Spondylo-epiphysial dysplasia tarda with progressive arthropathy. A new disorder of autosomal recessive inheritance," *Journal of Bone and Joint Surgery B*, vol. 64, no. 4, pp. 442–445, 1982.

[4] S. Laundau, *International Dictionary of Medicine and Biology*, John Wiley & Sons, New York, NY, USA, 1st edition, 1986.

[5] P. E. Boyle, *Kronfeld's Histopathology of the Teeth and Their Surrounding Structures*, Lea & Febiger, Philadelphia, Pa, USA, 3rd edition, 1955.

[6] W. G. Shafer, M. K. Hine, and B. M. Levy, *A Textbook of Oral Pathology*, WB Saunders, Philadelphia, Pa, USA, 1st edition, 1958.

[7] P. Rubin, *Dynamic Classification of Bone Dysplasias*, Year Book Medical Publishers, Chicago, Ill, USA, 1st edition, 1964.

[8] A. V. Pathare, M. A. Kothari, A. A. Chikhalikar, S. G. Dalvi, and I. M. Vora, "Spondylo-epiphyseal dysplacea tarda (a case report)," *Journal of Postgraduate Medicine*, vol. 37, no. 2, pp. 105–108, 1991.

[9] A. Villa, A. Albonico, and F. Villa, "Hypodontia and microdontia: clinical features of a rare syndrome," *Journal of Canadian Dental Association*, vol. 77, article b115, 2011.

[10] S. D. Bargale and S. D. P. Kiran, "Non-syndromic occurrence of true generalized microdontia with mandibular mesiodens—a rare case," *Head and Face Medicine*, vol. 7, no. 1, article 19, 2011.

[11] I. Thesleff, "Genetic basis of tooth development and dental defects," *Acta Odontologica Scandinavica*, vol. 58, no. 5, pp. 191–194, 2000.

[12] J. W. Osborn and A. R. T. Cate, *Advanced Dental Histology*, vol. 6 of *Dental Practitioner Handbook*, John Wright & Sons, Bristol, UK, 3 edition, 1976.

[13] V. Alexandersen and O. V. Nielsen, "Generalized microdontia probably associated with intrauterine growth retardation in a medieval skeleton," *American Journal of Physical Anthropology*, vol. 33, no. 3, pp. 389–401, 1970.

32

Nonsyndromic Facial Asymmetry with Unilateral Condylar Aplasia

Ranganadh Nallamothu, Rama Mohan Kodali, N. Koteswara Rao, Leela krishna Guttikonda, and U. Vijayalakshmi

Department of Oral and Maxillofacial Surgery, Drs. Sudha & Nageswara Rao Siddhartha Institute of Dental Sciences, Chinoutpalli, Gannavaram, Krishna District, Andhra Pradesh 521 286, India

Correspondence should be addressed to Ranganadh Nallamothu; drranganadh@gmail.com

Academic Editors: Y. S. Khader and S. R. Watt-Smith

Introduction. The temporomandibular joint (TMJ) is the most complex elegantly designed joint in the human body. Abnormal development and growth of TMJ may lead to condyle aplasia present in several syndromes expressions, but it is extremely rare when not connected to any underlying pathological disorder or in conjunction with any syndrome. *Objective.* A rare case of aplasia of the mandibular condyle is presented, along with 3D computed tomography (3D CT) findings. *Conclusion.* Based on clinical and radiological findings we suggest the abnormal development of the TMJ as the origin. The 3D CT has provided high-quality images, which made diagnosis and a prompt treatment plan possible.

1. Introduction

The temporomandibular joint (TMJ) is the most complex elegantly designed joint in the human body [1]. It is a ginglymoarthrodial joint, a term that is derived from ginglymus, meaning a hinge joint, allowing motion only backward and forward in one plane, and arthrodia, meaning a joint which permits a gliding motion of the surfaces [2].

The right and left TMJ form a bicondylar articulation and ellipsoid variety of the synovial joints similar to knee articulation [3]. The most important functions of the TMJ are mastication and speech and are of great interest to dentists, orthodontists, clinicians, and radiologists. This interest stems from the standpoints of structure, function, adaptability, symptomatology, pathology, and imaging [4].

TMJ develops from separate temporal and condylar bronchial arches that grow towards each other at eighth week of fetal stage, with the ossification process starting at tenth week. The TMJ initial functions start at twentieth week during the fetal stage, when mouth opening movements appears it is before the development of the definitive joint. The development process will not be complete until twelfth year of life [5]. Varying degrees of condylar hypoplasia, from minimal to complete absence named as condylar aplasia, may occur due to abnormal development and growth of TMJ [5].

The most common causes of condyle alterations are inflammatory process in the area, rheumatoid arthritis, and radiotherapy [6]. The parathyroid hormone-related protein also affects the bone formation and chondrocyte differentiation and, consequently, the condyle formation [7, 8]. We are presenting a rare case of aplasia of the mandibular condyle, along with 3D computed tomography (3D CT) findings.

2. Case Report

A 10-year-old female presented with a chief complaint of asymmetry of left half of the face, which was first noticed during early childhood and had gradually progressed. At the anamnesis there was a history of forceps delivery. Her family history and personal history were noncontributory. No abnormalities were noted on general physical examination and her vital signs were within normal limits. Extraoral clinical examination revealed facial asymmetry (Figures 1 and 2) and affected side external ear (helix, antihelix, tragus, antitragus, concha scaphoid fossa, and lobule) was normal; a scar was noticed on the left side of the face and it was located well below the ala-tragal line and 1 to 2 cm away from the corner of the mouth, upon dwelling the history regarding scar it was revealed that patient gives history of fall while playing at school. Few months later the wound healed

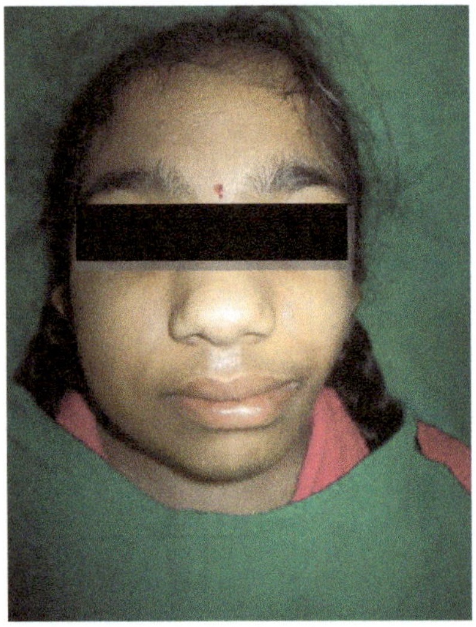

Figure 1: Frontal view.

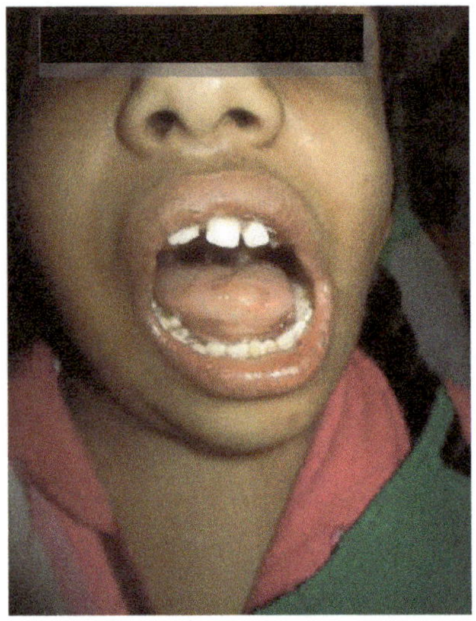

Figure 3: Deviation of the jaw to the left side.

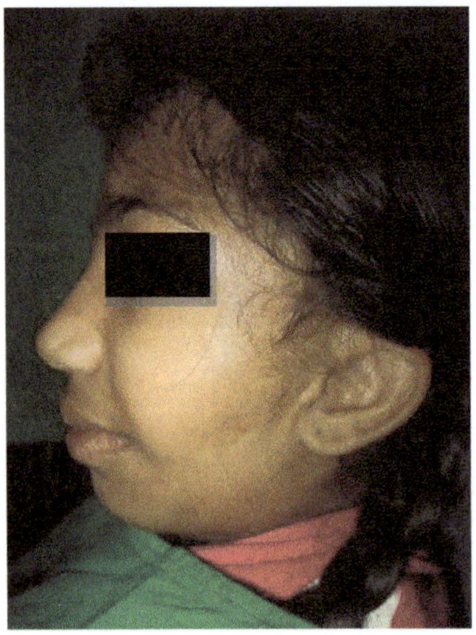

Figure 2: Lateral view.

uneventfully and no developmental defects were noticed and there was a deviation of the mandible to the left side on opening (Figure 3).

On temporomandibular examination the left condyle is not palpable. Besides that no other important clinical findings were observed. Intraorally she had mixed dentition (Figures 4(a) and 4(b)) and hence the severity of malocclusion was not assessed. For detailed information, the patient was submitted to CT scan (3D). The images revealed complete condylar aplasia with missing condylar neck and glenoid fossa (Figures 5 and 6).

3. Discussion

Alterations, including condyle aplasia, are present in several syndromes expressions as observed in hemifacial microsomia, the Goldenhar syndrome, the Treacher Collins syndrome, the Proteus syndrome, the Morquio syndrome, and auriculocondylar syndrome. But the condyle aplasia is extremely rare when not connected to any syndrome [9, 10].

Facial asymmetry, deviation of the midline, and malocclusion are the consequences of the TMJ abnormality [9], as a syndrome expression (Figures 1 and 2). Our case shows the condyle aplasia without connection to any syndrome, and that highlights the rarity of the case.

The condyle malformation occurred due to abnormal development of the TMJ, probably at the fetal stage, before the tenth week. The trauma during delivery, as related, may not be the cause of the malformation in the present case; otherwise, there would not be a complete absence of the condyle, since its formation and ossification start at fetal stage. More often forceps delivery is correlated with TMJ ankylosis. With the arrival of 3D computed tomography (CT) and magnetic resonance imaging (MRI), diagnostic imaging of the TMJ has improved tremendously [11].

The 3D CT examination enables accurate surgical planning and provides quantitative information from skeletal and muscular parameters [12]. The present case needs a multidisciplinary approach including a team of maxillofacial surgeon, pedodontist, general surgeon, and orthodontist [13–15]. The treatment options for this situation are use of costochondral graft [16, 17], orthognathic surgery, and distraction osteogenesis [18, 19] based on the growth spurt concept.

Hence costochondral grafting procedure for the left temporomandibular joint was preferred before the growth spurt. Once the growth spurt ceases, either orthognathic surgery or the distraction osteogenesis will be preferred. Orthodontic treatment will be supported at all the stages of the treatment.

In summary, we report a rare case of unilateral condyle aplasia with no underlying pathological disorder or in conjunction with any syndrome. Based on clinical and radiological (3D CT) findings we suggest the abnormal development of the TMJ as the origin. Early recognition, accurate diagnosis,

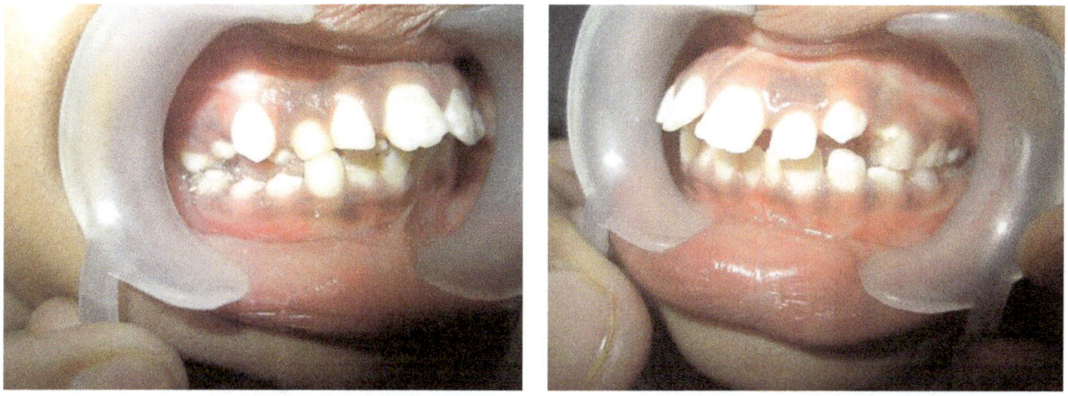

(a) (b)

FIGURE 4: Intraoral right and left occlusal views showing mixed dentition.

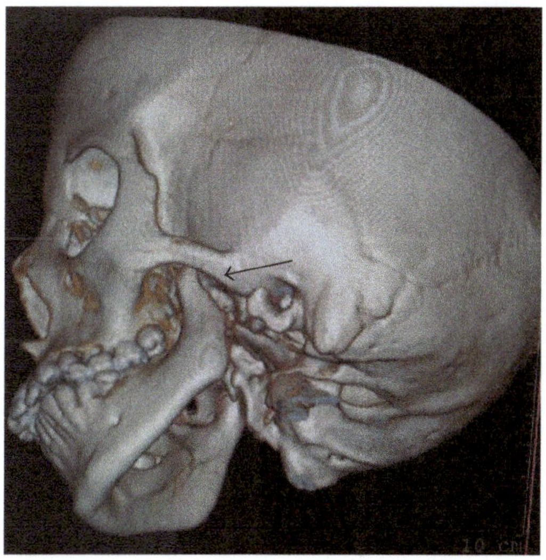

FIGURE 5: 3D CT scan of affected side (left) with missing condyle and glenoid fossa.

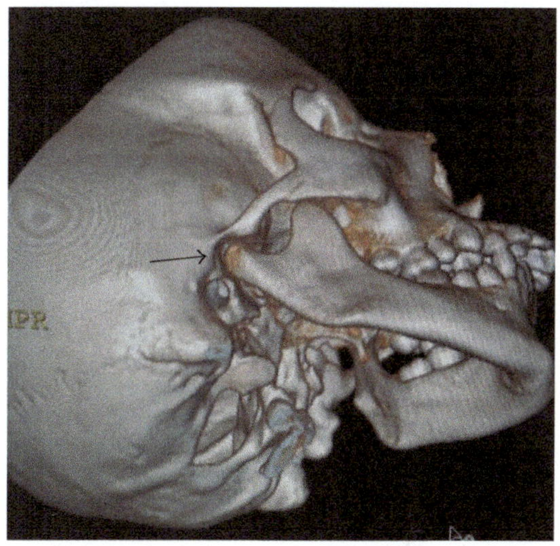

FIGURE 6: 3D CT scan of normal side (right) with normal condyle and glenoid fossa.

and multidisciplinary approach regarding the treatment will reduce the morbidity and provide better prognosis to these patients.

References

[1] J. K. Potter and E. J. Dericks, "Vascularized options for reconstruction of the mandibular condyle," *Seminars in Plastic Surgery*, vol. 22, no. 3, 2008.

[2] W. A. Dorland, *Medical Dictionary*, WB Saunders, Philadelphia, Pa, USA, 1957.

[3] P. L. Williams, "Gray's anatomy," in *Skeletal System*, pp. 578–582, Churchill Livingstone, London, UK, 38th edition, 1999.

[4] X. Alomar, J. Medrano, J. Cabratosa et al., "Anatomy of the Temporomandibular Joint," *Seminars in Ultrasound, CT and MRI*, vol. 28, no. 3, pp. 170–183, 2007.

[5] G. H. Speber, "Temporomandibular joint," in *Craniofacial Development*, G. H. Speber, Ed., pp. 139–143, BC Deker, Hamilton, Canada, 2001.

[6] B. W. Neville, D. D. Damm, C. M. Allen, and J. E. Bouquot, "Developmental defects of the oral and maxillofacial region," in *Oral and Maxillofacial Pathology*, B. W. Neville, D. D. Damm, C. M. Allen, and J. E. Bouquot, Eds., pp. 17–18, WB Saunders, Philadelphia, Pa, USA, 2nd edition, 2002.

[7] S. Shibata, N. Suda, K. Fukada, K. Ohyama, Y. Yamashita, and V. E. Hammond, "Mandibular coronoid process in parathyroid hormone-related protein-deficient mice shows ectopic cartilage formation accompanied by abnormal bone modeling," *Anatomy and Embryology*, vol. 207, no. 1, pp. 35–44, 2003.

[8] M. Ishii-Suzuki, N. Suda, K. Yamazaki et al., "Differential responses to parathyroid hormone-related protein (PTHrP) deficiency in the various craniofacial cartilages," *The Anatomical Record*, vol. 255, pp. 452–457, 1999.

[9] O. Krogstad, "Aplasia of the mandibular condyle," *European Journal of Orthodontics*, vol. 19, no. 5, pp. 483–489, 1997.

[10] K. C. P. Santos, M. E. P. Dutra, C. Costa, C. A. Lascala, C. E. Lascala, and J. X. De Oliveira, "Aplasia of the mandibular

condyle," *Dentomaxillofacial Radiology*, vol. 36, no. 7, pp. 420–422, 2007.

[11] T. Sano, M. Otonari-Yamamoto, T. Otonari, and A. Yajima, "Osseous abnormalities related to the temporomandibular joint," *Seminars in Ultrasound, CT and MRI*, vol. 28, no. 3, pp. 213–221, 2007.

[12] J. L. Kahn, P. Bourjat, and P. Barrière, "Imaging of mandibular malformations and deformities," *Journal de Radiologie*, vol. 84, no. 9, pp. 975–981, 2003.

[13] O. Krogstad, "Aplasia of the mandibular condyle," *European Journal of Orthodontics*, vol. 19, no. 5, pp. 483–489, 1997.

[14] E. M. Canger and P. Çelenk, "Aplasia of the mandibular condyle associated with some orthopaedic abnormalities: a case report," *Dentomaxillofacial Radiology*, vol. 41, no. 3, pp. 259–263, 2012.

[15] K. Vargervik and L. B. Kaban, "Hemifacial microstomia diagnosis and management," in *Modern Practice in Orthognathic and Reconstructive Surgery*, W. H. Bell, Ed., vol. 2, pp. 1533–1560, WB Saunders, Philadelphia, Pa, USA, 1992.

[16] A. A. Shaker, "The use of costochondral grafts in the management of temporomandibular joint ankylosis," *Egyptian Journal of Plastic and Reconstructive Surgery*, vol. 27, no. 1, pp. 73–83, 2003.

[17] L. Villanueva-Alcojol, F. Monje-Gil, R. González-García et al., "Costochondral graft with green-stick fracture used in reconstruction of the mandibular condyle: experience in 13 clinical cases," *Medicina Oral, Patologia Oral y Cirugia Bucal*, vol. 14, no. 12, pp. e663–e667, 2009.

[18] E. W. Ko, K.-F. Hung, C. S. Huang, and P. K. T. Chen, "Correction of facial asymmetry with multiplanar mandible distraction: a one-year follow-up study ," *Cleft Palate-Craniofacial Journal*, vol. 41, no. 1, pp. 5–12, 2004.

[19] H.-J. Yoon and H.-G. Kim, "Intraoral mandibular distraction osteogenesis in facial asymmetry patients with unilateral temporomandibular joint bony ankylosis," *International Journal of Oral and Maxillofacial Surgery*, vol. 31, no. 5, pp. 544–548, 2002.

Papilliferous Keratoameloblastoma: An Extremely Rare Case Report

Neeta Mohanty,[1] Varun Rastogi,[2] Satya Ranjan Misra,[3] and Susant Mohanty[4]

[1] *Department of Oral and Maxillofacial Pathology, Institute of Dental Sciences, Bhubaneswar, Odisha 751003, India*
[2] *Department of Oral and Maxillofacial Pathology, Kalka Dental College, Meerut, Uttar Pradesh 250 006, India*
[3] *Department of Oral Medicine and Radiology, Institute of Dental Sciences, Bhubaneswar, Odisha 751003, India*
[4] *Department of Paediatric Dentistry, Institute of Dental Sciences, Bhubaneswar, Odisha 751003, India*

Correspondence should be addressed to Satya Ranjan Misra; drsatyaranjanmds@gmail.com

Academic Editors: P. G. Arduino and M. J. Wahl

Odontogenic tumors develop in the jaw bones from the odontogenic tissue-oral epithelium in tooth germ, enamel organ, dental papilla, reduced enamel epithelium, remnants of Hertwig's root sheath or dental lamina, and so forth. Hence, a bewildering variety of tumors are encountered in the maxilla and mandible. Ameloblastoma is the second most common odontogenic neoplasm after odontomes, and it has numerous clinical and histologic variants. We report a very rare histologic variant: the papilliferous keratoameloblastoma which is the fifth reported case in the English literature.

1. Introduction

Ameloblastoma is a true neoplasm of enamel organ-type, tissue which does not undergo differentiation to the point of enamel formation. It has been described very aptly by Robinson as being a tumor that is usually "unicentric, nonfunctional, intermittent in growth, anatomically benign, and clinically persistent" [1].

Ameloblastoma is the most common odontogenic epithelial tumor of the jaw bones [2], and it is characterized by a substantial number of histologic subtypes [3]. Recognition of the various histomorphic patterns is thus only of diagnostic significance and is especially important for histopathologists, despite the fact that they are generally considered to be locally aggressive and destructive, exhibiting various rates of recurrences.

Variations of ameloblastoma that exhibit keratinization in their parenchyma are the Acanthomatous ameloblastoma, Keratoameloblastoma (KA), and Papilliferous Keratoameloblastoma (PKA). Of these, Keratoameloblastoma and Papilliferous Keratoameloblastoma are extremely rare tumors, and despite the similarity of the names, Keratoameloblastoma and Papilliferous Keratoameloblastoma are distinct morphologically [4].

Pindborg [5] first proposed the term "Keratoameloblastoma" for use as a diagnostic entity. In his 1970 report, Pindborg described a histologic variant of ameloblastoma, which he termed Papilliferous Keratoameloblastoma. Subsequently, 3 additional cases of ameloblastoma with a Papilliferous component were reported in 1991 [3], 1994 [6], and 2002 [7], bringing the number of case reports of PKA in the English Language literature to four. We report a case of Papilliferous Keratoameloblastoma which is the 5th case to document in the English literature.

2. Case Report

A 46-year male patient reported to the dental hospital with the complaint of swelling in the right side of the lower jaw since 1 year. The swelling progressed slowly to the present side with no history of toothache, and the past medical history is noncontributory.

On examination, a single localized swelling was seen in the right side body of the mandible, ovoid in shape, about 2 cm in greatest diameter, nontender, bony hard in consistency, and fixed to the underlying bone. Intraorally, a swelling was seen having bicortical expansion extending

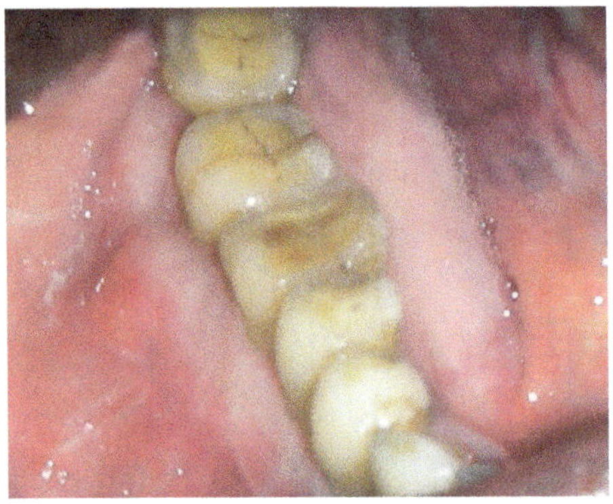

FIGURE 1: Intraoral swelling with bicortical expansion extending from 44 to 48 region.

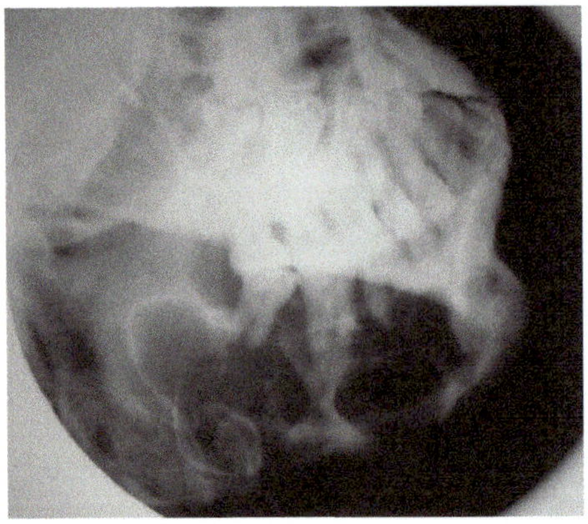

FIGURE 2: Lateral oblique projection of the body of the mandible showing a multilocular radiolucency, extending from first premolar to the angle of the mandible.

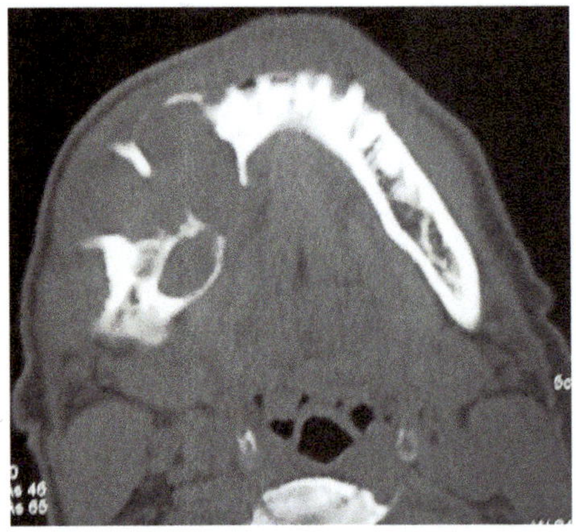

FIGURE 3: Axial view CT scan showing bicortical expansion with perforation of the buccal and lingual cortices on the right side.

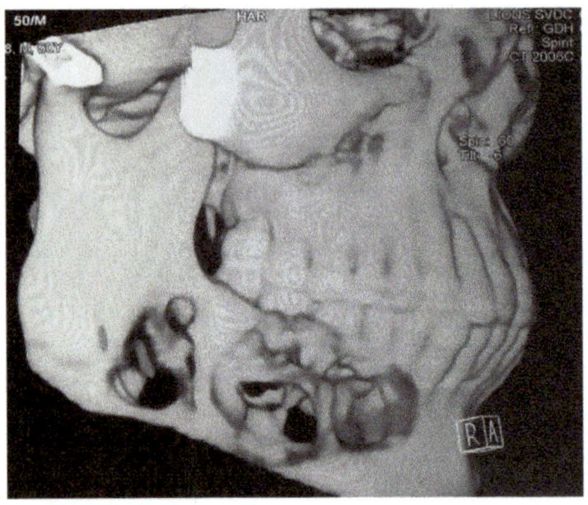

FIGURE 4: 3D reformatted CT scan showing perforation of the mandible from 44 to angle region on right side.

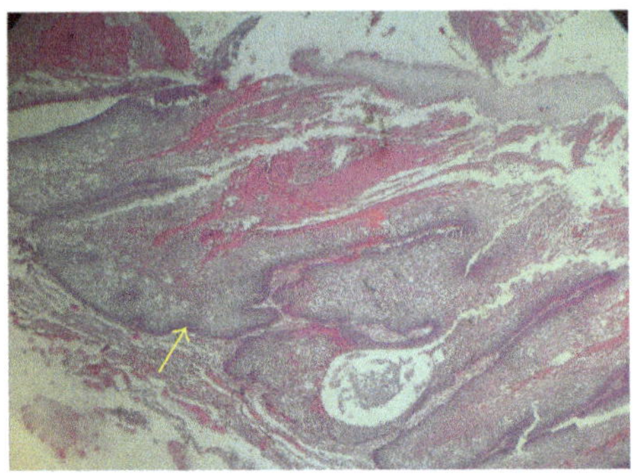

FIGURE 5: H & E section (10X) showing cystic spaces filled with the necrotic debris and lined by papillary (Yellow arrow) keratin lined infolding of odontogenic epithelium resembling ameloblastoma with connective tissue cores.

from 44 to 48 region (Figure 1). It was nontender and firm in consistency, and it obliterates the buccal vestibule. A provisional diagnosis of benign bony neoplasm was made, and the patient subjected to radiologic investigations.

Periapical, occlusal, and lateral oblique projections of the mandible revealed a multilocular radiolucency, extending from the first premolar to the angle of the mandible (Figure 2); there is bicortical expansion with perforation of both the buccal and lingual cortex. There is root resorption of the involved teeth. Computer Tomography scans also revealed bicortical expansion and cortical perforation (Figures 3 and 4).

An incisional biopsy of the lesion was done, and, microscopically, the lesion consisted of cystic spaces filled with the necrotic debris and lined by papillary keratin lined infolding of odontogenic epithelium resembling ameloblastoma with connective tissue cores (Figures 5 and 6). The cystic spaces also showed squamous metaplasia and presence of keratin squames (Figure 7). The odontogenic epithelium consisted of loosely arranged polygonal or angular cells resembling stellate reticulum of the enamel organ (Figure 8) and basal layer of tall columnar ameloblast-like cells showing palisading and reversal of polarity (Figures 8 and 9). Correlating the histopathological features, a definitive diagnosis of Papilliferous keratoameloblastoma of the mandible was made, and the patient was referred to the oral surgery department for management.

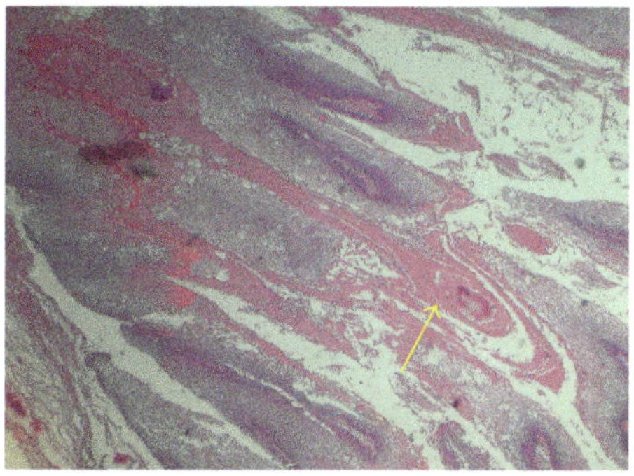

FIGURE 6: H & E section (10X) showing cystic spaces lined by papillary keratin lined infolding (Yellow arrow) of odontogenic epithelium.

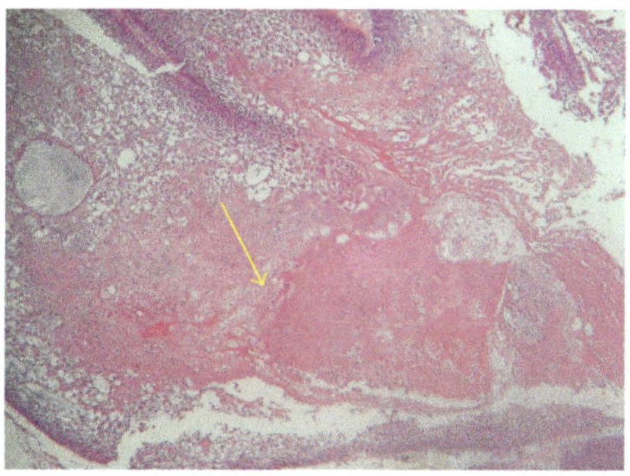

FIGURE 7: Cystic spaces showing squamous metaplasia (Yellow arrow) and presence of keratin squames (H & E 10X).

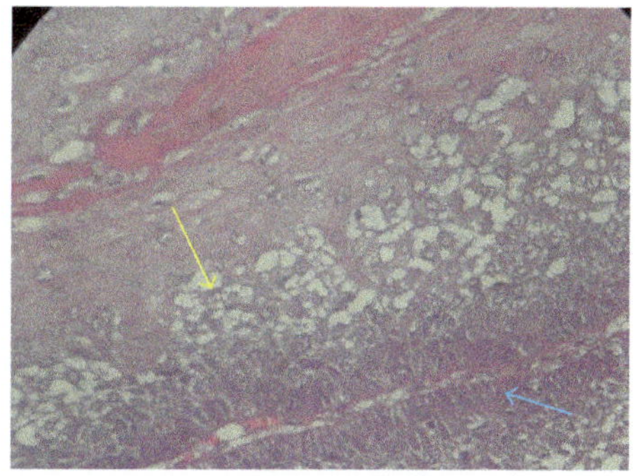

FIGURE 8: Odontogenic epithelium consisting of loosely arranged polygonal/angular cells resembling stellate reticulum (Yellow arrow) of the enamel organ and basal layer of tall columnar ameloblast-like cells (Blue arrow) showing palisading and reversal of polarity (H & E 40X).

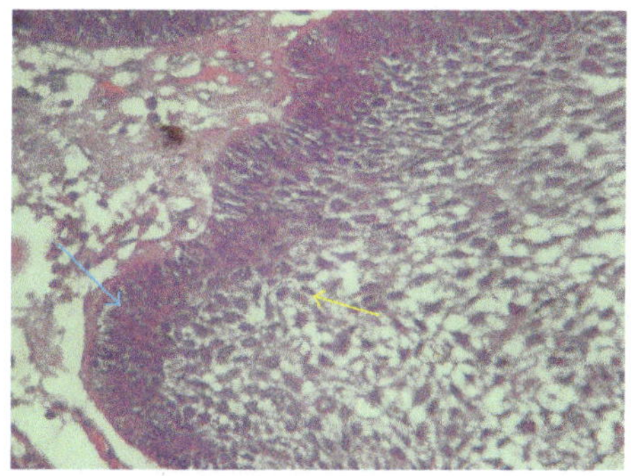

FIGURE 9: Loosely arranged polygonal/angular cells resembling stellate reticulum (Yellow arrow) of the enamel organ and basal layer of tall columnar ameloblast-like cells (Blue arrow) showing palisading and reversal of polarity (H & E 40X).

3. Discussion

Ameloblastomas undergo different forms of metaplasia and are therefore highly polymorphic benign odontogenic tumors, giving rise to the histologic variants like acanthomatous, granular cell, desmoplastic, basal cell, keratoameloblastoma, and clear-cell ameloblastoma. The cause or the stimulus for these metaplasias is unknown; however, it is generally attributed to the multipotentiality of odontogenic epithelium [8, 9].

Histopathologically, ameloblastoma recapitulates the morphology of the prematrix stage of the enamel organ and may assume a variety of histological configurations. Clinically, no behavioural difference has been observed among histological and cytological variants.

Papilliferous keratoameloblastoma and Keratoameloblastoma are extremely rare variants of ameloblastoma [10]. Papilliferous keratoameloblastoma was first described as a subtype of ameloblastoma by Pindborg and Weinmann [11]. In 1970, Pindborg [5] produced a radiograph and three photomicrographs of an unusual type of ameloblastoma consisting partly of keratinizing cysts and partly of tumor islands with Papilliferous appearance, and the term Papilliferous keratoameloblastoma was then suggested [12]. Later, Altini et al. [3] described a similar tumor that differed from the one described by Pindborg in that it did not show the Papilliferous epithelium nor the extensive necrosis and debris in the follicles.

Since only one of the four cases showed convincing evidence of ameloblastoma, there is minimal evidence that they are ameloblastoma and may represent a separate entity. This finding is consistent with our case which showed histopathological features of ameloblastoma.

The Papilliferous nature of the epithelium seems to have occurred as result of intercellular adherence and different rates of necrosis of individual cells [13]. The necrotic cells separate from the remainder of the epithelium resulting in the formation of numerous pseudopapillary structures which project into the lumina of the cystic follicles.

Keratoameloblastoma, Papilliferous Keratoameloblastoma, or a possible hybrid lesion of the two is an extremely rare neoplasm, and an accurate evaluation of the clinical spectrum, radiology, and behavioural potential must await further case accrual.

References

[1] W. G. Shafer, M. K. Hine, and B. M. Levy, *A Textbook of Oral Pathology*, WB Saunders, Philadelphia, Pa, USA, 4th edition, 1983.

[2] Y. Takeda, M. Satoh, S. Nakamura, and T. Ohya, "Keratoameloblastoma with unique histological architecture: an undescribed variation of ameloblastoma," *Virchows Archiv*, vol. 439, no. 4, pp. 593–596, 2001.

[3] M. Altini, H. D. Slabbert, and T. Johnston, "Papilliferous keratoameloblastoma," *Journal of Oral Pathology and Medicine*, vol. 20, no. 1, pp. 46–48, 1991.

[4] J. C. Whitt, C. L. Dunlap, J. L. Sheets, and M. L. Thompson, "Keratoameloblastoma: a tumor sui generis or a chimera?" *Oral Surgery, Oral Medicine, Oral Pathology, Oral Radiology and Endodontology*, vol. 104, no. 3, pp. 368–376, 2007.

[5] J. J. Pindborg, *Pathology of the Dental Hard Tissues*, WB Saunders, Philadelphia, Pa, USA, 1970.

[6] E. J. Norval, I. O. Thompson, and C. W. van Wyk, "An unusual variant of keratoameloblastoma," *Journal of oral Pathology & Medicine*, vol. 23, no. 10, pp. 465–467, 1994.

[7] P. Collini, N. Zucchini, G. Vessecchia, and M. Guzzo, "Papilliferous keratoameloblastoma of mandible: a papillary ameloblastic carcinoma: report of a case with a 6-year follow-up and review of the literature," *International Journal of Surgical Pathology*, vol. 10, no. 2, pp. 149–155, 2002.

[8] D. G. Gardner, "Some current concepts on the pathology of ameloblastomas," *Oral Surgery, Oral Medicine, Oral Pathology, Oral Radiology, and Endodontics*, vol. 82, no. 6, pp. 660–669, 1996.

[9] L. J. van Rensburg, I. O. C. Thompson, H. E. C. Kruger, and E. J. G. Norval, "Hemangiomatous ameloblastoma: clinical, radiologic, and pathologic features," *Oral Surgery, Oral Medicine, Oral Pathology, Oral Radiology, and Endodontics*, vol. 91, no. 3, pp. 374–380, 2001.

[10] I. R. H. Kramer, J. J. Pindborg, and M. Shear, *Histological Typing of Odontogenic Tumors*, Springer, New York, NY, USA, 2nd edition, 1992.

[11] J. J. Pindborg and J. P. Weinmann, "Squamous cell metaplasia with calcification in ameloblastomas," *Acta pathologica et microbiologica Scandinavica*, vol. 44, no. 3, pp. 247–252, 1958.

[12] P. A. Reichart and H. P. Philipsen, *Odontogenic Tumors and Allied Lesions*, Quintessence, Chicago, Ill, usa, 1st edition, 2004.

[13] L. Barnes, *Surgical Pathology of the Head and Neck*, vol. 3, Marcel Dekker, New York, NY, USA, 2001.

34

Histological Features and Biocompatibility of Bone and Soft Tissue Substitutes in the Atrophic Alveolar Ridge Reconstruction

Carlo Maiorana,[1] Mario Beretta,[2] Davide Rancitelli,[2] Giovanni Battista Grossi,[2] Marco Cicciù,[3] and Alan Scott Herford[4]

[1] *Center for Edentulism and Jawbone Atrophies, Fondazione IRCCS Policlinico, Department of Oral Sciences, University of Milan, 20141 Milan, Italy*
[2] *Oral Surgery and Implantology, Fondazione IRCCS Policlinico, University of Milan, 20141 Milan, Italy*
[3] *Human Pathology Department, School of Dentistry University of Messina, 98100 Messina, Italy*
[4] *Oral and Maxillofacial Surgery, Loma Linda University School of Dentistry, Loma Linda, CA 95231, USA*

Correspondence should be addressed to Marco Cicciù; acromarco@yahoo.it

Academic Editor: Miguel de Araújo Nobre

The reconstruction of the atrophic alveolar ridges for implant placement is today a common procedure in dentistry daily practice. The surgical reconstruction provides for the optimization of the supporting bone for the implants and a restoration of the amount of keratinized gingiva for esthetic and functional reasons. In the past, tissue regeneration has been performed with autogenous bone and free gingival or connective tissue grafts. Nowadays, bone substitutes and specific collagen matrix allow for a complete restoration of the atrophic ridge without invasive harvesting procedures. A maxillary reconstruction of an atrophic ridge by means of tissue substitutes and its histological features are then presented.

1. Introduction

Prosthetically guided implantology provides for the creation of an optimal bone support to dental implants in order to guarantee an adequate prosthetic restoration. Moreover, the reconstruction of the soft tissues around the implant is essential, in order to reduce the risk of peri-implant mucositis and peri-implantitis [1, 2]. Such sophisticated and multiple stepped treatments include three to four surgical phases usually from 12 to 18 months to be concluded. With the purpose of reducing the invasiveness of the treatment, bone substitutes have been used within the last 20 years to avoid autogenous bone harvesting [3, 4]. In the last five years, even soft tissue substitutes have been tested to avoid the use of autogenous free gingival or connective tissue grafts [5, 6]. The association of bone regeneration techniques, soft tissues reconstruction, and devices able to maintain the biomaterials in site for at least six to eight months prior to implant placement is nowadays a widely documented approach. The purpose of this paper was to show a paradigmatic clinical case of an upper jaw alveolar atrophy, in which a titanium mesh, xenogeneic bone, and a collagen porcine matrix were used to restore the anatomic integrity of the deficient ridge as well as the soft tissues around the implants.

2. Materials and Methods

A 56-years-old. female patient, in good general health status, was examined at the Department of Implantology, Fondazione IRCCS Cà Granda, Ospedale Maggiore Policlinico, Milan, Italy. The patient was asking for the rehabilitation of the upper left edentulous maxilla with a fixed implant-supported prosthesis. The clinical appearance of the edentulous ridge showed a vertical and horizontal contraction with a cross bite intermaxillary relationship. On the right side, an extended sinus could be appreciated in the edentulous posterior area. The radiographic examination, carried out by means of a panoramic radiograph and a CBCT scan, confirmed the atrophy, characterized by a narrow knife-edge ridge in the bicuspid area and a residual ridge 3 mm in height associated with an expanded maxillary sinus in the molar area. Patient undersigned an informed consent and the treatment was performed accordingly with the declaration of Helsinki rules.

The rehabilitation plan consisted in a three-step surgical treatment:

(i) bone reconstruction of the atrophic ridge with autogenous chips, xenogeneic bone, titanium mesh, and bilateral sinus elevation with xenogeneic bone,

(ii) titanium mesh removal after seven months and soft tissues reconstruction with a collagen matrix,

(iii) implant placement,

(iv) prosthetic rehabilitation with acrylic temporary prosthesis followed by a gold ceramic bridge.

Firstly the patient underwent a full mouth disinfection session, and proper home oral hygiene instructions were given. Sinus was prepared 15 days prior to surgery with mometasone nasal spray (Nasonex® Merck, Sharp and Dhome, Ch), twice a day. During the first surgical session, under general anesthesia, a full thickness flap from upper left canine to the maxillary tuberosity was reflected, a sinus elevation procedure with a lateral approach was conducted, and the subantral cavity was filled with xenogeneic bone (Bio-Oss, Geistlich®, Wohlusen, Ch). The ridge reconstruction was performed with a 1 : 1 ratio mixture of autogenous bone harvested with a bonescraper from the tuberosity and xenogeneic bone particles. The mix was maintained in place with a titanium mesh (OMNIA S.p.A., Fidenza (Parma), Italy) screwed to the recipient site with bone screws. A collagen resorbable membrane (BioGide, Geistlich, Wolhusen, Chiasso) was adapted over the mesh in order to limit the soft tissue cells migration in the grafted area and to promote soft tissues creeping in case of wound dehiscence and early exposure of the mesh.

Rehrmann periosteal incisions were performed at the buccal flap and a two-layer suture with a 4-0 polyglactin (Vycril®, Ethicon, USA) wire was done to seal the tissues. On the right side, a lateral approach sinus elevation was done at the first molar site and the regeneration was done with xenogenic bone. Sutures were removed after 15 days. The healing preceded uneventfully and after seven months the second surgery for mesh removal and soft tissues reconstruction was carried out. Under local anesthesia, the titanium mesh was exposed to a midcrestal incision and then removed. After the titanium mesh removal a sample of the regenerated tissue was taken by means of a trephine bur for the histological evaluation.

The buccal flap was apically repositioned to the underlying connective tissue to recreate the vestibule and the exposed tissue was covered with a porcine collagen matrix (Mucograft®, Geistlich, Wolhusen, Chiasso), which was secured to the recipient site with 5-0 polyglactin sutures. Forty days after the surgery, a complete healing of the soft tissue was observed and the third step for implant placement was executed. A full thickness flap was elevated both at the right and left sites and five implants (Camlog Screw line®, Camlog AG, Ch) were placed. After implant placement in the prosthetically driven position, a small horizontal bony defect was present at the canine level and the correction was done by means of Bio-Oss and Biogide®.

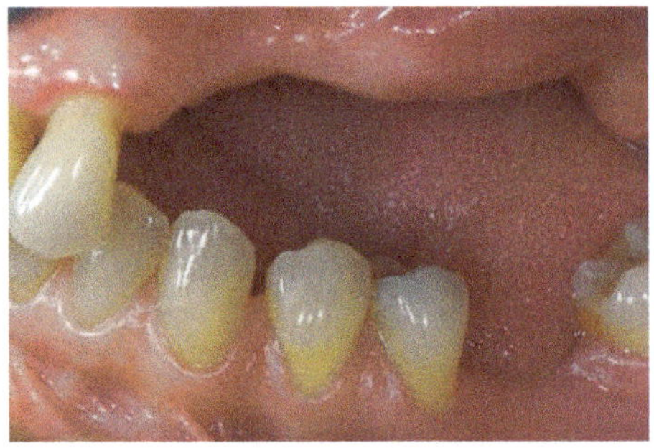

FIGURE 1: Clinical view of the left upper maxilla atrophic ridge.

Four months later, implants uncovering and healing abutment connection were done with a simple straight incision at the first right upper molar and a straight incision plus papillae reconstruction according to Palacci [7] technique was performed at the left side. Two months later, impressions were taken, and temporary crowns were placed after two weeks. After five months, impressions for final rehabilitation were taken and a gold ceramic bridge was given. The two-year X-ray orthopantomography showed a physiological contour of the bone levels and the soft tissue appeared clinically stable (Figures 1–13).

2.1. Histological Analysis. For the augmented area, one cylindrical bone biopsy was taken using a trephine bur with an inner diameter of 2.6 mm. The biopsy was fixed in 10% neutrally buffered formalin for at least 48 h and processed for light microscopy without demineralization by using the Donath and Breuner method [8].

Dehydration was accomplished by increasing ethanol concentrations using a dehydration system with agitation and vacuum. The blocks were embedded in Kulzer Technovit 7200 VLC-resin and sliced longitudinally on an Exakt cutting unit (Exakt, Norderstedt, Germany). Each analyzed slice was reduced by a microgrinding process and then polished using an Exakt grinding unit to an even thickness of 20 mm. These were stained with toluidine blue/pyronine G. Histomorphometric measurements of the tissue fractions (DBBM, autologous bone, newly formed bone and marrow, and/or connective tissue, resp.) were performed only in the augmented area. The sections were digitally photographed using a Leica camera DFC480 fixed on a Leica MZ16 stereomicroscope (Leica, Heerbrugg, Switzerland) using Image Access software (Imagic®, Glattbrugg, Switzerland). The sections were digitally photographed using a Leica camera DFC480 fixed on a Leica MZ16 stereomicroscope (Leica, Heerbrugg, Switzerland) using Image Access software (Imagic, Glattbrugg, Switzerland). Using the same software, the areas were measured by digitally surrounding the contours of the objects. In cases of uncertainty, the areas were compared with the live image using a measured by digitally surrounding the contours of the objects. In this way, the used system is able to clarify the images overlapping the analyzed images with

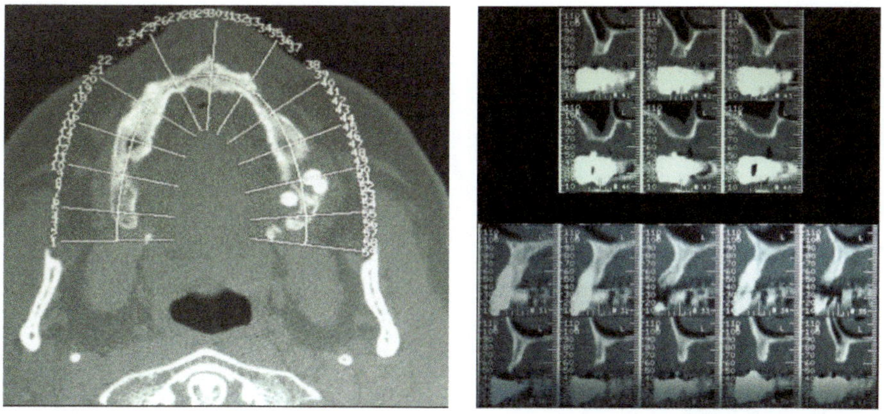

(a) (b)

Figure 2: The CT dental scan confirms the clinical view showing atrophic maxillary ridge with important horizontal bone defect. (a) It is possible to underline all the atrophies of the upper maxilla; (b) a particular of the axial section of the area involved in the grafting procedures.

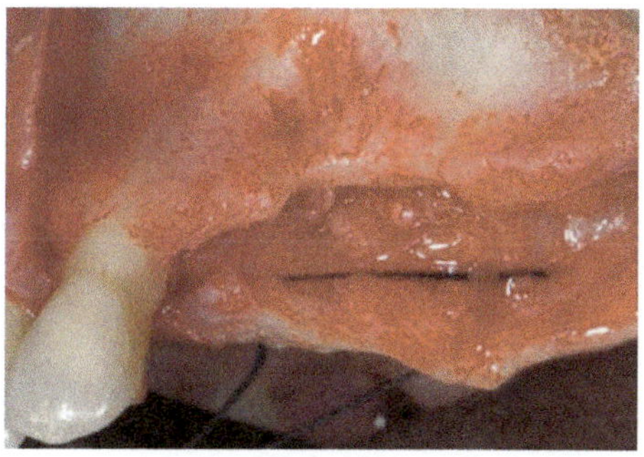

Figure 3: Clinical view of the bone after the elevation of the mucoperiosteal flap.

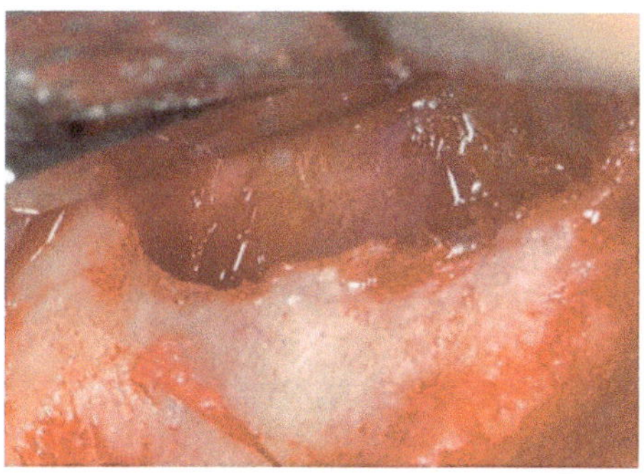

Figure 4: Sinus lift was performed in order to increase the volume of the bone height.

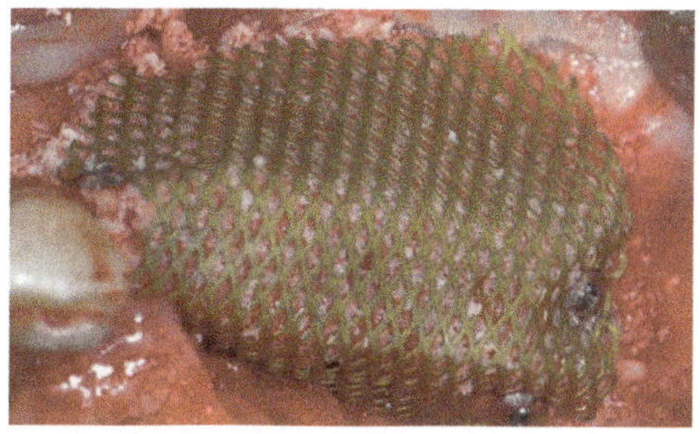

Figure 5: A titanium mesh has been placed for increasing the vertical and horizontal defect.

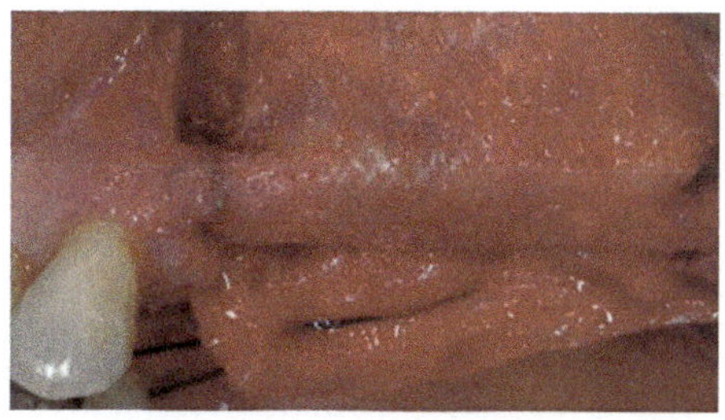

Figure 6: The time titanium mesh removal showed a good healing and the bone volume recovering.

previous acquired data. In cases of uncertainty, the areas were compared with the live image using a Leica DM6000B light microscope at a higher magnification. The results of the histological evaluation underline part from mature cancellous bone, and granules from the Bio-Oss coverage (BO) embedded in newly formed bone are present in the upper part of the biopsy (Figure 11).

3. Discussion

A successful implant treatment is determined by taking into account a number of factors: the management of hard and soft tissues, the quality of the prosthetic restoration, and the response to the aesthetic patient's demand.

The combined use of multiple biomaterials and reconstructive techniques could be required in order to obtain the desired result.

The reestablishment of an adequate amount of bone and a proper contour of the alveolar ridge has consequently become

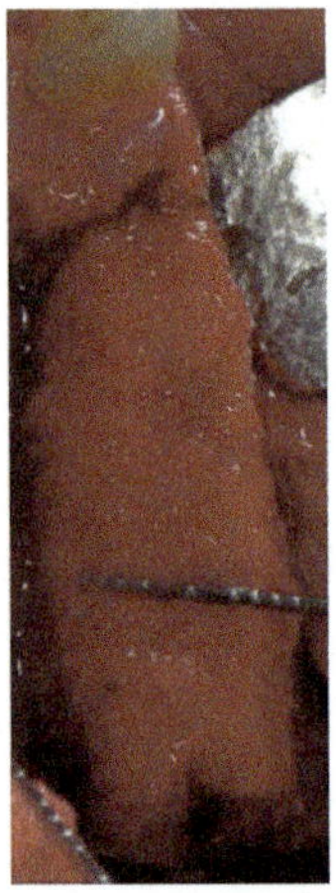

Figure 7: Occlusal view of the increased bone after the bone regeneration procedure with the applied titanium mesh.

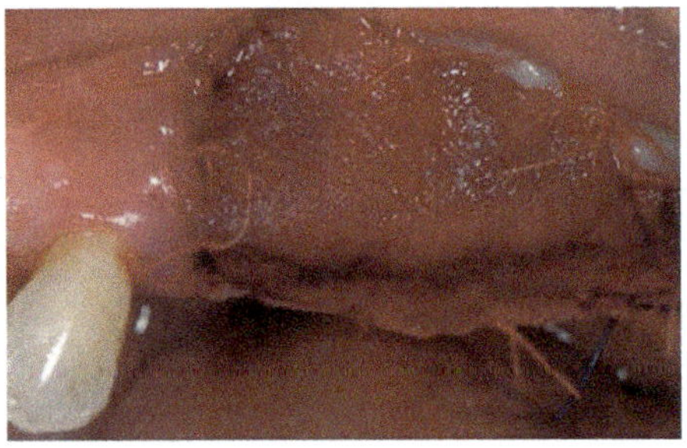

Figure 8: A collagen membrane has been placed in order to favor the soft tissue healing.

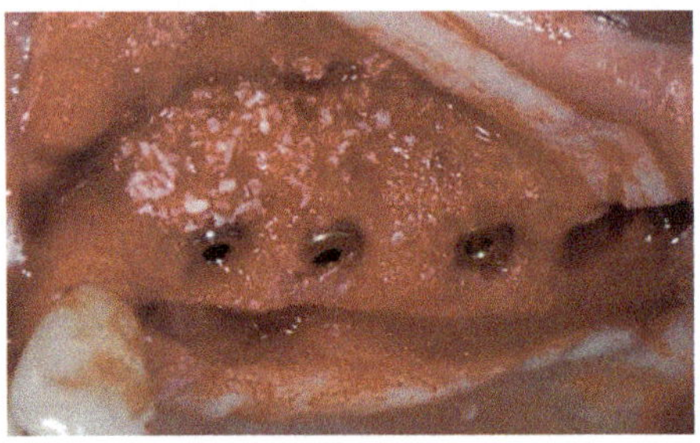

Figure 9: At the time of dental implants the healed bone has been removed and analyzed in order to perform the histologic analysis.

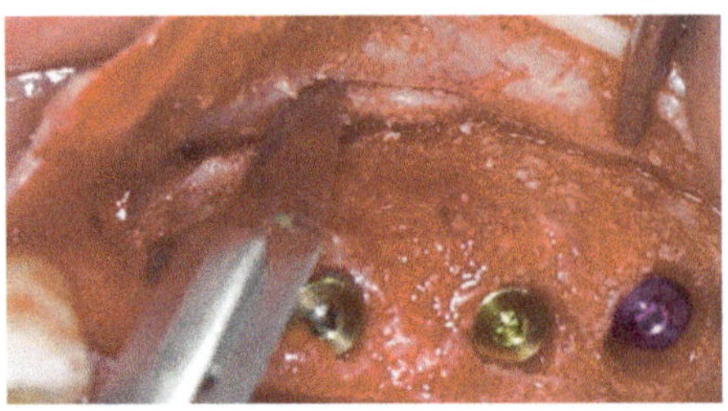

Figure 10: Dental implant was placed and periosteal incision has to be made in order to have a complete soft tissue covering of the dental implants placed.

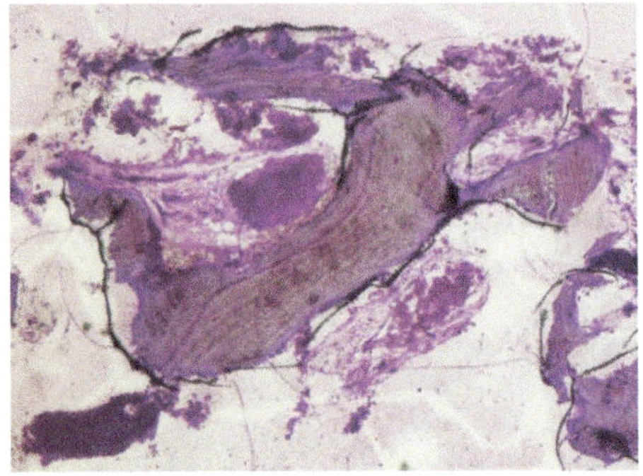

Figure 11: Histological image 40x magnification underlines the presence of new bone cells and some residual particles of the substitute material.

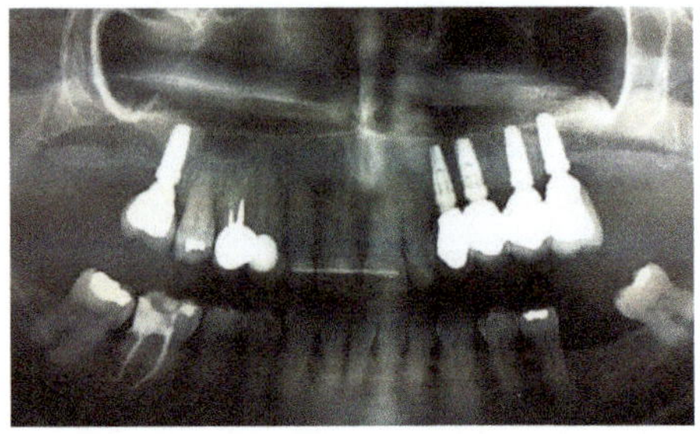

Figure 12: Two-year postoperative X-ray control evidences the integration of the dental implants for support of a fixed prosthetic rehabilitation.

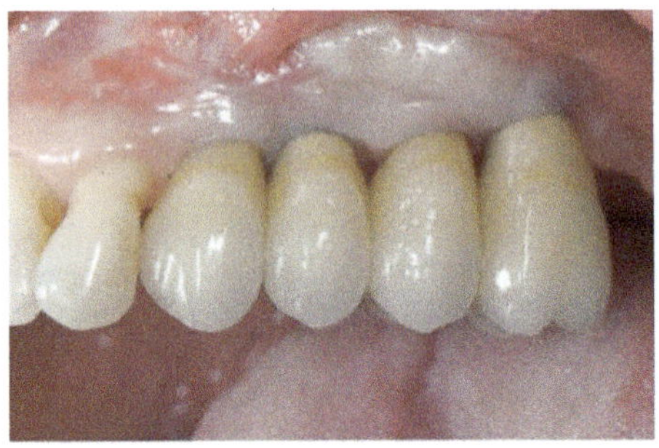

Figure 13: Two-year clinical analyses show a good healing of the soft tissue.

mandatory to allow a prosthetically driven implant placement.

Guided bone regeneration has become one of the most proper techniques to achieve this goal. A recent retrospective study on 192 implants placed in augmented bone stated that the cumulative survival rate of the sample was 96% ± 2% over 6-year mean follow-up period and no statistically significant difference was found between type of graft and membrane [9].

A different and valuable treatment option for maxillary atrophic ridge is related to the use of zygomatic dental implants. Zygomatic implants have been introduced as an alternative to conventional grafting and rehabilitation of severely resorbed maxilla. High success rates and longevity have been documented with zygomatic implant; however, its use is related with a high surgical skill and, at the same time, the prosthodontics final rehabilitation is only a full arch overdenture because a prosthodontics ceramic cemented crown restoration over zygomatic implant is not currently documented [10]. Moreover, the limited evidence of using zygomatic implants in partial rehabilitations with short follow-up times compared to the existing evidence for bone grafts is well documented in the current literature [11, 12].

In the presented clinical case the authors opted for the bone regeneration technique by means of a titanium mesh plus mixed autologous and xenogenic bone mineral particles. The real advantage of this device, as well documented in literature, is the rare risk of superinfection in case of exposure. In a recent systematic review only in 20% of the cases the mesh removal was necessary, while in the remaining cases, it was sufficient to treat the dehiscence with a topical application of chlorhexidine gel, not jeopardizing the final implant rehabilitation despite the less quantity of regenerated bone [13]. A recent work of Lizio et al. found a significant correlation between lack of regenerated bone and time and extent of early exposure [14].

The rationale of mixing autogenous bone with deproteinized bovine bone mineral (DBBM) is to combine the scaffold properties of the xenograft to the osteogenic and osteoinductive properties of the autograft [15, 16].

Moreover, the use of this combination allows for a reduction of the amount of autogenous bone harvested, subsequently decreasing the morbidity related to the technique, the surgical time required to complete the graft, and postoperative discomfort of the patient.

In the presented clinical case, at mesh removal, a connective tissue layer was present in some of the specimens between the mesh and the regenerated bone. This periosteal-like tissue has been described in literature [17] and has been shown particularly evident when titanium meshes are employed for alveolar ridges reconstruction instead of e-PTFE membranes.

Simion et al. [18] conducted an histological and histomorphometrical evaluation of the 1:1 mixture of deproteinized bovine bone mineral and autogenous bone graft associated with an expanded-polytetrafluoroethylene (e-PTFE) membrane for vertical ridge augmentation in the human. The histological analysis showed new bone formation and ongoing remodeling of the autogenous bone and the DBBM particles. Both in simultaneous and staged surgical approach, the regenerated bone led to proper osseointegration of dental implants inserted. The authors observed that histologically DBBM underwent very slow resorption and substitution with new bone. Both the autogenous bone and the DBBM particles undergo evident resorption during the healing period from 6 to 9 months. This is demonstrated by the observed mean DBBM density of 8.63% and the autogenous bone density of 6.23% in the 1:1 mixture group starting from a hypothetical density of about 25–50% for each material (considering the space between the particle occupied by the blood clot) at the time of the regenerative surgery. Additional evidence regarding the resorbability of DBBM comes from the occasional observation of typical bright beams with adjacent osteoclasts around the particles, indicating active demineralization and remineralization with a physiological remodeling pattern [18].

The peculiarity of DBBM resorption pattern could represent an advantage for the long-term stability of regenerated bone.

One of the problems that the clinician has to deal with, after a regenerative bone procedure, is the deepening of the vestibule and the recreation of the adequate quantity of keratinized mucosa.

As a matter of fact the coronally advanced flap used to obtain a primary wound closure often causes an inadequate vestibular depth at the moment of the second stage surgery. Moreover, the emergence of the implant would appear in the mucosa with aesthetic and functional consequences.

In those cases, a vestibuloplasty is the treatment of choice. This surgical procedure is primarily used to optimize the jaws for prosthesis integration [19].

The secondary aim is to increase the height of the residual alveolar ridge or to generate a sufficient band of keratinized mucosa around teeth or dental implants [20]. In the present clinical case a porcine collagen matrix has been adopted (Mucograft, Geistlich, Wolhusen, Chiasso). The current literature on the role of peri-implant tissue is conclusive to support augmenting peri-implant soft tissues or increasing the width of peri-implant keratinized mucosa [21].

Current studies have demonstrated that sufficient peri-implant keratinized mucosa prevented peri-implant plaque accumulation and buccal soft tissue recessions and therefore reduced the risk of peri-implant mucositis and peri-implantitis [21, 22].

A prospective clinical trial conducted by Schmitt et al. compared the autogenous free gingival grafts with the graft of collagen matrix. In this work authors concluded that the groups showed similar healing with increased peri-implant keratinized mucosa after surgery and therefore are both suitable for the regeneration of the peri-implant keratinized mucosa with a sufficient long-term stability. Moreover, tissue harvesting procedures with Mucograft are less invalid, surgery time can be reduced, and regenerated tissues have a more esthetic appearance [23, 24].

After getting the new vestibule, in this case report an apical reposition flap plus the papillae reconstruction technique was adopted [25–27] in order to obtain a soft tissue architecture similar to natural teeth morphology. The attached masticatory mucosa is displaced buccally, thereby increasing the tissue volume at the buccal side of the implants. The excess buccal tissue allows for a dissection and rotation of pedicles with the purpose of filling the interimplant space with a papilla like soft tissue. In the end, the soft conditioning has been obtained through screw retained temporary resin crowns.

4. Conclusions

The case report showed a wide overview of the most advanced techniques adopted in oral surgery to manage hard and soft tissues in order to achieve the prepathologic conditions for a prosthetically driven implant rehabilitation.

The combined use of the autologous bone and biomaterials could represent the treatment of choice for a complete and less invasive treatment.

Conflict of Interests

The authors declare that there is no conflict of interests regarding the publication of this paper.

References

[1] J. L. Wennström and J. Derks, "Is there a need for keratinized mucosa around implants to maintain health and tissue stability?" *Clinical Oral Implants Research*, vol. 23, supplement 6, pp. 136–146, 2012.

[2] A. Bouri Jr., N. Bissada, M. S. Al-Zahrani, F. Faddoul, and I. Nouneh, "Width of keratinized gingiva and the health status of the supporting tissues around dental implants," *The International Journal of Oral & Maxillofacial Implants*, vol. 23, no. 2, pp. 323–326, 2008.

[3] M. Cicciù, A. S. Herford, E. Stoffella, G. Cervino, and D. Cicciù, "Protein-signaled guided bone regeneration using titanium mesh and Rh-BMP2 in oral surgery: a case report involving left mandibular reconstruction after tumor resection," *The Open Dentistry Journal*, vol. 6, no. 1, pp. 51–55, 2012.

[4] A. S. Herford, L. Akin, M. Cicciu, C. Maiorana, and P. J. Boyne, "Use of a porcine collagen matrix as an alternative to autogenous tissue for grafting oral soft tissue defects," *Journal of Oral and Maxillofacial Surgery*, vol. 68, no. 7, pp. 1463–1470, 2010.

[5] S. Yamada, N. Shima, H. Kitamura, and H. Sugito, "Effect of porous xenographic bone graft with collagen barrier membrane on periodontal regeneration," *International Journal of Periodontics and Restorative Dentistry*, vol. 22, no. 4, pp. 389–397, 2002.

[6] M. Barbeck, S. E. Udeabor, J. Lorenz et al., "Induction of multinucleated giant cells in response to small sized bovine bone substitute (Bio-Oss™) results in an enhanced early implantation bed vascularization," *Annals of Maxillofacial Surgery*, vol. 4, no. 2, pp. 150–157, 2014.

[7] P. Palacci, "Aesthetic treatment of the anterior maxilla: soft and hard tissue considerations," *Oral and Maxillofacial Surgery Clinics of North America*, vol. 16, no. 1, pp. 127–137, 2004.

[8] K. Donath and G. Breuner, "A method for the study of undecalcified bones and teeth with attached soft tissues. The Säge-Schliff (sawing and grinding) technique," *Journal of Oral Pathology*, vol. 11, no. 4, pp. 318–326, 1982.

[9] M. Beretta, M. Cicciù, P. P. Poli et al., "A retrospective evaluation of 192 implants placed in augmented bone: long-term follow-up study," *The Journal of Oral Implantology*, vol. 41, no. 6, pp. 669–674, 2015.

[10] J. G. Rodríguez-Chessa, S. Olate, H. D. Netto, J. Shibli, M. de Moraes, and R. Mazzonetto, "Treatment of atrophic maxilla with zygomatic implants in 29 consecutives patients," *International Journal of Clinical and Experimental Medicine*, vol. 7, no. 2, pp. 426–430, 2014.

[11] R. Davó, C. Malevez, and O. Pons, "Immediately loaded zygomatic implants: a 5-year prospective study," *European Journal of Oral Implantology*, vol. 6, no. 1, pp. 39–47, 2013.

[12] C. Aparicio, W. Ouazzani, A. Aparicio et al., "Immediate/early loading of zygomatic implants: clinical experiences after 2 to 5 years of follow-up," *Clinical Implant Dentistry and Related Research*, vol. 12, supplement 1, pp. e77–e82, 2010.

[13] M. Rasia-dal Polo, P.-P. Poli, D. Rancitelli, M. Beretta, and C. Maiorana, "Alveolar ridge reconstruction with titanium meshes: a systematic review of the literature," *Medicina Oral, Patologia Oral y Cirugia Bucal*, vol. 19, no. 6, pp. e639–e646, 2014.

[14] G. Lizio, G. Corinaldesi, and C. Marchetti, "Alveolar ridge reconstruction with titanium mesh: a three-dimensional evaluation of factors affecting bone augmentation," *The International Journal of Oral & Maxillofacial Implants*, vol. 29, no. 6, pp. 1354–1363, 2014.

[15] C. E. Misch and F. Dietsh, "Bone-grafting materials in implant dentistry," *Implant dentistry*, vol. 2, no. 3, pp. 158–167, 1993.

[16] M. Yildirim, H. Spiekermann, S. Handt, and D. Edelhoff, "Maxillary sinus augmentation with the xenograft Bio-Oss and autogenous intraoral bone for qualitative improvement of the implant site: a histologic and histomorphometric clinical study in humans," *The International Journal of Oral & Maxillofacial Implants*, vol. 16, no. 1, pp. 23–33, 2001.

[17] R. K. Schenk, D. Buser, W. R. Hardwick, and C. Dahlin, "Healing pattern of bone regeneration in membrane-protected defects: a histologic study in the canine mandible," *The International Journal of Oral & Maxillofacial Implants*, vol. 9, no. 1, pp. 13–29, 1994.

[18] M. Simion, F. Fontana, G. Rasperini, and C. Maiorana, "Vertical ridge augmentation by expanded-polytetrafluoroethylene membrane and a combination of intraoral autogenous bone graft and deproteinized anorganic bovine bone (Bio Oss)," *Clinical Oral Implants Research*, vol. 18, no. 5, pp. 620–629, 2007.

[19] B. J. Costello, N. J. Betts, H. D. Barber, and R. J. Fonseca, "Preprosthetic surgery for the edentulous patients," *Dental Clinics of North America*, vol. 40, no. 1, pp. 19–38, 1996.

[20] S. Heberer and K. Nelson, "Clinical evaluation of a modified method of vestibuloplasty using an implant-retained splint," *Journal of Oral and Maxillofacial Surgery*, vol. 67, no. 3, pp. 624–629, 2009.

[21] M. Esposito, M. G. Grusovin, E. Martinis, P. Coulthard, and H. V. Worthington, "Interventions for replacing missing teeth: 1-versus 2-stage implant placement," *The Cochrane Database of Systematic Reviews*, no. 3, Article ID CD006698, 2007.

[22] B.-S. Kim, Y.-K. Kim, P.-Y. Yun et al., "Evaluation of peri-implant tissue response according to the presence of keratinized mucosa," *Oral Surgery, Oral Medicine, Oral Pathology, Oral Radiology, and Endodontology*, vol. 107, no. 3, pp. e24–e28, 2009.

[23] S. Speroni, M. Cicciù, P. Maridati, G. B. Grossi, and C. Maiorana, "Clinical investigation of mucosal thickness stability after soft tissue grafting around implants: a 3-year retrospective study," *Indian Journal of Dental Research*, vol. 21, no. 4, pp. 474–479, 2010.

[24] C. M. Schmitt, T. Moest, R. Lutz, F. Wehrhan, F. W. Neukam, and K. A. Schlegel, "Long-term outcomes after vestibuloplasty with a porcine collagen matrix (Mucograft) versus the free gingival graft: a comparative prospective clinical trial," *Clinical Oral Implants Research*, 2015.

[25] A. S. Herford, M. Lu, L. Akin, and M. Cicciù, "Evaluation of a porcine matrix with and without platelet-derived growth factor for bone graft coverage in pigs," *The International Journal of Oral & Maxillofacial Implants*, vol. 27, no. 6, pp. 1351–1358, 2012.

[26] P. Palacci and H. Nowzari, "Soft tissue enhancement around dental implants," *Periodontology 2000*, vol. 47, no. 1, pp. 113–132, 2008.

[27] C. Maiorana, M. Beretta, G. B. Grossi et al., "Histomorphometric evaluation of anorganic bovine bone coverage to reduce autogenous grafts resorption: preliminary results," *Open Dentistry Journal*, vol. 5, no. 1, pp. 71–78, 2011.

35

Management of Grossly Decayed Mandibular Molar with Different Designs of Split Cast Post and Core

Rashmi Bansal, Nakul Mehrotra, Priyanka Chowdhary, and Anuraag Gurtu

Department of Conservative Dentistry & Endodontics, Institute of Dental Sciences, Bareilly, India

Correspondence should be addressed to Rashmi Bansal; drrashmirajeshbansal@gmail.com

Academic Editor: Tatiana Pereira-Cenci

Mandibular molar with extensive loss of tooth structure, especially where no cavity wall is remaining, and insertion of posts in both the roots appear necessary so as to achieve proper retention for the core material. A single unit metal casting with two posts, one in the mesial root and the other in the distal divergent root, is difficult to fabricate due to difference in the path of insertion of the two posts. Multisection post and core or single cast post and core with auxiliary post can be an effective design to manage grossly decayed mandibular molars.

1. Introduction

Comprehensive treatment plan is required before the start of endodontic treatment. When the decision is made to treat the teeth endodontically consideration must be given to the placement of the subsequent restoration. Endodontically treated posterior teeth are often mutilated due to caries and access requirement, sometimes to the extent that all the walls of coronal structure are missing and only the radicular portion is present. In such cases if ferrule is available and coronal retention core buildup is not sufficient then intraradicular retention may be used by custom made post and core which replaces any lost coronal tooth structure [1]. Relatively long post with circular cross sections provides good retention and support in anterior teeth but should be avoided in posterior teeth, which often have curved roots and elliptical or ribbon shaped canals. For these teeth, retention is better provided by two or more relatively short posts in divergent canals [2]. This can be achieved by multisection post and core with each section having its own path of withdrawal or single piece post and core with a separate auxiliary post.

This paper presents two case reports on post endodontic management of badly mutilated mandibular molars: one with two-section post and core and one with single post and core with separate auxiliary post. A review of custom post and core in posterior teeth is listed in Table 1 [3–6].

2. Case Presentation

Case 1 (multisection post and core). A 21-year-old male patient reported to the Department of Conservative Dentistry and Endodontics, Institute of Dental Sciences Bareilly, with the chief complaint of pain in lower left tooth region. Extraoral examination revealed no significant findings. Intraoral examination revealed grossly decayed 36 (Figure 1(a)). The tooth was not tender on percussion. The tooth was not mobile and nonresponsive to any pulp sensitivity tests. Intraoral sinus tract was present on the buccal aspect in left quadrant. Path of this sinus tract was traced with gutta percha using periapical radiograph. On radiographic examination, radiolucency was observed involving both the mesial and distal root of 36 (Figure 1(b)).

Chronic periapical abscess was diagnosed. A comprehensive treatment plan was made consisting of two phases: endodontic phase and restorative phase.

2.1. Endodontic Phase. After excavation of caries unsupported tooth structure was removed. Access cavity was refined and working length was established (distal: 13 mm, mesiobuccal and mesiolingual: 11 mm). Biomechanical preparation was completed by Mtwo files up to 6% taper number 25. During preparation canals were irrigated with normal saline (0.9% W/V) and metronidazole (0.5% W/V). A final

TABLE 1: Review of literature.

S number	Author	Technique	Drawbacks
1	Bass 2002 [3]	Single post and core with auxiliary post Distal-single cast post Mesiolingual-prefabricated screw post	As the mesial canal had prefabricated post the precision was less than what could have been achieved by the custom made cast post.
2	Gogna et al. 2009 [4]	Single post and core with auxiliary post Distal-single cast post Mesiobuccal-post with core	Since mesiobuccal canal was chosen to place the post there are more chances of root perforation.
3	Kumar et al. 2013 [5]	Single post and core with auxiliary post Distal-single cast post Mesiolingual-post with core	Core was not encasing the coronal tooth structure; instead it was wedged within the coronal tooth structure.
4	Dăguci et al. 2014 [6]	Multisection post and core (lock and key arrangement) Distobuccal-single post with core Palatal-single post with core	Technique sensitive procedure.
5	Mattoo et al. 2014 [9]	Multisection post and core (lock and key arrangement) Distolingual-single post with core Mesiolingual-single post with core	Indirect pattern was used to prepare the posts that will not be as accurate.
6	Deenadayalan et al. 2015 [10]	Multisection post and core (lock and key arrangement) Distolingual-single post with core Mesiolingual-single post with core	

rinse with 2% chlorhexidine solution was done after completion of biomechanical preparation. Triple antibiotic paste (ciprofloxacin 200 mg, metronidazole 500 mg, and minocycline 100 mg) was placed in the canal and patient was recalled after two weeks.

At second appointment patient was asymptomatic, and sinus tract was healed so obturation was completed with 6% taper number 25 single cone gutta percha using AH plus as a sealer. Patient was recalled after three weeks; there were no clinical signs and symptoms. Restorative phase was planned.

2.2. Restorative Phase. Using peeso reamer numbers 1–3 (1.1 mm diameter) post space of length 5 mm (leaving 6 mm of gutta percha apically) was prepared in the mesiobuccal canal taking care that at least minimum of 1 mm of dentin remains around the canal. Similarly post space was prepared in the distal canal using peeso reamer numbers 1–4 (1.3 mm diameter) of length 6 mm (leaving 7 mm of gutta percha apically).

Following this ferrule preparation was completed. Wax pattern of post in mesiobuccal canal with part of its core was prepared. Any undercut adjacent to another half was removed (Figure 1(c)). Casting of the mesial portion was done and the fit was checked. Direct wax pattern of the distal section of post and core was prepared with the casting of mesial section of post and core in place (Figure 1(d)). Distal section wax pattern was casted and fit was checked by keeping mesial casting in place. Dovetail to interlock the mesial and distal section was not prepared as final buildup was to be held together by the fixed cast restoration. Both the castings were luted with type II GIC (Figure 1(g)). Core preparation was finished for all metal crown. Rubber base impression was taken and was temporized for 3 weeks. All metal crown was fabricated and cemented in the next appointment. At 1-year clinical follow-up, the prosthesis exhibited no evidence of failure and the patient was satisfied with the function and esthetics.

Case 2 (single piece core with auxiliary post). A 23-year-old male patient reported to the Department of Conservative Dentistry and Endodontics, with the chief complaint of decayed tooth in lower left tooth region. Extraoral examination revealed no significant findings. On intraoral examination 37 was grossly decayed (Figure 2(a)) and tender on percussion. Intraoral periapical radiograph revealed deep caries involving pulp space with no periapical changes (Figure 2(b)). There was more divergence between mesial and distal root as compared to Case 1. The tooth was nonresponsive to any pulp sensitivity tests. Endodontic therapy was planned for the tooth followed by post and core to rehabilitate the occlusal portion.

2.3. Endodontic Phase. Since there was no periapical change a single sitting root canal treatment was planned which was commenced by excavating all the caries and refining the access preparation. Working length was determined (distal: 13 mm, mesiobuccal and mesiolingual: 11 mm). Biomechanical preparation with Mtwo rotary files was completed up to 6% taper number 25 with concomitant irrigation using metronidazole (0.5% W/V) and normal saline (0.9% W/V). Single cone obturation was completed with 6% gutta percha number 25 using AH plus as a sealer. Patient was recalled after 1 week for restorative phase.

2.4. Restorative Phase. Since the divergence between the mesial and distal root was more a single core with small post

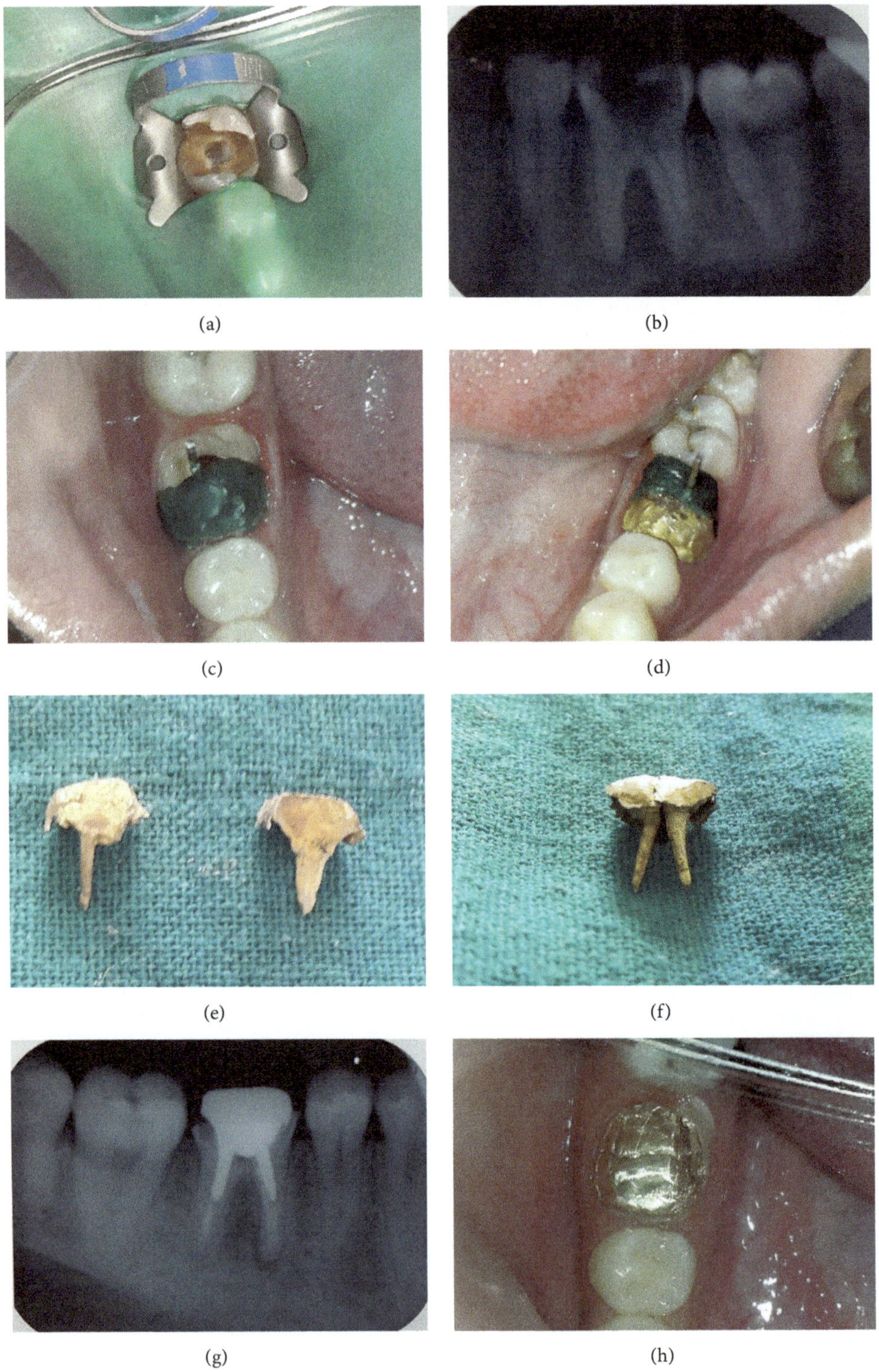

Figure 1: (a) Preoperative intraoral photograph showing grossly carious tooth. (b) Preoperative IOPAR showing grossly decayed molar with roots showing parallel configuration. (c) Fabrication of wax pattern in mesiolingual canal involving mesial half of the tooth. (d) Wax pattern fabrication of the distal half with mesial post and core in place. (e) Mesial and distal sections of split cast post and core. (f) Assembly of mesial and distal sections of split cast post and core. (g) IOPAR of luted and finished split cast post and core. (h) Luted and finished split cast post and core.

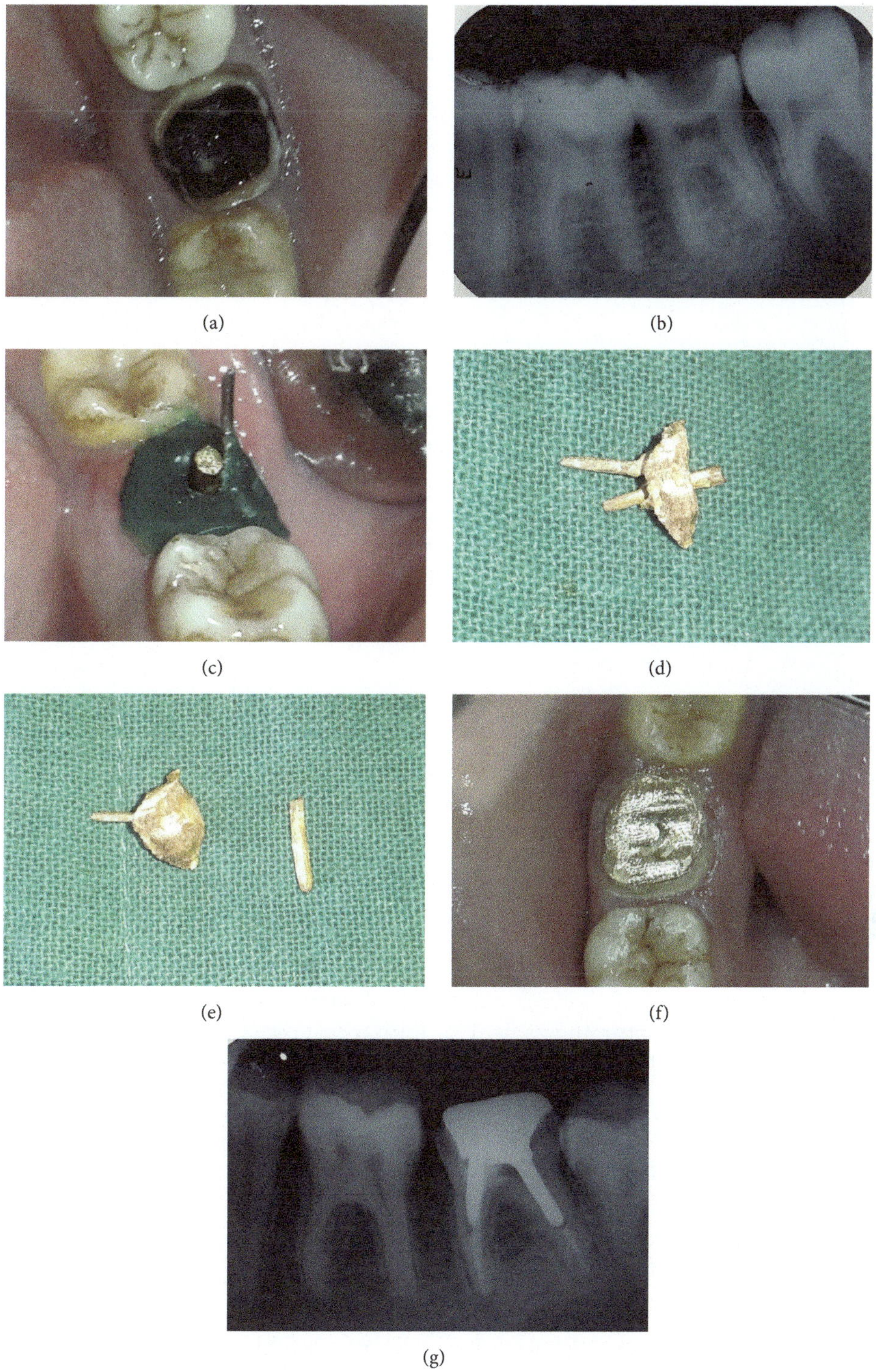

FIGURE 2: (a) Preoperative intraoral photograph showing grossly decayed molar. (b) Preoperative IOPAR showing grossly decayed molar with divergent root configuration. (c) Wax pattern fabrication of mesiolingual canal and core with distal casting in place. (d) Assembly of mesial and distal sections of split cast post and core. (e) Mesial and distal sections of split post and core. (f) Luted and finished split cast post and core. (g) IOPAR of luted and finished split cast post and core.

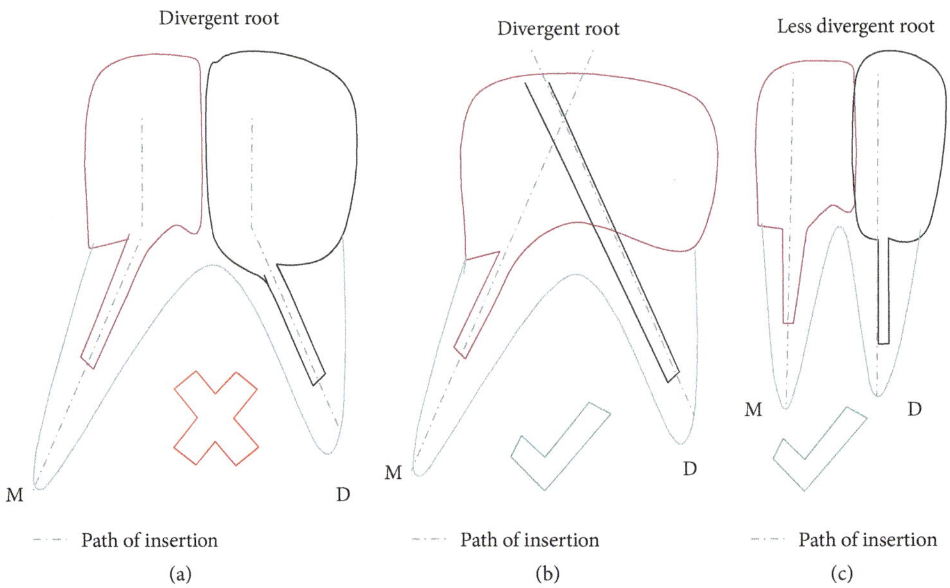

FIGURE 3: Line diagram showing different type of designs made according to the anatomy of root. In teeth with divergent roots the paths of insertion of the two posts (a) coincide with each other, so it is difficult to prepare the wax pattern. Hence in such cases the design in (b) is suggested, while in teeth with lesser divergence design in (c) is suggested.

in mesial root and a separate auxiliary post in distal root was planned.

Using pesso reamer numbers 1–3 (1.1 mm diameter) post space of length 4 mm (leaving 7 mm of gutta percha apically) was prepared in the mesiobuccal canal, taking care that at least minimum of 1 mm of dentin remains around the canal. Similarly post space was prepared in the distal canal using pesso reamer numbers 1–4 (1.3 diameter) of length 6 mm (leaving 7 mm of gutta percha apically).

Ferrule preparation was completed followed by the auxiliary post preparation in distal canal and single post with core preparation in the mesial canal.

2.5. Auxiliary Post Preparation. K file number 40 was used and its handle was removed. Green inlay wax was added to the file and impression of the distal canal was taken for auxiliary post. Post length should extend coronally beyond the actual preparation. Then impression was removed and reseated back into the canal several times while it was still soft; it was then invested and casted.

2.6. Single Core with Single Auxiliary Post. Wax pattern of short post in mesiobuccal canal and single core was prepared with casted auxiliary distal post in place (Figure 2(c)).

Auxiliary post was gripped with forceps and removed. Wax pattern of single short post with core was removed and casting was done. The hole for the auxiliary post was refined with the appropriate twist drill. The casting of core with post was checked with the auxiliary post through the hole into the canal. During luting of the castings, the single core and post of the mesial root was luted first followed by the immediate sliding of the distal auxiliary post through the hole in the core which was held by locking tweezer for fast and comfortable insertion (Figure 2(f)). The finishing and refining of the axial walls were done after 10 mins so that the cement is fully set (Figure 2(f)).

3. Discussion

The mandibular molars in the two cases presented were not having sufficient coronal tooth structure to provide retention for crown. More conservative approach was planned instead of extraction of the teeth followed by implant or fixed partial denture. Decision for cast post and core was taken as fiber or prefabricated metal post with GIC, composite, or amalgam core could have increased the chances of failure at the interface of post and core. Single cast post and core in largest and straightest canal was also not considered as single post in the distal canal may lead to either rotation of the core or inadequate retention. Further a long post also increases the chances of perforation of the root leading to failure. Internal stresses are more by placing one long post as compared to two short posts.

In both the cases, decision was made to place one long post in distal canal and one short post in the mesiobuccal canal. Mesiobuccal canal was selected instead of mesiolingual canal as more amount of dentin is present at the danger zone area in mesiobuccal canal.

Divergence of mesial and distal root does not allow fabrication of the two posts with core as single unit since path of withdrawal for the two posts will be different. So it was decided to prepare multisection post and core with each section having separate path of withdrawal in Case 1 (Figure 3). In Case 2 divergence between the roots was more as compared to Case 1, so long axis of post and core in each section of multisection post and core will not be in a straight line. This will cause interference during wax pattern fabrication for both the castings due to the undercut formed. Further the stresses will not be evenly distributed. Hence single post and core with auxiliary post was planned in Case 2. In both the cases two units were fabricated in separate appointments.

Preparation of dowel space within 3–5 mm of the apical seal is not considered nowadays as post length equal to the length of expected crown is thought to be sufficient. When two posts are placed in divergent roots even this length is not required and much shorter posts can provide adequate retention [7].

Multisection cast post and core reported in the literature is one in which lock and key arrangement was provided in the core of two sections [6]. This design is more technique sensitive and may require more appointments. As both the sections were resting on ferrule and are encased by full coverage crowns interlock was not required. Success in such cases was also reported in the literature previously [5].

Literature search reveals case reports in which custom cast post and core with prefabricated auxiliary post was used for restoration of badly mutilated teeth [8]. Since custom cast auxiliary post is better adapted according to canal anatomy it was also fabricated in Case 2.

Advantages of Split Cast Post and Core. Consider the following:

(i) Preservation of more tooth structure.

(ii) Provision of antirotation preparation.

(iii) Core retention as it is an inherent part of at least one post.

(iv) Retention of core.

Disadvantages. Consider the following:

(i) Placing the custom cast post and core requires additional operative and lab procedures. It is technique sensitive.

(ii) Preparing the tooth to accommodate the post requires removal of additional tooth structure.

(iii) The post can complicate or prevent future endodontic retreatment if this becomes necessary.

4. Conclusion

Grossly decayed mandibular molars with all walls missing can also be successfully restored by split cast post and core. Depending on the amount of divergence between mesial and distal root which affects the straight line path of withdrawal of wax pattern, multisection split post and core or single post and core with auxiliary post can be fabricated for retention of crown. Direct wax pattern technique results in precise casting. Two short posts in divergent root are sufficient to provide retention instead of one long post.

Competing Interests

The authors declare that they have no competing interests.

References

[1] I. Peroz, F. Blankenstein, K.-P. Lange, and M. Naumann, "Restoring endodontically treated teeth with posts and cores—a review," *Quintessence International*, vol. 36, no. 9, pp. 737–746, 2005.

[2] S. F. Rosensteil, M. F. Land, and J. Fujimoto, *Contemporary Fixed Prosthodontics*, Mosby, St. Louis, Mo, USA, 3rd edition, 2001.

[3] E. V. Bass, "Cast post and core foundation for the badly broken down molar tooth," *Australian Dental Journal*, vol. 47, no. 1, pp. 57–62, 2002.

[4] R. Gogna, S. Jagadish, K. Shashikala, and K. Prasad, "Restoration of badly broken, endodontically treated posterior teeth," *Journal of Conservative Dentistry*, vol. 12, no. 3, pp. 123–128, 2009.

[5] L. Kumar, R. Gupta R, and A. Yadav, "A systematic approach to restore grossly decayed multirooted teeth: split cast post and core," *International Journal of Prosthodontics and Restorative Dentistry*, vol. 2, no. 1, pp. 16–18, 2013.

[6] C. Dăguci, L. Dăguci, M. Bătăiosu et al., "Restoration of molar morphology with a split cast post and core," *Romanian Journal of Morphology and Embryology*, vol. 55, no. 2, pp. 401–405, 2014.

[7] A. Sadan, R. Elliot, and A. J. Raigrodski, "Treatment planning extensively broken-down mandibular molars for post and core fabrication," *Quintessence International*, vol. 29, no. 6, pp. 351–355, 1998.

[8] M. R. Spector, "A cast core system with interlocking posts," *The Journal of Prosthetic Dentistry*, vol. 56, no. 1, pp. 16–19, 1986.

[9] K. Mattoo, R. Garg, and V. Arora, "Sliding cast post core system—prosthodontic solution for divergent root canal configuration," *Journal of Medical Science And Clical Research*, vol. 2, no. 11, pp. 3001–3004, 2014.

[10] E. Deenadayalan, A. Kumar, R. K. Tewari, S. K. Mishra, and S. Alam, "Management of grossly destroyed endodontically treated teeth with lock and key custom modified cast post and core design. A case series," *Contemporary Clinical Dentistry*, vol. 6, no. 1, pp. 88–93, 2015.

36

Management of Oehler's Type III Dens Invaginatus Using Cone Beam Computed Tomography

Jaya Ranganathan, Mohan Kumar Rangarajan Sundaresan, and Srinivasan Ramasamy

Department of Conservative Dentistry and Endodontics, Priyadarshini Dental College & Hospital, Pandur, Thiruvallur, Chennai 631203, India

Correspondence should be addressed to Jaya Ranganathan; endojaya@gmail.com

Academic Editor: Jiiang H. Jeng

Dens Invaginatus is a dental malformation that poses diagnostic difficulties in the clinical context. This anomaly may increase the risk of pulp disease and can potentially complicate endodontic procedure due to the aberrant root canal anatomy. Compared to conventional radiographs, three-dimensional images obtained with Cone Beam Computed Tomography (CBCT) are invaluable in the diagnosis of the extent of this anomaly and in the appropriate treatment planning. Oehler's classification (1957) for Dens Invaginatus (DI) into three types depending on the depth of the invagination has been used for treatment planning. Of the three types Type III DI is characterized by infolding of the enamel into the tooth up to the root apex and is considered as the most severe variant of DI and hence the most challenging to treat endodontically, due to the morphological complexities. This report describes a case of Oehler's Type III DI in a necrotic permanent maxillary lateral incisor in which CBCT images played a key role in diagnosis and treatment planning. The case was managed successfully by a combination of nonsurgical and surgical endodontic therapy with orthograde and retrograde thermoplastic gutta percha obturation.

1. Introduction

Dens Invaginatus is a developmental anomaly which arises as a result of an invagination into the surface of the tooth crown before calcification has occurred [1].

Dens Invaginatus (DI) in a human tooth was first described by Socrates in 1856 [2]. The term Dens Invaginatus was proposed by Oehler in 1957 and is the most widely accepted. Synonyms for this anomaly reported in literature are dens in dente (Busch 1897), invaginated odontome, dilated gestant odontome, dilated composite odontome (Hunter 1951), tooth inclusion, telescopic tooth, and gestant anomaly [2–5].

The teeth most affected are the maxillary lateral incisors. Bilateral occurrence as high as 43% has been reported by Hülsmann [2]. There are rare case reports of DI in the posterior, deciduous, and supernumerary teeth [2, 3, 6]. The reported prevalence of adult teeth affected by DI is between 0.3 and 10%. This variation in reported prevalence is attributed to methodological differences in cohort studies, the identification criteria used, and diagnostic difficulties [2, 6, 7].

The most widely accepted classification of this anomaly is that proposed by Oehler (1957) who categorized it based on the enamel invagination depth observed radiographically. Type I describes an enamel lined invagination confined to the coronal part of the tooth; Type II represents extension of the invagination beyond the cementoenamel junction ending as a blind sac. Type III includes permeation of the root by the invagination to form an additional canal opening on lateral side of root [8]. This invaginated tract which usually has no direct communication with the pulp has been termed pseudo canal by Gonçalves et al. [4]. The invagination may be completely lined with enamel but frequently cementum may be found lining the invagination in the apical portion [2]. Amongst the three types Type I and Type II are considered as incomplete invagination and their incidence is 79% and 15%, respectively. Type III as reported in the present case is a complete invagination with the lowest incidence at 5% [3, 6].

There is a lack of consensus on the aetiology of DI. Various proposed theories are embryological cause with proliferation of enamel organ cells into dental papilla (Rushton 1937),

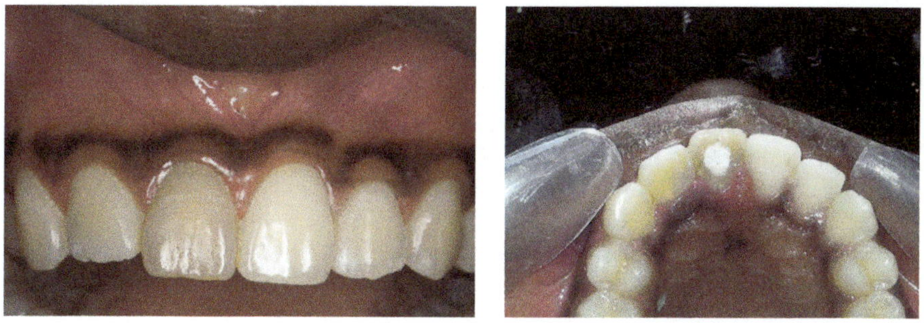

(a) (b)

FIGURE 1: (a) Labial view. (b) Palatal view.

retardation of focal group of cells (Kronfeld 1934), external forces (Atkinson 1943), trauma (Gustafson & Sundberg 1950), infection (Fischer 1936), and genetic factors as reported by Hülsmann, Alani, and Coriani [2, 3, 6].

Even though DI is one of the most common developmental anomalies, it is easily overlooked as very often there is absence of significant clinical signs of the anomaly and it is only detected on routine radiographs. Clinically, an unusual crown morphology (dilated/peg shaped), grooving of the palatal enamel, exaggerated/bifid cingulum, or a deep foramen cecum may be hints of the anomaly though the affected tooth may show no obvious clinical signs of the malformation. Due to the high incidence of bilateral occurrence, the contralateral tooth should also be investigated [2, 9]. The presence of DI predisposes the entry of bacteria into the invagination. If undetected in the early stages this leads to pulp/periodontal pathosis as there are channels between the invagination and the pulp space. The presence of hypomineralized enamel surrounding the invagination predisposes to early involvement of the pulp space through the invagination [2, 4, 5, 7, 10–12].

Clinically, severe pulpal (loss of vitality) and periodontal alterations as well as presence of sinus tracts can be associated with an untreated DI with pulp involvement [13].

Conventional radiographs are insufficient in most cases of DI as they show only a 2D view of a complex anatomy. The use of CBCT (Cone Beam Computed Tomography) images as was done in our case report, obtained in 3 orthogonal planes (axial, sagittal, and coronal), is invaluable to observe the extent of the invagination and the relationship of the invaginated portion and the root canal with high precision [6, 13, 14]. The use of CBCT images was crucial in our treatment planning.

Treatment of a tooth with DI and pulp pathosis is a challenge to an endodontist owing to the irregular shape of the root canal systems and invaginated tract [2]. The problems are further compounded if part of the invagination is obliterated or if the invagination encroaches into the pulp space at some level as was also observed in our case.

This case report describes Oehler's Type III DI in a necrotic permanent maxillary lateral incisor with periapical lesion managed successfully with a nonsurgical and surgical endodontic therapy with orthograde and retrograde backfilling of thermoplastic gutta percha. The use of CBCT images in this case was vital in diagnosis and treatment planning.

2. Case Presentation

A 14-year-old female reported to the dental hospital with complaints of pain and occasional swelling in relation to her right upper front tooth for past 6 months. Pain was aggravated by taking hot foods and mastication. History revealed that maxillary right central incisor was "filled" eight months earlier in a private dental hospital but no relevant treatment details or documents were available. Medical history was noncontributory.

Intraoral examination revealed a slight discoloration of the maxillary first central incisor and a diffuse swelling of the vestibular region adjacent to maxillary right central and lateral incisor. There was pain on percussion. The mesiodistal width of the maxillary right lateral incisor was slightly larger than that of the contralateral tooth; this difference was more prominent in the palatal view (Figures 1(a) and 1(b)).

Pulp sensibility tests of the tooth (thermal test with heated gutta percha and electric pulp testing (Parkell Electronics Division, Farmingdale, NY)) revealed irreversible pulpitis of maxillary central and lateral incisors.

On radiological examination (intraoral periapical and OPG) a radioopaque material was seen in coronal part of maxillary right central incisor with incomplete obturation and a diffuse radiolucency in relation to the periapical region of central and lateral incisor (Figures 2 and 3).

Endodontic retreatment was initiated in central incisor. Access cavity revealed a restorative material obstructing the access to the main canal. The patient was referred for CBCT (Cone Beam Computed Tomography) scanning to locate the main canal of right central incisor and to study the abnormal root anatomy of maxillary lateral incisor prior to initiating endodontic treatment procedures. The CBCT imaging was done with Kodak 9500 Cone Beam 3D system, Carestream Health Inc., Rochester, NY, USA, with exposure parameters of 90 kVp tube voltage and 10 mA tube current. The images were obtained with a voxel size of 0.20 mm × 0.20 mm × 0.20 mm with exposure time of 10.8 seconds. The images were

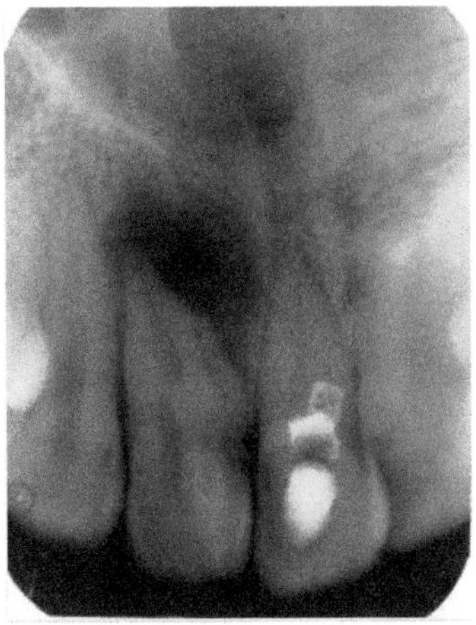

FIGURE 2: Intraoral periapical image.

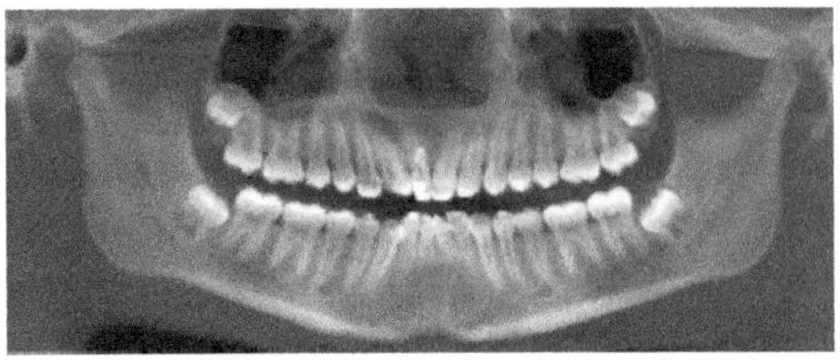

FIGURE 3: OPG.

examined with Carestream 3D Imaging software (Atlanta, GA, USA).

CBCT images of maxillary right central revealed restorative material extending from the cervical to the midroot region labially, suggesting an attempt to repair an improperly directed access opening. The access cavity was reentered; the obstructing cement was removed with GG drill number 3 (Dentsply, Maillefer, Ballaigues, Switzerland) with slow speed drill. The access was refined with CBCT image guidance to locate the main canal. After working length determination with apex locator (Root ZX mini apex locator, J. Morita Corp; Tokyo, Japan) chemomechanical preparation was done with Pro-Taper rotary files (Dentsply Tulsa) up to F3 using 2.5% NaOCl and 17% EDTA as irrigants. Canal projection technique was done using F3 Pro-Taper cone (Dentsply Maillefer) to repair the previous defective access attempt defect with ProRoot MTA (Dentsply Tulsa Dental Specialties, Tulsa, Oklahoma, USA). After the canal was dried with absorbent points (Dentsply, Maillefer) the canal was obturated by lateral condensation technique using 2% gutta percha (Dentsply, Maillefer, Ballaigues, Switzerland) and AH plus root canal sealer (Dentsply De Trey, Konstanz, Germany). The access cavity was restored with composite resin (3M ESPE, St. Paul, MN, USA).

The right lateral incisor showed a continuous main canal and an invaginated portion mesially in the CBCT images. Axial images in CBCT revealed the invaginated tract to be obliterated in the coronal third and midroot area and compressing the main canal (Figures 4(a) and 4(b)).

The patency of the invagination was observed in the apical third only in the axial and sagittal CBCT images (Figures 4(c) and 5).

Based on these images the case was diagnosed as Oehler's Type III Dens Invaginatus in a nonvital maxillary lateral incisor with periapical lesion. It was planned to do conventional orthograde nonsurgical treatment for the root canal followed by surgical retrograde approach to negotiate and obturate the apical patent portion of the invagination.

CBCT assisted access cavity of lateral incisor was prepared. Access cavity was prepared and the root canal was located distolingually. The orifice of the invaginated portion was not visible. Working length of the canal was determined by apex locater (Root ZX mini apex locator, J. Morita Corp; Tokyo, Japan) and confirmed radiographically with intraoral periapical. The main canal was negotiated and chemomechanical preparation was completed by crown down technique using rotary Pro-Taper Nickel-Titanium Rotary files (Dentsply Maillefer) up to F3 using 2.5% NaOCl and 17% EDTA as root canal irrigants. Calcium Hydroxide was injected in the canal (Calcicur; Voco, Cuxhaven, Germany) as an intracanal medicament for a period of three weeks to promote healing of the periapical lesion. The access was sealed with temporary restoration of Cavit (3M ESPE Norristown; PA, USA).

For the surgical approach, after administration of local anaesthesia using 2% lidocaine with 1 : 1,00,000 epinephrine, a labial full thickness rectangular mucoperiosteal flap was elevated to expose the area of the periapical lesion. The existing pathological cortical bone window was widened with surgical burs to expose the lesion adequately. The granulomatous soft tissue surrounding the root tip was curetted with surgical curettes. Root resection was not done to maintain original root length to help tooth stability.

The main canal of the lateral incisor was obturated by thermoplastic gutta percha backfilling technique using the Elements System (Sybron Endo) of size 30-gauge tip with AH plus as root canal sealer. A retro preparation was done in the apical root portion of the invagination using precurved K files (Dentsply; Mailefer) in a step back manner from number 10 to number 25K file and using 1% NaOCl. The retro preparation was obturated using AH plus (Maillefer, Dentsply, Konstanz, Germany) as sealer and by thermoplastic backfilling with gutta percha (Elements Sybron Endo) using 15-gauge tip and then cold burnished. The coronal access was sealed with glass ionomer cement (Fuji II, GC Corp.). Surgical site was irrigated with normal saline 0.9%, flap repositioned, and sutured with 4-0 nylon suture (Ethicon; Johnson & Johnson). Antibiotics and nonsteroidal inflammatory drugs as well as 2% chlorhexidine mouthwash was prescribed. Patient was called for a follow-up the next day when the soft tissue healing was found to be satisfactory. The sutures were removed after 5 days.

Follow-up after one year showed satisfactory healing on the radiograph (Figure 6).

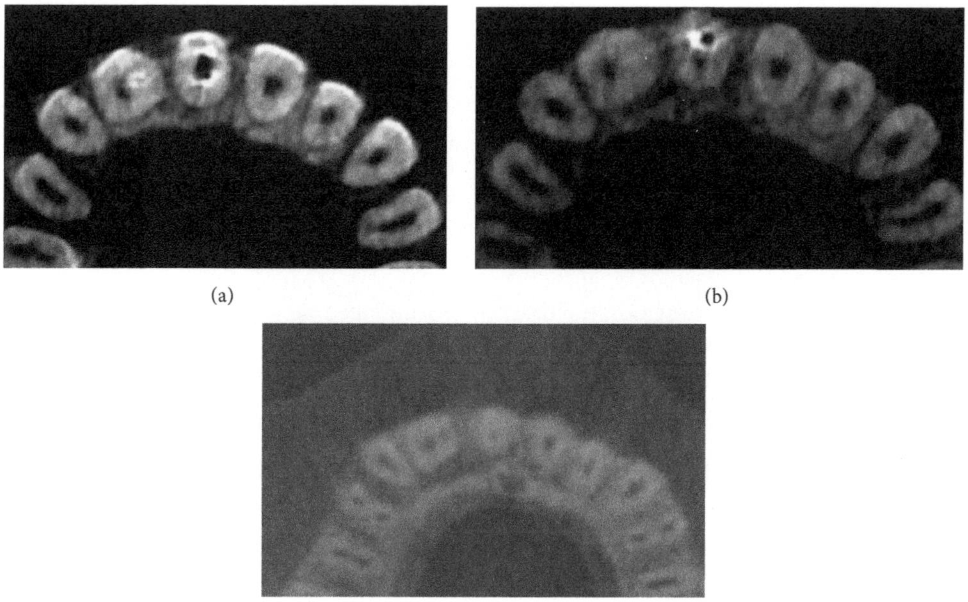

(a) (b) (c)

FIGURE 4: (a) Axial image coronal third of root. (b) Axial image middle third root. (c) Axial image apical third root.

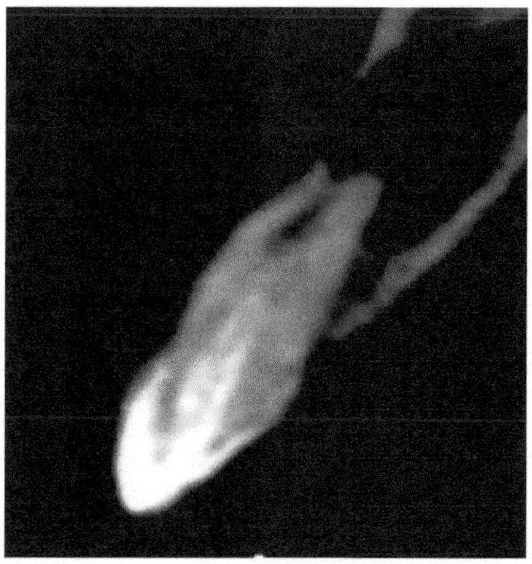

FIGURE 5: Sagittal view.

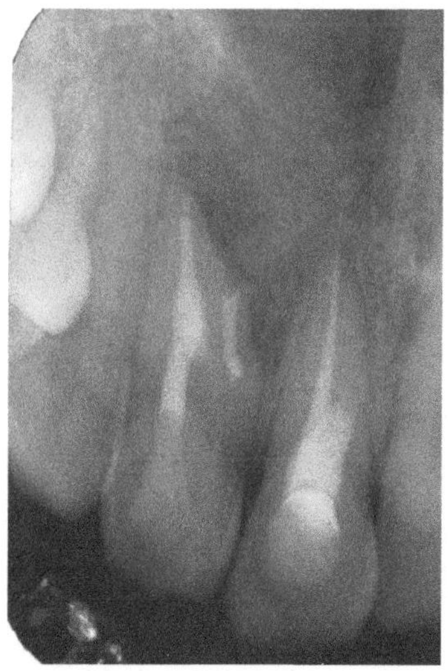

FIGURE 6: 1-year postoperative IOPA.

3. Discussion

Dens Invaginatus (DI) as a dental anomaly shows a broad spectrum of morphologic variations and predisposes the tooth to dental caries and in more severe invaginations to pulpitis and apical periodontitis [2, 3, 8, 12]. Oehler's Type III Dens Invaginatus as reported in this case is considered as the most severe variant of the anomaly wherein the affected tooth shows a deep infolding of the enamel and dentin extending into the root and communicating laterally with the periodontal space through a pseudo foramen [1, 8].

The enamel lining in these defects is often hypomineralized and incomplete with various channels that communicate with the pulp thereby allowing easy access for irritants from the invagination to reach the pulp space [12, 14].

Varied treatment options for Oehler's Type III DI have been mentioned in the literature. Suggested treatment modalities range from periodic observation to prophylactic sealing of the invaginated pit in asymptomatic teeth. In cases with pulp necrosis, endodontic therapy of only the invaginated portion [4] or of both the invaginated portion as well as the root canal has been suggested [15]. Surgical endodontics in addition to conventional endodontics should be considered only for large periapical lesions not resolved nonsurgically or in cases which cannot be treated nonsurgically due to failure to gain a coronal access. Surgery will provide a disinfection and retrograde seal to the apical portion of the invagination and/root canal which will otherwise retain a source of infection [2, 5–7, 9, 10, 16–18]. The surgical endodontic procedures include apical resection, apical curettage, and retrograde restoration. Extraction of the teeth is proposed only for those teeth that cannot be salvaged surgically [2, 4, 6, 7, 9, 14, 15]. Complete removal of the invaginated portion to create a large canal space as well as intentional replantation to treat Type III DI has been reported in literature [2, 9].

Type III DI is often associated with changes in the morphology of the root canal itself; thereby endodontic procedures are a challenging task due to the aberrant anatomy in both the pulp space and the invaginated track. Also, there can be an absence of a true apical constriction if the invagination opens into the periodontal space (as reported in this case) (Figure 5) which further contributes to making endodontic procedures complicated [2, 3, 7, 9, 15, 17]. The invaginated portion may compress the main canal at different levels as reported by Fregnani et al. [16] and as was seen in CBCT images in this case report (Figures 4(a) and 4(b)).

Cases of DI with its complex anatomy always pose a diagnostic and treatment challenge to the clinician. Due to the intrinsic limitations of the conventional radiographs, they are unable to reveal the details of the DI three-dimensionally. The introduction of CBCT in the 1990s with its 3D images has revolutionized the imaging of dental malformations and contributes in a large way to diagnosis and treatment planning of these cases. In cases of DI, CBCT images show the details in terms of type, extension, and morphologic changes in the tooth [7, 13, 19, 20]. CBCT uses low effective radiation dose and besides generating undistorted 3D reconstruction of the teeth and surrounding soft tissues provides interrelational images in three orthogonal planes: axial, sagittal, and coronal [21, 22].

We have presented a challenging case of Oehler's Type III DI in a maxillary lateral incisor associated with necrotic pulp and periradicular lesion. The use of Cone Beam Computed Tomography (CBCT) images was invaluable in diagnosis and treatment planning. The CBCT axial images revealed that in the coronal third of root the invagination was nearly obliterated and compressing the main canal outline (Figure 4(a)). In the midroot region the invaginated portion was partially patent towards the apical end while the apical portion of the invagination was wide open at its exit portal (Figure 5). As compared with the contralateral incisor the larger cross section of the invaginated tooth was evident (Figures 4(a), 4(b), and 4(c)). The invaginated canal seemed to be lined with enamel in the coronal and midroot region (Figure 5). Based on these CBCT images we decided to treat the main root canal with nonsurgical endodontic therapy and do a surgical endodontic approach with retrograde filling for the patent apical portion of the invagination (Figures 4(c) and 5). Due to the risk of lateral perforation with burs, conventional access to the obliterated portion of the invaginated portion was not made, nor was an attempt to join the invagination with the root canal done. A similar combination of conventional and surgical endodontics has also been reported in a case report by Vier-Pelisser et al. [7].

Calcium Hydroxide was used as an intracanal medicament in the root canal for a period of two weeks as its high alkalinity facilitates healing in necrotic teeth with periapical lesion.

Even though MTA has been the preferred root end material, our choice of gutta percha for the orthograde and retrograde obturation was based on its ability to be heat softened thereby allowing it to penetrate all parts of the aberrant canal anatomy of the DI (Figure 6). The advantage of the thermoplasticized gutta percha obturation has been well documented for both orthograde and retrograde fillings [2, 10, 15, 18].

The use of the CBCT images in this case was important in treatment planning and for successfully treating a case of Oehler's Type III DI with nonvital pulp and periapical lesion with combined nonsurgical and surgical endodontic therapy.

4. Conclusion

Teeth with Oehler's Dens Invaginatus Type III and with periapical pathosis are a challenge to the endodontist considering their aberrant anatomy. The use of CBCT was an important tool in our case to provide relevant details of the internal anatomy of the invaginated tooth and thereby played a vital role in treatment planning. The combination of nonsurgical and surgical treatments was an effective approach in our case.

Conflict of Interests

The authors declare that there is no conflict of interests regarding the publication of this paper.

References

[1] W. G. Shafer, M. K. Hine, and B. M. Levy, *Shafer's Textbook of Oral Pathology*, section I, Elsevier, 6th edition, 2009.

[2] M. Hülsmann, "Dens invaginatus: aetiology, classification, prevalence, diagnosis, and treatment considerations," *International Endodontic Journal*, vol. 30, no. 2, pp. 79–90, 1997.

[3] A. Alani and K. Bishop, "Dens invaginatus. Part 1: classification, prevalence and aetiology," *International Endodontic Journal*, vol. 41, no. 12, pp. 1123–1136, 2008.

[4] A. Gonçalves, M. Gonçalves, D. P. Oliveira, and N. Gonçalves, "Dens invaginatus type III: report of a case and 10-year radiographic follow-up," *International Endodontic Journal*, vol. 35, no. 10, pp. 873–879, 2002.

[5] J. C. Jefferson Marion, L. Maria Mesquita, T. M. Duque, and F. J. Souza Filho, "Endodontic treatment of three types of dens invaginatus: report of four cases," *Dental Press Endodontics*, vol. 2, no. 2, pp. 71–79, 2012.

[6] C. Coraini, T. Mascarello, C. M. de Palma et al., "Endodontic and periodontal treatment of dens invaginatus: report of 2 clinical cases," *Giornale Italiano di Endodonzia*, vol. 27, no. 2, pp. 86–94, 2013.

[7] F. V. Vier-Pelisser, R. D. Morgental, G. Fritscher, A. C. Ghisi, M. G. de Borba, and R. K. Scarparo, "Management of type III dens invaginatus in a mandibular premolar: a case report," *Brazilian Dental Journal*, vol. 25, no. 1, pp. 73–78, 2014.

[8] F. A. C. Oehlers, "Dens invaginatus (dilated composite odontome): I. Variations of the invagination process and associated

anterior crown forms," *Oral Surgery, Oral Medicine, Oral Pathology*, vol. 10, no. 11, pp. 1204–1218, 1957.

[9] K. Bishop and A. Alani, "Dens invaginatus. Part 2: clinical, radiographic features and management options," *International Endodontic Journal*, vol. 41, no. 12, pp. 1137–1154, 2008.

[10] U. X. da Silva Neto, V. H. G. Hirai, V. Papalexiou et al., "Combined endodontic therapy and surgery in the treatment of dens invaginatus type 3: case report," *Journal of the Canadian Dental Association*, vol. 71, no. 11, pp. 855–858, 2005.

[11] L. George, A. Mohan, and J. Mathew, "Oeler׳s type III dens invaginatus: a case report with 1-year follow-up," *European Journal of General Dentistry*, vol. 3, no. 2, pp. 155–157, 2014.

[12] M. Yamada, M. Nagayama, A. Katsumata et al., "Hypomineralized Enamel of Dens Invaginatus: its distinct images and pathogenesis of the type III invagination using micro-focusing computed tomography," *Journal of Hard Tissue Biology*, vol. 23, no. 4, pp. 449–453, 2014.

[13] F. S. Neves, L. C. Bastos, S. M. de Almeida, F. N. Boscolo, F. Haiter-Neto, and P. S. F. Campos, "Dens Invaginatus: a cone beam computed tomography case report," *Journal of the Health Sciences Institute*, vol. 28, no. 3, pp. 249–250, 2010.

[14] K. T. Ceyhanli, D. Çelik, S. H. Altintas, T. Taşdemir, and Ö. Sezgin, "Conservative treatment and follow-up of type III dens invaginatus using cone beam computed tomography," *Journal of Oral Science*, vol. 56, no. 4, pp. 307–310, 2014.

[15] A. H. Borges, A. S. Segundo, M. R. Nadalin, F. L. M. Pedro, A. M. D. Filho, and M. D. Sousa-Neto, "Conventional treatment of maxillary incisor type III dens Invaginatus with periapical lesion: a case report," *ISRN Dentistry*, vol. 2011, Article ID 257609, 5 pages, 2011.

[16] E. R. Fregnani, L. F. B. Spinola, J. R. O. Sônego, C. E. S. Bueno, and A. S. De Martin, "Complex endodontic treatment of an immature type III dens invaginatus. A case report," *International Endodontic Journal*, vol. 41, no. 10, pp. 913–919, 2008.

[17] H. Ozbas, "Rustem Kemal Subay, Melike Ordulu, Surgical Retreatment of an invaginated maxillary central incisor following overfilled endodontic treatment," *European Journal of Dentistry*, vol. 4, p. 324, 2010.

[18] G. Sauveur, F. Roth, M. Sobel, and Y. Boucher, "Surgical treatment of a periradicular lesion on an invaginated maxillary lateral incisor (dens in dente)," *International Endodontic Journal*, vol. 30, no. 2, pp. 145–149, 1997.

[19] H. Kato, "Non-surgical endodontic treatment for dens Invaginatus type III using cone beam computed tomography and dental operating microscope: a case report," *The Bulletin of Tokyo Dental College*, vol. 54, no. 2, pp. 103–108, 2013.

[20] D. D. A. Decurcio, J. A. Silva, R. D. A. Decurcio, R. G. Silva, and J. D. Pécora, "Influence of cone beam computed tomography on dens invaginatus treatment planning," *Dental Press Endodontics*, vol. 1, no. 1, pp. 87–93, 2011.

[21] C. William Scarfe, M. D. Levin, D. Gane, and G. Allan Farman, "Use of cone beam computed tomography in endodontics," *International Journal of Dentistry*, vol. 2009, Article ID 634567, 20 pages, 2009.

[22] S. Patel, A. Dawood, T. Pitt Ford, and E. Whaites, "The potential applications of cone beam computed tomography in the management of endodontic problems," *International Endodontic Journal*, vol. 40, no. 10, pp. 818–830, 2007.

37

Implant-Prosthetic Rehabilitation in Bilateral Agenesis of Maxillary Lateral Incisors with a Mini Split Crest

M. M. Figliuzzi,[1] A. Giudice,[1] S. Pileggi,[1] D. Pacifico,[1] M. Marrelli,[2] M. Tatullo,[2,3] and L. Fortunato[1]

[1]*Department of Periodontics and Oral Sciences, "Magna Graecia" University, 88100 Catanzaro, Italy*
[2]*Biomedical Section, Stem Cells Unit, Tecnologica Research Institute, 88900 Crotone, Italy*
[3]*Biomedicine Unit, Calabrodental Clinic, Via E. Fermi, 88900 Crotone, Italy*

Correspondence should be addressed to M. M. Figliuzzi; michelefigliuzzi@libero.it

Academic Editor: Giovanna Orsini

The reported clinical case describes the surgical procedure of ridge augmentation by using a "split crest" technique with a partial thickness flap and a subsequent implant-prosthetic rehabilitation aimed at treating a bilateral agenesis of the upper lateral incisors. In such cases with vestibule-palatal and mesial-distal scarce bone thicknesses associated with the need of a proper functional and aesthetic rehabilitation, the split crest technique is particularly suitable. In the case we reported, because of the poor bone thicknesses, we performed a minimally invasive split crest which allowed a correct insertion of the fixtures. This technique allowed us to achieve an optimal functional and aesthetic rehabilitation; moreover, we obtained a good emergency profile, ensuring the vitality of the close teeth and ensuring a good primary stability and the following osseointegration of dental implants.

1. Introduction

Tooth agenesis is one of the most frequent dental anomalies. Dental agenesis is clinically apparent because of the lack of one or more teeth: for this reason such alteration is one of the best candidates for implant-prosthetic rehabilitation. The literature reports that lateral incisors are affected by agenesis in 2.2% of cases [1].

When the agenesis affects the lateral incisors, besides the functional issues, the greater inconvenience is represented by the aesthetic reasons.

The most suitable solution for these clinical conditions is, of course, an implant-prosthetic rehabilitation, but this surgical approach is not always feasible.

We well know that the critical condition for a good osseointegration is to have an amount of at least 2 mm of healthy bone around the implant [2, 3].

It is also necessary to ensure a good dental emergence profile, to obtain a correct prosthetic rehabilitation from both aesthetic and functional points of view [4].

These conditions are not always possible and the presence of an exiguous bone thickness forces the surgeon to change the axis of insertion of the implants, exposing the prosthetic restoration to the concrete risk of failure.

2. Split Crest

During the last years, several methods were offered to solve the problem of scant bone thickness in those cases requiring an implant-prosthetic rehabilitation.

Indeed, thanks to several GBR (Guided Bone Regeneration) strategies, the idea to place the implants where the bone amount is abundant turned into an inclined bone guided arrangement [5].

Many authors proposed the use of bone grafts taking samples from oral tissues (mandibular branch); others preferred instead the extra-oral tissues (e.g., iliac crest bone) [6]. These methods usually led to good results, but they are very aggressive and cannot exclude complications such as additional surgical procedures. To find an alternative solution for increasing the thickness of the crest, a split crest approach between vestibular and lingual cortical layers was proposed, in order to induce new bone formation in the inner area.

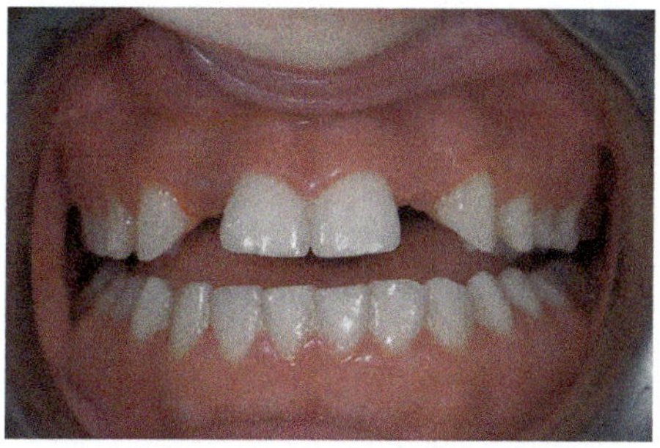

FIGURE 1: Preoperative clinical condition.

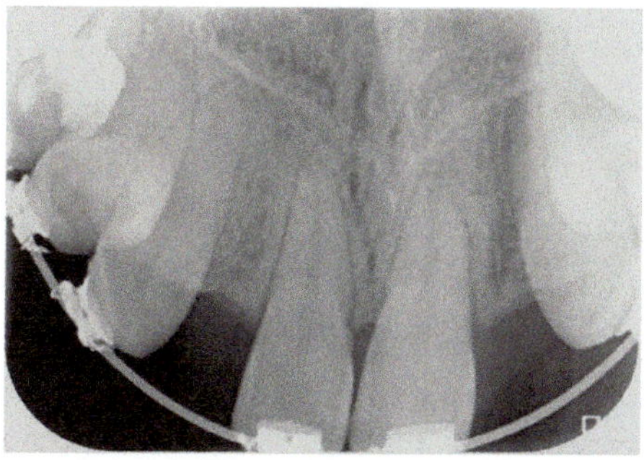

(a)

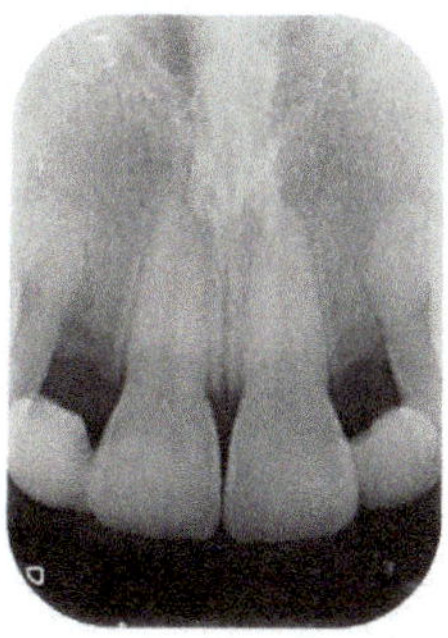

(b)

FIGURE 2: Radiographic preoperative condition.

The first original study by Osborn is dated 1985: it reported the green-stick fracture technique [7].

This technique was furtherly modified by Bruschi and Scipioni who used partial thickness flaps, obtaining great results [8, 9]. Since the partial flaps preserve periosteum integrity, it allows maintaining the vascular supply of the bone, thus enhancing its repairing capacities. Also hybrid methods were proposed: they coupled the advantages of partial flap approach to synthetic biomaterials use, to extend the high regenerating capacities of the periosteum [10].

3. Clinical Case

The patient here reported was 26 y/o: she showed a bilateral agenesis of the upper lateral incisors (Figure 1).

The agenesis of teeth 1.2 and 2.2 caused a mesial shifting of the teeth close to the space left empty by the missing elements.

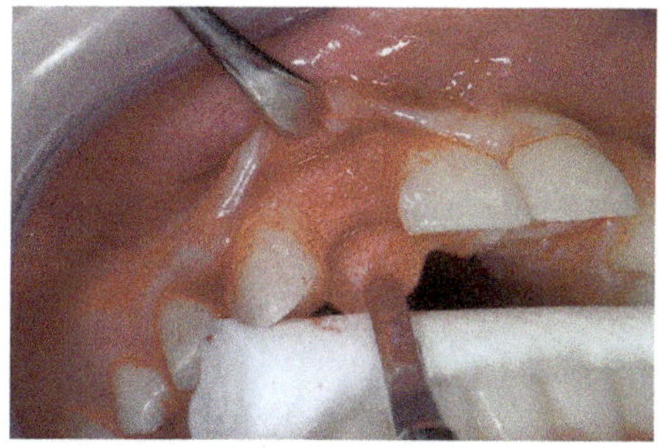

FIGURE 3: Flap incision in site to the left.

Consequently, an orthodontic treatment was performed to gain the space required to allow the insertion of dental implants. After the orthodontic treatment, a dental "Maryland" bridge was placed as a temporary rehabilitation, in order to ensure the stability of the occlusion, the proper function, and acceptable esthetics [11].

The newly obtained spaces were carefully evaluated to properly plan the implantology in such sites.

The bone showed a thin thickness both in vestibular-palatal and mesial-distal directions.

After oral and extra-oral clinical inspections and radiography examinations, the bone thickness was about 3 mm in crest in vestibule-lingual direction (Figures 2(a) and 2(b)).

The lacking bone depths impeded the right allocation of the implants and thus affected the prognosis.

Therefore, it was decided to proceed with a split crest surgical technique, to gain the necessary space for the implants insertion. For both the sites the procedure was performed as follows:

(i) local anesthesia,

(ii) incision of the partial thickness flap,

(iii) crestal osteotomy with Beaver 64 blade,

(iv) distraction of vestibular cortical plate,

(v) preparation of the implant site with the proper burs,

(vi) parallelism verification,

(vii) implant insertion,

(viii) suture of the flap with underlying periosteum anchorage.

4. Flap Incision

After having anesthetized the surgical site, a partial thickness trapezoidal flap was made through the blade Beaver 64. The incision was performed at the bone crest, with mesial and distal releasing cuttings (Figures 3 and 4).

The cuts were sharp and divergent to ensure an adequate blood supply and therefore an optimal healing.

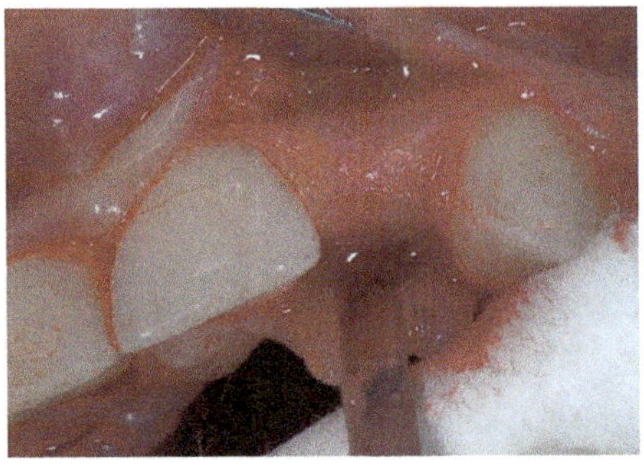

FIGURE 4: Flap incision in site to the right.

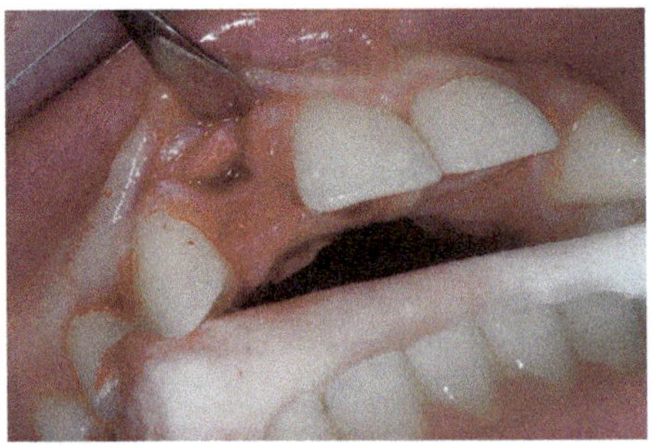

FIGURE 5: Crestal osteotomy and bone window creation in site to the left.

5. Crestal Osteotomy and Bone Window Creation

The Beaver 64 blade was positioned at the top of the crest and was sunk for 4 mm of the cortical bone by a surgical mallet, so as to make a proper bony fracture.

In the same way two other fractures involving mesial-distal release were realized, to mobilize the bone fragment and to shape an operculum. The operculum must have smaller dimensions than the flap to ensure an optimal healing and to avoid dehiscence and infections.

6. Osteodistraction

Using the Bard Parker and then a straight dental elevator, the last bone fragment was displaced (Figures 5 and 6). The surgeons must be careful during this step not to interfere with the apical anchorage of the bone fragment; taking into account this suggestion, the partial thickness flap holds the periosteum on the bone fragment.

7. Site Preparation and Implant Insertion

After the dislocation of the bone fragment, we proceeded to the insertion of a series of burs to prepare the implant site.

This operation was performed paying great attention to avoid the risk of injury to the closest dental roots.

Soon after the insertion of the first guiding bur, an X-ray examination verified the correct inclination and position of

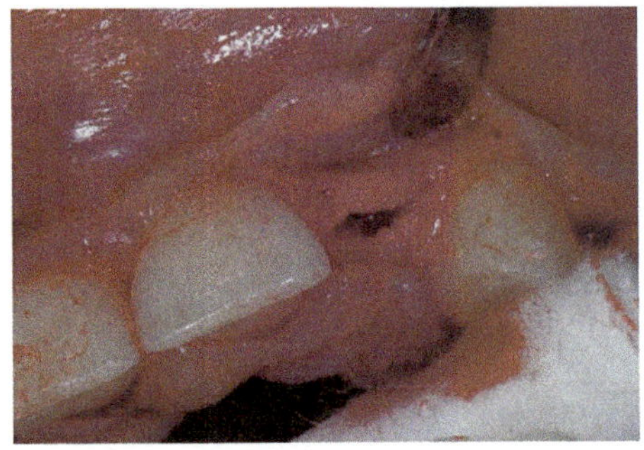

FIGURE 6: Crestal osteotomy and bone window creation in site to the right.

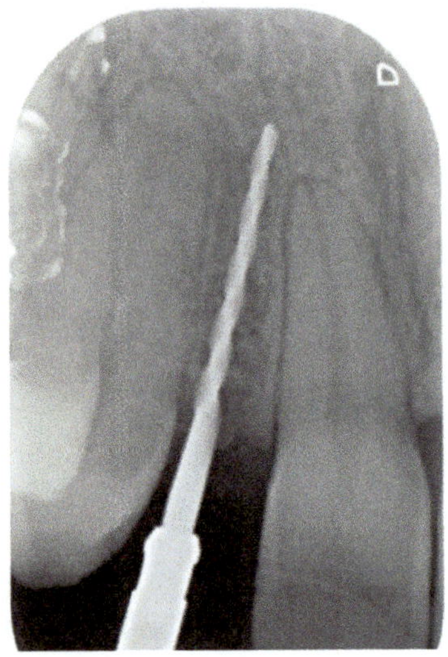

FIGURE 7: Radiographic examination of the correct inclination in site to the left.

the bur inside the bone (Figures 7, 8, and 9). After having inserted the dental implant (Figures 10 and 11) with size of 3.4 × 10.0 mm (Intra-Lock® International, Boca Raton, USA), we performed testing W-rays (Figures 12 and 13). The bone operculum was finally repositioned in the right position and the flap was properly closed with single stitches linking the periosteum.

Three months later, the abutments and the crowns were added (Figures 14(a), 14(b), and 15). The next check was done one year after the prosthesization (Figures 16 and 17).

8. Discussion

The choice of the surgical approach detailed above was due to functional and especially esthetic needs concerning the young age of the patient.

The orthodontic treatment has led to obtaining the necessary space where the dental implants will be placed; later an orthodontic appliance of Maryland type has been placed, to ensure acceptable stability, function, and aesthetics, as clearly demonstrated in the scientific literature [11]. Reaching

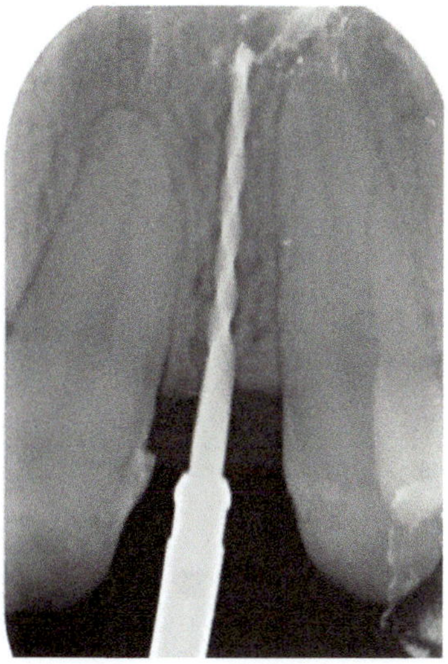

FIGURE 8: Radiographic examination of the correct inclination in site to the right.

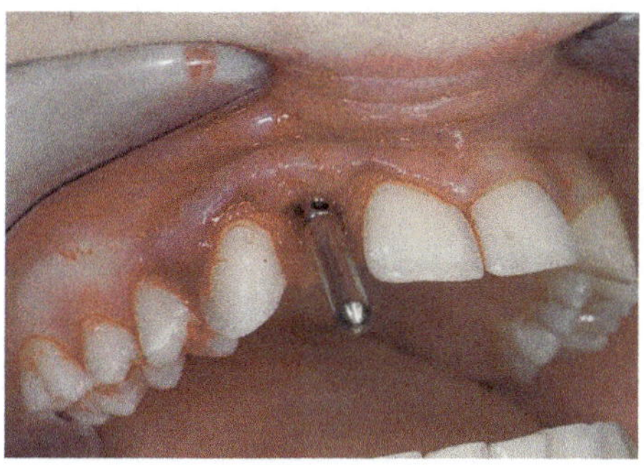

FIGURE 9: Clinical examination of the correct inclination.

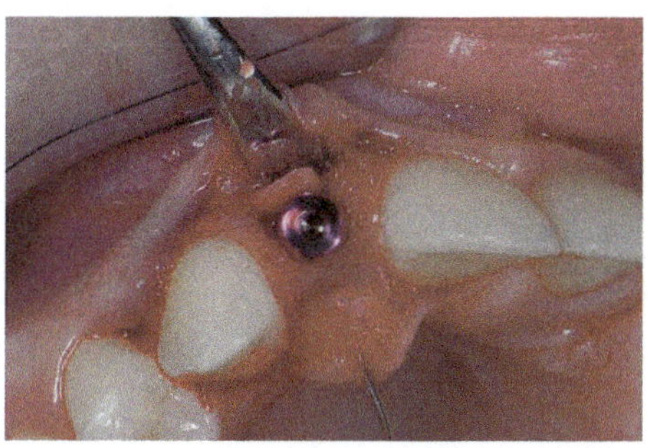

FIGURE 10: Implant placement in site to the left.

a suitable age, the treatment changed to an implant-prosthetics one, even with the difficulties represented by the lacking of vestibular-palatal bone depth and by the small mesial-distal space.

We know indeed that the distance between the implant and the center of the adjacent teeth should be about 7-8 mm.

A proper position towards the mesial-distal way enables the formation of an adequate contact-point.

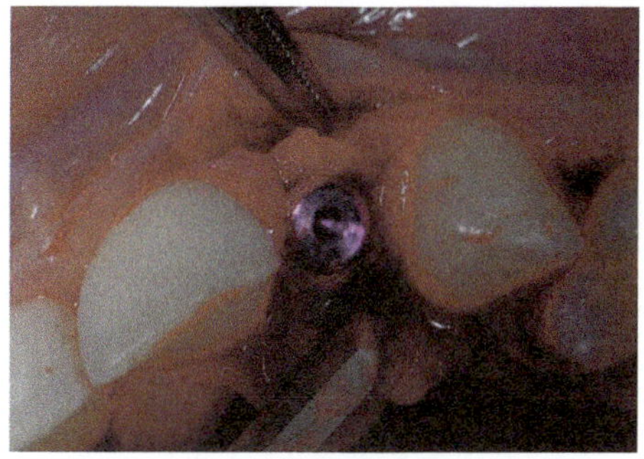

FIGURE 11: Implant placement in site to the right.

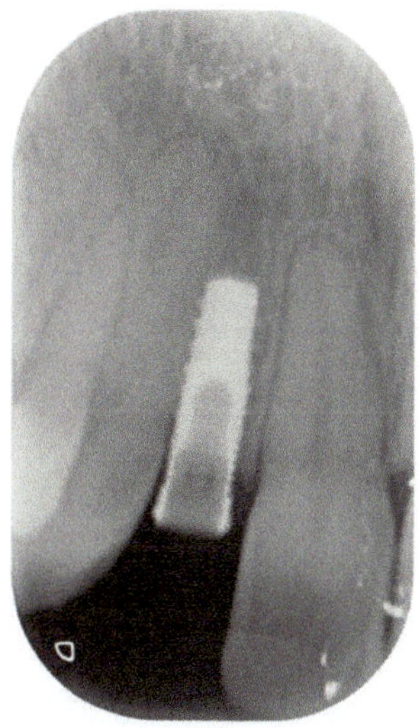

FIGURE 12: Radiographic control after implant placement in site to the left.

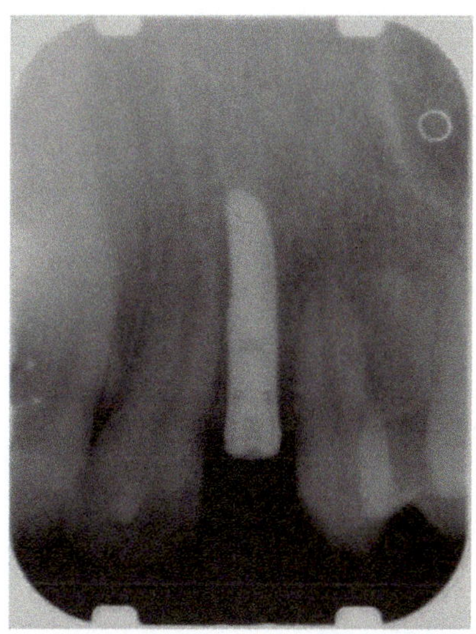

FIGURE 13: Radiographic control after implant placement in site to the right.

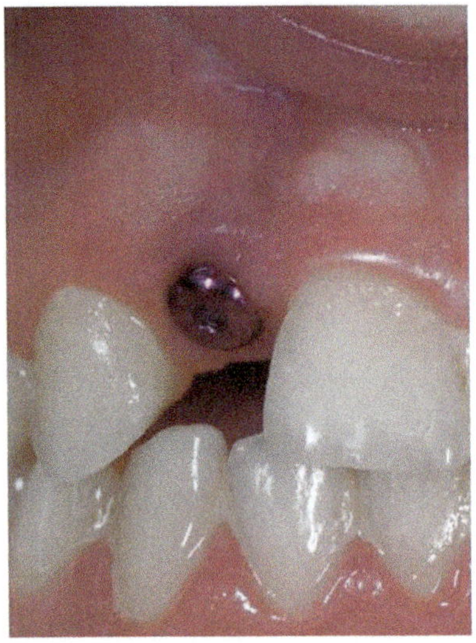

(a)

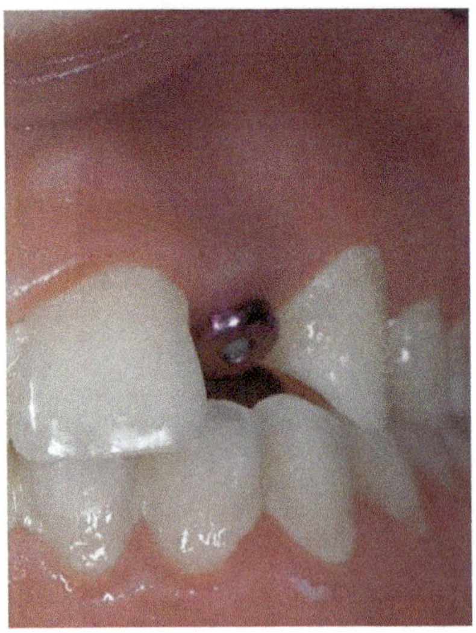

(b)

Figure 14: Clinical control after three months.

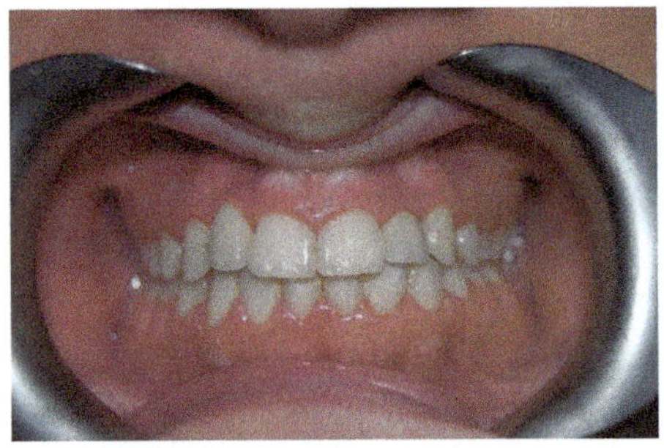

Figure 15: Implant prosthesization.

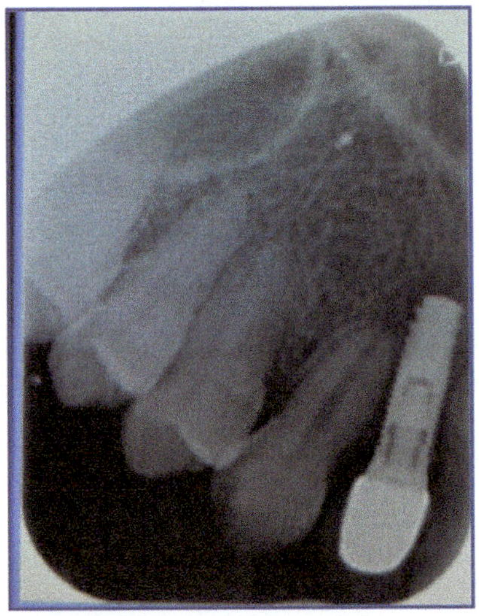

Figure 16: Radiographic control after one year in site to the left.

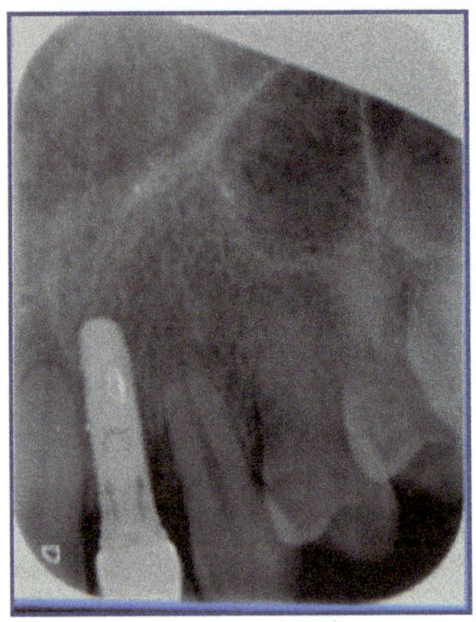

Figure 17: Radiographic control after one year in site to the right.

The implant should be placed along the oral-lingual direction 1 mm behind the buccal bone in order to obtain a correct distribution of the interdental soft tissues.

The use of this procedure has been allowed to expand not only the dimension of the crest along vestibular-palatal direction but also an increased control on the implant insertion, improving the prognosis.

Thanks to the split crest approach we also obtained an emergence profile resulting as appropriate to the high esthetic requirements, with a good prosthetic rehabilitation.

Competing Interests

The authors declare that they have no competing interests.

Authors' Contributions

M. Tatullo and L. Fortunato equally contributed to this paper.

References

[1] A. L. Symons, F. Stritzel, and J. Stamation, "Anomalies associated with hypodontia of the permanent lateral incisor and second premolar," *The Journal of Clinical Pediatric Dentistry*, vol. 17, no. 2, pp. 109–111, 1993.

[2] P. I. Brånemark, R. Adell, U. Breine, B. O. Hansson, J. Lindström, and A. Ohlsson, "Intra-osseous anchorage of dental prostheses: I. Experimental studies," *Scandinavian Journal of Plastic and Reconstructive Surgery*, vol. 3, no. 2, pp. 81–100, 1969.

[3] P. I. Brånemark, B. O. Hansson, R. Adell et al., "Osseointegrated implants in the treatment of the edentulous jaw. Experience from a 10-year period," *Scandinavian Journal of Plastic and Reconstructive Surgery, Supplementum*, vol. 16, pp. 1–132, 1977.

[4] P. S. Wohrle, "La sinergia tra forma e diametro: l'arte e la scienzaimplantolofia migliorata con il sistema implantare replace," *Quintessenza Int*, vol. 5-6, pp. 151–157, 1998.

[5] M. B. Hürzeler, C. R. Quiñones, and P. Schüpbach, "Guided bone regeneration around dental implants in the atrophic alveolar ridge using a bioresorbable barrier," *Clinical Oral Implants Research*, vol. 8, no. 4, pp. 323–331, 1997.

[6] C. M. Misch, "Comparison of intraoral donor sites for onlay grafting prior to implant placement," *International Journal of Oral and Maxillofacial Implants*, vol. 12, no. 6, pp. 767–776, 1997.

[7] J. F. Osborn, "Die alveolar-extensionplastic," *Quintessenza Int*, vol. 36, pp. 239–246, 1985.

[8] G. B. Bruschi and A. Scipioni, "Alveolar augmentation: new application for implants," in *Osseo-Integrated Implants*, G. Heimke, Ed., vol. 2, chapter 2, pp. 35–61, CRC Press, Boca Raton, Fla, USA, 1990.

[9] G. B. Bruschi, A. Scipioni, G. Calesini, and E. Bruschi, "Localized management of sinus floor with simultaneous implant placement. A clinical report," *International Journal of Oral and Maxillofacial Implants*, vol. 13, no. 2, pp. 219–226, 1998.

[10] C. Mg, M. Figliuzzi, and M. Giudice, "Pre-implanted atropi ridge augmentation: osseo-periosteum distraction and Biomaterial grafting. Tyhe Periosteum as a natural membrane: our experience," *Annali di Stomatologia*, vol. 3, pp. 119–124, 2004.

[11] O. El-Mowafy and M. H. M. Rubo, "Resin-bonded fixed partial dentures—a literature review with presentation of a novel approach," *International Journal of Prosthodontics*, vol. 13, no. 6, pp. 460–467, 2000.

Adalimumab: Another Medication Related to Osteonecrosis of the Jaws?

Andrea Cassoni, Umberto Romeo, Valentina Terenzi, Marco Della Monaca, Oriana Rajabtork Zadeh, Ingrid Raponi, Maria Teresa Fadda, Antonella Polimeni, and Valentino Valentini

Odontostomatological Science and Maxillo facial Surgery Department, "Sapienza" University of Rome, 00161 Rome, Italy

Correspondence should be addressed to Valentina Terenzi; v.terenzi@libero.it

Academic Editor: Luis M. J. Gutierrez

Objective. The acronym MRONJ has been created in order to identify "Medication-Related Osteonecrosis of the Jaw," observed after the use of Bisphosphonates, RANK ligand inhibitor, and antiangiogenic medications. Only a case of osteonecrosis of the jaw in a Chron's disease patient following a course of Bisphosphonate and Adalimumab therapy has been recently described, so that it has been supposed that also this medication could promote manifestation of osteonecrosis. *Clinical Case.* On August, 2014, a 63-year-old female with a history of idiopathic arthritis treated with medical treatment with Adalimumab from 2010 to 2013 presented referring pain in the right mandible. *Results.* This patient presented with nonexposed osteonecrosis of the jaw after placement, on September, 2010, of four titanium fixtures in the mandible. *Conclusions.* The authors suggest that the biologic therapy with an anti-TNF-α antibody might promote the manifestation of osteonecrosis and compromise oral healing capacity of the bone.

1. Introduction

Osteonecrosis of the jaw related to Bisphosphonate (BRONJ) and, recently, Denosumab related osteonecrosis of the jaws (DRONJ) and other medicaments such as antiangiogenic agents (MRONJ) has been described [1–3]. Adalimumab (Humira®, Human Monoclonal Antibody in Rheumatoid Arthritis) is a human monoclonal TNF-α antibody used to threat rheumatoid arthritis, juvenile idiopathic arthritis, psoriatic arthritis, ankylosing spondylitis, plaque psoriasis, and Chron's disease in case of other drugs' failure. Adalimumab binds to tumor necrosis factor-alpha (TNF-α). TNF-α normally binds to TNF-α receptors, which leads to the inflammatory response of autoimmune diseases. By binding to TNF-α, Adalimumab reduces this inflammatory response. Common side effects include redness, itching, pain, or swelling at the injection site (it is administered by subcutaneous injection), and because TNF-α is part of the immune system that protects the body from infection, treatment with Adalimumab may increase the risk of infections such as tuberculosis, while rarely worsening or initiation of congestive heart failure or of a multiple sclerosis/neurological disease, a lupus-like syndrome, a promotion of lymphoma, and pancytopenia have been reported [4]. Just one case of osteonecrosis of the jaw in a Crohn's disease patient following a course of Bisphosphonate and Adalimumab therapy has been recently described, so that it has been supposed that this medication could promote manifestation of osteonecrosis [5]; to the best of our knowledge, we describe the first case of osteonecrosis of the jaws that could be consequent to the use of Adalimumab to treat idiopathic arthritis in a woman.

2. Case Report

A 63-year-old female presented to our center on August 2014 referring pain in the right mandible. No history of smoking or alcohol abuse was referred. Comorbidities include obesity and idiopathic arthritis treated with medical treatment with Salazopyrin on 2009 and with Adalimumab (1 injection every two weeks) from 2010 to 2013: during this period, improvement of symptoms has been referred by the patient. Her physician also proposed a treatment with glucocorticoids, but she refused because of side effects. She referred 4.7 (caries) and 4.8 (impacted tooth) extraction on 2008, before starting

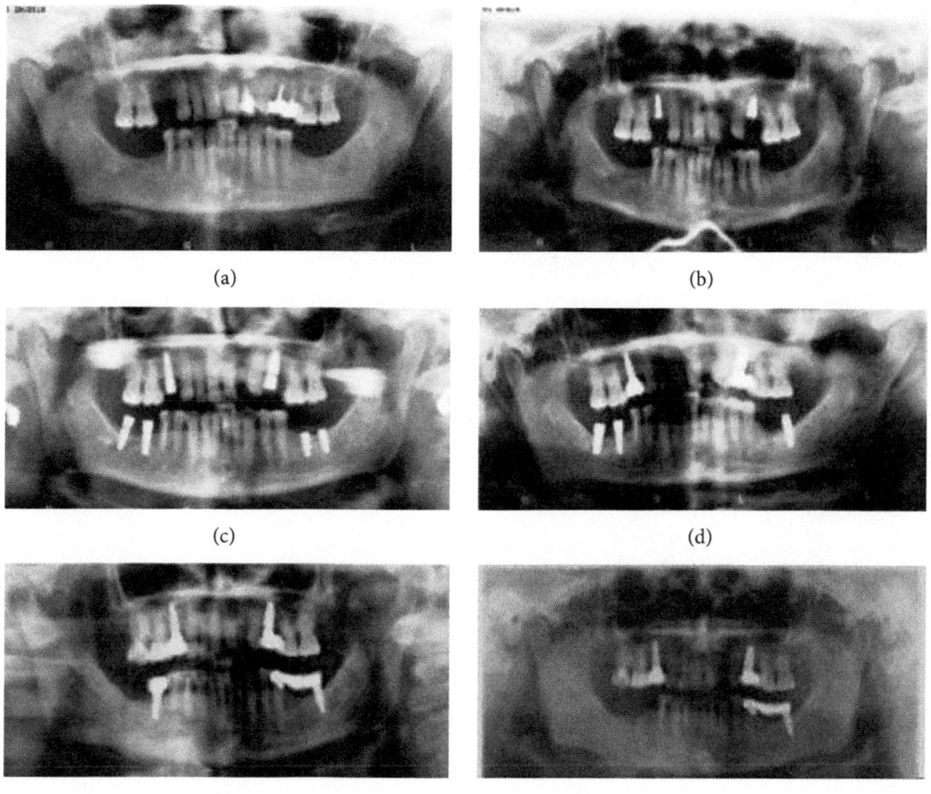

(a) (b) (c) (d) (e) (f)

Figure 1: Orthopantomography (OPT) performed on 2009 (a), on May, 2010 (b), on September, 2010 (c), on May, 2011 (d), on August, 2011 (e), and on August, 2014 (f). The last one revealed osteosclerosis, osteolysis, and subperiosteal bone deposition and persistence of extraction socket.

any treatment for idiopathic arthritis. An orthopantomography (OPT) performed on 2009, before starting treatment with Humira, did not show bone alterations (Figure 1(a)). On May, 2010, two titanium fixtures were positioned in the maxilla (1.5 and 2.5) (Figure 1(b)) and, on September-October, 2010, four titanium fixtures were put in the mandible by her dentist (3.6, 3.7, 4.6, and 4.7) (Figure 1(c)). On June, 2011, the one positioned in the region of 4.7 was lost, and it was decided to reposition it about 1 month later. On May, 2011, the fixture positioned in the region of 3.6 was lost too (Figure 1(d)), and, moreover, one month later, after appearance of pain in the right mandible, the fixture in the region of 4.7 was removed (Figure 1(e)). A CT scan was performed (Figure 2); because of difficult healing, patient underwent curettage medications with local antibiotics (Rifocin) for about 2-3 months. Patient referred persistence of pain, partially resolved after systemic antibiotic therapy (amoxicillin + clavulanic acid 1 gr twice a day) (Figure 1(e)). A static whole body bone scintigraphy revealed an intensive trace uptake at the right mandible (Figure 3). Nevertheless, no remission of pain was referred and patient underwent systemic therapy with paracetamol and eventually ketorolac in order to control it. Occasionally systemic antibiotic therapy was administered in order to control swelling of the right mandible, and partial resolution of pain has been described. On May, 2014, fixture removal (the one positioned in the site of 4.6) was performed and temporary remission of pain was referred; on July, 2014, due to the persistence of pain, extraction of 4.5 was performed. Orthopantomography revealed osteosclerosis, osteolysis, and subperiosteal bone deposition and persistence of extraction socket (Figure 1(f)). Nevertheless, the patient came to our attention on August 2014 referring recurrence of pain; on the basis of clinical history (Figure 4) and radiological imaging, such as CT scan showing sequestrum, diagnosis of MRONJ with nonexposed necrotic bone was suspected (Figure 5). We considered the patient to be at Stage 0 (nonexposed bone variant) because she presented with no clinical evidence of necrotic bone but presented with nonspecific symptoms and clinical and radiographic findings [1] (odontalgia not explained by an odontogenic cause and aching bone pain in the body of the mandible, loosening of teeth not explained by chronic periodontal disease, alveolar bone loss or resorption not attributable to chronic periodontal disease, changes to trabecular pattern dense woven bone, and persistence of unremodeled bone in extraction sockets and regions of osteosclerosis involving the alveolar bone and/or the surrounding basilar bone) (Figure 6).

The patient reported good pain control using medical therapy consisting in FANS and antibiotics up to March, 2015.

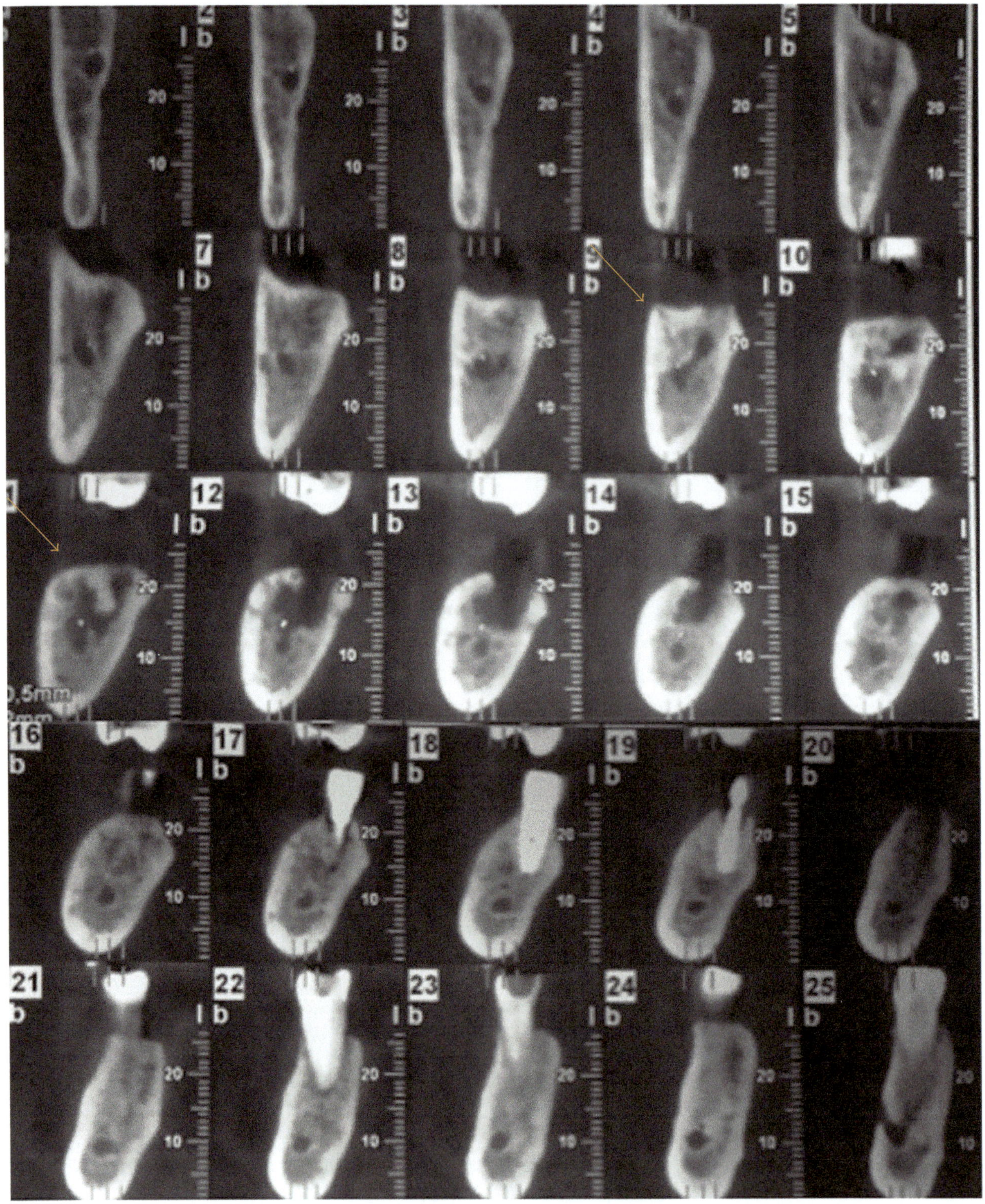

Figure 2: CT Dentascan scan performed on July, 2011, showing sequestrum.

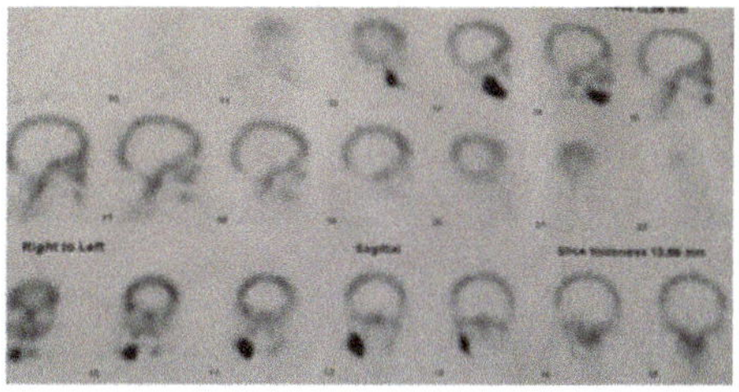

FIGURE 3: Static whole body bone scintigraphy performed on October, 2013, revealed an intensive trace uptake at the right mandible.

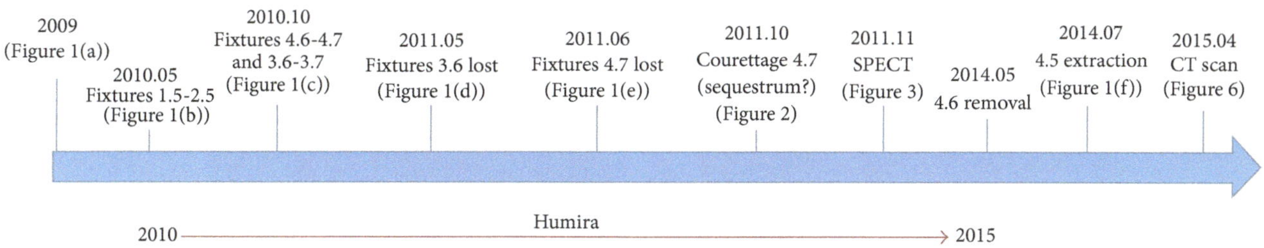

FIGURE 4: Schematic view of disease progression.

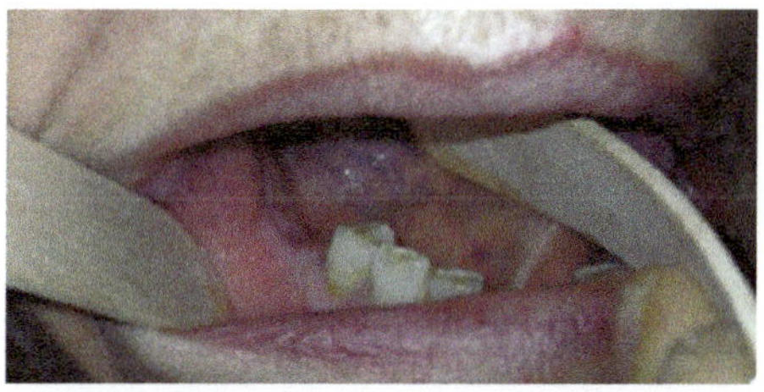

FIGURE 5: Postoperative control in 2015 showing the healing of the mucosa after extraction of tooth 4.5 and curettage of the bone.

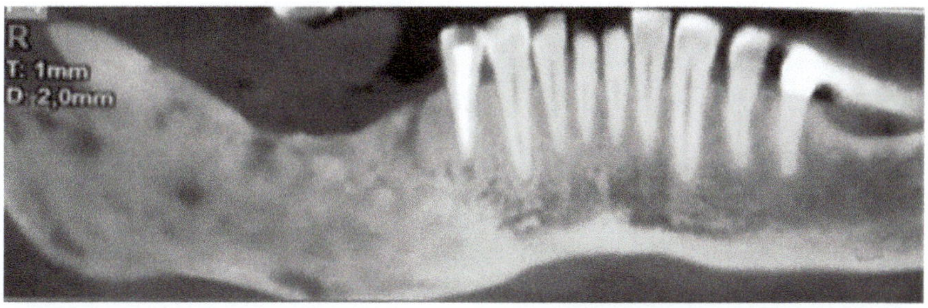

(a)

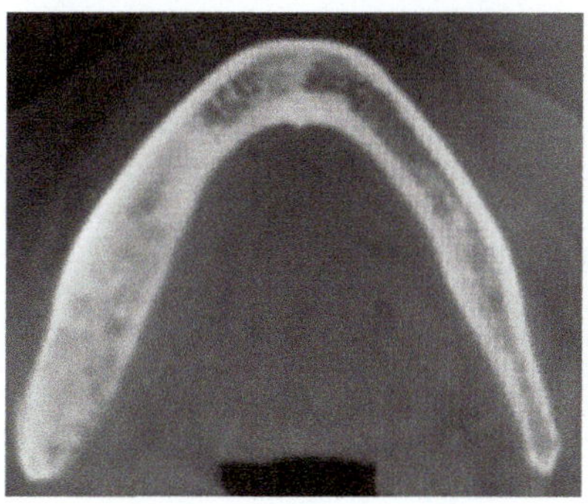

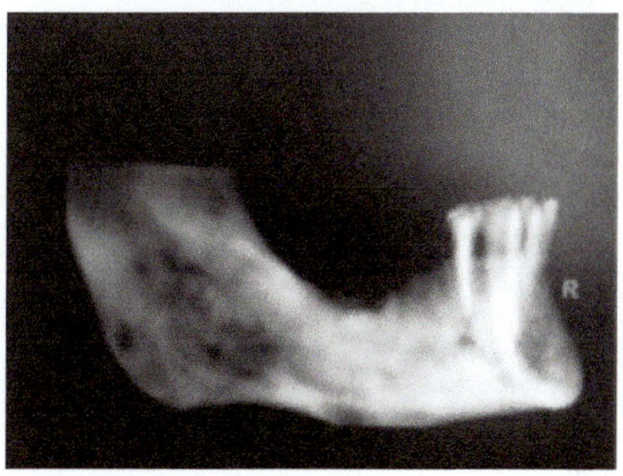

(b) (c)

FIGURE 6: CT scan performed on April, 2015. (a) Panorex view showing sequestrum, (b) axial view, and (c) 3D reconstruction.

3. Discussion

Osteonecrosis of the jaw can be usually observed as an adverse reaction to some medications or to radiotherapy: histologically, it appears similar to osteomyelitis, and it is not clear whether infection is the cause or consequence of bone exposure [6–8]. The term MRONJ has been created in order to identify "Medication-Related Osteonecrosis of the Jaw," observed after the use of antiresorptive (Denosumab) and antiangiogenic therapies, other than Bisphosphonates [1]. In particular, in the last 2014 AAOMS Position Paper [1], it has been assessed that diagnosis of MRONJ can be done if the following are present:

(i) Current or previous treatment with antiresorptive or antiangiogenic agents.

(ii) Exposed bone or bone that can be probed through an intraoral or extraoral fistula(e) in the maxillofacial region that has persisted for longer than 8 weeks.

(iii) No history of radiation therapy to the jaws or obvious metastatic disease of the jaws.

Nevertheless, some cases of medication-related ONJ without bone exposure have been described [9]. It is largely reported that BRONJ is caused by apoptosis of osteoclasts, disturbance of osteoclast progenitor cell differentiation and enzyme activity, antineovascularization, and destruction of bone microstructure caused by bone deposition [9, 10]. DRONJ is related to inhibition of the receptor activator of nuclear factor kappa-B ligand (RANKL), resulting in osteoclast function inhibition. Differently from Bisphosphonate, the return of bone turnover to normal can be evidenced about six months after drug injection [2]. The use of glucocorticoids has been demonstrated to lead to osteoblast inhibition and to bone resorption [11]. Also, antiangiogenic medications, such as Bevacizumab and Rituximab, have been found to be implicated in the pathogenesis of ONJ [1, 12, 13].

TNF inhibitors, such as Adalimumab, seem to be able to arrest systemic bone loss assessed by bone mineral density and bone turnover markers in rheumatoid arthritis; nevertheless, evidences of the effect of anti-TNF treatment in preventing fractures are still scarce [14].

It has been described that TNF-α has an important effect on systemic bone loss in rheumatoid arthritis, since it enhances osteoclasts activity, differentiation and activation, and osteoblasts production and proliferation resulting in an inhibition on bone turnover markers demonstrated by some studies [14].

Nevertheless, no cases related to the use of other drugs have been described, except one in which the use of Adalimumab has been hypothesized to improve necrosis caused by Bisphosphonates. It has been supposed that anti-TNF-α treatment could cause an inhibition of bone turnover mediated by a reduction of RANKL which could already be shown in patients with rheumatoid arthritis and anti-TNF-α therapy [5]. Another hypothesis is the fact that the induced apoptosis of activated human monocytes can lead to worsening of bone repair after jaw necrosis. Nevertheless, since one of the side effects described after Adalimumab treatment are infectious complications due to immunosuppression, it can be proposed that osteonecrotic lesions of the jaws can "occur because of spreading ongoing infections" [5, 15].

Local factors related to ONJ are dentoalveolar surgery, denture use, and preexisting inflammatory dental disease [1]. In case of nonexposed Bisphosphonate-related osteonecrosis and asymptomatic patients (no clinical evidence of infection and radiographic findings can be present), only follow-up is advocated [10]; in our case, only pain was referred, and FANS associated with systemic antibiotics were administered in order to control it. A chronic infection was also present, and patient referred multiple local medications to gain healing after fixture removal. Radiological signs include osteosclerosis, cortical disruption, osteolysis, subperiosteal bone deposition, thickening of lamina dura, and widening of periodontal ligament; in addiction, surface irregularity and persistent sockets strictly correlate with ONJ [16, 17]. Osteosclerosis is due to mineralization in the absence of balanced bone resorption, and the persistence of extraction sockets results from marked inhibition of remodeling following removal of the tooth [17]. In our case report, CT scan showed signs of bone sequestrum and analyzing previous OPT signs of osteosclerosis and subperiosteal bone deposition were present. Delayed healing after fixture removal and persistence of pain, associated with these radiological findings and bone scintigraphy, showed positive tracer led us to suspect diagnosis of MRONJ related to Adalimumab [18]. Nevertheless, further case reports are required in order to confirm the hypothesis but this clinical case suggests that a dental exam is indicated before prescription of biological drugs like Adalimumab. In those patients, periodic dental checkup can be recommended too.

Competing Interests

The authors declare that they have no competing interests.

References

[1] S. L. Ruggiero, T. B. Dodson, J. Fantasia et al., "American Association of Oral and Maxillofacial Surgeons position paper on medication-related osteonecrosis of the jaw—2014 update," *Journal of Oral and Maxillofacial Surgery*, vol. 72, no. 10, pp. 1938–1956, 2014.

[2] W.-X. Qi, L.-N. Tang, A.-N. He, Y. Yao, and Z. Shen, "Risk of osteonecrosis of the jaw in cancer patients receiving denosumab: a meta-analysis of seven randomized controlled trials," *International Journal of Clinical Oncology*, vol. 19, no. 2, pp. 403–410, 2014.

[3] S. Kühl, C. Walter, S. Acham, R. Pfeffer, and J. T. Lambrecht, "Bisphosphonate-related osteonecrosis of the jaws—a review," *Oral Oncology*, vol. 48, no. 10, pp. 938–947, 2012.

[4] N. Scheinfeld, "Adalimumab: a review of side effects," *Expert Opinion on Drug Safety*, vol. 4, no. 4, pp. 637–641, 2005.

[5] R. H. M. Preidl, T. Ebker, M. Raithel, F. Wehrhan, F. W. Neukam, and P. Stockmann, "Osteonecrosis of the jaw in a Crohn's disease patient following a course of Bisphosphonate and Adalimumab therapy: a case report," *BMC Gastroenterology*, vol. 14, no. 1, article 6, 2014.

[6] D. Carmagnola, E. Canciani, D. Sozzi, F. Biglioli, L. Moneghini, and C. Dellavia, "Histological findings on jaw osteonecrosis associated with bisphosphonates (BONJ) or with radiotherapy (ORN) in humans," *Acta Odontologica Scandinavica*, vol. 71, no. 6, pp. 1410–1417, 2013.

[7] E. Merigo, M. Manfredi, M. Meleti et al., "Bone necrosis of the jaws associated with bisphosphonate treatment: a report of twenty-nine cases," *Acta Biomedica de l'Ateneo Parmense*, vol. 77, no. 2, pp. 109–127, 2006.

[8] M. Capocci, U. Romeo, F. Cocco, I. Bignozzi, S. Annibali, and L. Ottolenghi, "The 'CROMa' project: a care pathway for clinical management of patients with bisphosphonate exposure," *International Journal of Dentistry*, vol. 2014, Article ID 719478, 8 pages, 2014.

[9] S. Patel, S. Choyee, J. Uyanne et al., "Non-exposed bisphosphonate-related osteonecrosis of the jaw: a critical assessment of current definition, staging, and treatment guidelines," *Oral Diseases*, vol. 18, no. 7, pp. 625–632, 2012.

[10] K. Niibe, T. Ouchi, R. Iwasaki, T. Nakagawa, and N. Horie, "Osteonecrosis of the jaw in patients with dental prostheses being treated with bisphosphonates or denosumab," *Journal of Prosthodontic Research*, vol. 59, no. 1, pp. 3–5, 2015.

[11] E. Lespessailles, "Bisphosphonates and glucocorticoid-induced osteoporosis: efficacy and tolerability," *Joint Bone Spine*, vol. 80, no. 3, pp. 258–264, 2013.

[12] D. Pakosch, D. Papadimas, J. Munding, D. Kawa, and M. S. Kriwalsky, "Osteonecrosis of the mandible due to anti-angiogenic agent, bevacizumab," *Oral and Maxillofacial Surgery*, vol. 17, no. 4, pp. 303–306, 2013.

[13] A. Allegra, G. Oteri, A. Alonci et al., "Association of osteonecrosis of the jaws and POEMS syndrome in a patient assuming rituximab," *Journal of Cranio-Maxillofacial Surgery*, vol. 42, no. 4, pp. 279–282, 2014.

[14] M. Manara and L. Sinigaglia, "Bone and TNF in rheumatoid arthritis: clinical implications," *RMD Open*, vol. 1, Article ID e000065, 2015.

[15] I. C. Lawrance, G. L. Radford-Smith, P. A. Bampton et al., "Serious infections in patients with inflammatory bowel disease receiving anti-tumor-necrosis-factor-alpha therapy: an Australian and New Zealand experience," *Journal of Gastroenterology and Hepatology*, vol. 25, no. 11, pp. 1732–1738, 2010.

[16] M. Hutchinson, F. O'Ryan, V. Chavez et al., "Radiographic findings in bisphosphonate-treated patients with stage 0 disease in the absence of bone exposure," *Journal of Oral and Maxillofacial Surgery*, vol. 68, no. 9, pp. 2232–2240, 2010.

[17] N. Treister, N. Sheehy, E. H. Bae, B. Friedland, M. Lerman, and S. Woo, "Dental panoramic radiographic evaluation in bisphosphonate-associated osteonecrosis of the jaws," *Oral Diseases*, vol. 15, no. 1, pp. 88–92, 2009.

[18] F. S. O'Ryan, S. Khoury, W. Liao et al., "Intravenous bisphosphonate-related osteonecrosis of the jaw: bone scintigraphy as an early indicator," *Journal of Oral and Maxillofacial Surgery*, vol. 67, no. 7, pp. 1363–1372, 2009.

Mucoepidermoid Carcinoma in a Minor Salivary Gland in a Child

Fatih Sengul,[1] Sera Simsek,[1] and Binali Cakur[2]

[1] *Department of Pedodontics, Faculty of Dentistry, Ataturk University, 25240 Erzurum, Turkey*
[2] *Department of Oral, Dental And Maxillofacial Radiology, Faculty of Dentistry, Ataturk University, 25240 Erzurum, Turkey*

Correspondence should be addressed to Fatih Sengul; fatihs@gmail.com

Academic Editors: D. W. Boston, A. C. B. Delbem, A. Kasaj, T. Lombardi, and P. Lopez Jornet

Mucoepidermoid carcinoma (MEC), one of the most common salivary gland malignancies, is rare in children. MEC mainly occurs in the parotid gland, along with minor glands being the second common site, particularly in palate. Clinical, histological, and radiological findings of palatal MEC in a 12-year-old girl are presented with three-year follow-up. Pathologic lesions must be considered in differential diagnoses of intraoral asymptomatic lesions, and their detailed inspection should be taken into consideration.

1. Introduction

Mucoepidermoid carcinoma (MEC) is one of the most common salivary gland malignancies. As its name implies, MEC is composed of a mixture of cells, including mucus-producing, epidermoid or squamous, and intermediate types [1]. When MEC appears as asymptomatic swellings in minor salivary glands, being the second most common site of occurrence after the parotid gland, it can be located on palate, in retromolar area, floor of mouth, buccal mucosa, lips, and tongue [2–5].

Few series or case reports describing salivary gland tumors in the pediatric population have been published [6–8]. This report describes an additional case of a low-grade MEC affecting the palate of a 12-year-old girl.

2. Case Report

A 12-year-old girl patient visited the Department of Pediatric Dentistry, Ataturk University, Erzurum, Turkey, complaining of the pain in maxillar left central incisor (no. 11) and mandibular left lateral incisor (no. 22). She had a history of untreated Ellis II trauma and grade two mobility in these teeth for two years. Also, clinical examination revealed enlargement of the soft tissue in left posterior hard palate, with 8 mm diameter (Figure 1). During physical examination she had a firm, painless, and nontender mass, near the teeth 24 and 27, overlying the palate with normal color of mucosa, and the median palatal raphe was clearly identified. She denied any symptoms attributed to the mass. Adjacent teeth had no mobility or displacement, and electrical pulp test results were positive. In panoramic and periapical radiographs the alveolar bone had no resorption and the floor of the maxillary sinus appeared intact. Axial plain CT examination showed a moderately enhancing soft-tissue density lesion extending posteriorly and inferiorly destroying the hard palate and the alveolar process (Figure 2). No other abnormalities, including palpable submandibular and cervical lymph nodes, were found. Since fine needle aspiration yielded no fluid, a local oral surgeon performed an open biopsy and noticed a sinus opening near the foramen palatinum majus. Microscopic analysis revealed a low-grade mucoepidermoid carcinoma (Figure 3). By the end of the third year CT and oral examination showed no problem.

3. Discussion

Epithelial salivary gland neoplasms are rare both in adults and children, accounting for less than 3% of all head and neck tumors. 5% of these tumors occur in patients younger than 18 years old with girls mostly affected, while its occurrence in newborns is exceedingly rare [6, 9–11]. Malignancy seen in

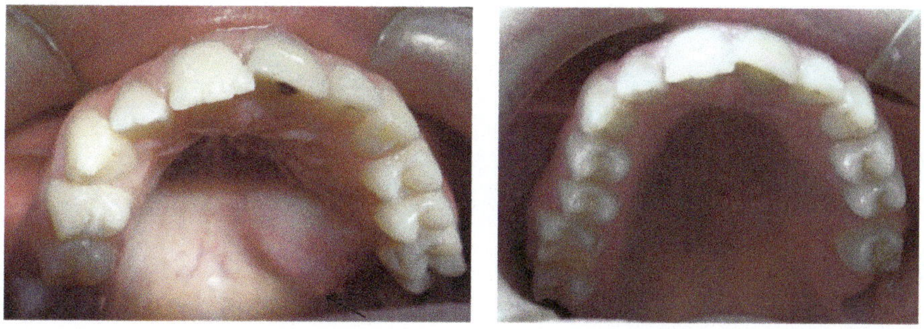

(a) (b)

FIGURE 1: (a) Preoperative intraoral image of a mucoepidermoid carcinoma of the left posterior hard palate with 8 mm diameter and fistula opening (black arrow). (b) Postoperative (3 years) image of a reconstructed palate.

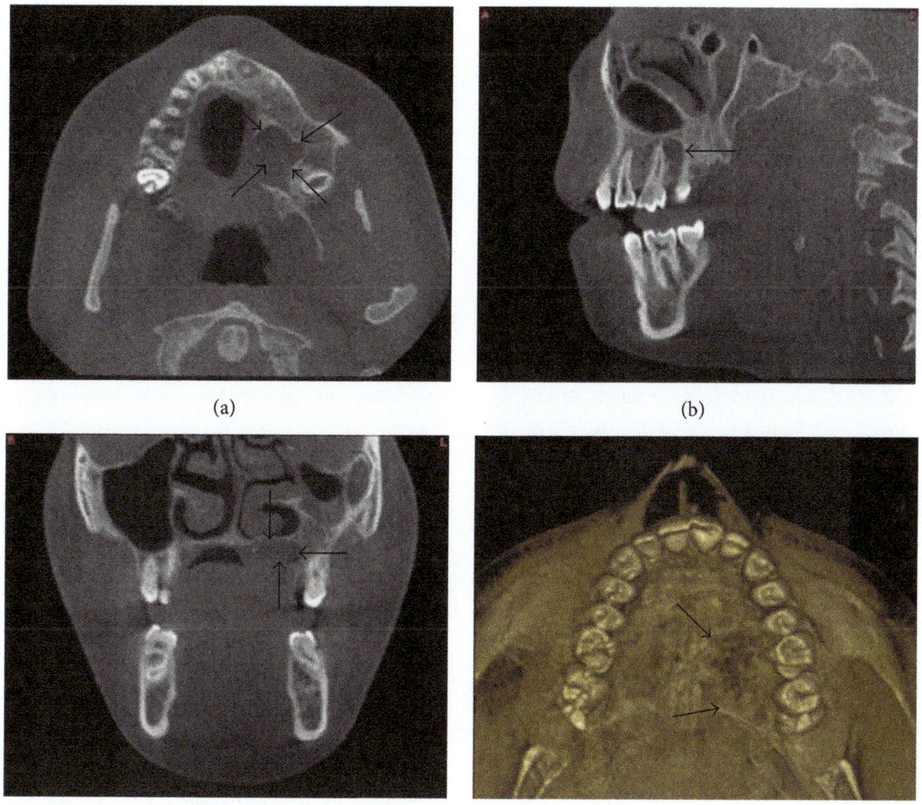

(a) (b) (c) (d)

FIGURE 2: Dental volumetric tomography images of MEC (black arrows); (a) axial, (b) sagittal, (c) coronal, and (d) 3D image.

salivary gland tumors is 50% in children and 15–25% in adults [12].

As a typical intraoral presentation this malignancy has a painless and persistent enlargement, which lasts for about a year. Paresthesia, pain, and difficulty with swallowing are noted frequently when major salivary glands and tongue are involved. Intraoral lesions are observable as a localized fluctuant nodule with a bluish or reddish-purple, smooth, mucosal surface. Like in our study, mucus may be discharged from the tumor through a small sinus tract [8]. High-grade MEC epithelial cells are predominantly squamous whereas in low-grade, mucous cells predominate [13, 14]. Low-grade tumors are soft and compressible whereas, high-grade lesions may be quite firm and accompanied with ulceration, resorption of bone, and numbness of adjacent teeth [8].

Radiographically low-grade MECs are similar to benign mixed tumors. They demonstrate smooth margins and are characterized by cystic components containing mucin. On the other hand high-grade MECs have poorly defined margins, local infiltrations, and solid appearances [15].

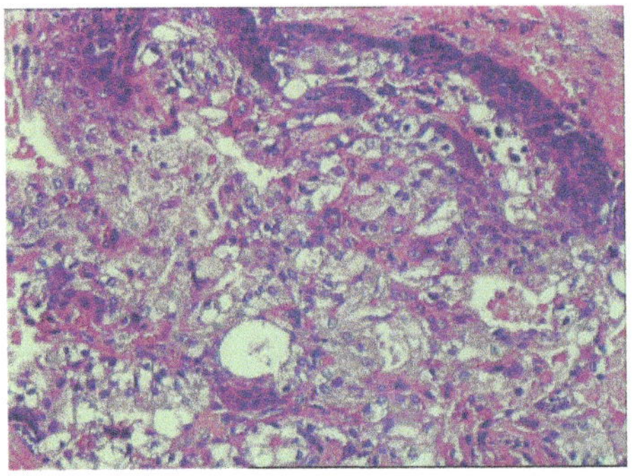

FIGURE 3: Histopathology showing mucous secreting cells and intermediate cells.

The clinical and radiographic differential diagnosis of a palatal mass includes reactive and neoplastic lesions. In children, the most common of these entities is the palatal space abscess derived from pulpal necrosis. They are differentiated by tooth mobility, diffuse, erythematous swelling of sudden onset, suppuration, fluctuation in lesion size, and radiographic evidence of inflammatory pulpal disease. Mucocele is a frequently seen fluctuant reactive lesion of salivary glands, with transparent blue swelling including mucin. Deep mucoceles, often surrounded by a fibrous tissue wall, do not fluctuate, and if located at sites other than the lower lip cannot clinically and reliably be differentiated from salivary gland tumors. Our case was not similar to a mucocele because mucin discharged from a sinus opening. Palatal region vascular malformations like hemangiomas are differentiated by clinical examination and imaging. Neurofibroma and schwannoma are occasionally encountered as compressible or firm asymptomatic nodules and pink in color unless they are secondarily traumatized [8, 15].

The tumor is dissected down to the periosteum to obtain adequate tumor-free margins [10]. But, if there is any evidence of bony involvement, removal of a portion of the jaw is necessary. Overall survival rate has been linked to histocytologic grade with 95%–100% in low-grade and 25%–43% in high-grade tumors [14]. Also, it should be considered that micromarsupialization, cryosurgery, and laser therapy are contraindicated in management of an intraoral submucosal mass/nodules in children particularly if the palate is involved [16–18]. These kinds of treatments may result in local spread of the tumor, and more aggressive surgery may be needed [8]. Based on low recurrence and mortality rates in surgical treatment of low-grade MEC, it seems that the treatment of our patient is adequate.

Radiation therapy should be used judiciously in pediatric patients with high-grade histology, positive margins, and lymph node involvement, due to its long-term consequences as facial deformity, trismus, xerostomia, osteoradionecrosis, and risk of secondary malignancy. Chemotherapy was not used as an adjuvant therapy in our patient and does not currently have a role in the standard treatment of MEC patients [19].

There is a potential risk of the development of a mucoepidermoid carcinoma in parotid and minor salivary glands of children who have received chemotherapy and cranial irradiation [6, 20]. Moreover, survivors of the childhood cancer must be followed closely throughout their lifetime for the risk of developing a secondary malignancy following the treatment of childhood cancer [21].

4. Conclusions

In this case it is noteworthy that swellings in the palatal area which could resemble a dental abscess can cause unnecessary treatments, waste of time, and delay in diagnosis. Although mucoepidermoid carcinoma and other tumors in this region are exceedingly rare, patients with these kinds of swellings must be considered cautiously, and multidisciplinary approach can lead to successful treatment.

References

[1] B. W. Neville, "Salivary gland pathology," in *Oral and Maxillofacial Pathology*, W. B. Neville, D. D. Damm, C. M. Allen, and J. E. Bouquot, Eds., pp. 420–422, Saunders, Edinburgh, Scotland, 2002.

[2] M. S. Brookstone and A. G. Huvos, "Central salivary gland tumors of the maxilla and mandible: a clinicopathologic study of 11 cases with an analysis of the literature," *Journal of Oral and Maxillofacial Surgery*, vol. 50, no. 3, pp. 229–236, 1992.

[3] B. Wedell, P. Burian, R. Dahlenfors, G. Stenman, and J. Mark, "Cytogenetical observations in a mucoepidermoid carcinoma arising from heterotopic intranodal salivary gland tissue," *Oncology Reports*, vol. 4, no. 3, pp. 515–516, 1997.

[4] S. Noda, S. Sundaresan, and E. N. Mendeloff, "Tracheal mucoepidermoid carcinoma in a 7-year-old child," *Annals of Thoracic Surgery*, vol. 66, no. 3, pp. 928–929, 1998.

[5] M. S. Brandwein, K. Ivanov, D. I. Wallace et al., "Mucoepidermoid carcinoma: a clinicopathologic study of 80 patients with special reference to histological grading," *American Journal of Surgical Pathology*, vol. 25, no. 7, pp. 835–845, 2001.

[6] J. Hicks and C. Flaitz, "Mucoepidermoid carcinoma of salivary glands in children and adolescents: assessment of proliferation markers," *Oral Oncology*, vol. 36, no. 5, pp. 454–460, 2000.

[7] D. E. da Cruz Perez, F. R. Pires, F. A. Alves, O. P. Almeida, and L. P. Kowalski, "Salivary gland tumors in children and adolescents: a clinicopathologic and immunohistochemical study of fifty-three cases," *International Journal of Pediatric Otorhinolaryngology*, vol. 68, no. 7, pp. 895–902, 2004.

[8] C. M. Flaitz, "Mucoepidermoid carcinoma of the palate in a child," *Pediatric Dentistry*, vol. 22, no. 4, pp. 292–293, 2000.

[9] M. A. Luna, J. G. Batsakis, and A. K. El-Naggar, "Salivary gland tumors in children," *Annals of Otology, Rhinology and Laryngology*, vol. 100, no. 10, pp. 869–871, 1991.

[10] P. L. Auclair and G. L. Ellis, "Mucoepidermoid carcinoma," in *Surgical Pathology of the Salivary Glands*, G. L. Ellis, P. L. Auclair, and D. R. Gnepp, Eds., pp. 269–298, WB Saunders, Philadelphia, Pa, USA, 1991.

[11] S. A. Kumar and M. Ramakrishnan, "Mucocele in lower lip as a result of improper use of feeding bottle: a case report," *Case Reports in Dentistry*, vol. 2013, Article ID 520425, 3 pages, 2013.

[12] S. R. Baker and B. Malone, "Salivary gland malignancies in children," *Cancer*, vol. 55, no. 8, pp. 1730–1736, 1985.

[13] C. M. Bower and R. A. Dyleski, "Diseases of the salivary glands," in *Pediatric Otolaryngology*, C. D. Bluestone, Ed., pp. 1251–1267, Saunders, Philadelphia, Pa, USA, 2003.

[14] R. G. Khadaroo, J. M. Walton, J. A. Ramsay, M. J. Hicks, and S. D. Archibald, "Mucoepidermoid carcinoma of the parotid gland: a rare presentation in a young child," *Journal of Pediatric Surgery*, vol. 33, no. 6, pp. 893–895, 1998.

[15] P. M. Som and M. S. Brandwein, "Anatomy and pathology of the salivary glands," in *Head and Neck Imaging*, P. M. Som and H. D. Curtin, Eds., pp. 2448–2609, Mosby Elsevier, St. Louis, Mo, USA , 2011.

[16] A. C. B. Delbem, R. F. Cunha, A. E. de Mello Vieira, and L. L. G. Ribeiro, "Treatment of mucus retention phenomena in children by the micro-marsupialization technique: case reports," *Pediatric Dentistry*, vol. 22, no. 2, pp. 155–158, 2000.

[17] S. Twetman and S. Isaksson, "Cryosurgical treatment of mucocele in children," *American Journal of Dentistry*, vol. 3, no. 4, pp. 175–176, 1990.

[18] R. A. Neumann and R. M. Knobler, "Treatment of oral mucous cysts with an argon laser," *Archives of Dermatology*, vol. 126, no. 6, pp. 829–830, 1990.

[19] M. E. Kupferman, G. O. de la Garza, A. A. Santillan et al., "Outcomes of pediatric patients with malignancies of the major salivary glands," *Annals of Surgical Oncology*, vol. 17, no. 12, pp. 3301–3307, 2010.

[20] L. Prasannan, A. Pu, P. Hoff, R. Weatherly, and V. Castle, "Parotid carcinoma as a second malignancy after treatment of childhood acute lymphoblastic leukemia," *Journal of Pediatric Hematology/Oncology*, vol. 21, no. 6, pp. 535–538, 1999.

[21] S. L. Savelli, K. J. Klopfenstein, and A. M. Termuhlen, "Mucoepidermoid carcinoma of the parotid gland as a second malignant neoplasm," *Pediatric Blood and Cancer*, vol. 45, no. 7, pp. 997–1000, 2005.

40

Complex Odontoma: A Case Report with Micro-Computed Tomography Findings

L. A. N. Santos,[1] L. J. Lopes,[2] G. D. Roque-Torres,[2] V. F. Oliveira,[3] and D. Q. Freitas[4]

[1]*Department of Oral Diagnosis, Division of Oral Radiology, State University of Montes Claros, Avenida Dr. Ruy Braga, N/N, Vila Mauriceia, 39401-089 Montes Claros, MG, Brazil*
[2]*Piracicaba Dental School, State University of Campinas, Avenida Limeira 901, Areião, 13414-903 Piracicaba, SP, Brazil*
[3]*Department of Maxillofacial Surgery, State University of Montes Claros, Avenida Dr. Ruy Braga, N/N, Vila Mauriceia, 39401-089 Montes Claros, MG, Brazil*
[4]*Department of Oral Diagnosis, Division of Oral Radiology, State University of Campinas, Avenida Limeira 901, Areião, 13414-903 Piracicaba, SP, Brazil*

Correspondence should be addressed to L. J. Lopes; lu_jacome@hotmail.com

Academic Editor: Luis M. J. Gutierrez

Odontomas are the most common benign tumors of odontogenic origin. They are normally diagnosed on routine radiographs, due to the absence of symptoms. Histopathologic evaluation confirms the diagnosis especially in cases of complex odontoma, which may be confused during radiographic examination with an osteoma or other highly calcified bone lesions. The micro-CT is a new technology that enables three-dimensional analysis with better spatial resolution compared with cone beam computed tomography. Another great advantage of this technology is that the sample does not need special preparation or destruction in the sectioned area as in histopathologic evaluation. An odontoma with CBCT and microtomography images is presented in a 26-year-old man. It was first observed on panoramic radiographs and then by CBCT. The lesion and the impacted third molar were surgically excised using a modified Neumann approach. After removal, it was evaluated by histopathology and microtomography to confirm the diagnostic hypothesis. According to the results, micro-CT enabled the assessment of the sample similar to histopathology, without destruction of the sample. With further development, micro-CT could be a powerful diagnostic tool in future research.

1. Introduction

The term odontoma was first described by Broca [1] as a benign odontogenic tumor of epithelial and mesenchymal origin characterized by slow growth and dental contents (enamel, dentin, cementum, and pulp) [2]. It is considered a tumor-like malformation (hamartoma), not a true neoplasm, in which all of the dental tissues are represented [3, 4]. Although odontomas are usually asymptomatic, there are some clinical indicators such as retention of deciduous teeth, no eruption of permanent teeth, expansion of cortical bone, and displacement of teeth. Other symptoms include numbness in the lower lip and swelling in the affected area [5].

Odontomas are usually small in size [3, 4, 6, 7]. The age at diagnosis is commonly in the second decade of life without gender predilection, occurring more often in the posterior region of the mandible [8]. Based on radiographic and microscopic characteristics, odontomas are subdivided into compound and complex types. The compound type is characterized by tooth-like structures arranged in an orderly fashion and the complex type is characterized by dental tissues in a disorderly pattern without any anatomic resemblance to a tooth [3, 9–14]. Odontomas are the most common benign tumors of odontogenic origin. They are normally diagnosed on routine radiographs, mainly due to the absence of symptoms [7]. Histopathologic evaluation confirms the diagnosis especially [15] in cases of complex odontoma, which may be confused with an osteoma or another highly calcified bone lesion on radiographs [6, 7].

The diagnosis could be established by radiography (panoramic radiography and/or intraoral radiographs) but

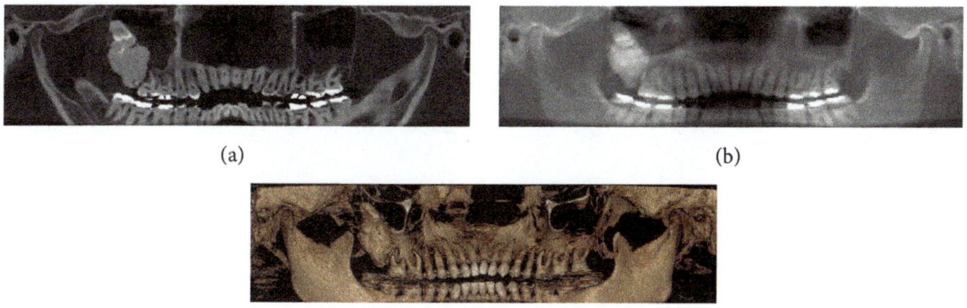

(a) (b) (c)

FIGURE 1: Panoramic radiograph reconstructed of CBCT. (a) With a thickness of 1 mm. (b) With a thickness of 10 mm. (c) 3D panoramic reconstructed.

cone beam computed tomography (CBCT) has played an important role in the diagnosis and identification of lesions [16, 17], thereby helping in treatment planning [8].

Modern high-resolution micro-computed tomography (micro-CT) is increasingly used in dental research. This new technology enables three-dimensional analysis with better spatial resolution compared with CBCT. In addition, a great advantage of micro-CT is that the sample needs no special preparation; the only demand is that it is small enough to be mounted in the scanner [18]. A wide range of specimens may be examined directly including mineralized tissues, such as teeth and bone and materials such as ceramics, polymers, and biomaterial scaffolds [19, 20]. The morphological characteristics provided by micro-CT include the assessment of the mineral concentration of teeth with high accuracy (coefficient of variation < 1%), resolution of 5–30 μm [21–23], and assessment of mineral density, all without sample destruction unlike the histopathological exam.

This paper presents a case report of a complex odontoma focusing on the micro-CT findings and highlighting the advantages of this new technology.

2. Case Report

A 26-year-old man was referred to the Department of Maxillofacial and Oral Surgery, Montes Claros University, with the chief complaint of pain in the region of the posterior right maxilla. Clinical examination revealed a swelling in the region of the upper right third molar shrouded by a large yellowish-brown hard mass, which resembled dentin, and a secretion-draining tract.

Panoramic radiographs reconstructed of CBCT showed an irregular radiopaque mass surrounded by a distinct radiolucent rim associated with the upper right third molar, which was dislocated into the maxillary sinus (Figure 1). The first diagnostic hypothesis was a complex odontoma, but osteoma and other calcified bone lesions were not ruled.

In anticipation of surgical excision of the lesion, CBCT images were obtained. The CBCT images revealed a 3.2 × 2.3 × 2.2 cm hyperdense mass interspersed with areas of hypodensity. The lesion extended superiorly from the alveolar ridge to the middle third of the right maxillary sinus, displacing the upper right third molar to the top. Laterally, the lesion extended toward the infratemporal fossa and a slight displacement of the medial wall of the right maxillary sinus was noted. Hyperdense areas resembling teeth were observed in the lesion. Thickening of the soft tissues with obstruction of the drainage pathways of the maxillary sinus was also observed. Coronal images demonstrated the extent of the internal epithelium of the maxillary sinus swelling suggesting sinusitis. The presence of fluid levels was seen in the left maxillary sinus, diagnostic of a sinus pathology (mucosa thickening) (Figure 2). The diagnostic hypothesis of a complex odontoma remained.

Under local anesthesia, the lesion and the impacted third molar were surgically excised using a modified Neumann approach (Figure 3).

The specimen was sent for histopathological and micro-CT evaluation. Histologic sections revealed a mixture of radiopaque material composed mainly of dental tissues, consisting of immature dentin, enamel, enamel matrix, cementum, and pulp tissue. Histopathologic examination confirmed the diagnosis of complex odontoma (Figure 4(a)) [24].

A micro-CT scan of the sample (approximately 30 mm × 47 mm) was obtained using a SkyScan 1172 machine (Bruker SkyScan, Aartselaar, Belgium). A greater amount of hyperdense material in the periphery of the lesion was observed (Figures 4(b) and 4(c), white arrows), which is compatible with tooth enamel. Hypodense areas (Figures 4(b) and 4(c), black arrows) are compatible with areas of pulp tissue. The definitive diagnosis was complex odontoma.

In addition to the visual evaluation of the micro-CT images, we evaluated the density, volume, and surface. For this purpose, the sample was scanned at 50 kV, 800 μA beam intensity, 30 μm image pixel size, a 0.4° rotation step, 3-frame averaging, and a 411 ms exposure time at each step. A 0.5-mm aluminum filter was used during the scans. The images were reconstructed with NRecon (Bruker SkyScan, Aartselaar, Belgium). Polynomial correction was used to reduce smoothing, ring, and beam-hardening effects during the reconstructions [25–27].

The odontoma was assessed qualitatively with CTAn software (SkyScan, v. 1.4). The volume of interest (VOI) was designed by drawing polygons interactively on the two-dimensional gray images. Polygons were drawn in five

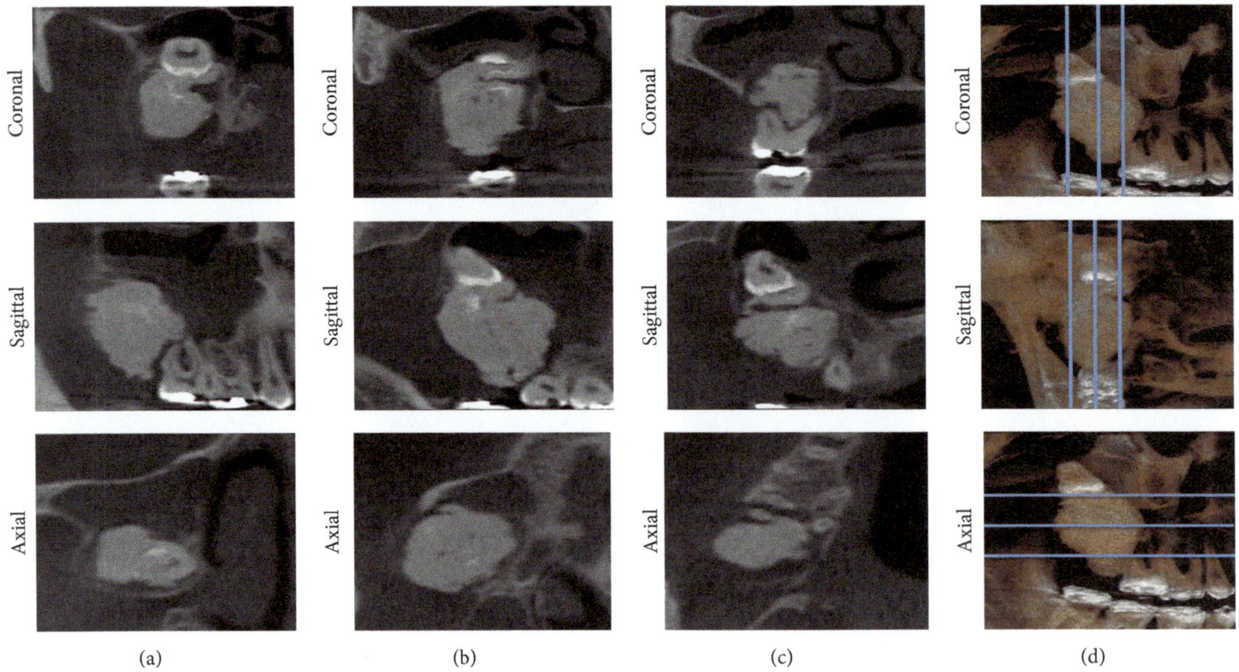

FIGURE 2: Multiplanar reconstruction of CBCT in three different regions from each view.

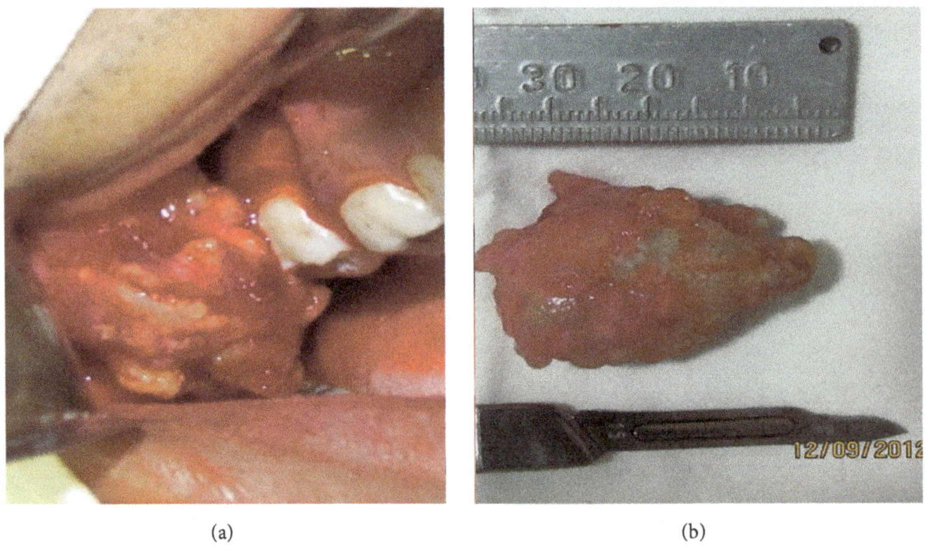

FIGURE 3: (a) Odontoma removal. (b) Complex odontoma.

sections (i.e., all the sample), and a routine utility calculated all the intermediary masks by interpolation. The VOI comprised only odontoma tissue and the following parameters were evaluated: tissue volume, bone volume, tissue surface, bone surface, bone surface density (hard tissue surface/tissue volume), total porosity, total volume of pore space, mineral concentration, density of the whole sample, and the value gray scale.

In the present case, the evaluation of the sample by micro-CT showed the parameters and values in Table 1.

3. Discussion

Odontomas are common odontogenic tumors and are usually asymptomatic [17]; however, in this case, the patient experienced pain in the region of the third molar, probably due to the presence of inflammatory component of the lesion with exudate drainage. Odontomas rarely erupt [24] but when this occurs, they are different from a normal tooth because of the lack of the periodontal ligament. The increase in size leads to sequestration of the overlying bone, causing pressure

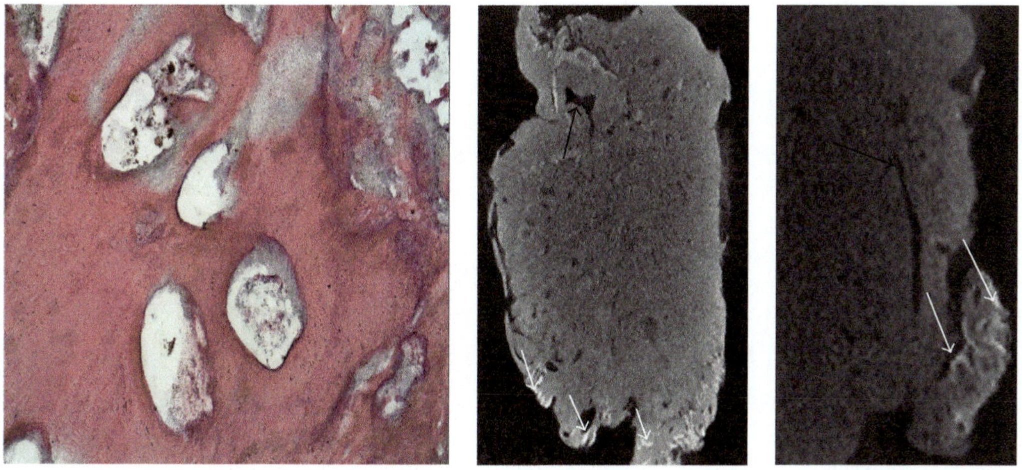

(a) (b) (c)

FIGURE 4: (a) Histopathology of the odontoma showing dense acellular eosinophilic dentin; basophilic dentin; prominent tubular array and minimal loose mesenchyme (hematoxylin and eosin stain). (b-c) Micro-CT images of the complex odontoma. White arrows, hyperdense areas; black arrows, hypodense areas. (b) Without zoom. (c) With zoom.

TABLE 1: Parameters and values of the micro-CT findings.

Parameters	Values
Tissue volume (TV)	6506.8 mm^3
Bone volume (BV)	5719.3 mm^3
Percent bone volume (BV/TV)	87.9%
Tissue surface (TS)	3193.1 mm^2
Bone surface (BS)	9758.8 mm^2
Bone surface density (BS/TV)	1.49979 1/mm
Total porosity (percent) (Po(tot))	12.1%
Total volume of pore space (Po.V(tot))	787.593.38 mm^3
Mineral concentration	0.69 g/cm^3
Density	0.92 (0.27)
Gray scale	93.38 (15.80)

and possible movement in the occlusal direction, leading to eruption.

In this case, the tumor led to retention of the right third molar, which is a common characteristic in odontomas, although not reported in clinical cases with tuberosity of the maxilla [12], because there is high predilection of complex odontoma in the posterior region of the mandible [12, 24]. Most complex odontomas reported in the literature typically measure around 1-2 cm [3]. A large complex odontoma as in this case (3 × 4.7 cm) is rare [4, 7, 14].

The diagnosis of compound odontoma can usually be established by conventional radiographic examination (intraoral or panoramic radiographs) performed for another reason when the lesion is small [17]. However, this is not usually the case with complex odontomas, because they may be confused with other tumors, such as cementoid tumors and several other bone lesions [8]. For that reason, CBCT was performed, which also aided surgical planning. The scan was very useful to visualize the precise relationship between the lesion and the third molar [5, 17]. As demonstrated by other studies, early diagnosis of odontomas allows for less complex treatment, guaranteeing a better prognosis [17].

As a relatively new method of high-resolution three-dimensional imaging, micro-CT has been widely used in many academic fields. Many studies have presented the current state of micro-CT imaging [18, 27–30]. The images represent spatial distribution maps of linear attenuation coefficients determined by the energy of the X-ray source and the atomic composition of the material sample, without preparation or destruction of the sample in the area to be sectioned [27]. Micro-CT has become more and more used for the analysis of mineral concentrations of teeth. Accurate and detailed images of the morphological characteristics of teeth are provided by micro-CT scans in dental research; the mineral concentration of teeth can be measured with high accuracy, images at a resolution of 5–30 μm are obtained, and mineral density can be indirectly assessed [23].

In this case, the sample had 957 slices, the total tissue volume was 6506.8 mm^3 (100%), and the hard tissue volume was 5719.3 mm^3 (87.9%). The soft tissue surface was 3193.1 mm^2 and the hard tissue surface was 9758.8 mm^2. The density of the sample was 0.92 g/cm^3 (0.27 g/cm^3); this density is close to the density of circumpulpal dentin (1.3 g/cm^3) and the mineral concentration of the sample was 0.69 g/cm^3, similar to demineralized dentin (0.55 g/cm^3). The gray scale value of the sample was found 93.38 (15.80), similar to that of rigid dentin [31].

Histopathologically, complex odontomas are composed of a mixture of dental tissues, mainly forming a single homogeneous mass of immature dentin, enamel, enamel matrix, cement, and pulp tissue in a random fashion. The micro-CT images of this case showed results consistent with histopathological evaluation, with a large volume of hard tissue and a mineral density similar to human immature dentin [31, 32]. This case report also demonstrates the possibility of clinical application of this imaging modality with good visualization. However, more studies are necessary to elucidate whether micro-CT analysis is valuable in the management of the odontoma.

4. Conclusions

This case report demonstrates the use of advanced diagnostic imaging, such as CBCT, which allowed a more appropriate treatment plan for excision of the lesion. In addition, micro-CT enabled the assessment of the sample similar to histopathology, without destruction of the sample. With further development, micro-CT could be a powerful diagnostic tool in future research.

Competing Interests

The authors deny any competing interests.

References

[1] P. P. Broca, *Traite des Tumeurs*, P. Asselin, Paris, France, 1866.

[2] L. Barnes, L. EveBarnes, J. W. Eveson, P. Reichart, and D. Sidransky, *Pathology and Genetics of the Head and Neck Tumors. World Health Organization Classification of Tumors*, IARC, Lyon, France, 2005.

[3] H. Lehman, J. Lustmann, and E. Regev, "Removal of an extensive mandibular odontoma using an intraoral approach," *Quintessence International*, vol. 44, no. 6, pp. 425–428, 2013.

[4] G. S. P. Reddy, G. V. Reddy, B. Sidhartha, K. Sriharsha, J. Koshy, and R. Sultana, "Large complex odontoma of mandible in a young boy: a rare and unusual case report," *Case Reports in Dentistry*, vol. 2014, Article ID 854986, 4 pages, 2014.

[5] S. C. Isler, S. Demircan, M. Soluk, and Z. Cebi, "Radiologic evaluation of an unusually sized complex odontoma involving the maxillary sinus by cone beam computed tomography," *Quintessence International*, vol. 40, no. 7, pp. 533–535, 2009.

[6] B. Neville, D. D. Damm, C. M. Allen, and J. Bouquot, *Oral and Maxillofacial Pathology*, WB Saunders, Philadelphia, Pa, USA, 2007.

[7] C. J. Perumal, A. Mohamed, A. Singh, and C. E. Noffke, "Sequestrating giant complex odontoma: a case report and review of the literature," *Journal of Maxillofacial and Oral Surgery*, vol. 12, no. 4, pp. 480–484, 2013.

[8] T. M. Soluk, S. Pehlivan, V. Olgac, N. Aksakallı, and C. Alatli, "Clinical and histopathological investigation of odontomas: review of the literature and presentation of 160 cases," *Journal of Oral and Maxillofacial Surgery*, vol. 70, no. 6, pp. 1358–1361, 2012.

[9] M. Kaneko, M. Fukuda, T. Sano, T. Ohnishi, and Y. Hosokawa, "Microradiographic and microscopic investigation of a rare case of complex odontoma," *Oral Surgery, Oral Medicine, Oral Pathology, Oral Radiology, and Endodontics*, vol. 86, no. 1, pp. 131–134, 1998.

[10] C. H. Lee and G. J. Park, "Complex and compound odontomas are clinico-pathological entities," *Basic and Applied Pathology*, vol. 1, no. 1, pp. 30–33, 2008.

[11] J. T. Korpi, V. T. Kainulainen, G. K. B. Sándor, and K. S. Oikarinen, "Removal of large complex odontoma using Le Fort I osteotomy," *Journal of Oral and Maxillofacial Surgery*, vol. 67, no. 9, pp. 2018–2021, 2009.

[12] P. Boffano, E. Zavattero, F. Roccia, and C. Gallesio, "Complex and compound odontomas," *Journal of Craniofacial Surgery*, vol. 23, no. 3, pp. 685–688, 2012.

[13] S. Ezirganli, U. Tasdemir, and U. Gurer, "Compound odontoma associated with mandibular impacted permanent central incisor: a case report," *Cumhuriyet Dental Journal*, vol. 15, no. 2, pp. 162–165, 2012.

[14] A. M. D'Cruz, S. Hegde, and U. A. Shetty, "Large complex odontoma: a report of a rare entity," *Sultan Qaboos University Medical Journal*, vol. 13, no. 2, pp. 342–345, 2013.

[15] P. K. S. Virk, U. Sharma, and J. S. Rajput, "Intraosseous and erupted compound odontoma: a report of two cases," *Indian Journal of Dentistry*, vol. 3, no. 4, pp. 243–246, 2012.

[16] B. Anuraag, M. Choudhary, B. Chaudhary, M. B. Motwani, S. M. Chaudhary, and P. J. Banode, "Utility of cone beam CT in maxillo-facial radiology," *International Journal of Dentistry*, vol. 3, pp. 134–145, 2013.

[17] K. S. Kannan, R. Prabhakar, R. Saravanan, Karthikeyan, and Rajvikram, "Composite compound odontoma—a case report," *Journal of Clinical and Diagnostic Research*, vol. 7, no. 10, pp. 2406–2407, 2013.

[18] F. J. Rühli, G. Kuhn, R. Evison, R. Müller, and M. Schultz, "Diagnostic value of micro-CT in comparison with histology in the qualitative assessment of historical human skull bone pathologies," *American Journal of Physical Anthropology*, vol. 133, no. 4, pp. 1099–1111, 2007.

[19] I. S. Tamminen, H. Isaksson, A. S. Aula, E. Honkanen, J. S. Jurvelin, and H. Kröger, "Reproducibility and agreement of micro-CT and histomorphometry in human trabecular bone with different metabolic status," *Journal of Bone and Mineral Metabolism*, vol. 29, no. 4, pp. 442–448, 2011.

[20] L. H. E. Karssemakers, J. W. Nolte, D. B. Tuinzing, G. E. J. Langenbach, P. G. Raijmakers, and A. G. Becking, "Microcomputed tomographic analysis of human condyles in unilateral condylar hyperplasia: increased cortical porosity and trabecular bone volume fraction with reduced mineralisation," *British Journal of Oral and Maxillofacial Surgery*, vol. 52, no. 10, pp. 940–944, 2014.

[21] H. Hamba, T. Nikaido, A. Sadr, S. Nakashima, and J. Tagami, "Enamel lesion parameter correlations between polychromatic micro-CT and TMR," *Journal of Dental Research*, vol. 91, no. 6, pp. 586–591, 2012.

[22] J.-T. Hsu, S.-P. Wang, H.-L. Huang, Y.-J. Chen, J. Wu, and M.-T. Tsai, "The assessment of trabecular bone parameters and cortical bone strength: a comparison of micro-CT and dental cone-beam CT," *Journal of Biomechanics*, vol. 46, no. 15, pp. 2611–2618, 2013.

[23] G. Dong, Q. Dong, Y. Liu et al., "High-resolution micro-CT scanning as an innovative tool for evaluating dental hard tissue development," *Journal of Applied Clinical Medical Physics*, vol. 15, no. 4, pp. 49–56, 2014.

[24] S. Govindrajan, J. Muruganandhan, S. Shamsudeen, N. Kumar, M. Ramasamy, and S. Prasad, "Complex composite odontoma with characteristic histology," *Case Reports in Dentistry*, vol. 2013, Article ID 157614, 5 pages, 2013.

[25] M. Kovács, R. Danyi, M. Erdélyi, P. Fejérdy, and C. Dobó-Nagy, "Distortional effect of beam-hardening artefacts on microCT: a simulation study based on an in vitro caries model," *Oral Surgery, Oral Medicine, Oral Pathology, Oral Radiology and Endodontology*, vol. 108, no. 4, pp. 591–599, 2009.

[26] W. Zou, N. Hunter, and M. V. Swain, "Application of polychromatic μCT for mineral density determination," *Journal of Dental Research*, vol. 90, no. 1, pp. 18–30, 2011.

[27] M. V. Swain and J. Xue, "State of the art of Micro-CT applications in dental research. State of the art of Micro-CT applications in dental research," *International Journal of Oral Science*, vol. 1, no. 4, pp. 177–188, 2009.

[28] M. D. Bentley, M. C. Ortiz, E. L. Ritman, and J. Carlos Romero, "The use of microcomputed tomography to study microvasculature in small rodents," *American Journal of Physiology—Regulatory Integrative and Comparative Physiology*, vol. 282, no. 5, pp. R1267–R1279, 2002.

[29] G. Plotino, N. M. Grande, R. Pecci, R. Bedini, C. H. Pameijer, and F. Somma, "Three-dimensional imaging using microcomputed tomography for studying tooth macromorphology," *Journal of the American Dental Association*, vol. 137, no. 11, pp. 1555–1561, 2006.

[30] A. Parsa, N. Ibrahim, B. Hassan, P. Van der Stelt, and D. Wismeijer, "Bone quality evaluation at dental implant site using multislice CT, micro-CT, and cone beam CT," *Clinical Oral Implants Research*, vol. 26, no. 1, pp. e1–e7, 2015.

[31] D. R. Schwass, M. V. Swain, D. G. Purton, and J. W. Leichter, "A system of calibrating microtomography for use in caries research," *Caries Research*, vol. 43, no. 4, pp. 314–321, 2009.

[32] J. C. Elliott, F. S. L. Wong, P. Anderson, G. R. Davis, and S. E. P. Dowker, "Determination of mineral concentration in dental enamel from X-ray attenuation measurements," *Connective Tissue Research*, vol. 38, no. 1–4, pp. 61–72, 1998.

A New Multi-Ingredient Recipe for the Treatment of Localized Advanced Periodontal Disease following the Surgical Removal of Impacted Wisdom Teeth

Nabil Khzam,[1] Adam Fell,[2] Anthony Fisher,[3] Paul Kim,[4] Usman A. Khan,[5] and Mahmoud M. Bakr[6]

[1] *DB Dental, BDS, MPhil, DClinDent, MRACDS (Perio), Perth, WA 6159, Australia*
[2] *DB Dental, BSc, BDent, MJDF RCS, Perth, WA 6011, Australia*
[3] *PerioHEALTH and Implants Practice, BDSc, DClinDent, Brisbane, QLD 4059, Australia*
[4] *Benowa Mansions Periodontal Practice, BPharm, BDSc, DClinDent, Gold Coast, QLD 4217, Australia*
[5] *Dalby Dental Clinic, BDS, MDS, PhD, Western Downs, QLD 4405, Australia*
[6] *General Dental Practice, School of Dentistry and Oral Health, BDS, MDS, Griffith University, Gold Coast, QLD 4222, Australia*

Correspondence should be addressed to Mahmoud M. Bakr; m.bakr@griffith.edu.au

Academic Editor: Gilberto Sammartino

Periodontal disease is a chronic inflammation of the tooth supporting structures. It leads to bone and attachment loss which is irreversible. Extraction of horizontally impacted lower third molar (L3M) teeth may result in localized periodontal pockets at the distal aspect of the adjacent lower second molars (L2M). We present a case of a 21-year-old male who suffered from a swelling and pain around his lower right second molar following surgical removal of a mesioangular impacted lower right third molar. We showed that oral hygiene measures, surgical access, mixture of autogenous and synthetic bone graft, and guided tissue regeneration (GTR) were enough to control the problem.

1. Introduction

The presence of horizontally impacted L3M often leads to localized periodontal disease next to the extracted tooth which often needs surgical procedure to resolve [1, 2]. Conservative periodontal treatment in terms of scaling and root planning on the distal root surface of the tooth adjacent to the impacted wisdom tooth after the extraction may result in small benefit [3]. Some studies showed that various flap designs for the surgical removal of wisdom teeth can lead to positive outcomes in terms of periodontal pocket reduction on the distal surface of the adjacent L2M [4]. On the other hand, GTR technique utilizing bone graft and barrier membranes were shown to be the treatment of choice in the prevention of these periodontal defects [5, 6]. Bone grafts to fill the periodontal defect on the distal root surface of L2M adjacent to the extracted horizontally impacted L3M have long been discussed and revealed some good results [7, 8].

In this study, a combination of autogenous bone chips harvested from the external oblique ridge and bovine porous bone mineral Bio-Oss (Geistlich Biomaterials) were used to fill the advanced periodontal pocket on the distal side of the L2M. This mixture was used to support and maintain the space that is essential for bone regeneration as well as in the support of the overlying double bioabsorbable membrane. A collagen membrane (Bio-Gide, Geistlich Biomaterials) was used to cover the bony mixture.

The innovative technique used in this case report aimed to evaluate the efficacy of using autogenous bone chips mixed with bovine bone particles plus double layer of absorbable membrane for the treatment of advanced periodontal defect on the distal root surface of L2M adjacent to the extracted mesioangular impacted L3M.

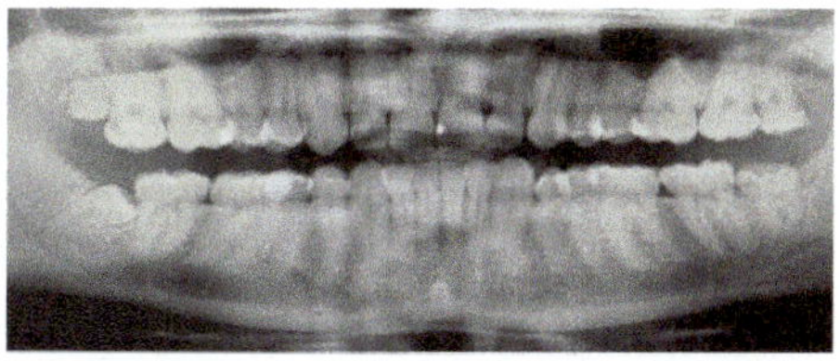

FIGURE 1: Preoperative orthopantograph (OPG) demonstrating the mesioangular impaction of the lower right third molar.

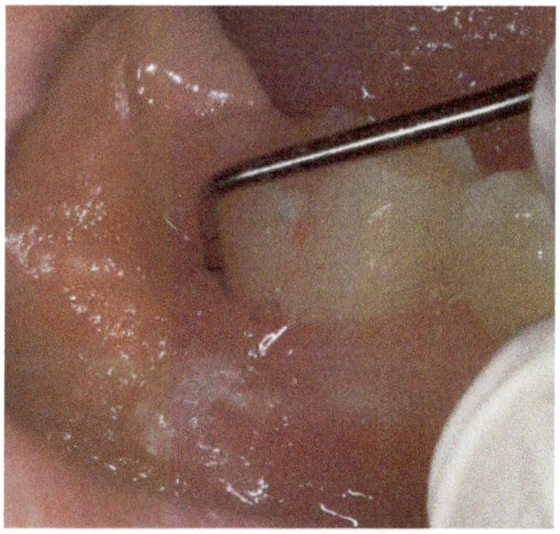

FIGURE 2: Preoperative clinical photograph of the lower right second molar.

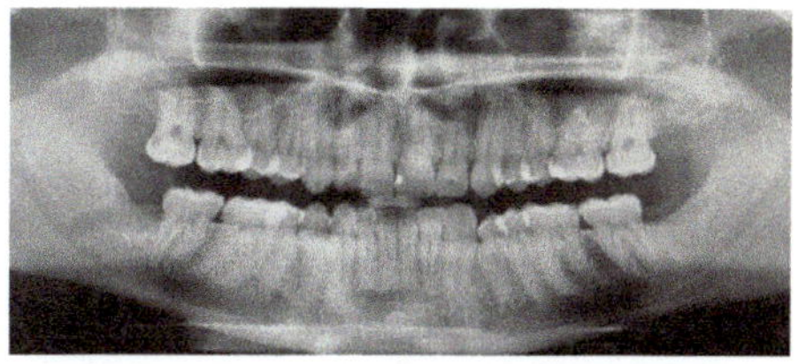

FIGURE 3: Postoperative orthopantograph (OPG) showing the extraction socket of the lower right third molar.

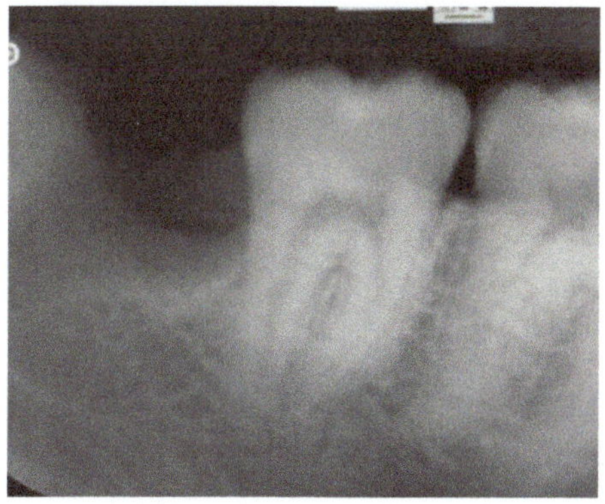

FIGURE 4: Preoperative periapical X-ray of the lower right second molar.

2. Case Presentation

A healthy 21-year-old male, nonsmoker, was referred to a specialist periodontist (NK) for a consultation regarding a swelling and associated halitosis, which started three months after surgical extraction of right L3M tooth that was impacted in a mesioangular position as shown in the orthopantograph (OPG) (Figure 1). Clinical examination revealed an eight-millimeter-deep periodontal pocket, bleeding on probing, and suppuration on the distal root surface of the right L2M adjacent to the mesioangular impacted right L3M that was extracted three months ago (Figure 2). A new OPG and a periapical radiograph were taken to explore the distal root of L2M before surgery planning. Both radiographs showed incomplete healing and poor bone fill in the extraction socket of the right L3M, as well as vertical bone loss distal to the L2M (Figures 3 and 4).

GTR technique was conducted under local anesthesia. A full thickness mucoperiosteal flap was raised around the distal side of L2M. Chronically inflamed tissue was removed using piezo tips on a piezo surgery unit. Debridement of the distal root surface of L2M was performed using a combination of ultrasonic tips and 13/14 Gracey Curettes. A bone scraper was used to harvest bone from the external oblique ridge. A mixture of autogenous bone chips and Bio-Oss particles was used to fill the intrabony defects distal to L2M. Double layer of Bio-Gide membrane was used to cover the bone mixture, Vicrly sutures 5-0 (Ethicon GmbH, Germany) were used to secure the membrane. Prolene 5-0 sutures (Ethicon GmbH, Germany) were used to achieve primary closure. Postoperative and oral hygiene instructions were given. A period of five months was allowed for healing before reviewing the case. Upon review, the pocket depth was reduced to 3 mm with complete absence of bleeding upon probing and suppuration on the distal root surface of L2M. Patient was informed to attend regular review appointments for monitoring. Both clinical photograph and periapical X-ray were taken to confirm the good result after 4 months from the day of surgery (Figures 5, 6, and 7).

3. Discussion

Extraction of impacted L3M often results in increased risk for caries and periodontal intrabony defects adjacent to the distal surface of the L2M [1, 9]. A retrospective study revealed that 43% of the cases had periodontal pocket of ≥7 mm on the distal side of the adjacent L2M two years after the surgical removal of the impacted wisdom molar [2, 10]. In this retrospective report of 215 cases, the investigators were able to show that the initial periodontal defect, the angle of the impacted molar, and the age of the patient were important factors that influenced the incidence of localized advanced periodontal disease. In our case report, the advanced periodontal disease developed within 4 weeks after tooth extraction despite the lack of preexisting periodontal disease on the distal side of the L2M.

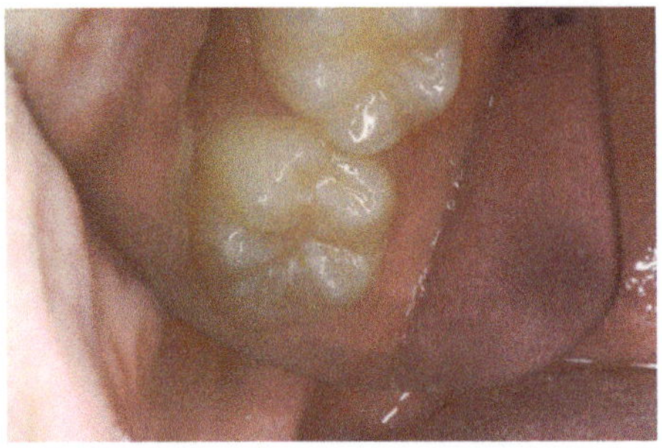

FIGURE 5: Postoperative clinical photograph of the lower right second molar.

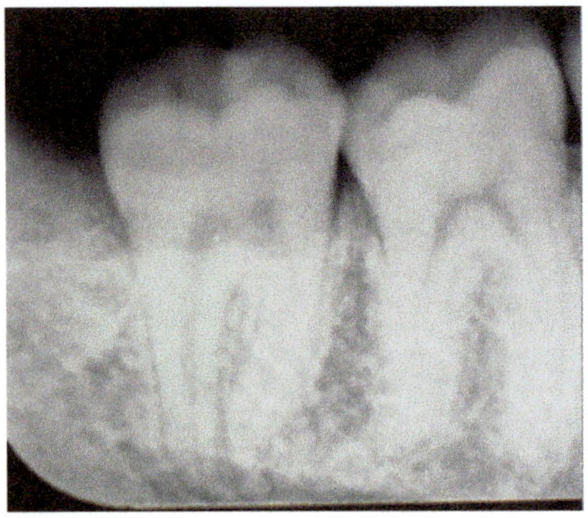

FIGURE 6: Postoperative periapical X-ray of the lower right second molar.

Some studies aimed to prevent the formation of future periodontal defects around the L2M by grafting the extraction socket of the removed impacted L3M. In a study by Sammartino and his associates, they used autologous platelet-rich plasma to promote healing, which reduced the incidence of possible periodontal complications on the L2M [11]. In another investigation, the regeneration technique showed that the use of bovine porous bone mineral with or without a collagen membrane can be a viable and stable treatment to alleviate the periodontal defects that are often associated with impacted L3M extractions [12]. The best clinical results were noted in the bovine porous bone mineral plus collagen membrane group. A literature review concluded that flap design does not influence probing depth or attachment level on the distal aspect of the L2M following surgery of the L3M. Curettage of the radicular surface of L2M together with oral hygiene control reduces these clinical parameters. Bone regeneration techniques with bone graft are recommended in cases of prior periodontal defect distal to L2M [13].

Reports provide evidence of increased attachment levels when using GTR technique for the treatment of periodontal defects that occur on the distal aspect of L2M which are next to an extracted mesioangular impacted L3M with oral communication. A study was conducted by Oxford et al. to test if the use of GTR can enhance probing attachment levels following extraction of mesioangular impacted third molars. 12 patients with bilateral soft tissue impacted L3M entered this split mouth study. After extractions, the previously exposed distal root surface of L2M was debrided. The defects on the randomly selected experimental sites were covered with expanded polytetrafluoroethylene membrane and the tissue was replaced to cover the membrane. Membranes were removed after 6 weeks. Control sites were treated identically except that no membrane was placed. The use of barrier material did not provide statistically significant differences in probing attachment levels when comparing experimental versus control sites. Nevertheless, probing attachment levels gain was consistently greater at 3 and 6 months when GTR techniques were used in sites with deep impactions [6]. All the above procedures dealt with the advanced bone loss on the distal side of the L2M at the time of L3M extraction.

A randomized clinical trial was carried out to evaluate the healing of periodontal intrabony defects at the distal aspect of L2M using a resorbable polylactic acid barrier and a nonresorbable polytetrafluoroethylene barrier and to compare the therapeutic effect of the bioresorbable barrier versus the nonresorbable barrier. 19 patients with intrabony defects distal to L2M of > or =4 mm (on radiographs) were included in the study. The defects remained 5 years after surgical removal of impacted L3M. Following flap elevation and defect debridement, the defects were randomly covered with either a resorbable or a nonresorbable barrier. Treatment was evaluated clinically after 1 year by measurements of probing depth, probing attachment level, and probing bone level and radiographically by measurements of bone levels on radiographs taken immediately before and 1 year after surgery.

Both treatments resulted in significant pocket reduction, attachment gain, and radiographic bone fill. It was concluded that the GTR treatment of deep intrabony defects distal to L2M using resorbable barriers resulted in significant improvement at least equivalent to the results obtained using nonresorbable barriers [14]. The efficacy of platelets-rich plasma combined with bovine hydroxyapatite bone graft and resorbable membrane was investigated both clinically and radiographically for the treatment of intrabony pockets on the distal aspect of L2M following the surgical extraction of fully impacted L3M. The study concluded that the combined use of platelet-rich plasma with bovine hydroxyapatite bone graft materials for the treatment of intrabony defects might be an appropriate approach when the main goal is providing earlier bone regeneration [15]. Another combination that included platelet-rich plasma and a resorbable membrane of procaine origin (Bio-Gide; Geistlich Biomaterials, Wolhusen, Switzerland) was investigated in a randomized controlled trial in 2009. From a clinical point of view, it was not evident that the above-mentioned combination was superior to using platelet-rich plasma alone. However, histological analysis showed earlier onset of bone maturation [16].

In our present case, Bio-Oss was selected for its safety, excellent compatibility, and high porosity which can promote cell adhesion and differentiation. To enhance this effect, autogenous chips of bone were mixed with the Bio-Oss and the mix was covered with Bio-Gide barrier; to our knowledge this is the first case report of this kind using this mixture which resulted in a quicker healing time and excellent bone fill as can be seen in the postoperative X-ray.

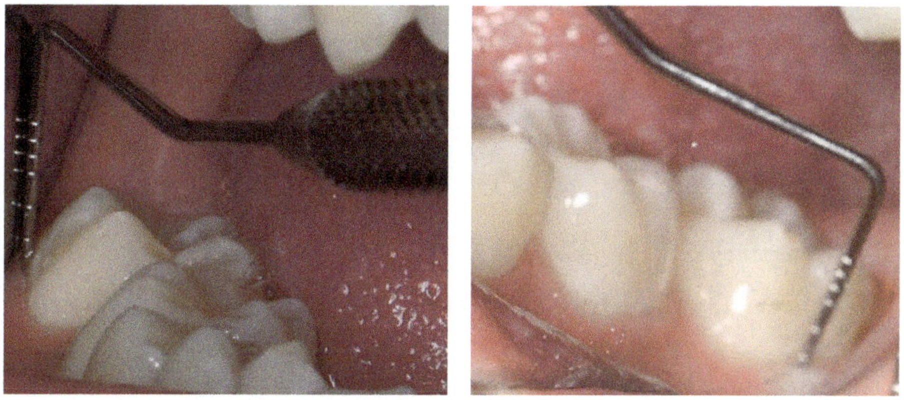

FIGURE 7: Postoperative clinical photograph of the lower right second molar confirming the pocket depth after the successful treatment.

Competing Interests

The authors declare that they have no competing interests.

Acknowledgments

The authors would like to thank Mrs. Stephanie Grundy for her contribution to the clinical examination.

References

[1] A. Inocêncio Faria, M. Gallas-Torreira, M. López-Ratón, E. Crespo-Vázquez, I. Rodríguez-Núñez, and G. López-Castro, "Radiological infrabony defects after impacted mandibular third molar extractions in young adults," *Journal of Oral and Maxillofacial Surgery*, vol. 71, no. 12, pp. 2020–2028, 2013.

[2] C. F. Kugelberg, U. Ahlström, S. Ericson, and A. Hugoson, "Periodontal healing after impacted lower third molar surgery. A retrospective study," *International Journal of Oral Surgery*, vol. 14, no. 1, pp. 29–40, 1985.

[3] R. E. LaBelle, "The influence of third molars on periodontal health," *The Minneapolis District Dental Journal*, vol. 53, no. 2, pp. 25–28, 1969.

[4] B. J. Groves and J. R. Moore, "The periodontal implications of flap design in lower third molar extractions," *The Dental Practitioner and Dental Record*, vol. 20, no. 9, pp. 297–304, 1970.

[5] M. Aimetti, E. Pigella, and F. Romano, "Clinical and radiographic evaluation of the effects of guided tissue regeneration using resorbable membranes after extraction of impacted mandibular third molars," *International Journal of Periodontics & Restorative Dentistry*, vol. 27, no. 1, pp. 51–59, 2007.

[6] G. E. Oxford, G. Quintero, C. B. Stuller, and M. E. Gher, "Treatment of 3rd molar-induced periodontal defects with guided tissue regeneration," *Journal of Clinical Periodontology*, vol. 24, no. 7, pp. 464–469, 1997.

[7] T. Irinakis and M. Tabesh, "Preserving the socket dimensions with bone grafting in single sites: an esthetic surgical approach when planning delayed implant placement," *The Journal of Oral Implantology*, vol. 33, no. 3, pp. 156–163, 2007.

[8] J. D. Keith Jr. and M. A. Salama, "Ridge preservation and augmentation using regenerative materials to enhance implant predictability and esthetics," *Compendium of Continuing Education in Dentistry*, vol. 28, no. 11, pp. 614–624, 2007.

[9] V. Irja, "Impacted third molars increase the risk for caries and periodontal pathology in neighboring second molars," *Journal of Evidence-Based Dental Practice*, vol. 14, no. 2, pp. 89–90, 2014.

[10] C. F. Kugelberg, U. Ahlstrom, S. Ericson, A. Hugoson, and H. Thailander, "The influence of anatomical, pathophysiological and other factors on periodontal healing after impacted lower third molar surgery," *Journal of Clinical Periodontology*, vol. 18, no. 1, pp. 37–43, 1997.

[11] G. Sammartino, M. Tia, G. Marenzi, A. Espedito Di Lauro, E. D'Agostino, and P. P. Claudio, "Use of autologous Platelet-Rich Plasma (PRP) in periodontal defect treatment after extraction of impacted mandibular third molars," *Journal of Oral and Maxillofacial Surgery*, vol. 63, no. 6, pp. 766–770, 2005.

[12] G. Sammartino, M. Tia, T. Bucci, and H.-L. Wang, "Prevention of mandibular third molar extraction-associated periodontal defects: a comparative study," *Journal of Periodontology*, vol. 80, no. 3, pp. 389–396, 2009.

[13] A. Aloy-Prósper, B. García-Mira, C. Larrazabal-Morón, and M. Peñarrocha-Diago, "Distal probing depth and attachment level of lower second molars following surgical extraction of lower third molars: a literature review," *Medicina Oral, Patologia Oral y Cirugia Bucal*, vol. 15, no. 5, pp. e755–e759, 2010.

[14] S. Karapataki, A. Hugoson, H. Falk, L. Laurell, and C. F. Kugelberg, "Healing following GTR treatment of intrabony defects distal to mandibular 2nd molars using resorbable and non-resorbable barriers," *Journal of Clinical Periodontology*, vol. 27, no. 5, pp. 333–340, 2000.

[15] M. C. DurmuŞlar, C. Alpaslan, G. Alpaslan, and M. Çakır, "Clinical and radiographic evaluation of the efficacy of platelet-rich plasma combined with hydroxyapatite bone graft substitutes in the treatment of intra-bony defects in maxillofacial region," *Acta Odontologica Scandinavica*, vol. 72, no. 8, pp. 948–953, 2014.

[16] G. Sammartino, M. Tia, E. Gentile, G. Marenzi, and P. P. Claudio, "Platelet-rich plasma and resorbable membrane for prevention of periodontal defects after deeply impacted lower third molar extraction," *Journal of Oral and Maxillofacial Surgery*, vol. 67, no. 11, pp. 2369–2373, 2009.

Radiographic Follow-Up during Orthodontic Treatment for Early Diagnosis of Sequential Supernumerary Teeth

Selma Sano Suga, Paula de Castro Kruly, Talissa Mayer Garrido, Marise Sano Suga Matumoto, Uhana Seifert Guimarães Suga, and Raquel Sano Suga Terada

State University of Maringá, Avenida Mandacaru, 1550 Bairro Mandacaru, 87080-000 Maringá, PR, Brazil

Correspondence should be addressed to Raquel Sano Suga Terada; rssterada@uem.br

Academic Editor: Hüsamettin Oktay

Most supernumerary teeth are impacted and asymptomatic. *Objective.* The aim of this paper is to describe two cases of sequential development of supernumerary teeth in the mandibular premolar region, identified during orthodontic treatment. *Reports.* The first case describes the radiographic follow-up of a female patient that presented a supernumerary tooth at the age of 9 years and 10 months in the right mandibular premolar region, followed by a further supernumerary tooth in the left mandibular premolar region identified at the age of 11 years and 3 months. In the second case, the radiographic follow-up of a male patient demonstrated 3 supernumerary teeth in the premolar region at the age of 16 years. During orthognathic surgery planning at the age of 20 years and 5 months, a supplemental supernumerary tooth was found in the left mandibular region. *Conclusion.* Considering the late developing of supernumerary premolars, appropriate follow-up with panoramic radiographs of patients with previous experience of supernumerary teeth is essential for early diagnosis of supplemental premolars to prevent possible complications.

1. Introduction

Supernumerary teeth can affect the development of occlusion [1, 2], cause root resorption of adjacent teeth, and induce pathological changes such as cysts [3]. The prevalence of third premolars is relatively low (0.29% of the population), representing between 8 and 9.1% of all supernumerary teeth [4]. Approximately 75% of all third premolars remain impacted [5]. As they tend to remain trapped and are almost always asymptomatic, radiographic diagnosis is usually incidental [6]. Therefore, early diagnosis performed with routine radiographic examinations before, during, and after clinical or orthodontic treatment is essential to identify these alterations, which can negatively affect the normal development of occlusion [2, 7].

There are few reports in the literature on sequential supernumerary teeth in the premolar region [8]. Because they tend to occur after the normal tooth development period, they can interfere with orthodontic treatment.

Although not clearly defined in the literature, supernumerary teeth have been reported as being "nonsequential," when diagnosed on a single occasion, and as "sequential," when they are found at different times over a period of an individual's life [9, 10]. The incidence of supernumerary teeth in the permanent dentition has been reported to range between less than 1% and 4% [9] and 1% and 3.5% [3], while in the deciduous dentition it ranges between 0.3% and 0.8% [9] and 0.3% and 0.6% [3]. Supernumerary teeth are more frequently reported in males than in females in a proportion of 2 : 1 [7]. In previous reviews of the literature on supernumerary teeth, the mandibular premolar region was found to be the most common site of occurrence [5, 11].

Therefore, the aim of this paper is to report on two cases of sequential development of supernumerary teeth in the mandibular premolar region and discuss the importance of the clinical and radiographic follow-up during orthodontic treatment.

2. Case Reports

Case 1. A female, leucoderma, Brazilian patient, aged 7 years and 3 months, presenting mouth breathing and skeletal

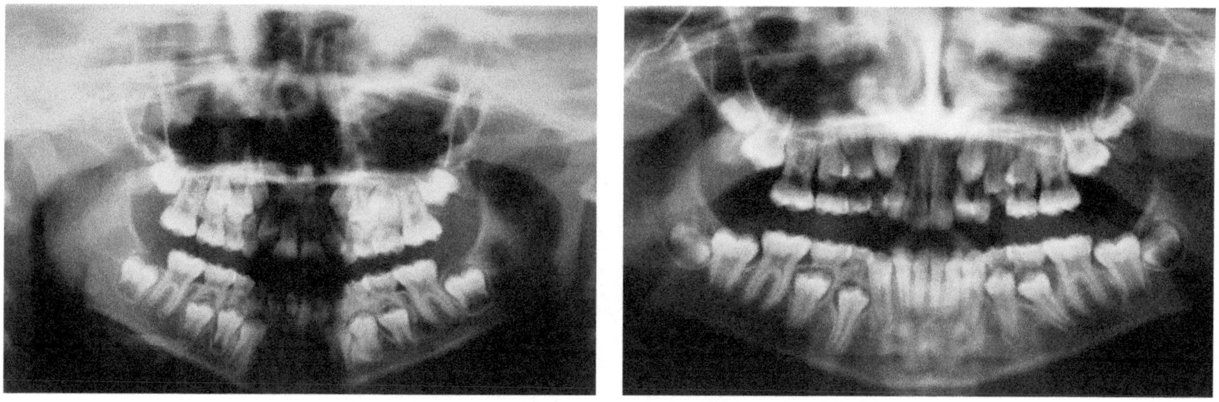

(a) (b)

FIGURE 1: (a) Panoramic radiograph of the patient aged 7 years and 3 months and (b) 9 years and 4 months with no evidence of supernumerary teeth.

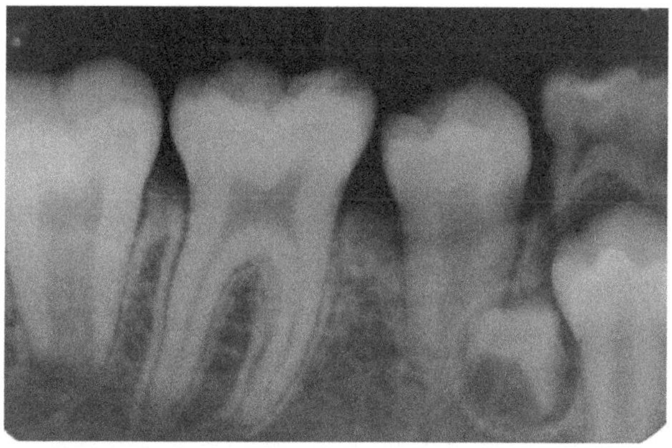

FIGURE 2: Periapical radiograph of the patient aged 9 years and 10 months showing early formation of a supernumerary tooth in the right mandibular premolar region.

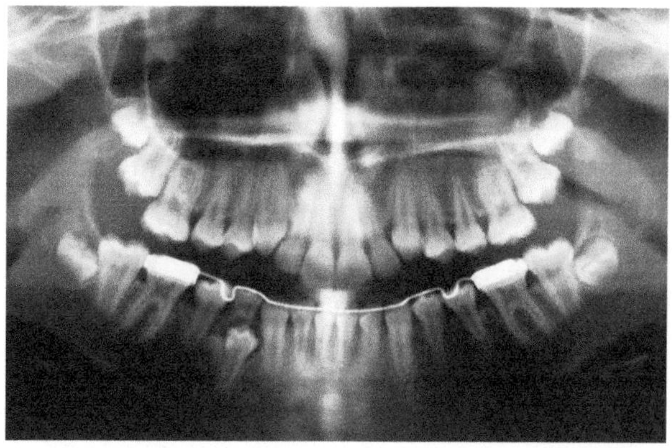

FIGURE 3: Panoramic radiograph of the patient aged 10 years 5 months showing early formation of a supernumerary tooth in the right mandibular premolar region.

Class II, division 2 malocclusion, sought a private clinic for orthodontic treatment. The initial panoramic radiograph revealed no abnormalities in the dentition (Figure 1).

Orthodontic treatment started two years later, when the patient was aged 9 years and 4 months. The corrective phase of the treatment occurred after the interceptive phase. For the treatment of the Class II malocclusion, an orthopedic expansion device across the upper and lower arches was placed over a period of 12 months. After this period, a lingual bar was adapted, and a follow-up radiograph was required because tooth 84 exhibited no physiological mobility and was the last deciduous teeth to remain in the oral cavity. Control radiographs obtained at 31 and 38 months after the first initial radiographic assessment revealed the early formation of a supernumerary tooth in the right mandibular premolar region (Figures 2 and 3). There were no reports of supernumerary teeth in the family. Due to its location, surgical removal was indicated.

Before beginning the second phase of the treatment, additional tests and a new panoramic radiograph were requested, which revealed the formation of a supplemental supernumerary tooth, this time in the left mandibular premolar region (Figure 4), which was also surgically removed.

Control panoramic radiographs taken at two different moments along the orthodontic treatment demonstrated no evidence of further supernumerary teeth (Figure 5).

Case 2. A male, leucoderma, Brazilian patient, aged 9 years and 11 months, presenting Class 3 malocclusion, sought a private clinic for orthodontic treatment, which was planned in two phases (interceptive and corrective), to be completed with orthognathic surgery. Similarly to Case 1, the initial panoramic radiographs revealed no abnormalities in the dentition (Figures 6 and 7).

In the first phase of the orthodontic treatment, a modified HAAS expander associated with a facial mask was used for 8 months. Two years later, a new expander and facial mask were recommended for further 6 months.

During the planning of the second phase of the treatment, with complete permanent dentition, an orthodontic/surgical

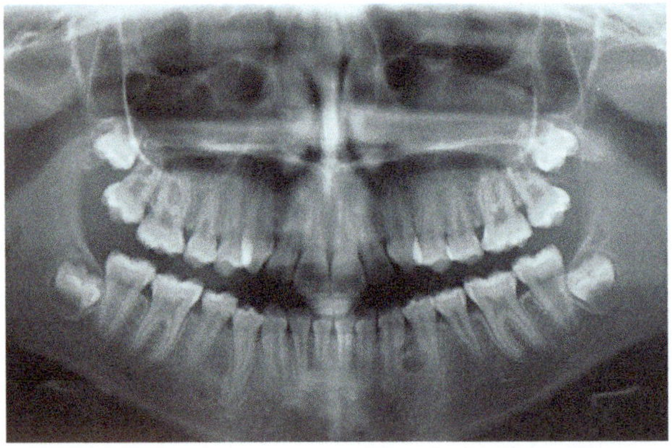

FIGURE 4: Panoramic radiograph of the patient aged 11 years and 3 months showing the early formation of a supplemental supernumerary tooth in the left mandibular premolar region.

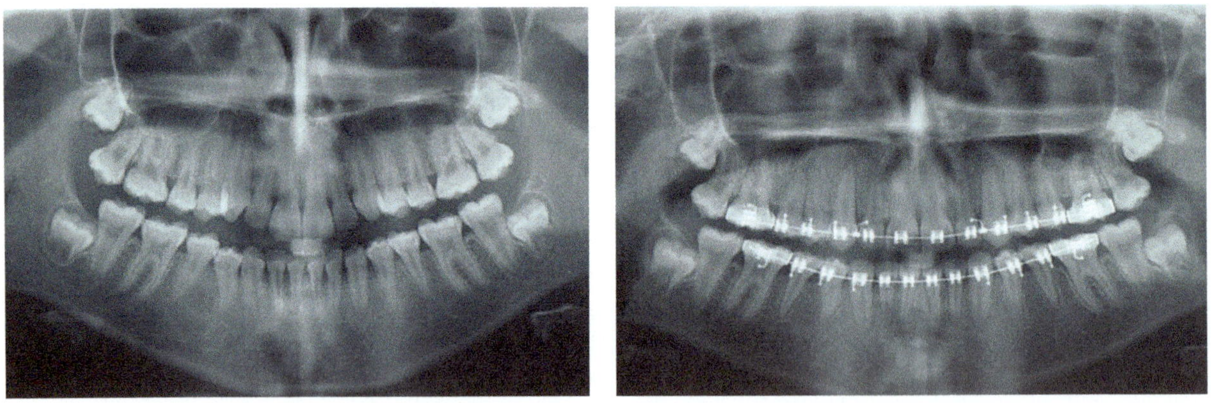

(a) (b)

FIGURE 5: Panoramic radiographs of the patient aged (a) 12 years and 5 months and (b) 13 years and 7 months with no evidence of further supernumerary teeth.

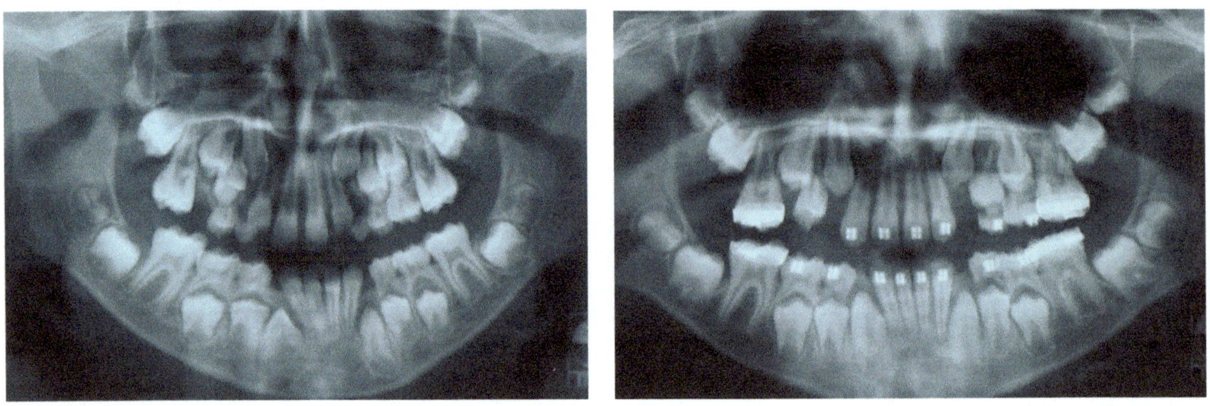

(a) (b)

FIGURE 6: Panoramic radiographs of the patient aged (a) 9 years and 11 months and (b) 10 years and 4 months with no evidence of supernumerary teeth.

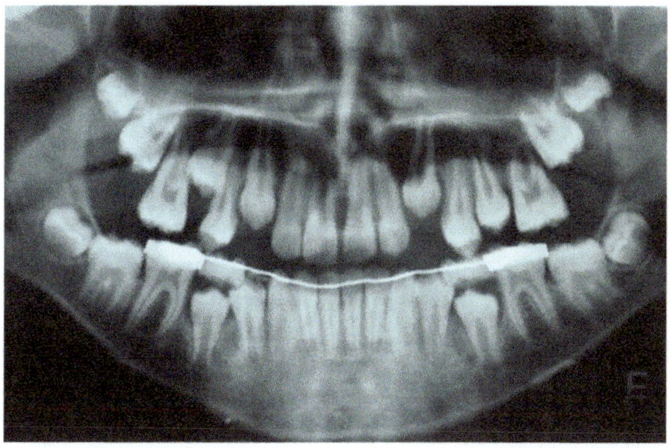

Figure 7: Panoramic radiograph of the patient aged 11 years and 10 months with no evidence of supernumerary teeth.

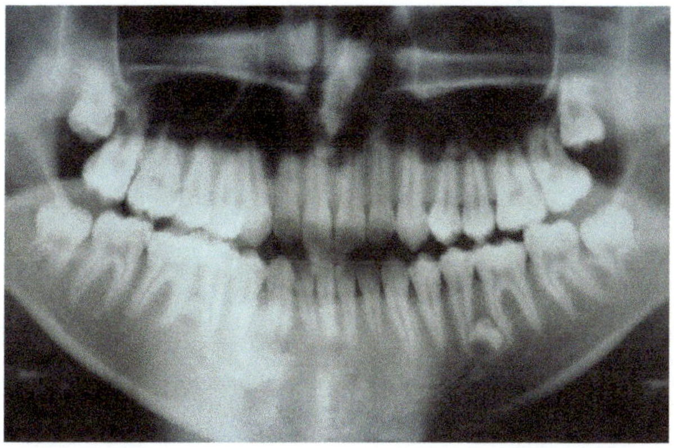

Figure 8: Panoramic radiograph of the patient aged 16 years showing the early formation of 3 supernumerary teeth in the right and left mandibular premolar region and in the left maxillary premolar region.

approach was deemed necessary after facial growth had been completed. When additional tests were performed, the radiographic follow-up revealed the presence of three supernumerary teeth in the premolar region (Figures 8 and 9). Surgical removal of all third molars as well as the 3 supernumerary teeth was performed in a hospital setting under general anesthesia, along with the surgery for the correction of deviated nasal septum (Figure 10).

At 20 years and 5 months, during orthognathic surgery planning, a new radiographic image showed a supplemental supernumerary tooth in the left mandibular premolar region (Figure 11), which was also surgically removed.

3. Discussion

Supernumerary teeth may cause several disorders, such as the displacement, rotation or impaction of permanent teeth, crowding, abnormal or premature diastema, space closure, abnormal or delayed root development, and root resorption, and also lead to the formation of follicular primordial cysts [2, 5, 9, 10, 12, 13].

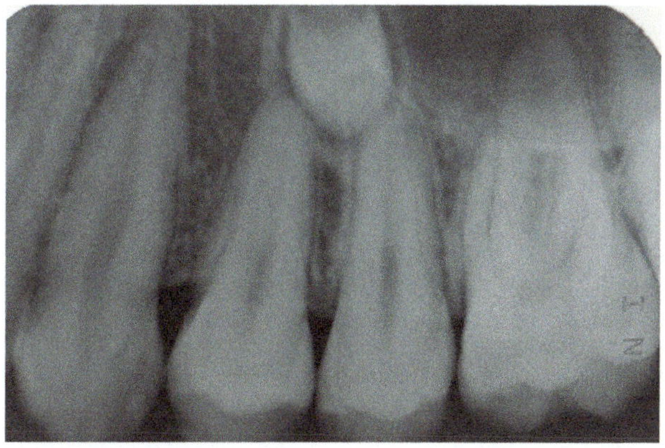

Figure 9: Periapical radiograph of the patient showing a supernumerary tooth in the left maxillary region.

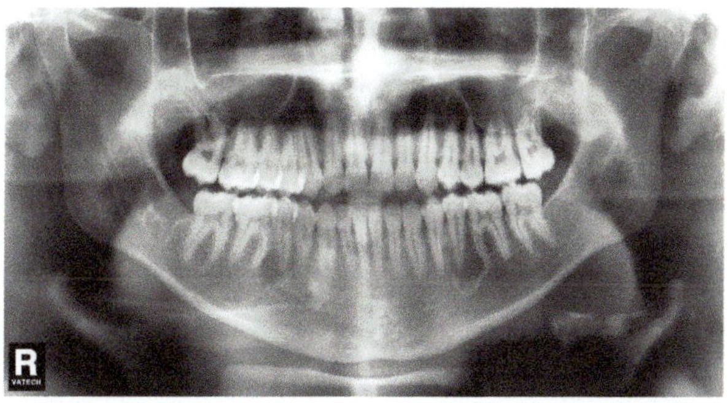

Figure 10: Panoramic radiograph of the patient aged 18 years after the extraction of all supernumerary teeth and third molars.

Currently, the most accepted theory regarding the etiology of supernumerary teeth is localized hyperactivity of the dental lamina [1, 4, 5, 7, 14]. The mobility of the facial process during facial growth can result in the rupture of the dental lamina. If these structures penetrate a region that allows their development, an enamel organ may be formed, resulting in the emergence of a supernumerary tooth. Other theories include genetic factors [15], gender and racial inheritance [5, 9, 10, 12, 13], and the combination of genetic and environmental factors [16]. More than 20 syndromes and developmental conditions appear to be associated with single and multiple supernumerary teeth such as Gardner's syndrome or Cleidocranial Dysplasia [2, 17]. However, the occurrence of supernumerary teeth associated with systemic conditions or syndromes is a rare event [11].

The most common type of supernumerary teeth to sequentially develop is the mandibular premolars [9]. Although supernumerary premolars have been reported bilaterally in both the mandible and maxilla, they occur almost three times more in the mandible than in the maxilla [5]. Supernumerary mandibular teeth tend to maintain their normal shape and size. However, in the maxilla, they are more likely to present alterations, with the conical shape being the most prevalent. Although supernumerary premolars may emerge buccally, they are usually located lingually or centrally in the alveolar

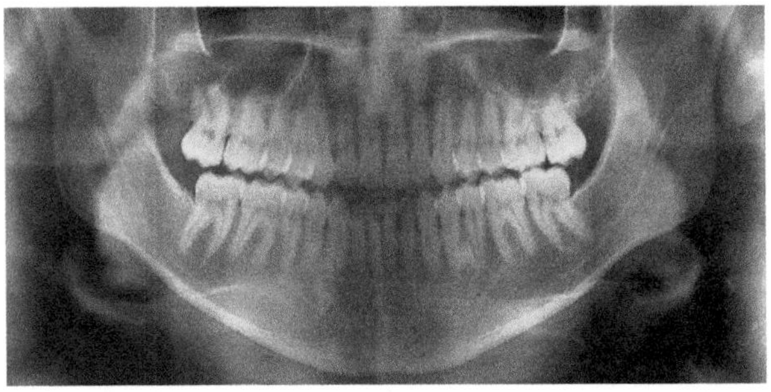

Figure 11: Panoramic radiograph of the patient aged 20 years and 5 months showing a supplemental supernumerary tooth in the left mandibular premolar region.

ridge, which explain the reason why they tend to stay trapped [1].

Third premolars usually develop until the age of 13-14 years [1], that is, 7–11 years after the development of the normal premolars [4]. However, the root formation of third premolars has been reported to occur until the age of 23 years [1]. Although two cases of sequential supernumerary teeth have been reported in the first decade of life [9], the first sequential supernumerary premolars were identified only in the second decade [10].

When a supernumerary tooth is diagnosed, a decision must be made concerning its removal or monitoring. The possible risks and benefits of preserving or surgically extracting a supernumerary tooth must be carefully assessed in each case. Extraction of supernumerary premolars is justified due to the possibility of root resorption of adjacent teeth and the induction of pathological changes, such as cysts [3]. However, in cases when spontaneous eruption is likely, extraction should be delayed to facilitate the surgical procedure and reduce risks [1].

The recurrence of supernumerary teeth may be explained by the incomplete resorption of the dental lamina and the reactivation of a dental follicle portion at the moment when the crown of the permanent tooth is being formed [5]. The late development of supplemental teeth may also be due to the presence of supernumerary teeth crypts that were not detected in the initial radiographs [9].

In a literature review by Solares & Romero [5], the authors reported that recurrence of supernumerary premolars after their surgical removal was 8% and that patients with a previous history of supernumerary teeth in the anterior region were 24% more likely to develop supplemental premolars later. The authors also reported that 75% of all supernumerary premolars remain impacted and asymptomatic, with a 5 : 1 unerupted/erupted ratio [5]. As a result, early diagnosis of supernumerary premolar development is unlikely without timely radiographic assessment [5, 10]. Thus, clinical and radiographic monitoring of patients with previous experience of supernumerary teeth is essential for early diagnosis of supplemental premolars.

It has been previously proposed that radiographic monitoring of patients who develop supernumerary teeth should be periodically performed between 3 and 5 years. However, due to the possible complications mentioned above, it is suggested that this period is reduced to 6 to 12 months, especially in cases where the decision to keep supernumerary teeth in situ is made [5, 10].

4. Conclusion

Considering the late developing of supernumerary premolars, appropriate follow-up with panoramic radiographs of patients with previous experience of supernumerary teeth is essential for early diagnosis of supplemental premolars.

Competing Interests

The authors declare that there are no competing interests regarding the publication of this paper.

References

[1] O. G. Silva Filho, V. D. Picolli, G. A. G. Oliveira, and F. A. Bertoz, "Pré-molares supranumerários tardios: intercorrência remota no período pós-tratamento ortodôntico," *Revista Clínica de Ortodontia Dental Press*, vol. 8, no. 6, pp. 52–59, 2010.

[2] E. Vahid-Dastjerdi, A. Borzabadi-Farahani, M. Mahdian, and N. Amini, "Supernumerary teeth amongst Iranian orthodontic patients. A retrospective radiographic and clinical survey," *Acta Odontologica Scandinavica*, vol. 69, no. 2, pp. 125–128, 2011.

[3] H.-K. Hyun, S.-J. Lee, B.-D. Ahn et al., "Nonsyndromic multiple mandibular supernumerary premolars," *Journal of Oral and Maxillofacial Surgery*, vol. 66, no. 7, pp. 1366–1369, 2008.

[4] R. T. Anegundi, A. Tavargeri, K. R. Indushekar, and P. Sudha, "Sequential development of multiple supplemental premolars. Four-year follow-up report," *The New York State Dental Journal*, vol. 74, no. 1, pp. 46–49, 2008.

[5] R. Solares and M. I. Romero, "Supernumerary premolars: a literature review," *Pediatric Dentistry*, vol. 26, no. 5, pp. 450–458, 2004.

[6] A. Açikgöz, G. Açikgöz, U. Tunga, and F. Otan, "Characteristics and prevalence of non-syndrome multiple supernumerary teeth: a retrospective study," *Dentomaxillofacial Radiology*, vol. 35, no. 3, pp. 185–190, 2006.

[7] A. V. L. Segundo, D. L. B. Faria, U. H. Silva, and I. T. A. Vieira, "Epidemiologic study of supernumerary teeth diagnosed by panoramic radiography," *Revista de Cirurgia e Traumatologia Buco-Maxilo-Facial*, vol. 6, pp. 53–56, 2006.

[8] J. Alvira-González and C. Gay-Escoda, "Non-syndromic multiple supernumerary teeth: meta-analysis," *Journal of Oral Pathology and Medicine*, vol. 41, no. 5, pp. 361–366, 2012.

[9] C. de Oliveira Gomes, B. C. Jham, B. Q. Souki, T. J. Pereira, and R. A. Mesquita, "Sequential supernumerary teeth in nonsyndromic patients: report of 3 cases," *Pediatric Dentistry*, vol. 30, no. 1, pp. 66–69, 2008.

[10] S. R. Moore, D. F. Wilson, and J. Kibble, "Sequential development of multiple supernumerary teeth in the mandibular premolar region—a radiographic case report," *International Journal of Paediatric Dentistry*, vol. 12, no. 2, pp. 143–145, 2002.

[11] W. Z. Yusof, "Non-syndrome multiple supernumerary teeth: literature review," *Journal of the Canadian Dental Association*, vol. 56, no. 2, pp. 147–149, 1990.

[12] L. D. Rajab and M. A. M. Hamdan, "Supernumerary teeth: review of the literature and a survey of 152 cases," *International Journal of Paediatric Dentistry*, vol. 12, no. 4, pp. 244–254, 2002.

[13] M. I. L. Berrocal, J. F. M. Morales, and J. M. M. González, "An observational study of the frequency of supernumerary teeth in a population of 2000 patients," *Medicina Oral, Patología Oral y Cirugía Bucal*, vol. 12, no. 2, pp. E134–E138, 2007.

[14] Y. T. Lin, S. W. Chang, and Y. T. J. Lin, "Delayed formation of multiple supernumerary teeth," *Journal of Dental Sciences*, vol. 4, no. 3, pp. 159–164, 2009.

[15] M. Bozkurt, T. Bezgin, A. T. Öncül, R. Göçer, and F. Sarı, "Late developing supernumeraries in a case of nonsyndromic multiple supernumerary teeth," *Case Reports in Dentistry*, vol. 2015, Article ID 840460, 6 pages, 2015.

[16] M. Hopcraft, "Multiple supernumerary teeth. Case report," *Australian Dental Journal*, vol. 43, no. 1, pp. 17–19, 1998.

[17] H. Sasaki, J. Funao, H. Morinaga, K. Nakano, and T. Ooshima, "Multiple supernumerary teeth in the maxillary canine and mandibular premolar regions: a case in the postpermanent dentition," *International Journal of Paediatric Dentistry*, vol. 17, no. 4, pp. 304–308, 2007.

43

Clinical and Radiological Findings of Autosomal Dominant Osteopetrosis Type II

Priyanka Kant,[1] Neelkamal Sharda,[1] and Rahul R. Bhowate[2]

[1] *Department of Oral Medicine and Radiology, Manav Rachna Dental College, Sector 43, Aravalli Hills, Delhi-Surajkund Road, Faridabad, Haryana 121001, India*
[2] *Department of Oral Medicine and Radiology, Sharad Pawar Dental College and Hospital, Sawangi, Wardha, Maharashtra 442001, India*

Correspondence should be addressed to Priyanka Kant; drpriyankakant@gmail.com

Academic Editors: D. W. Boston, R. S. Brown, M. B. D. Gaviao, M. A. d. A. M. Machado, and S. R. Watt-Smith

Osteopetrosis is a rare inherited genetic disease characterized by sclerosis of the skeleton caused by the absence or malfunction of osteoclasts. Three distinct forms of the disease have been recognized, autosomal dominant osteopetrosis being the most common. Autosomal dominant osteopetrosis exhibits a heterogeneous trait with milder symptoms, often at later childhood or adulthood. The aim of this case report is to present the clinical and radiographic features of a 35-year-old female patient with autosomal dominant osteopetrosis type II who exhibited features of chronic generalised periodontitis, and the radiographs revealed generalised osteosclerosis and hallmark radiographic features of ADO type II, that is, "bone-within-bone appearance" and "Erlenmeyer-flask deformity."

1. Introduction

The term osteopetrosis is derived from the Greek word "osteo" meaning bone and "petros" meaning stone. Osteopetrosis is referred to as "marble bone disease" and "Albers-Schönberg disease", after the German radiologist credited with the first description of the condition in 1904 [1]. Osteopetrosis comprises a clinically and genetically heterogeneous group of conditions that share the hallmark of increased bone density on radiographs. The increase in bone density results from abnormalities in osteoclast differentiation or function [2]. In healthy bone, a steady state is achieved in which production of bone by cells called osteoblasts is balanced by bone resorption by osteoclasts. Dysfunctional osteoclasts that are observed in osteopetrosis result in bony overgrowth, leading to bones that are abnormally dense and brittle. It is believed that osteoclasts fail to release the necessary lysosomal enzymes for bone resorption into the extracellular space [3, 4].

Defects in different genes have been described that lead to a phenotype with osteopetrosis, and mutations in at least 10 genes have been identified as causative in humans. These defects include mutations in the gene encoding carbonic anhydrase II, the proton pump gene, and the chloride channel gene [5, 6]. Recently, the immune response has been incriminated in the pathogenesis of various metabolic bone diseases, including osteopetrosis. Both cytotoxic T lymphocyte-associated antigen 4 and programmed death-1, a newly identified immunoregulatory receptor, have been shown to negatively regulate immune responses and to affect osteoclastogenesis and bone remodeling [7].

This disease has been reported in three clinical forms: (1) malignant infantile form with poor prognosis and autosomal recessive inheritance, (2) benign/adult osteopetrosis with autosomal dominant inheritance and with fewer symptoms, (3) autosomal recessive intermediate form with clinical manifestations similar to malignant form and lowest incidence rate [8–10].

The overall incidence of this condition is difficult to estimate, but autosomal recessive osteopetrosis has an incidence of 1 in 250,000 births [11], and autosomal dominant osteopetrosis has an incidence of 1 in 20,000 live births [8].

Osteopetrotic conditions vary greatly in their presentation and severity, ranging from neonatal onset with life-threatening complications such as bone marrow failure (e.g., classic or "malignant" ARO) to the incidental finding of osteopetrosis on radiographs (e.g., osteopoikilosis) [12]. Table 1 shows a summary of the key clinical manifestations, onset, severity, treatment, and prognosis of the main types of osteopetrosis [12].

Adult osteopetrosis is the most common type of osteopetrosis; it is usually discovered later in life and has a less severe manifestation. In most patients, this pattern is inherited as an autosomal dominant trait and has been termed benign osteopetrosis. Approximately 40% of those affected are asymptomatic, and marrow failure is rare, and most of patients are diagnosed only when osteomyelitis occurs in the mandible. Other symptoms include bone pain, recurrent fractures, back pain, and degenerative arthritis [13]. Bollerslev and Andersen Jr. described two subtypes of benign autosomal dominant osteopetrosis (ADO) on the basis of radiological and clinical differences; these include ADO type I and ADO type II [8].

ADO type I is generally very mild with a diffuse sclerosis without alterations in the bone turnover. Genetic mutations of low-density lipoprotein receptor related protein 5 gene are identified to be responsible for ADO type I thus causing an increased bone formation rather than decreased bone resorption [14, 15]. This phenotype is not associated with an increased fracture rate and is reported to be fully penetrant [8]. Radiographs reveal sclerosis of the skull, which mainly results in increased thickness of the cranial vault; however, the spine does not show much sclerosis. Cranial nerve compression is common in type I [13].

Autosomal dominant osteopetrosis type II was the first type of osteopetrosis recognized and described by Albers-Schonberg in 1904 [1]. In 75% of the cases, osteoclast chloride (CLC7) gene mutation is responsible for the clinical manifestations [12]. ADO type II is the most common form and has an extremely heterogeneous course ranging from an asymptomatic to a severe phenotype. Early death in patients with ADO type II is rare, but some patients can experience a very poor quality of life [16].

Clinical manifestations of ADO type II include hip osteoarthritis caused by excessive toughness of the subchondral bone, facial nerve palsy, mandibular osteomyelitis caused by dental caries and abscesses, and fractures of the long-bones with or without trauma in 75% of the patients. Cranial nerve compression is rare, hearing loss and visual loss occur in fewer than 5% of the affected patients. Many patients undergo several orthopaedic procedures that are often complicated owing to the hardness and the brittleness of their skeletons. However, 20%–40% of the patients remain asymptomatic [17, 18].

Skeletal alterations of patients with ADO type II are so dramatic that the diagnosis is usually easy to ascertain by standard radiographs. Radiographically, sclerosis predominates, in several sites, including the spine (vertebral end-plate thickening, or Rugger-Jersey spine), the pelvis ("bone-within-bone" structures), and the cranial base. Erlenmeyer-shaped femoral metaphysis and transverse bands of osteosclerosis are observed in the long bones. However, the radiological penetrance is only 60%–90% [12].

Due to therarity of the disease and paucity of reported cases of autosomal dominant osteopetrosis type II in the literature, the purpose of this paper is to report a case of ADO type II in a 35-year-old female patient.

2. Case Description

A 35-year-old female patient reported with the chief complaint of deposits on teeth from the past 6-7 months. While recording the case history, the patient complained of intermittent mild pain in the lower back region from the past three months which aggravated on daily activity and was relieved by rest, and pain was radiating to both the lower limbs. Patient gave no history of previous fractures or swellings elsewhere in the body. There was no history of trauma and fractures in any other part of the body.

General examination revealed a short stature, thin built with normal skin and gait. There was pallor present in the palpebral conjunctiva, nails, and the palms. On extraoral examination hypertelorism, exophthalmos, depressed nasal bridge, broad face, and a prognathic mandible were noted.

Intraoral examination revealed generalised gingival inflammation, generalised shallow pockets, and gingival recession with lower anterior teeth. No caries, mobility, attrition, abrasion, and so forth were noted in any of the teeth. A provisional diagnosis of chronic generalised periodontitis was made.

Panoramic radiograph showed signs of early periodontitis with generalised mild to moderate bone loss around teeth. Generalised marked increase in the bone density, lack of distinct lamina dura, and altered trabecular pattern were noted in both jaws; the trabeculae were coarse, dense, and increased in number. Right side of the mandible showed obliteration of the inferior alveolar canal, and cotton wool appearance of the trabeculae was noted at the right angle of the mandible. Left side of the mandible was comparatively less affected, showing an increase in bone density but no cotton wool appearance and no frank obliteration of the inferior alveolar canal. The trabeculae were dense in both sides of the maxilla, the zygomatic complex appeared hyper dense on both the sides, and the maxillary sinus was hypoplastic bilaterally (Figure 1).

After noting these features, the patient was subjected to further radiographic examination to study the skull, paranasal sinuses and the cervical spine (PNS, submentovertex, lateral skull, and cervical spine) which revealed increased bone density of all the bones of the skull, face, and the cervical spine. These views revealed thickening of the cortical boundaries of all the bones with obliteration of the marrow spaces. Lateral skull view revealed thickening of the inner and outer cortical tables and widening of the diploic space (Figure 2). The base of the skull appeared highly radiodense with loss of trabecular pattern, and there was hypoplasia of foramen magnum, and other foramina were obliterated (Figure 3). The nasal cavity and the sinuses were also hypoplastic showing high areas of radiodensity

Table 1: Summary of the key clinical manifestations, onset, severity, treatment, prognosis, and recurrence risks of the main types of osteopetrosis.

Osteopetrosis subtype	Autosomal recessive osteopetrosis (ARO)			X-linked osteopetrosis, lymphedema, anhidrotic ectodermal dysplasia, and immunodeficiency (OLEDAID)	Intermediate osteopetrosis (IRO)	Autosomal dominant osteopetrosis (Alber's Schönberg disease)
	Classic	Neuropathic	ARO with RTA			
Genetic basis	TCIRG	CLCN7, OSTM1	Carbonic anhydrase II	IKBKG (NEMO)	CLCN7, PLEKHM1	CLCN7
Skeletal manifestations	Increased bone density, diffuse and focal sclerosis of varying severity Modelling defects at metaphyses Pathologic fractures Osteomyelitis Dental abnormalities: tooth eruption defects and dental caries					
Other manifestations	Pancytopenia, extramedullary hematopoiesis, hepatosplenomegaly, cranial nerve compression (II, VII, and VIII), hydrocephalus, and hypocalcemia	As for classic ARO, but primary neurodegeneration, including retinal atrophy	Renal tubular acidosis, developmental delay, intracranial calcification, cranial nerve compression, and rare bone marrow impairement	Anhidrotic ectodermal dysplasia, lymphedema, and immunodeficiency resulting in overwhelming infection	Anaemia and extramedullary hematopoiesis, occasional optic nerve compression	Moderate haematological failure, cranial nerve compression
Onset	Perinatal	Perinatal	Infancy	Infancy	Childhood	Late childhood or adolescence
Severity	Severe	Severe	Moderate	Severe	Mild to moderate	Mild to moderate, occasionally severe
Treatment	Supportive HSCT	Supportive	Supportive May benefit from HSCT	Supportive	Supportive	Supportive
Prognosis	Poor Fatal in Infancy	Poor Fatal in Infancy	Variable	Poor Fatal in early childhood	Variable	Normal life expectancy

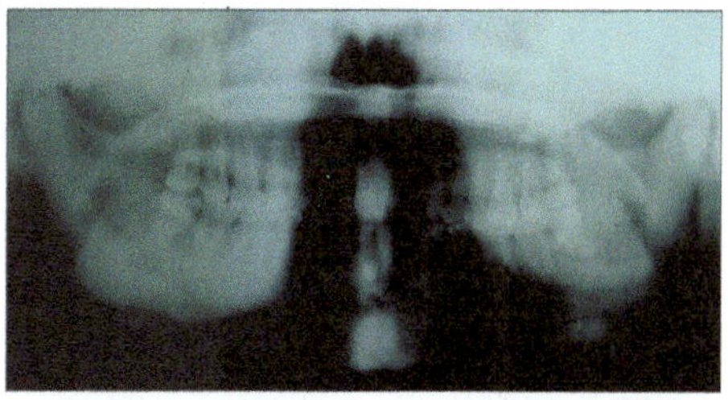

FIGURE 1: Panoramic radiograph showing signs of early periodontitis and sclerosis of the mandible and maxilla.

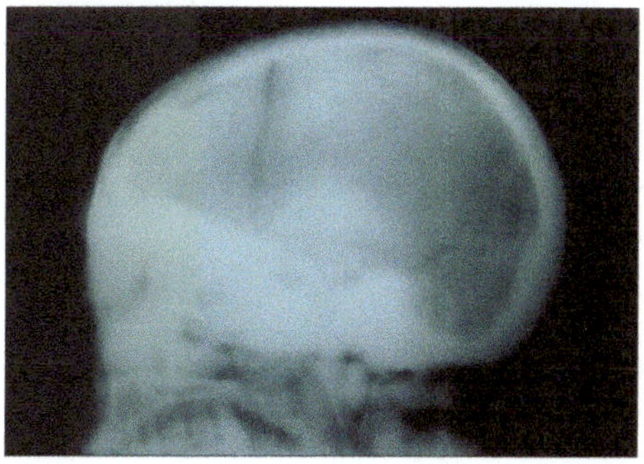

FIGURE 2: Lateral skull view showing thickening of the inner and outer cortical tables and widening of the diploic space.

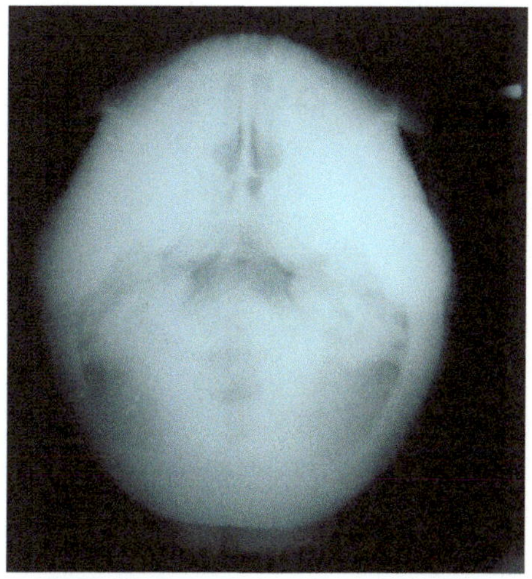

FIGURE 3: Submentovertex view showing increased radiodensity of the base of the skull, hypoplasia of foramen magnum, and obliteration of other foramina.

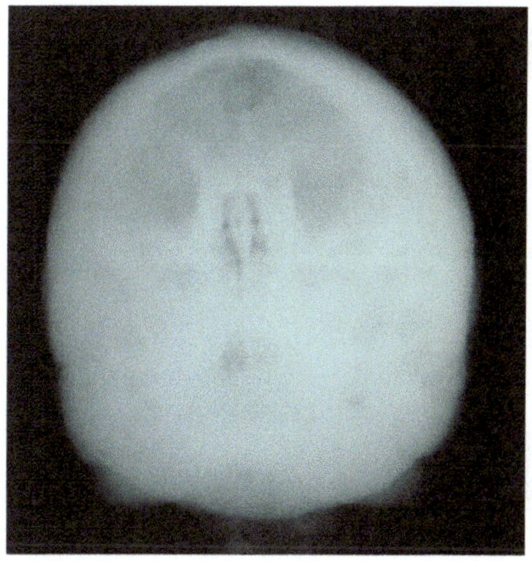

FIGURE 4: PNS view showing osteosclerosis and hypoplasia of sinuses and the nasal cavity.

(Figure 4). Anteroposterior view of cervical spine showed increased radiodensity in all the cervical vertebrae (Figure 5).

Following these findings, the patient was subjected to whole body radiographic survey to rule out the presence of pathological fractures in the bones. Posteroanterior chest radiograph showed a generalised increase in the bone density throughout the thoracic cage and both clavicular bones with normal heart shadow and normal lung fields (Figure 6). Radiograph of the lumbar spine AP and lateral view showed sclerosis at all the levels and "bone-in-bone appearance." Normal spinous processes, normal height, and morphology of the individual vertebrae were noted (Figures 7 and 8). Radiograph of the pelvis showed expanding osteosclerosis of the pelvic bone and the iliac wings (Figure 9). Radiograph of the hip joint showed generalised sclerosis of the pelvic rami and the femur bone (Figure 10). Radiograph of the humerus showing dense sclerosis of the humerus and scapula and "funnel-like appearance" in the humerus (Figure 11). AP view of radius and ulna showed increased radiodensity in all the bones, smoothening of the bone surfaces, and cylindrical metacarpals (Figure 12).

Hematologic investigations showed Hb of 10.8 g/dL, white blood cells 6.5 k/uL, and platelet count 130 k/uL, and ESR was in the normal range. Red cell indices and iron profile were normal. Peripheral smear showed normocytic and normochromic anemia. Renal function and serum electrolytes were within normal limits (creatinine 0.61 mg/dL, sodium 136 mEq/L, and potassium 3.9 mEq/L). Liver function tests were normal (serum bilirubin 0.75 mg/dL, SGOT 20 IU/L, SGPT 18.3 IU/L, alkaline phosphatase 80 IU/L, total protein 7 gms/L, albumin 4.6 gms/L, globulin 3 gms/L), and serum calcium was 8.9 mg/dL, and serum phosphorus was 3.0 mg/dL.

Family history of the patient was unclear. Panoramic radiograph of the patient's brother was also performed, which was normal (Figure 13).

Considering the history, along with clinical, radiological, and laboratory findings and orthopaedician's opinion, a final diagnosis of autosomal dominant osteopetrosis type II was given.

Supragingival, subgingival scaling, and root planning were done for the patient. Patient was also advised to rinse her mouth with 0.2% chlorhexidine gluconate mouth wash twice daily, and topical fluoride application was done. To combat lower back pain, patient was prescribed a topical

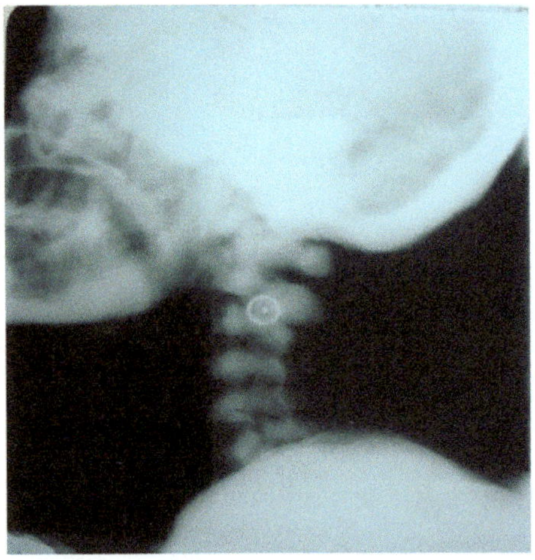

FIGURE 5: Anteroposterior view of the cervical vertebra showing increased radiodensity in all the cervical vertebrae.

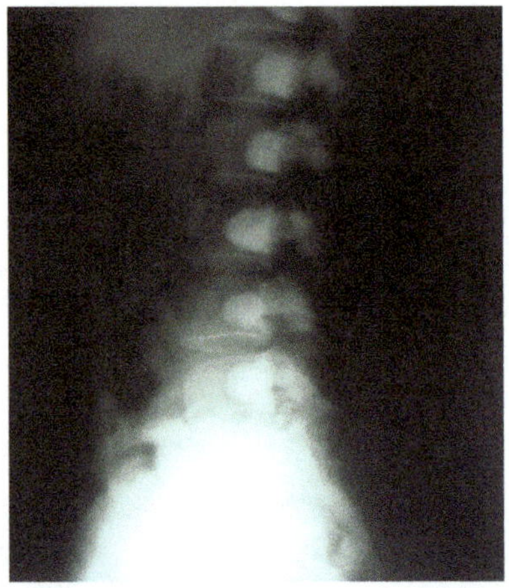

FIGURE 8: Lateral view of the lumbar spine showing "bone-within-bone appearance."

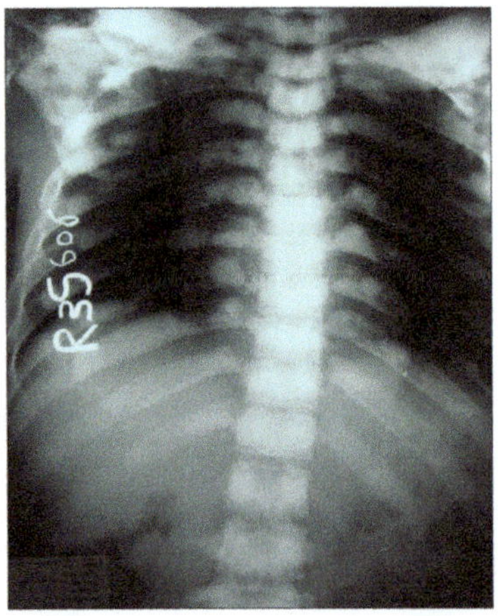

FIGURE 6: PA chest showing generalised osteosclerosis in the thoracic cage and both clavicular bones.

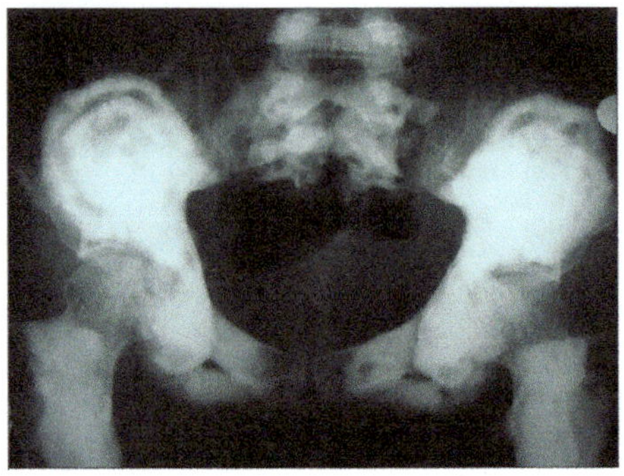

FIGURE 9: Anteroposterior view of the pelvis showing expanding osteosclerosis of the pelvic bone and the iliac wings.

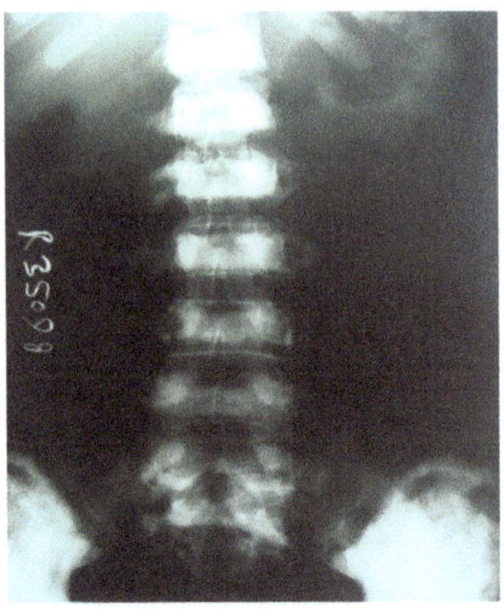

FIGURE 7: Anteroposterior view lumbar spine showing sclerosis at all the levels and "bone-in-bone appearance."

muscle relaxant and analgesic for SOS use. On regular follow-up visits for 6 months, the patient showed no evidence of fractures and osteomyelitis affecting any bone, no signs of cranial nerve involvement and no dental caries and abscesses. The patient also maintained a good oral hygiene. The patient was lost to follow up after 6 months.

3. Discussion

ADO type II is caused by mutation in gene encoding chloride channel 7. Del Fattore et al. reported ClCN7 mutation in 77.8% of the patients [19]. Cleiren et al. reported 7 distinctive mutations in ClCN7 gene in 12 unrelated families with ADO type II [20].

ADO type II is the most common form of osteopetrosis with an estimated prevalence of 1 in 20,000 births. Age of onset of ADO type II is late childhood or adolescence [12]. Del Fattore et al. studied 20 patients with type II autosomal dominant osteopetrosis, the youngest patient being 3 years old and the oldest patient being 63 years old [19]. Waguespack et al. discussed 62 cases with ADO type II, among these 19

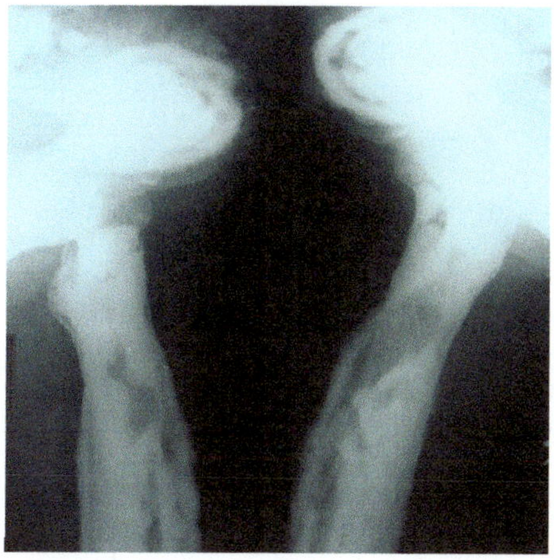

FIGURE 10: Anteroposterior view of the hip joint showed generalised sclerosis of the pelvic rami and the femur bone.

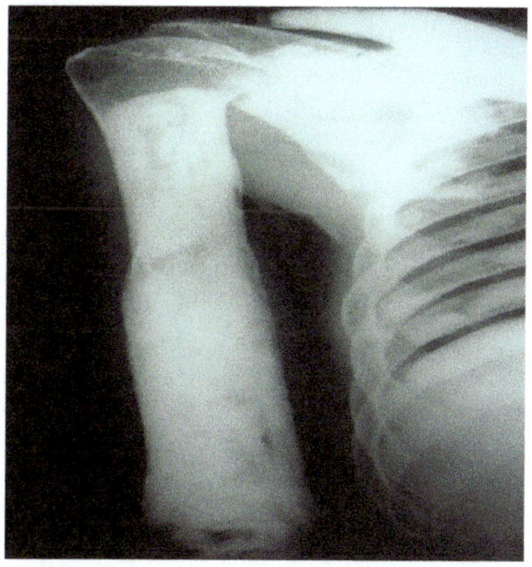

FIGURE 11: Radiograph of the humerus showing osteosclerosis of the humerus and scapula and typical "funnel-like appearance" (Erlenmeyer-flask deformity) in the humerus.

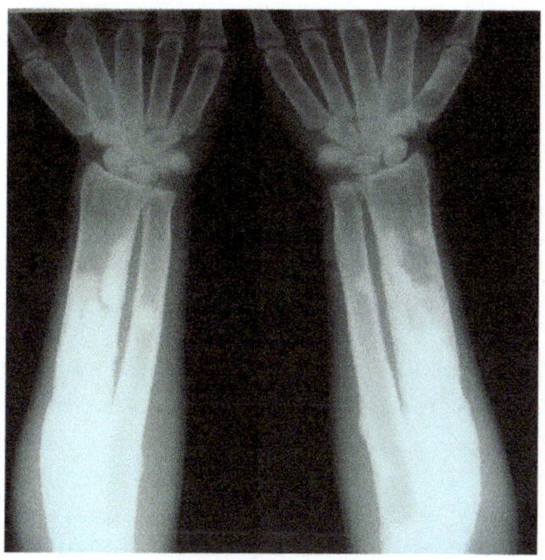

FIGURE 12: Anteroposterior view of radius and ulna showing increased radiodensity in all the bones, smoothening of the bone surfaces, and cylindrical appearance of the metacarpals.

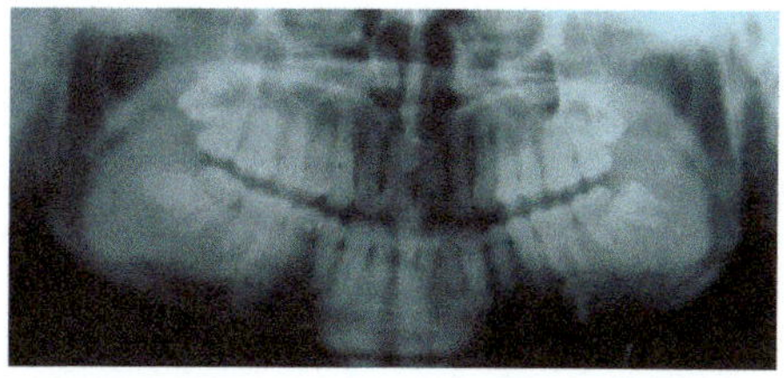

FIGURE 13: Panoramic radiograph of the patient's brother.

patients were ≤18 years of age and 43 patients were >18 years of age [21].

The incidence of autosomal dominant osteopetrosis type II is reported to be the same for males and females. However, 55% of the patients reported by Del Fattore et al. were males and 45% of the patients were females [19]. Waguespack et al. reported a male predominance in their study too [21]. Our patient was a 35-year-old female.

Most individuals diagnosed with autosomal dominant osteopetrosis type II have an affected parent, although in our case the family history was unclear, and a panoramic radiograph of the patient's brother was performed which was normal.

ADO type II has an extremely heterogeneous course ranging from an asymptomatic to a severe phenotype [22]. Clinical manifestations of ADO type II are dominated by long-bone fractures [19]. Other classic manifestations of ADO type II include hip osteoarthritis, scoliosis, and osteomyelitis, particularly affecting the mandible. Cranial nerve compression is a rare complication [23].

Clinical manifestation in the form of diffuse pain was reported in 30% of the patients by Del Fattore et al. with ADO type II and fractures in ≤3 bones was reported in 20% of the patients. 10% of the patients reported fractures in 4–10 bones, and more than 10 bones were fractured in 15% of the patients [19]. Fracture was the most prevalent clinical manifestations occurring in 84% of all ADO type II subjects reported by Waguespack et al., fractures of the pelvis, hip, and femur being most the common (84%) [21]. Clinical manifestations were experienced in 81% of the patients with ADO type II as reported by Bénichou et al. and fractures of femur and ribs being the most common (76%) [16]. El-Tawil and Stoker reported a fracture rate of 62% (femur most common) [24]. 67% fractures most commonly in the appendicular skeleton was reported by Bollerslev and Andersen Jr. [25]. In our case, the patient reported mild pain in the lower back region which was radiating to both the lower limbs, but there was no history of fractures reported in any of the bones, and full body radiographic survey of our patient showed no evidence of fracture in any of the other bones.

Visual impairment and central nervous system involvement is rare in autosomal dominant osteopetrosis type II [12]. Severe visual loss was reported in 19% of the patients by Waguespack et al. [21]. Bénichou et al. reported visual loss in 5% of the patients [16]. There were no signs of visual loss and central nervous system involvement in our case.

Osteomyelitis is the common clinical manifestation in patients with autosomal dominant osteopetrosis type II. Waguespack et al. reported osteomyelitis of the femur in 2 individuals after surgical repair of the fracture [21]. Bénichou et al. [16] reported osteomyelitis in 11% of the patients. Our case had no signs and symptoms of osteomyelitis affecting any of the bones.

The dental changes reported to be associated with osteopetrosis include disturbance of tooth eruption, hypodontia, malformed teeth, multiple caries, enamel dysplasia, abnormal pulp chambers, and hypercementosis [12, 13]. The main complication in patients with autosomal dominant osteopetrosis type II is osteomyelitis, particularly affecting the mandible in association with dental caries and abscess [12]. Waguespack et al. reported osteomyelitis affecting either the maxilla and or mandible in 13% of the patients [21]. Our case showed no abnormalities associated with the teeth, and there was no evidence of osteomyelitis affecting either the maxilla or mandible, but in our case there was early periodontitis with generalised gingival inflammation, shallow pockets, and gingival recession with lower anteriors.

Dental radiographs of patients with ADO type II reveal a generalized increase in radio density of the maxilla and mandible with abnormal trabecular pattern and diminished marrow spaces, constriction of the inferior alveolar nerve canal, and dental pulp canal as well as thickening of the lamina dura. Maxillary sinuses also appear hypoplastic [26]. Panoramic radiograph of our case showed generalised increase in the bone density, lack of distinct lamina dura, and absence of normal trabecular pattern involving both jaws, obliteration of the inferior alveolar nerve canal, cotton wool appearance on the right side of the mandible, and bilateral hypoplasia of the maxillary sinus.

In radiological manifestations of ADO type II, osteosclerosis of the spine predominates, with a "sandwich vertebra" appearance. Most individuals have a "bone-within-bone" appearance primarily in the iliac wings, but also in other bones. Transverse bands of sclerosis, perpendicular to the main axis, are often observed in long bones. Increase in the skull base density can also be seen [16]. Bollerslev and Andersen Jr. reported striking radiographic findings like diffuse systemic osteosclerosis, "rugger jersey spine," and "bone-within-bone appearance" in the pelvis in 15 patients autosomal dominant osteopetrosis type II patients, and the cranial vault was unaffected in almost all the patients [25]. Del Fattore et al. reported generalised osteosclerosis in 43% of the cases, rugger jersey spine was noted in 52.3% of the patients, and 33.3% patients had bone-in-bone appearance [19]. Our patient had hallmark diffuse sclerosis, affecting the skull, spine, pelvis, and appendicular bones; bone modelling defects at the metaphyses of long bones, such as funnel-like appearance ("Erlenmeyer-flask" deformity), and characteristic lucent bands; "bone-within-bone" appearance in the vertebrae.

The differential diagnosis that can be considered includes other sclerosing bone dysplasias, such as pycnodysostosis, craniometaphyseal dysplasia, diaphyseal dysplasia, melorheostosis, osteopoikilosis, and osteopathia striata. Fluoride poisoning and secondary hyperparathyroidism from renal osteodystrophy also may produce a diffuse osteosclerosis [4].

Bone marrow function in benign osteopetrosis is not compromised, and the hematological findings are often normal [12]. Waguespack et al. reported significant bone marrow failure necessitating haematological supportive care in 3% of the patients with ADO type II [21]. However, in our patient hemoglobin was 10.8 g/dL, and white blood cell count and platelet count were in the normal range. Peripheral smear showed normocytic normochromic anemia. Other investigations, that is, renal function test, liver function test, ESR, serum calcium, and serum phosphorus, were also within the normal limit.

The diagnosis of osteopetrosis is based on radiological and clinical features and these findings are sufficiently characteristic to make a definite diagnosis, and there is no need to perform a genetic study to confirm the disease. Furthermore, biopsy must be avoided because of a marked infection risk [26, 27].

At present, no effective medical treatment for osteopetrosis exists. Treatment is largely supportive and is aimed at providing multidisciplinary surveillance and symptomatic management of complications. Fractures and arthritis are common and require treatment by an experienced orthopaedic surgeon due to the brittleness of the bones, and the relatively frequent occurrence of secondary complications such as delayed union or nonunion of fractures and osteomyelitis [12].

Therefore, routine dental surveillance and maintenance of oral hygiene form an integral part of management and play an important role in preventing more severe complications such as osteomyelitis of the mandible [12]. Moreover, teeth should be endodontically treated, if possible, rather than extracted, due to the increased risk of infection. If osteomyelitis occurs, surgical intervention must be considered because antibiotics do not reach the compromised region [17].

In our case scaling, root planning, and topical fluoride application were done, and the patient was instructed to maintain good oral hygiene. The patient was also advised to rinse her mouth with 0.2% chlorhexidine gluconate mouth wash. The patient was prescribed Volini gel (diclofenac diethylamine 1.16%, methyl salicylate 10%, and linseed oil 3%) for topical application twice daily on the lower back. The patient was followed for 6 months, and during this period the patient showed no evidence of fractures and osteomyelitis affecting any bone. No signs of cranial nerve involvement, dental caries, and abscesses were noted. Patient was lost to follow up after 6 months.

4. Conclusion

Benign osteopetrosis is a rare disorder, which might be characterized by an asymptomatic clinical picture. Therefore, a proper clinical and radiographic investigation is essential for accurate diagnosis. Dental problems like delayed tooth eruption, ankylosis, abscesses, cysts, and fistulas are common in patients with benign osteopetrosis. Constriction of the inferior alveolar nerve canal and dental pulp canal and thickening of the lamina dura are routinely seen in dental radiographs because of increased bone density. Therefore, dental practitioners can play an important role in early diagnosis and treatment planning of the patients with benign osteopetrosis. Moreover, because of the high infection risk and increased susceptibility to jaw fracture in these patients, they should receive increased attention and prophylactic dental treatment to maintain their fragile oral health status. Continuous and vigorous preventive measures should be performed for patients to prevent any complications.

References

[1] H. E. Albers-Schonberg, "Rontgenbilder einer seltenen Knockenerkrankung," *Munchener Medizinische Wochenschrift*, vol. 5, pp. 365–368, 1904.

[2] A. Superti-Furga, S. Unger, and The Nosology Group of the International Skeletal Dysplasia Society, "Nosology and classification of genetic skeletal disorders: 2006 revision," *American Journal of Medical Genetics A*, vol. 143, no. 1, pp. 1–18, 2007.

[3] N. K. Wood and P. W. Goaz, *Differential Diagnosis of Oral and Maxillofacial Lesions*, Mosby, St. Louis, Mo, USA, 5th edition, 1991.

[4] S. C. White and M. J. Pharoah, *Oral Radiology Principles and Interpretataion*, Mosby, Philadelphia, Pa, USA, 6th edition, 2009.

[5] S. C. Marks Jr., "Pathogenesis of osteopetrosis in the *ia* rat: reduced bone resorption due to reduced osteoclast function," *The American Journal of Anatomy*, vol. 138, no. 2, pp. 165–189, 1973.

[6] B. H. Schofield, L. S. Levin, and S. B. Doty, "Ultrastructure and lysosomal histochemistry of *ia* rat osteoclasts," *Calcified Tissue Research*, vol. 14, no. 1, pp. 153–160, 1974.

[7] K. Nagahama, K. Aoki, K. Nonaka et al., "The deficiency of immunoregulatory receptor PD-1 causes mild osteopetrosis," *Bone*, vol. 35, no. 5, pp. 1059–1068, 2004.

[8] J. Bollerslev and P. E. Andersen Jr., "Radiological, biochemical and hereditary evidence of two types of autosomal dominant osteopetrosis," *Bone*, vol. 9, no. 1, pp. 7–13, 1988.

[9] D. K. Lam, G. K. B. Sándor, H. I. Holmes, R. P. Carmichael, and C. M. L. Clokie, "Marble bone disease: a review of osteopetrosis and its oral health implications for dentists," *Journal of the Canadian Dental Association*, vol. 73, no. 9, pp. 839–843, 2007.

[10] S. G. Kahler, J. A. Burns, and A. S. Aylsworth, "A mild autosomal recessive form of osteopetrosis," *American Journal of Medical Genetics*, vol. 17, no. 2, pp. 451–464, 1984.

[11] R. Loria Cortes, E. Quesada Calvo, and C. Cordero Chaverri, "Osteopetrosis in children: a report of 26 cases," *Journal of Pediatrics*, vol. 91, no. 1, pp. 43–47, 1977.

[12] Z. Stark and R. Savarirayan, "Osteopetrosis," *Orphanet Journal of Rare Diseases*, vol. 4, article 5, 2009.

[13] M. Öğütcen-Toller, M. Tek, I. Şener, C. Bereket, S. Inal, and B. Özden, "Intractable bimaxillary osteomyelitis in osteopetrosis: review of the literature and current therapy," *Journal of Oral and Maxillofacial Surgery*, vol. 68, no. 1, pp. 167–175, 2010.

[14] K. Henriksen, J. Gram, P. Hoegh-Andersen et al., "Osteoclasts from patients with autosomal dominant osteopetrosis type I caused by a T253I mutation in low-density lipoprotein receptor-related protein 5 are normal in vitro, but have decreased resorption capacity in vivo," *The American Journal of Pathology*, vol. 167, no. 5, pp. 1341–1348, 2005.

[15] E. Van Hul, J. Gram, J. Bollerslev et al., "Localization of the gene causing autosomal dominant osteopetrosis type I to chromosome 11q12-13," *Journal of Bone and Mineral Research*, vol. 17, no. 6, pp. 1111–1117, 2002.

[16] O. D. Bénichou, J. D. Laredo, and M. C. de Vernejoul, "Type II autosomal dominant osteopetrosis (Albers-Schonberg disease): clinical and radiological manifestations in 42 patients," *Bone*, vol. 26, no. 1, pp. 87–93, 2000.

[17] E. Tohidi and A. Bagherpour, "Clinicoradiological findings of benign osteopetrosis: report of two new cases," *Journal of Dental Research, Dental Clinics, Dental*, vol. 6, no. 4, pp. 152–157, 2012.

[18] K. Chu, R. Snyder, and M. J. Econs, "Disease status in autosomal dominant osteopetrosis type 2 is determined by osteoclastic properties," *Journal of Bone and Mineral Research*, vol. 21, no. 7, pp. 1089–1097, 2006.

[19] A. Del Fattore, B. Peruzzi, N. Rucci et al., "Clinical, genetic, and cellular analysis of 49 osteopetrotic patients: implications for diagnosis and treatment," *Journal of Medical Genetics*, vol. 43, no. 4, pp. 315–325, 2006.

[20] E. Cleiren, O. Bénichou, E. Van Hul et al., "Albers-Schönberg disease (autosomal dominant osteopetrosis, type II) results from mutations in the ClCN7 chloride channel gene," *Human Molecular Genetics*, vol. 10, no. 25, pp. 2861–2867, 2001.

[21] S. G. Waguespack, S. L. Hui, L. A. DiMeglio, and M. J. Econs, "Autosomal dominant osteopetrosis: clinical severity and natural history of 94 subjects with a chloride channel 7 gene mutation," *Journal of Clinical Endocrinology & Metabolism*, vol. 92, no. 3, pp. 771–778, 2007.

[22] B. M. Rashid, N. G. Rashid, A. Schulz, G. Lahr, and B. F. Nore, "A novel missense mutation in the CLCN7 gene linked to benign autosomal dominant osteopetrosis: a case series," *Journal of Medical Case Reports*, vol. 7, article 7, 2013.

[23] E. Cleiren, O. Bénichou, E. Van Hul et al., "Albers-Schönberg disease (autosomal dominant osteopetrosis, type II) results from mutations in the ClCN7 chloride channel gene," *Human Molecular Genetics*, vol. 10, no. 25, pp. 2861–2867, 2001.

[24] T. El-Tawil and D. J. Stoker, "Benign osteopetrosis: a review of 42 cases showing two different platterns," *Skeletal Radiology*, vol. 22, no. 8, pp. 587–593, 1993.

[25] J. Bollerslev and P. E. Andersen Jr., "Fracture patterns in two types of autosomal-dominant osteopetrosis," *Acta Orthopaedica Scandinavica*, vol. 60, no. 1, pp. 110–112, 1989.

[26] C. M. Garcia, M. A. P. Garcia, R. G. Garcia, and F. M. Gil, "Osteomyelitis of the mandible in a patient with osteopetrosis. Case report and review of literarure," *Journal of Oral and Maxillofacial Surgery*, vol. 3, no. 1, pp. 120–125, 2011.

[27] C. Krithika, R. S. Neelakandan, B. Sivapathasundaram, D. Koteeswaran, P. C. Rajaram, and G. S. Shetkar, "Osteopetrosis-associated osteomyelitis of the jaws: a report of 4 cases," *Oral Surgery, Oral Medicine, Oral Pathology, Oral Radiology and Endodontology*, vol. 108, no. 3, pp. e56–e65, 2009.

44

Recurrent Monostotic Fibrous Dysplasia in the Mandible

Nilton Alves,[1] Reinaldo José de Oliveira,[2] Denise Takehana,[2] and Naira Figueiredo Deana[3]

[1]*CIMA Research Group, Faculty of Dentistry, La Frontera University, 1145 Francisco Salazar Avenue, P.O. Box 54-D, 4780000 Temuco, Chile*
[2]*Faculty of Sciences of Guarulhos (FACIG), 1844 Guarulhos Avenue, 7196 Guarulhos, SP, Brazil*
[3]*Private Physical Therapist, 1171 Pasaje Frankfurt, 4780000 Temuco, Chile*

Correspondence should be addressed to Nilton Alves; niltonnalves@yahoo.com.br

Academic Editor: Giuseppe Colella

Fibrous dysplasia (FD) is a condition in which normal bone marrow is replaced by an abnormal proliferation of new fibrous connective tissue. Female patient, white, 20 years old, attended the dental clinic reporting a slow increase in volume in the right mandible region over the last 5 years. She was examined by imaging: the panoramic X-ray revealed a lesion with the appearance of ground glass while the cone-beam computed tomography showed an extensive lesion in the region of the right hemimandible. The histopathological examination was compatible with fibrous dysplasia. Bone gammagraphy was indicated, plus an endocrinological study to eliminate polyostotic forms, which produced a negative result. Monostotic fibrous dysplasia in the right hemimandible was diagnosed. Conservative surgery was carried out and after 1 year recurrence of the tumour was observed. We may conclude that conservative surgery might not be the best choice for treatment for monostotic fibrous dysplasia in the mandible and that other options must be considered, such as radical surgery or the use of bisphosphonates. In our study, we may also conclude that it is very important to explain to the patient the possibility of recurrence of the lesion and the need for monitoring with periodic imaging studies.

1. Introduction

Fibrous dysplasia (FD) is a condition in which normal bone marrow is replaced by an abnormal proliferation of new fibrous connective tissue [1, 2].

FD is caused by the genetic mutation of the cell-surface receptor guanine nucleotide protein (G protein) [3]. The α-subunit of the stimulatory G protein ($G_S\alpha$) activates the adenylyl cyclase, which in turn catalyzes the formation of cyclic adenosine monophosphate from ATP [4]. The gene for $G_S\alpha$ (GNAS1), when it suffers a mutation, is associated with the FD disorder spectrum. This mutation occurs in a somatic cell producing somatic mosaicism, in which the cells descending from the mutated cell produce abnormal characteristics, while the cells descending from the unaffected cells produce normal characteristics [5]. The increase in the activity of stimulatory G protein (G_S) in osteoblast progenitor cells is thought to be the result of an increase in their proliferation and abnormal differentiation. Studies have established a link between the $G_S\alpha$ mutation and the increased production of interleukin-6 stromal cells, which promotes osteoclast activity [6]. Thus, the complex of the FD pathogenesis arises from an imbalance between bone formation and destruction [7].

It generally appears in the first or second decade of life; it is asymptomatic, progresses slowly, and affects women twice as frequently as men [1, 2]. It affects the maxilla more frequently than the mandible and may involve one (monostotic) or less commonly two or more bones (polyostotic) [1]. The signs and symptoms vary depending on the type and location of the FD and include facial deformity and asymmetry, visual alteration, auditory disability, nasal congestion and/or obstruction, pain, paraesthesia, or malocclusion [8]. The dental arch is usually maintained, although tooth displacement, malocclusion, and interference with dental eruption may occur occasionally [1].

The object of this paper is to present a case of recurrent monostotic fibrous dysplasia in the mandible region, which

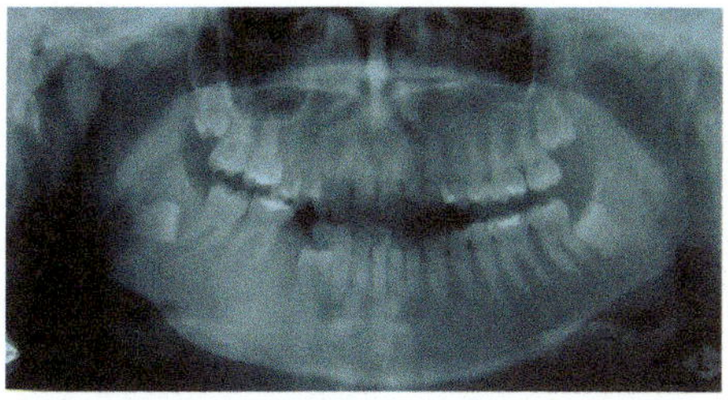

FIGURE 1: Panoramic X-ray (2005) showing alteration in the cancellous bone of the right hemimandible.

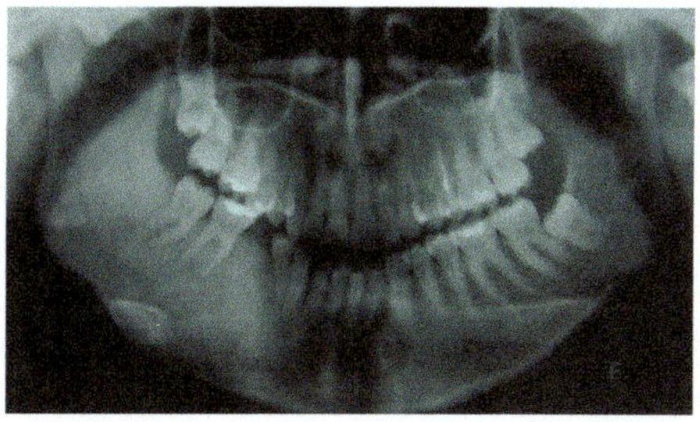

FIGURE 2: Panoramic X-ray (2009) showing radioopaque area of the image with the appearance of ground glass in the right hemimandible. It can be seen that pieces 4.5 and 4.8 have been removed.

was studied by imaging, with incisional biopsy for definitive diagnosis. Bone remodelling was carried out to improve the patient's facial contour.

2. Case Report

Female patient, white, 20 years old, with no systemic history, attended the dental clinic in 2005 reporting a slow, painless increase in volume in the mandible region (right side) over the last 5 years, producing facial deformity. During physical examination facial asymmetry was observed due to an increase in the size of the mandibular body on the right side, of solid consistency, pain-free, and without adenomegalies. Intraoral examination showed a hard-textured increase in the alveolar ridge on the right side; the adjacent mucous tissue was normal. A panoramic X-ray was done (Figure 1) in which alteration was observed in the pattern of the cancellous bone in the right hemimandible; it was then decided to do an incisional biopsy, resulting in a definitive diagnosis of fibrous dysplasia. Bone gammagraphy was indicated plus an endocrinological study to eliminate polyostotic forms which produced a negative result. Monostotic fibrous dysplasia in the right hemimandible was diagnosed. The treatment options were discussed jointly and it was decided to carry out monitoring with a sequence of imaging studies, with the patient being recalled for control.

When the patient returned for control four years later, in 2009, she expressed interest in treating the facial deformity produced by the pathology. She reported that she had received surgical treatment to remove two teeth which were retained in the mandible on the right side. After clinical examination, a panoramic X-ray was done (Figure 2) in which it was observed that pieces 4.5 and 4.8, which were retained, had been removed. Furthermore there was a radioopaque area of the image with the appearance of ground glass in the right hemimandible. A more detailed examination by cone-beam computed tomography (CBCT) not only confirmed the existence of the bone lesion in the right hemimandible (Figure 3), but also allowed the location and extent of the tumour to be determined precisely, from which the surgical procedure indicated could be planned correctly. A conservative surgical treatment was carried out, removing some bone (Figure 4) and remodelling the region affected by the deformity. The patient was asked to return for monitoring through a sequence of imaging studies. When the patient returned for control after four years, in 2013, clinical and X-ray examination revealed recurrence of the lesion. Figure 5 presents the panoramic X-ray showing a radioopaque area of the image with the appearance of ground glass in the right hemimandible. Figure 6 is the intraoral appearance in which an increase of the alveolar ridge on the right side can be observed. Figure 7 shows the 3D reconstruction by cone-beam computed tomography (anterior and lateral views) with an increase in the volume of the right hemimandible, confirming mandibular asymmetry. The patient has been advised to continue with monitoring by sequential imaging studies.

3. Discussion

Craniofacial bones are affected in approximately 30% of cases of FD [9]. In a retrospective study of 25 patients, the mandible was the primary site of the tumour in 76% of cases. It may appear in the premolar and molar region, that is, from the mental foramen towards the angle of the mandible; the anterior part of the mandible is least affected [2].

Asymmetry and oedema are the most common complaints when FD is found in the bones of the facial skeleton [2]. Other symptoms such as malocclusion of the teeth, pain, distortion of facial contour, alveolar abscess, and cellulitis in the face are also reported in the literature [2, 10]. In our case the patient's main complaint was facial asymmetry, but malocclusion of the teeth and distortion of facial contour were also present.

Tumours in young patients or recent tumours present a cyst-like appearance. The smallest mandibular tumour was 1.5 cm in diameter [2]. In general small tumours are unilocular while larger tumours are multilocular. The majority of lesions caused by FD presented large, irregular cancellous zones, with mottled appearance because of other masses of calcified material.

The preferred imaging examination is cone-beam computed tomography, since it offers a broader view of the extent and location of the lesion, which helps in planning the surgical procedure [11]. The most frequent X-ray characteristic of craniofacial FD is "ground glass" appearance with a fine cortex and no defined borders [12]; this was the kind of image found in examination of our patient. Ogunsalu et al.

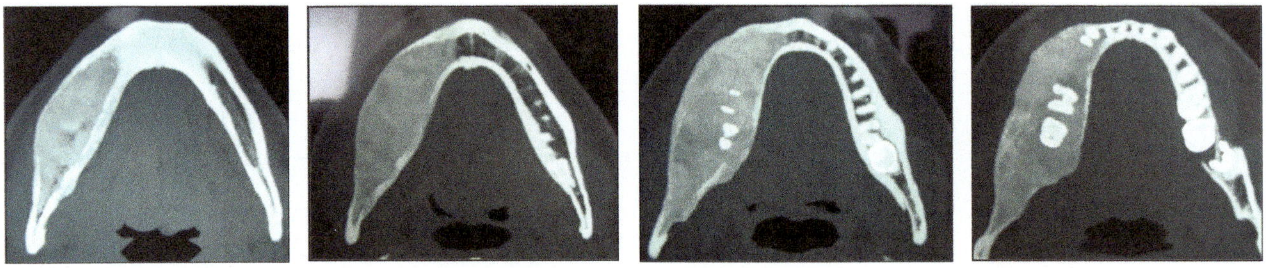

FIGURE 3: Axial sections by cone-beam computed tomography showing increase in the size of the mandibular body on the right side.

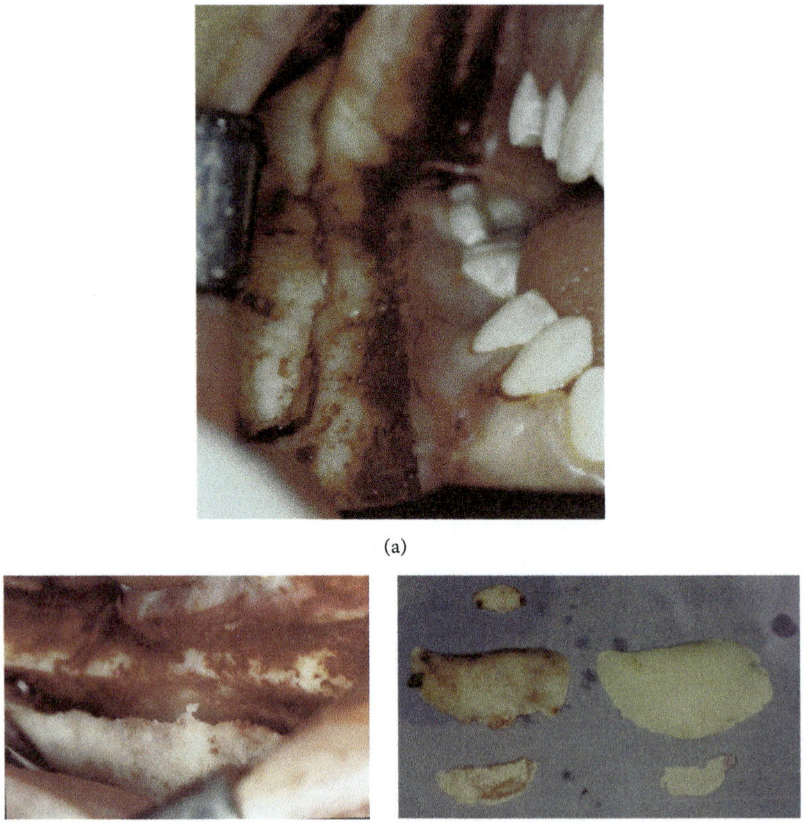

(a)

(b)

(c)

FIGURE 4: (a and b) Photographs of the surgical procedure; (c) photograph of surgical pieces removed.

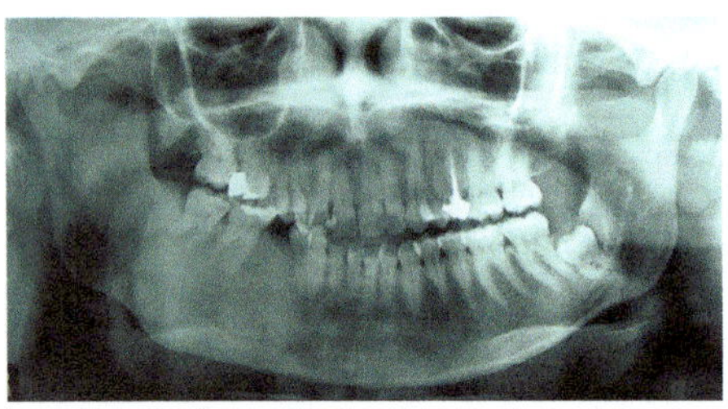

FIGURE 5: Panoramic X-ray (2013) showing radioopaque area of the image with the appearance of ground glass in the right hemi-mandible. Recurrence of the lesion.

[12] propose the following categories of X-ray appearance: (1) orange peel/ground glass appearance; (2) opacification of the antrum; (3) radiolucent lesion of the mandible; and (4) varying degrees of opacification (not ground glass and not orange peel).

Hart et al. [13], in a study of 266 bone gammagraphy images in 66 patients, showed that 90% of FD lesions, regardless of site, were present before the age of 15. However the literature reports cases of adults developing FD. Ogunsalu et al. [12] studied 15 cases of patients with FD in the maxilla and mandible, reporting that in 10 cases the lesions presented

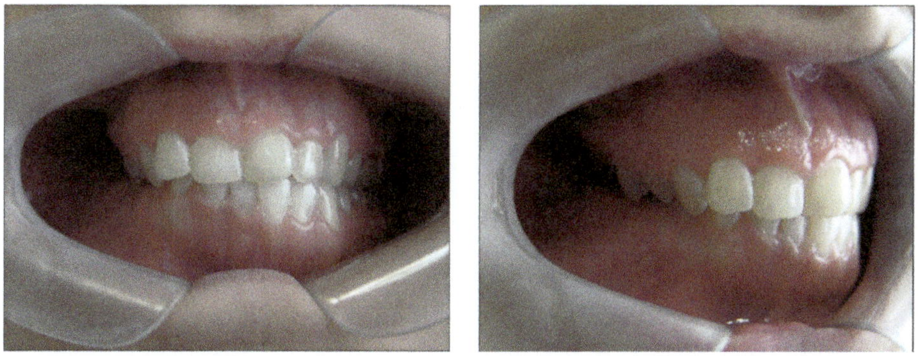

(a) (b)

FIGURE 6: (a) Anterior and (b) anterolateral view of the intraoral region showing an increase in the alveolar ridge in the right hemimandible.

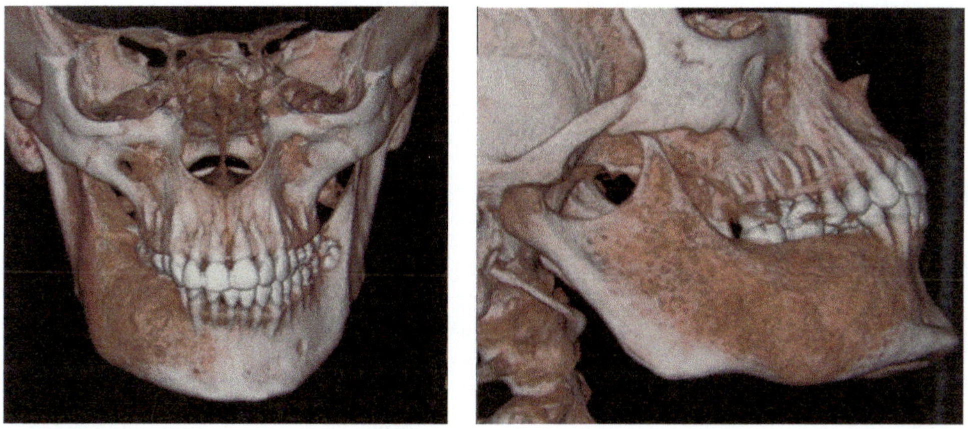

(a) (b)

FIGURE 7: 3D reconstruction by cone-beam computed tomography showing an increase in the volume of the right hemimandible. (a) Anterior view and (b) lateral view.

initially after the age of 20 and in 2 cases at the age of 47. Pinsolle et al. [14] studied 25 patients with FD of the craniofacial bone aged between 8 and 56 years. 70–80% of cases of monostotic FD occur in the second and third decade of life [15, 16]. In our study the patient presented the initial lesion before the age of 15.

Some authors report that growth of this lesion tends to stop around puberty [17]; however other studies indicate that its progression is continuous into adulthood [18]. In our study the patient reported that growth started at puberty, contradicting the literature. Another important fact is that approximately 20–25% of these tumours continue to grow after treatment, regardless of the type of therapy applied, except if they are extirpated radically, it is impossible to prognosticate whether the FD will recur or not [2, 19].

Primary treatment of mandibular lesions always includes correction of asymmetries and deformities and/or prevention of functional problems by conservative surgery which can be carried out regardless of the size of the lesion; this is the technique indicated by many authors [2, 9, 20]. In our case we performed excision of the tumour using a conservative procedure. After 1 year growth of the lesion was observed in the same region, from which we concluded that conservative treatment was insufficient in this case. In a retrospective study of 68 patients, including 19 cases of monostotic FD and 2 cases of polyostotic FD involving the mandible, Valentini et al. [21] reported that there was no case of recurrence when radical resection of the lesion was applied; further surgery due to recurrence of the tumour was necessary in only one case of FD in a mandible which had received conservative treatment. These authors consider that radical surgery prevents recurrence and is the only option for eliminating the disease. Treatment options apart from surgery and drugs for pain control are limited, but one alternative for the treatment of FD is the use of bisphosphonates. Bisphosphonates are drugs that reduce osteoclast activity when they bind to the bone surfaces, particularly those subjected to active resorption, which acts as a biochemical barrier for bone resorption [22]. Its use in adult patients has presented good results in the control of FD, inhibiting progression of the disease once treatment has begun [23]. The use of this drug promotes reduced bone pain, a decrease in biochemical markers of bone turnover, and a radiographically apparent "refilling of osteolytic sites" in some patients [24]. However, prolonged use must be monitored because it can cause an increase in bone mineral density [23]. One important side effect caused by the use of bisphosphonates is osteonecrosis of the jaw [25, 26]. In addition, it is known that the medication remains in the skeleton for a long time and caution is recommended for use in women of child-bearing age [27]. In our study the patient presented a good health condition, but as a young female patient the decision was made not to treat with bisphosphonates.

Considering that there was recurrence in our case and that similar cases are reported in the literature, we may conclude that conservative surgery may not be the best choice for treatment for monostotic fibrous dysplasia in the mandible and that other options must be considered, such as radical surgery or the use of bisphosphonates. It is important for the dentist to analyze each case of FD, taking aspects like gender, age, recurrence, extent of the lesion, and the involvement of adjacent structures into consideration in order to choose the best treatment for each patient. In our study we may also conclude that it is very important to explain to the patient the possibility of recurrence of the lesion and the need for monitoring with periodic imaging studies.

Competing Interests

The authors declare that they have no competing interests.

Acknowledgments

The authors want to thank Dr. Ricardo Wagner Modes for provided images.

References

[1] J. A. Regezi, J. J. Sciubba, and R. C. K. Jordan, *Oral Pathology: Clinical Pathologic Correlations*, Saunders, Philadelphia, Pa, USA, 4th edition, 2003.

[2] J. S. Lee, E. J. Fitzgibbon, Y. R. Chen et al., "Clinical guidelines for the management of craniofacial fibrous dysplasia," *Orphanet Journal of Rare Diseases*, vol. 7, supplement 1, article S2, 2012.

[3] M. M. Cohen Jr. and R. E. Howell, "Etiology of fibrous dysplasia and McCune–Albright syndrome," *International Journal of Oral and Maxillofacial Surgery*, vol. 28, no. 5, pp. 366–371, 1999.

[4] M. A. Levine, W. S. Modi, and S. J. O'Brien, "Mapping of the gene encoding the α subunit of the stimulatory G protein of adenylyl cyclase (GNAS1) to 20q13.2 $\rightarrow$ q13.3 in human by in situ hybridization," *Genomics*, vol. 11, no. 2, pp. 478–479, 1991.

[5] H. Youssoufian and R. E. Pyeritz, "Mechanisms and consequences of somatic mosaicism in humans," *Nature Reviews Genetics*, vol. 3, no. 10, pp. 748–758, 2002.

[6] M. Riminucci, S. A. Kuznetsov, N. Cherman, A. Corsi, P. Bianco, and P. Gehron Robey, "Osteoclastogenesis in fibrous dysplasia of bone: in situ and in vitro analysis of IL-6 expression," *Bone*, vol. 33, no. 3, pp. 434–442, 2003.

[7] K. Chao and L. Katznelson, "Use of high-dose oral bisphosphonate therapy for symptomatic fibrous dysplasia of the skull," *Journal of Neurosurgery*, vol. 109, no. 5, pp. 889–892, 2008.

[8] N. Alves, "Monostotic craniofacial fibrous dysplasia: how should it be diagnosed?" *International Journal of Odontostomatology*, vol. 7, no. 2, pp. 221–224, 2013.

[9] Y.-R. Chen, F.-H. Wong, C. Hsueh, and L.-J. Lo, "Computed tomography characteristics of non-syndromic craniofacial fibrous dysplasia," *Chang Gung medical journal*, vol. 25, no. 1, pp. 1–8, 2002.

[10] L. C. England, "Fibrous dysplasia of the mandible: case report and analysis (monostotic fibrous dysplasia)," *Oral Surgery, Oral Medicine, Oral Pathology*, vol. 1, no. 12, pp. 1085–1091, 1948.

[11] D. C. Zimmerman, D. C. Dahlin, and E. C. Stafne, "Fibrous dysplasia of the maxilla and mandible," *Oral Surgery, Oral Medicine, Oral Pathology*, vol. 11, no. 1, pp. 55–68, 1958.

[12] C. Ogunsalu, N. J. D. Smith, and A. Lewis, "Fibrous dysplasia of the jaw bone: a review of 15 new cases and two cases of recurrence in Jamaica together with a case report," *Australian Dental Journal*, vol. 43, no. 6, pp. 390–394, 1998.

[13] E. S. Hart, M. H. Kelly, B. Brillante et al., "Onset, progression, and plateau of skeletal lesions in fibrous dysplasia and the relationship to functional outcome," *Journal of Bone and Mineral Research*, vol. 22, no. 9, pp. 1468–1474, 2007.

[14] V. Pinsolle, J. Rivel, V. Michelet, C. Majoufre, and J. Pinsolle, "Treatment of fibrous dysplasia of the cranio-facial bones. Report of 25 cases," *Annales de Chirurgie Plastique et Esthétique*, vol. 43, no. 3, pp. 234–239, 1998.

[15] R. Tabrizi and B. T. Ozkan, "Craniofacial fibrous dysplasia of orbit," *Journal of Craniofacial Surgery*, vol. 19, no. 6, pp. 1532–1537, 2008.

[16] M. Keskin, F. E. Karabekmez, B. T. Ozkan, Z. Tosun, M. C. Avunduk, and N. Savaci, "Simultaneous occurrence of facial fibrous dysplasia and ameloblastoma," *Journal of Cranio-Maxillofacial Surgery*, vol. 37, no. 2, pp. 102–105, 2009.

[17] C. Ozek, H. Gundogan, U. Bilkay, C. Tokat, T. Gurler, and E. Songur, "Craniomaxillofacial fibrous dysplasia," *Journal of Craniofacial Surgery*, vol. 13, no. 3, pp. 382–389, 2002.

[18] M. R. Zenn and J. Zuniga, "Treatment of fibrous dysplasia of the mandible with radical excision and immediate reconstruction: case report," *Journal of Craniofacial Surgery*, vol. 12, no. 3, pp. 259–263, 2001.

[19] J. W. Choi, S. W. Lee, and K. S. Koh, "Correction of proptosis and zygomaticomaxillary asymmetry using orbital wall decompression and zygoma reduction in craniofacial fibrous dysplasia," *Journal of Craniofacial Surgery*, vol. 20, no. 2, pp. 326–330, 2009.

[20] E. Béquignon, C. Cardinne, X. Lachiver, I. Wagner, F. Chabolle, and B. Baujat, "Craniofacial fibrous dysplasia surgery: a functional approach," *European Annals of Otorhinolaryngology, Head and Neck Diseases*, vol. 130, no. 4, pp. 215–220, 2013.

[21] V. Valentini, A. Cassoni, T. M. Marianetti, V. Terenzi, M. T. Fadda, and G. Iannetti, "Craniomaxillofacial fibrous dysplasia: conservative treatment or radical surgery? a retrospective study on 68 patients," *Plastic and Reconstructive Surgery*, vol. 123, no. 2, pp. 653–660, 2009.

[22] S. Colucci, V. Minielli, G. Zambonin et al., "Alendronate reduces adhesion of human osteoclast-like cells to bone and bone protein-coated surfaces," *Calcified Tissue International*, vol. 63, no. 3, pp. 230–235, 1998.

[23] A. A. Mäkitie, J. Törnwall, and O. Mäkitie, "Bisphosphonate treatment in craniofacial fibrous dysplasia—a case report and review of the literature," *Clinical Rheumatology*, vol. 27, no. 6, pp. 809–812, 2008.

[24] R. D. Chapurlat, "Medical therapy in adults with fibrous dysplasia of bone," *Journal of Bone and Mineral Research*, vol. 21, no. 2, pp. P114–P119, 2006.

[25] T. Van den Wyngaert, M. T. Huizing, and J. B. Vermorken, "Osteonecrosis of the jaw related to the use of bisphosphonates," *Current Opinion in Oncology*, vol. 19, no. 4, pp. 315–322, 2007.

[26] S. L. Ruggiero, J. Fantasia, and E. Carlson, "Bisphosphonate-related osteonecrosis of the jaw: background and guidelines for diagnosis, staging and management," *Oral Surgery, Oral Medicine, Oral Pathology, Oral Radiology and Endodontology*, vol. 102, no. 4, pp. 433–441, 2006.

[27] B. Chan and M. Zacharin, "Maternal and infant outcome after pamidronate treatment of polyostotic fibrous dysplasia and osteogenesis imperfecta before conception: a report of four cases," *Journal of Clinical Endocrinology and Metabolism*, vol. 91, no. 6, pp. 2017–2020, 2006.

45

Treatment of Class II Division 2 Malocclusion Using the Forsus Fatigue Resistance Device and 5-Year Follow-Up

Ezgi Atik and Ilken Kocadereli

Department of Orthodontics, Faculty of Dentistry, Hacettepe University, 06100 Ankara, Turkey

Correspondence should be addressed to Ezgi Atik; ezgibaytorun@hotmail.com

Academic Editor: Jamil A. Shibli

This case report presents the treatment of a 14-year-and-8-month-old boy with Class II division 2 mandibular retrusion, severe deep bite, and concave profile. The Forsus fatigue resistance device (FRD) was effective in correcting both skeletal and dental parameters. At 5-year posttreatment follow-up, the teeth were well aligned and the occlusion was stable. FRD application with appropriate treatment time can result with prominent changes in the facial profile and dentition, and the outcomes can be maintained at the long-term follow-up periods.

1. Introduction

Class II malocclusion is one of the most frequent problems encountered in orthodontics [1]. This malocclusion is described as a distal relationship of the mandible related to the maxilla with a combination of different dental and skeletal components which can affect facial aesthetics and functional status adversely [2].

The most common characteristic of Class II malocclusion is mandibular retrognathia rather than maxillary protrusion according to McNamara [3]. Functional orthopedic appliances are mostly used to treat Class II malocclusion originated from mandibular retrusion [4, 5]. Appliance selection can involve removable or fixed functional appliances according to the existing anteroposterior discrepancy, cooperation, and growth period of the patient. Nongrowing patients with Class II mandibular retrusion are mostly treated with fixed functional appliances which do not require the patient's collaboration [6–8].

One of the most preferred compliance free fixed functional appliances is Forsus Fatigue Resistant Device (FRD, 3M Unitek, Monrovia, Calif) which is used for the correction of Class II malocclusion with permanent dentition stage [9]. FRD can apply consistent forces with nickel-titanium coil springs, and the force level can be modified by the clinician [10]. In the literature, favorable dentoalveoler effects have been presented during postpubertal growth period by interarch fixed functional appliances [9–11]. The main functions of the FRD appliance are restraining sagittal maxillary growth, stimulating mandibular growth, inducing mesial movement of the mandibular arch, and distal movement of the maxillary arch [6].

The aim of this case report is to present both the effects of the FRD and 5 years' posttreatment stability on Class II division 2 patient with mandibular retrusion, severe deep bite, and concave profile.

2. Case Presentation

A 14-year-and-8-month-old Caucasion boy referred to our clinic with a chief complaint of irregular anterior teeth and backward positioned mandibular arch. Extraoral clinical examination indicated concave profile with prominent chin, decreased anterior facial height, and deep labiomental sulcus. The intraoral examination showed cusp to cusp canine and Class II molar relationships in both right and left segments with severe overjet (7.8 mm) and deep bite (7.5 mm). The maxillary and mandibular arch-length deficiencies were 3.8 and 2.5 mm, respectively (Figure 1).

Examination of the lateral cephalometric radiograph indicated normal positioned maxilla (SNA: 81°), retrognathic

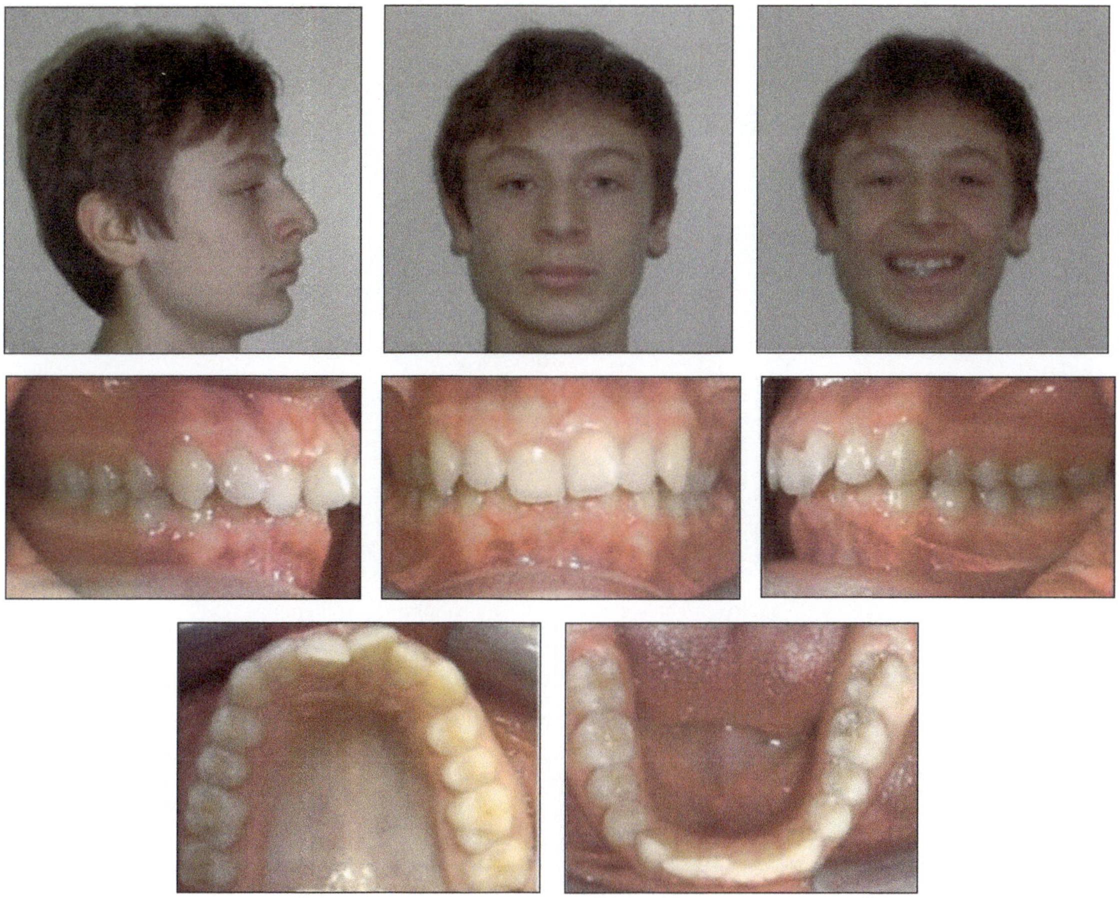

FIGURE 1: Pretreatment facial and intraoral photographs.

mandible (SNB: 75.6°), skeletal Class II malocclusion (ANB: 5.4°), and horizontal growth pattern (GoGnSN: 22.9°). The upper incisors were retroclined (U1-FH: 104.8°) and the lower incisors were proclined (IMPA: 101.1°). Panoramic radiographic evaluation showed permanent dentition with all teeth present including the third molars in all quadrants. Anteroposterior radiograph revealed no skeletal asymmetry (Figure 2).

2.1. Treatment Objectives. The treatment objectives were the following: (1) expansion of the dentally constricted maxillary arch; (2) protrusion of the severely retroclined upper incisors; (3) resolving the crowding of the maxillary and mandibular arch; (4) correction of severe deep bite; (5) establishing Class I canine and molar relationships; (6) obtaining normal overjet and overbite; and (7) improvement of the patient's facial esthetic.

2.2. Treatment Alternatives. The first treatment alternative was the orthognathic surgery with mandibular advancement and genioplasty. However the patient was unwilling to undergo the surgery. Therefore nonextraction orthodontic treatment protocol including interarch Class II mechanics was chosen for the treatment of the patient.

2.3. Treatment Progress. At the beginning of the orthodontic treatment, maxillary dentoalveolar constriction was treated with Quad-helix appliance. When the desired maxillary expansion was achieved, upper incisors were bonded, leveled, and protruded with leveling and protrusion utility arches. Afterwards, upper and lower arches were bonded with 0.018-inch Roth prescribed appliances (Forestadent, Pforzheim, Germany). Leveling and aligning stage started with 0.014-inch Ni-Ti and continued with 0.016-inch Ni-Ti, 0.016 × 0.016-inch Ni-Ti, 0.016 × 0.016-inch stainless steel (SS), 0.016 × 0.022-inch SS, and 0.017 × 0.025-inch SS archwires, respectively. In the upper arch, a transpalatal arch was applied to minimize the potential transverse side effects of the FRD appliance. After leveling and alignment were achieved, the FRD appliances with a 32 mm length of rod were inserted bilaterally when 0.017 × 0.025-inch SS archwires were inserted at both maxillary and mandibular arches (Figure 3). A lingual arch was placed and the SS archwire was cinched back in the lower arch at the stage of FRD insertion. In addition to these, extra buccal root torque was applied to the lower incisors to limit the buccal inclination of the lower incisors. The lower parts of the FRD appliance were placed on the distal to the mandibular canine teeth.

Activation of the FRD appliance was applied with 4-week intervals until a super Class I canine and molar relationships

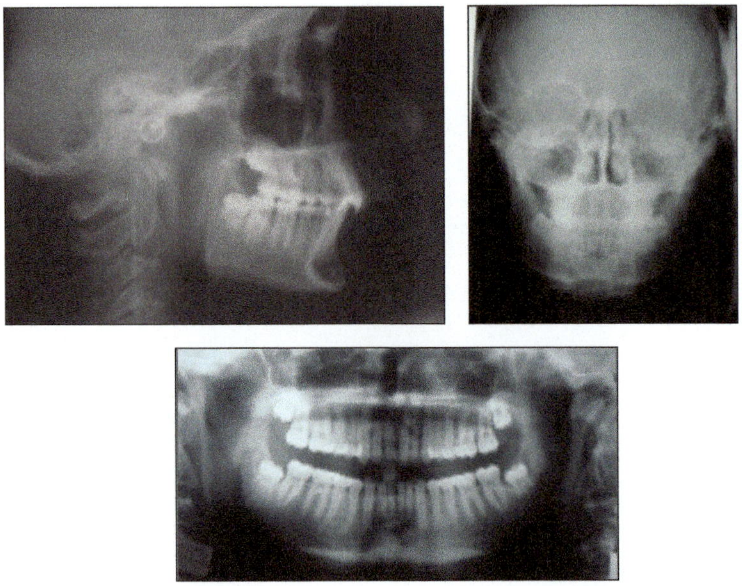

Figure 2: Pretreatment lateral, frontal, and panoramic radiographs.

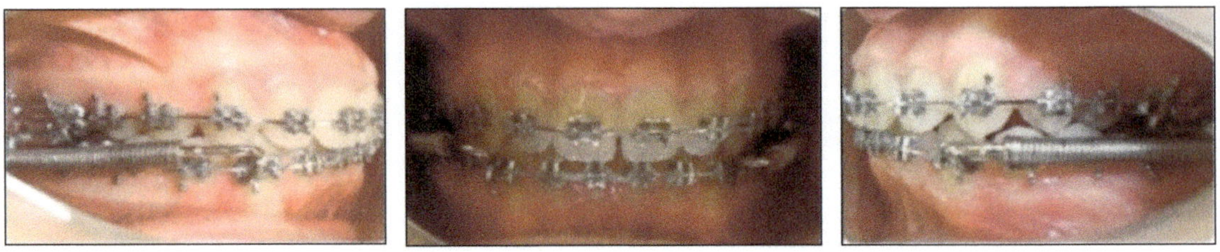

Figure 3: Progress intraoral photographs after application of the Forsus FRD.

were obtained and overjet was eliminated. Active FRD application took 4 months. Total active orthodontic treatment period was 16 months. After obtaining ideal overjet, overbite and a functional interdigitation, brackets were removed and the retention period began (Figure 4). Increase in the mentolabial angle was significant in posttreatment facial photograph (Figure 4).

During the retention period, the patient was instructed to wear Hawley retainer which had anterior bite plane in the maxillary arch and in the lower Hawley retainer with fixed mandibular lingual retainer for 12 months all day.

2.4. Treatment Results. Cephalometric measurements at the pretreatment, posttreatment and postretention (5 years' follow-up) periods are given in Table 1. The results indicated improvement in both skeletal and dental parameters. At the end of treatment, overjet was reduced from 7.8 mm to 2.6 mm and overbite reduced from 7.5 mm to 2.2 mm. Cephalometric superimposition indicated downward and forward movement of the mandibular dentoalveolar arch and backward movement of the maxillary dentoalveolar arch. ANB angle decreased from 5.4 degrees to 2.5 degrees. Convexity decreased and the prominency of labiomental fold diminished. The posttreatment panoramic radiograph showed no alveolar bone loss or apical root resorption (Figures 5 and 6).

Posttreatment follow-ups were carried out after 5 years (Figure 7). Intraoral photographs showed that teeth were well aligned and the occlusion was stable. Cephalometric measurements indicated that maxillary incisors were slightly labially inclined, however mandibular incisors were unchanged (Table 1). Third molars were in good positions as seen in the posttreatment panoramic radiograph; however the patient extracted both maxillary and mandibular third molars.

3. Discussion

In adult patients with Class II mandibular retrusion, either camouflage or orthognathic surgical treatment is carried out depending upon the severity of maxillomandibular discrepancy [12]. A surgical procedure was suggested to improve the facial esthetic; however the patient declined this approach. Extraction treatment was not suitable since the patient had both severe deep-bite and concave profile which could become worsen the occlusion and the profile. Therefore it was decided to apply nonextraction orthodontic treatment including Class II inter-arch mechanics.

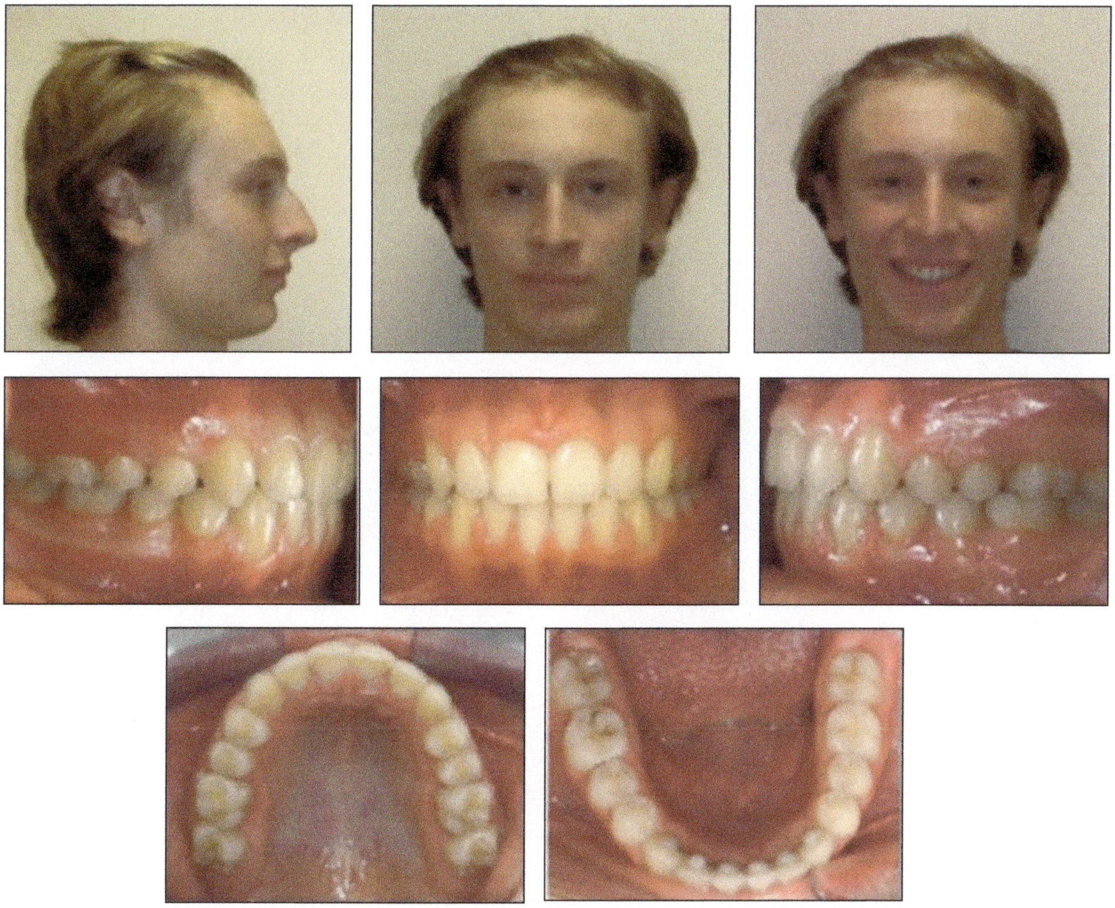

FIGURE 4: Posttreatment facial and intraoral photographs.

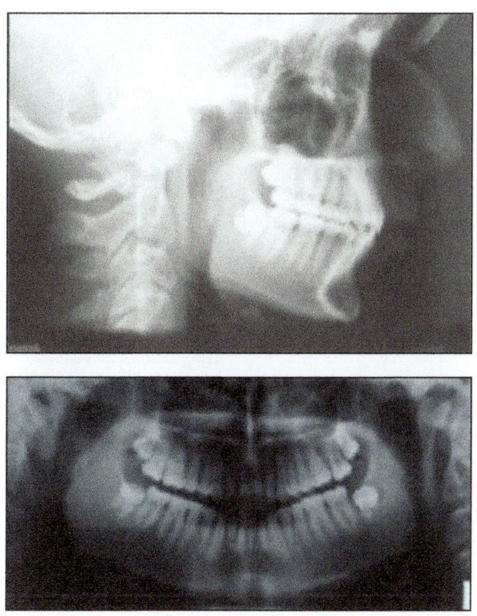

FIGURE 5: Posttreatment lateral and panoramic radiographs.

Table 1: Mean values of the measurements at pretreatment (T0), posttreatment (T1), and 5 years' after retention (T2).

Measurement	Norm	Pretreatment (T0)	Posttreatment (T1)	5 years' after retention (T2)
SNA°	82°	81°	81°	79.6°
SNB°	80°	75.6°	78.5°	77.2°
ANB°	2°	5.4°	2.5°	2.3°
Convexity (mm)	0.8 mm	3.2 mm	0.2 mm	−0.5 mm
GoGnSN°	32°	22.9°	21.6°	21.8°
U1-FH°	111°	104.8°	103.4°	111.3°
U1-NA°	22°	14.3°	17.9°	23.5°
IMPA°	90°	101.1°	106°	107°
L1-NB°	25°	19.5°	26.1°	26.7°
Interincisor angle°	130°	140.8°	130.7°	127.9°
U6-PTV (mm)	17.7 mm	22.1 mm	16.7 mm	19.4 mm
Overjet (mm)	2.5 mm	7.8 mm	2.6 mm	2.6 mm
Overbite (mm)	2.5 mm	7.5 mm	2.2 mm	2.6 mm
Low.Lip-E (mm)	−2.0 mm	−3.9 mm	−6 mm	−5.9 mm

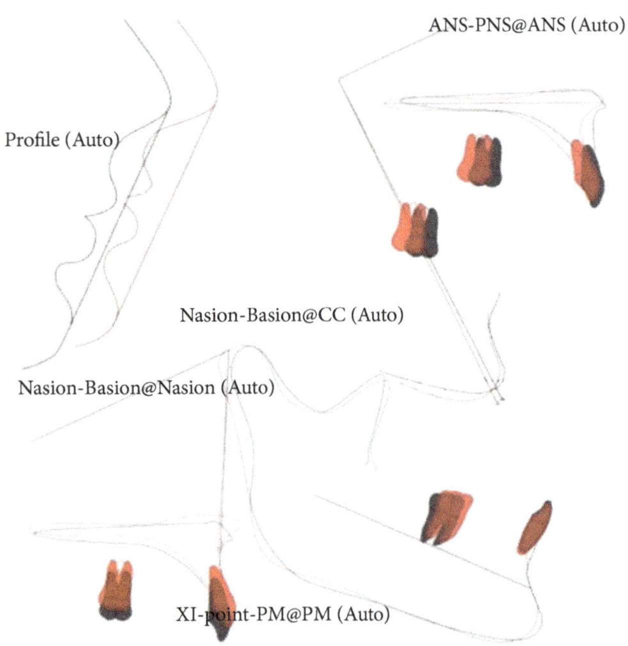

Figure 6: Superimposition (black line, pretreatment; red line, posttreatment).

FRD appliance is usually recommended for the Class II malocclusions especially in patients with mandibular dentoalveolar retrusion. This appliance can lead mandibular growth and favorable dentoalveolar changes in patients at or before the peak phase of pubertal growth [13, 14]. On the other hand, mostly dental changes are encountered for the patients at postpubertal period [15]. However, in this case report, the increase of the SNB angle was nearly 3 degrees and the patient showed slight forward mandibular displacement after the treatment. This result can be correlated with the minimal residual growth of the patient during orthodontic treatment.

The dentoalveolar changes were evident at both maxillary and mandibular arches (Table 1). Maxillary incisors and first molars demonstrated distal movement and intrusion. Mandibular first molars showed mesial movement and extrusion, and lower incisors exhibited proclination. The correction of the overjet was achieved by both retroclination of the upper incisors and protrusion of the lower incisors. Similar dental changes are also reported by the other studies [6, 10].

Application of negative torque to the lower incisors and a lingual arch did not eliminate the unfavorable lower incisor protrusion. Even with these anchorage mechanics, mandibular incisors were proclined by 5 degrees. Increase in the mandibular incisor inclination is a similar common finding of fixed functional appliances as shown by the other studies [9, 16]. To eliminate this side effect of the FRD appliance, it could be effective to use miniscrew anchorage as shown by Aslan et al. [17]. Furthermore, mandibular rectangular archwires of greater size and addition of negative torque in the lower incisor region can be considered.

The patient was followed up for 5 years. Stable treatment results were obtained with the FRD in this young adult patient, and this result was in accordance with the outcomes of the studies observing stability after fixed functional appliance systems. Bock et al. [12] reported stable molar and canine relationships in Class II adult patients treated with Herbst appliance. Ruf and Pancherz [18] found fewer relapse in postpeak patients treated with Herbst/multibracket appliance system. Gao et al. [19] evaluated the effects and the stability of FRD appliance treatment and concluded relatively stable results 2 years after treatment. In a case report, Zhang et al. [20] reported a stable and functional occlusion using Forsus FRD in a young patient with two congenitally missing mandibular incisors after 42 months of retention. The stable results in the long-term follow-up periods in our case report may be related with different factors including finishing the treatment with stable interdigitation in permanent dentition and the patient's postpeak growth.

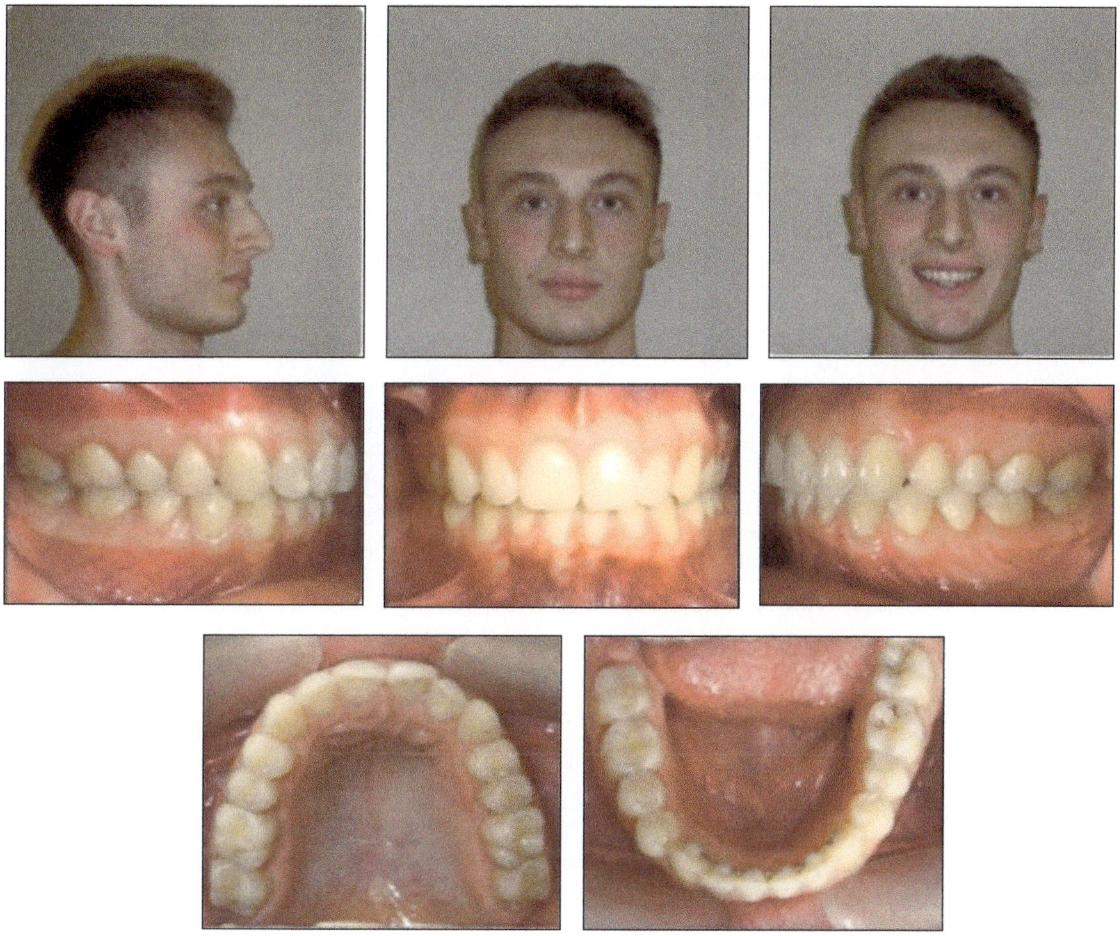

FIGURE 7: Facial and intraoral photographs after 5 years of retention.

4. Conclusion

Fixed functional appliance (FRD) application with appropriate treatment time resulted in prominent changes in the facial profile and dentition. The stability of the outcomes was maintained at the long-term follow-up periods.

Conflict of Interests

The authors declare that there is no conflict of interests related to the publication of this paper.

References

[1] W. R. Proffit, H. W. Fields Jr., and L. J. Moray, "Prevalence of malocclusion and orthodontic treatment need in the United States: estimates from the NHANES-III survey," *The International Journal of Adult Orthodontics and Orthognathic Surgery*, vol. 13, no. 2, pp. 97–106, 1998.

[2] M. Alarashi, L. Franchi, A. Marinelli, and E. Defraia, "Morphometric analysis of the transverse dentoskeletal features of class II malocclusion in the mixed dentition," *The Angle Orthodontist*, vol. 73, no. 1, pp. 21–25, 2003.

[3] J. A. McNamara Jr., "Components of class II malocclusion in children 8–10 years of age," *The Angle Orthodontist*, vol. 51, no. 3, pp. 177–202, 1981.

[4] C. Nelson, M. Harkness, and P. Herbison, "Mandibular changes during functional appliance treatment," *American Journal of Orthodontics and Dentofacial Orthopedics*, vol. 104, no. 2, pp. 153–161, 1993.

[5] P. Cozza, T. Baccetti, L. Franchi, L. De Toffol, and J. A. McNamara Jr., "Mandibular changes produced by functional appliances in Class II malocclusion: a systematic review," *American Journal of Orthodontics and Dentofacial Orthopedics*, vol. 129, no. 5, pp. 599.e1–599.e12, 2006.

[6] L. Franchi, L. Alvetro, V. Giuntini, C. Masucci, E. Defraia, and T. Baccetti, "Effectiveness of comprehensive fixed appliance treatment used with the Forsus Fatigue Resistant Device in Class II patients," *The Angle Orthodontist*, vol. 81, no. 4, pp. 678–683, 2011.

[7] V. F. Zymperdikas, V. Koretsi, S. N. Papageorgiou, and M. A. Papadopoulos, "Treatment effects of fixed functional appliances in patients with Class II malocclusion: a systematic review and meta-analysis," *The European Journal of Orthodontics*, 2015.

[8] O. Dalci, A. T. Altuğ, and U. T. Memikoglu, "Treatment effects of a twin-force bite corrector versus an activator in comparison

with an untreated Class II sample: a preliminary report," *Australian Orthodontic Journal*, vol. 30, no. 1, pp. 45–53, 2014.

[9] E. A. Gunay, T. Arun, and D. Nalbantgil, "Evaluation of the immediate dentofacial changes in late adolescent patients treated with the Forsus™ FRD," *European Journal of Dentistry*, vol. 5, no. 4, pp. 423–432, 2011.

[10] G. Jones, P. H. Buschang, K. B. Kim, and D. R. Oliver, "Class II non-extraction patients treated with the forsus fatigue resistant device versus intermaxillary elastics," *The Angle Orthodontist*, vol. 78, no. 2, pp. 332–338, 2008.

[11] N. Heinig and G. Goz, "Clinical application and effects of the Forsus spring. A study of a new Herbst hybrid," *Journal of Orofacial Orthopedics*, vol. 62, no. 6, pp. 436–450, 2001.

[12] N. C. Bock, J. von Bremen, and S. Ruf, "Occlusal stability of adult Class II Division 1 treatment with the Herbst appliance," *American Journal of Orthodontics and Dentofacial Orthopedics*, vol. 138, no. 2, pp. 146–151, 2010.

[13] F. Bilgiç, O. Hamamci, and G. Başaran, "Comparison of the effects of fixed and removable functional appliances on the skeletal and dentoalveolar structures," *Australian Orthodontic Journal*, vol. 27, no. 2, pp. 110–116, 2011.

[14] I. K. Mahamad, P. K. Neela, R. Mascarenhas, and A. Husain, "A comparision of Twin-block and Forsus (FRD) functional appliance—a cephalometric study," *International Journal of Orthodontics*, vol. 23, no. 3, pp. 49–58, 2012.

[15] M. Upadhyay, S. Yadav, K. Nagaraj, F. Uribe, and R. Nanda, "Mini-implants vs fixed functional appliances for treatment of young adult Class II female patients: a prospective clinical trial," *The Angle Orthodontist*, vol. 82, no. 2, pp. 294–303, 2012.

[16] A. Aras, E. Ada, H. Saracoğlu, N. S. Gezer, and I. Aras, "Comparison of treatments with the Forsus fatigue resistant device in relation to skeletal maturity: a cephalometric and magnetic resonance imaging study," *American Journal of Orthodontics and Dentofacial Orthopedics*, vol. 140, no. 5, pp. 616–625, 2011.

[17] B. I. Aslan, E. Kucukkaraca, C. Turkoz, and M. Dincer, "Treatment effects of the Forsus Fatigue Resistant Device used with miniscrew anchorage," *The Angle Orthodontist*, vol. 84, no. 1, pp. 76–87, 2014.

[18] S. Ruf and H. Pancherz, "Herbst/multibracket appliance treatment of Class II division 1 malocclusions in early and late adulthood. A prospective cephalometric study of consecutively treated subjects," *European Journal of Orthodontics*, vol. 28, no. 4, pp. 352–360, 2006.

[19] W. Gao, X. Li, and Y. Bai, "An assessment of late fixed functional treatment and the stability of Forsus appliance effects," *Australian Orthodontic Journal*, vol. 30, no. 1, pp. 2–10, 2014.

[20] R. Zhang, Y. Bai, and S. Li, "Use of Forsus fatigue-resistant device in a patient with Class I malocclusion and mandibular incisor agenesis," *American Journal of Orthodontics and Dentofacial Orthopedics*, vol. 145, no. 6, pp. 817–827, 2014.

Permissions

All chapters in this book were first published in CRID, by Hindawi Publishing Corporation; hereby published with permission under the Creative Commons Attribution License or equivalent. Every chapter published in this book has been scrutinized by our experts. Their significance has been extensively debated. The topics covered herein carry significant findings which will fuel the growth of the discipline. They may even be implemented as practical applications or may be referred to as a beginning point for another development.

The contributors of this book come from diverse backgrounds, making this book a truly international effort. This book will bring forth new frontiers with its revolutionizing research information and detailed analysis of the nascent developments around the world.

We would like to thank all the contributing authors for lending their expertise to make the book truly unique. They have played a crucial role in the development of this book. Without their invaluable contributions this book wouldn't have been possible. They have made vital efforts to compile up to date information on the varied aspects of this subject to make this book a valuable addition to the collection of many professionals and students.

This book was conceptualized with the vision of imparting up-to-date information and advanced data in this field. To ensure the same, a matchless editorial board was set up. Every individual on the board went through rigorous rounds of assessment to prove their worth. After which they invested a large part of their time researching and compiling the most relevant data for our readers.

The editorial board has been involved in producing this book since its inception. They have spent rigorous hours researching and exploring the diverse topics which have resulted in the successful publishing of this book. They have passed on their knowledge of decades through this book. To expedite this challenging task, the publisher supported the team at every step. A small team of assistant editors was also appointed to further simplify the editing procedure and attain best results for the readers.

Apart from the editorial board, the designing team has also invested a significant amount of their time in understanding the subject and creating the most relevant covers. They scrutinized every image to scout for the most suitable representation of the subject and create an appropriate cover for the book.

The publishing team has been an ardent support to the editorial, designing and production team. Their endless efforts to recruit the best for this project, has resulted in the accomplishment of this book. They are a veteran in the field of academics and their pool of knowledge is as vast as their experience in printing. Their expertise and guidance has proved useful at every step. Their uncompromising quality standards have made this book an exceptional effort. Their encouragement from time to time has been an inspiration for everyone.

The publisher and the editorial board hope that this book will prove to be a valuable piece of knowledge for researchers, students, practitioners and scholars across the globe.

List of Contributors

Kiran Kumar, Devi Charan Shetty and Raghu Dhanapal
Department of Oral & Maxillofacial Pathology, I.T.S-CDSR, Muradnagar, Ghaziabad 201206, India

Mahima Dua
Department of Oral & Maxillofacial Pathology, Inderprastha Dental College, Sahibabad, Ghaziabad 201010, India

Amit Dua
Department of Prosthodontics, Krishna Dental College, Mohannagar, Ghaziabad 201206, India

Shinji Yamaguchi, Madoka Inui, Takashi Takeoka, Kenya Okumura and Toshiro Tagawa
Department of Oral and Maxillofacial Surgery, Department of Clinical Sciences, Medical Life Sciences, Mie University, Graduate School of Medicine, 2-174 Edobashi, Tsu, Mie 514-8507, Japan

Amish Diwanji
Department of Pedodontics and Preventive Dentistry, Faculty of Dental Science, Nadiad, Gujarat, India

Preet Jain and Prakash Somani
2Department of Prosthodontics, Pacific Dental College, Udaipur, India

Jigar Doshi
Department of Orthodontics and Dentofacial Orthopedics, Darshan Dental College, Udaipur, India

Dhaval Mehta
Department of Oral Medicine and Radiology, Karnavati School of Dentistry, Gandhinagar, Gujarat, India

Sertan Ergun, Alp SaruhanoLlu and HakkJ Tanyeri
Department of Oral Medicine and Surgery, Faculty of Dentistry, Istanbul University, 34093 Istanbul, Turkey

Dante-AntonioMigliari
Department of Oral Diagnosis, School of Dentistry, University of Sao Paulo, 05508-900 Sao Paulo, SP, Brazil

Ilay Maden
Department of Periodontology, Istanbul Faculty of Medicine, Istanbul University, 34093 Istanbul, Turkey

Ravikumar S. Kulkarni, Amitabh Sarkar and Sandeep Goyal
Department of Oral Pathology, Surendera Dental College and Research Institute, H. H. Gardens, Sri Ganganagar, Rajasthan 335001, India

StefanoMastroberardino, Laura Strohmenger, Alessandro Villa and Maria Grazia Cagetti
Dental Clinic, San Paolo Hospital, University of Milan, 20142 Milan, Italy

Guglielmo Campus
Dental Institute, University of Sassari, 07100 Sassari, Italy

Ranganadh Nallamothu
Department ofOral andMaxillofacial Surgery, Drs. Sudha&Nageswarao Siddhartha Institute of Dental Sciences, Chinoutpalli, Gannavaram 521 286, Krishna District, Andhra Pradesh, India

Shanmukha Reddy Kallam
Sri Sai College of Dental Surgery, Shiv Nagar, Kotherapally, Range Reddy District, Vikarabad 501101, Andhra Pradesh, India

Srikanth Gunturu
A B Shetty Memorial Institute of Dental Sciences Medical Sciences Complex, P.O. Nityanandanagar, Deralakatte 575018, India

Sukumar Singh
Subharati Dental College, Meerut Subharati Puram, NH-58, Delhi-Haridwar Bypass Road, Meerut 250005, Uttar Pradesh, India

Vijay Kumar Rachalapally
S.V.S. Institute of Dental Sciences,Mahabubnagar 509 001, Andhra Pradesh, India

Vijay Shekhar and K. Shashikala
Department of Conservative Dentistry and Endodontics, D.A.P.M. R.V. Dental College and Hospital, Bangalore, Karnataka 560078, India

Mi-ae Jeong
Department of Dental Hygiene, Kangwon National University, Samcheok, Republic of Korea

Ah-hyeon Kim
Department of Preventive Dentistry and Public Oral Health, Research Center for Orofacial Hard Tissue Regeneration, College of Dentistry, Yonsei University, Seoul, Republic of Korea

Youn-soo Shim
Department of Dental Hygiene, Cheongju University, Cheongju, Republic of Korea

So-youn An
Pediatric Dentistry, College of Dentistry,Wonkwang University, Sanbon 435-040, Republic of Korea

M. P. V. Prabhat, Prasannasrinivas Deshpande, Sarat Gummadapu,
Raja Lakshmi Chintamaneni and Bhavana Sujanamulk

Department of OralMedicine and Radiology, Dr. Sudha and Nageswara Rao Siddhartha Institute of Dental Sciences, Chinnaoutpalli, Krishna District, Gannavaram, Andhra Pradesh 521286, India

Suresh Babburi
Department of Oral Pathology, Dr. Sudha and Nageswara Rao Siddhartha Institute of Dental Sciences, Chinnaoutpalli, Krishna District, Gannavaram, Andhra Pradesh 521286, India

Manish Agrawal and Banashree Sankeshwari
Department of Prosthodontics and Crown and Bridge, Bharati Vidyapeeth Dental College and Hospital, Sangli 416 416, India

Channaveer V. Pattanshetti
Department of Oral and Maxillofacial Surgery, Bharati Vidyapeeth Dental College and Hospital, Sangli 416 416, India

Francisco Ojeda-Gutierrez, Brenda Martinez-Marquez and Soraya Arteaga-Larios
General DentistryDepartment, Facultad de Estomatología, Universidad Autónoma de San Luis Potosí, 2 Dr. Manuel Nava, Zona Universitaria, 78290 San Luis Potosí, SLP, Mexico

M. Socorro Ruiz-Rodriguez and Amaury Pozos-Guillen
Pediatric Dentistry Posgraduate Program, Facultad de Estomatología, Universidad Autónoma de San Luis Potosí, 2 Dr. Manuel Nava, Zona Universitaria, 78290 San Luis Potosí, SLP, Mexico

Osamu Baba, Kenji Yamagata, Hiroyuki Itoh, Toru Yanagawa, Kojiro Onizawa and Hiroki Bukawa
Department of Oral and Maxillofacial Surgery, Faculty of Medicine, University of Tsukuba, 1-1-1 Tennodai, Ibaraki, Tsukuba City 305-8575, Japan

Yasushi Tomidokoro and Akira Tamaoka
Department of Clinical Pathophysiology of the Neurological Disorders, Faculty of Medicine, University of Tsukuba, Japan

Leila Atash biz Yeganeh,Mamak Adel, Reza Vahedi and Maryam Tofangchiha
Department of Endodontics, School of Dentistry, Qazvin University of Medical Sciences, Qazvin, Iran

Dhaval Mehta, Nilesh Raval, Sneha Udhani, Viral Parekh and ChintanModi
Department of Oral Medicine and Radiology, Karnavati School of Dentistry, 907/A Uvarsad, Gandhinagar, Gujarat 382422, India

Mohita Marwaha, Radhika Chopra, Payal Chaudhuri, Atul Gupta and Jayna Sachdev
Department of Pedodontics & Preventive Dentistry, SGT Dental College, Hospital & Research Institute, Budhera 123505, India

Siddarth Gupta
School of Dentistry, CardiffUniversity, Heath Park, Cardiff CF14 4XY, UK

Hashmat Popat
Applied Clinical Research and PublicHealth, School of Dentistry, Cardiff University,Heath Park, Cardiff CF14 4XY,UK

Muktishree Mahendra, Sanjeev Tyagi and Santosh Singh
Department of Conservative Dentistry & Endodontics, People's Dental Academy, Bhopal, Madhya Pradesh 462037, India

KapilMalviya, Ramit Chaddha and Anand Verma
Anand VermaDental Clinic, C/2-30, Civil Lines, Shamla Hill, Bhopal 462002, India

Rajat G. Panigrahi, Sanat K. Bhuyan and Abhishek Ranjan Pati
Department of Oral Medicine & Radiology, Institute of Dental Science, Siksha O Anusandhan University, K8 Kalinga Nagar, Bhubaneswar, Odisha 751003, India

Antarmayee Panigrahi
Department of Pedodontics & Preventive Dentistry, JSS Dental College, JSS University, Sri Shivarathreeshwara Nagara, Mysore, Karnataka 570 015, India

Poornima Vijayakumar
Department of Pedodontics & Preventive Dentistry, Tamil Nadu Dr. M. G. R. Medical University, Ragas Dental College & Hospital, No. 191 East Coast Road, Uthandi, Chennai, Tamil Nadu 600096, India

Priyadarshini Choudhury
Department of Oral Medicine & Radiology, Kalinga Institute of Dental Sciences, KIIT University, Bhubaneswar, Odisha 751024, India

Ruchi Bhuyan
Department of Oral Pathology, Institute of Dental Science, Siksha O Anusandhan University, K8 Kalinga Nagar, Bhubaneswar, Odisha 751003, India

G. Maragathavalli
Department ofOralMedicine & Radiology, Saveetha Dental College, Saveetha University, No. 162 Poonamalee High Road, Vellapanchavadi, Chennai, Tamil Nadu 600077, India

M. S. Rangareddy, Archana Daga and Y. Vishnu Vardhan
Panineeya Institute of Dental Sciences, Hyderabad, Andhra Pradesh 500060, India

M. Daneswari
Mamtha Dental College, Khammam, Andhra Pradesh 500060, India

María del Carmen González Galván, Rafael Martinez-Conde Llamosas and JoséManuel Aguirre-Urizar
Oral and Maxillofacial Pathology Unit, Dental Clinic Service, Stomatology II Department, UFI 11/25, University of the Basque Country (EHU/EHU), Vizcaya, 48940 Leioa, Spain

Abel García-García
University of Santiago of Compostela, 15782 Santiago of Compostela, Spain

Eduardo Anitua-Aldecoa
Private Practice, Eduardo Anitua Institute, 01005 Vitoria-Gasteiz, Spain

Ashwini Ramakrishna
Department of Oral Pathology and Microbiology, College of Dental Sciences, Room No. 7, Pavilion Road, Davangere-Karnataka 577004, India

Kiran B. Rajashekarappa
Sai Multispecialty Dental Clinic, Vidyanagar Main Road, Davangere, Karnataka 577005, India

N. Umashree
Department of Oral Medicine and Maxillofacial Radiology, Al-Badar Dental College and Hospital, Gulbarga, Karnataka, India

Avinash Kumar
Department of Orthodontics and Dentofacial Orthopedics, Al-Badar Dental College and Hospital, Gulbarga, Karnataka, India

Tejavathi Nagaraj
Department of Oral Medicine and Maxillofacial Radiology, Sri Rajiv Gandhi College of Dental Sciences and Hospital, Karnataka, India

Sezin Ozer
Department of Pediatric Dentistry, Faculty of Dentistry, Ondokuz Mayıs University, Atakum, 55139 Samsun, Turkey

Bora Ozden
Department of Oral and Maxillofacial Surgery, Faculty of Dentistry, Ondokuz Mayıs University, 55139 Samsun, Turkey

Feyza Otan Ozden
Department of Periodontology, Faculty of Dentistry, Ondokuz Mayıs University, Kurupelit, 55139 Samsun, Turkey

Kaan Gunduz
Department of Oral Diagnosis and Radiology, Faculty of Dentistry, Ondokuz Mayıs University, Kurupelit, 55139 Samsun, Turkey

Vincenzo Bruno, Mauro Badino, Francesco Riccitiello and Gianrico Spagnuolo
Department of Neurosciences, Reproductive and Odontostomatological Sciences, University of Naples Federico II, Naples, Italy

Massimo Amato
Medical School, University of Salerno, Salerno, Italy

Derya Demircioglu Guler and Emine Sen Tunc
Department of Pediatric Dentistry, Faculty ofDentistry,Ondokuz MayisUniversity, Kurupelit, 55139 Samsun, Turkey

Nursel Arici
Department ofOrthodontics, Faculty ofDentistry,Ondokuz MayisUniversity, Kurupelit, 55139 Samsun, Turkey

Nilüfer Ozkan
Department ofOral andMaxillofacial Surgery, Faculty ofDentistry,Ondokuz MayisUniversity, Kurupelit, 55139 Samsun, Turkey

Andrea Enrico Borgonovo
School of Oral Surgery, University of Milan, Via Festa del Perdono 7, 20122 Milano, Italy

Federica Rizza, Adele Dudaite and Dino Re
Department of Oral Rehabilitation, Istituto Stomatologico Italiano, University of Milan, Via Pace 21, 20122 Milano, Italy

Rachele Censi
Department of Periodontology and Implantology III, Istituto Stomatologico Italiano, Via Pace 21, 20122 Milano, Italy

Rathy Ravindran
Department of Oral and Maxillofacial Pathology, Azeezia College of Dental Science & Research, Diamond Hills, Meeyannoor, Kollam-691537, Kerala State, India

Anila Karunakaran
Department of Oral and Maxillofacial Pathology, Kannur Dental College, Anjarakandy, Mamba, Kannur-670611, Kerala State, India

P. Ramaswamy, Tanya Khaitan, B. Praveen Kumar and S. Sudhakar
Department of Oral Medicine and Radiology, St. Joseph Dental College and Hospital, Duggirala, Eluru, Andhra Pradesh 534003, India

A. Anuradha
Department of Oral and Maxillofacial Pathology, St. Joseph Dental College and Hospital, Duggirala, Eluru, Andhra Pradesh 534003, India

Sera SJmsek Derelioglu, Yücel YJlmaz and Sultan Keles
Department of Pedodontics, Faculty of Dentistry, Atat¨urk University, 25240 Erzurum, Turkey

Anita Singhal
Department of Oral Pathology and Microbiology, H.P. Government Dental College and Hospital, Shimla, Himachal Pradesh 171001, India

Parul Singhal
Department of Pedodontics and Preventive Dentistry, H.P. Government Dental College and Hospital, Shimla, Himachal Pradesh 171001, India

Ranjan Gupta
Department of Prosthodontics, H.P. Government Dental College and Hospital, Shimla, Himachal Pradesh 171001, India

Kush Dev Jarial
Department of Pediatrics, Indira Gandhi Medical College & Hospital, Shimla, Himachal Pradesh 171001, India

Ranganadh Nallamothu, Rama Mohan Kodali, N. Koteswara Rao, Leela krishna Guttikonda, and U. Vijayalakshmi
Department of Oral and Maxillofacial Surgery, Drs. Sudha & Nageswara Rao Siddhartha Institute of Dental Sciences, Chinoutpalli, Gannavaram, Krishna District, Andhra Pradesh 521 286, India

NeetaMohanty
Department of Oral and Maxillofacial Pathology, Institute of Dental Sciences, Bhubaneswar, Odisha 751003, India

Varun Rastogi
Department of Oral and Maxillofacial Pathology, Kalka Dental College, Meerut, Uttar Pradesh 250 006, India

Satya RanjanMisra
Department of Oral Medicine and Radiology, Institute of Dental Sciences, Bhubaneswar, Odisha 751003, India

SusantMohanty
Department of Paediatric Dentistry, Institute of Dental Sciences, Bhubaneswar, Odisha 751003, India

CarloMaiorana
Center for Edentulism and Jawbone Atrophies, Fondazione IRCCS Policlinico, Department of Oral Sciences, University of Milan, 20141 Milan, Italy

Mario Beretta, Davide Rancitelli and Giovanni Battista Grossi
Oral Surgery and Implantology, Fondazione IRCCS Policlinico, University of Milan, 20141 Milan, Italy

Marco Cicciù
Human Pathology Department, School of Dentistry University of Messina, 98100 Messina, Italy

Alan Scott Herford
Oral and Maxillofacial Surgery, Loma Linda University School of Dentistry, Loma Linda, CA 95231, USA

Rashmi Bansal, Nakul Mehrotra, Priyanka Chowdhary and Anuraag Gurtu
Department of Conservative Dentistry & Endodontics, Institute of Dental Sciences, Bareilly, India

Jaya Ranganathan, Mohan Kumar Rangarajan Sundaresan and Srinivasan Ramasamy
Department of Conservative Dentistry and Endodontics, Priyadarshini Dental College & Hospital, Pandur, Thiruvallur, Chennai 631203, India

M. M. Figliuzzi, A. Giudice, S. Pileggi, D. Pacifico and L. Fortunato
Department of Periodontics and Oral Sciences, "Magna Graecia" University, 88100 Catanzaro, Italy

M. Marrelli
Biomedical Section, Stem Cells Unit, Tecnologica Research Institute, 88900 Crotone, Italy

M. Tatullo
Biomedical Section, Stem Cells Unit, Tecnologica Research Institute, 88900 Crotone, Italy

Biomedicine Unit, Calabrodental Clinic, Via E. Fermi, 88900 Crotone, Italy

Andrea Cassoni, Umberto Romeo, Valentina Terenzi, Marco Della Monaca, Oriana Rajabtork Zadeh, Ingrid Raponi,Maria Teresa Fadda, Antonella Polimeni and Valentino Valentini
Odontostomatological Science and Maxillo facial Surgery Department, "Sapienza" University of Rome, 00161 Rome, Italy

Fatih Sengul and Sera Simsek
Department of Pedodontics, Faculty of Dentistry, Ataturk University, 25240 Erzurum, Turkey

Binali Cakur
Department of Oral, Dental And Maxillofacial Radiology, Faculty of Dentistry, Ataturk University, 25240 Erzurum, Turkey

L. A. N. Santos
Department of Oral Diagnosis, Division of Oral Radiology, State University of Montes Claros, Avenida Dr. Ruy Braga, N/N, Vila Mauriceia, 39401-089 Montes Claros, MG, Brazil

L. J. Lopes and G. D. Roque-Torres
PiracicabaDental School, StateUniversity of Campinas, Avenida Limeira 901, Arei˜ao, 13414-903 Piracicaba, SP, Brazil

V. F. Oliveira
Department of Maxillofacial Surgery, State University of Montes Claros, Avenida Dr. Ruy Braga, N/N, Vila Mauriceia, 39401-089 Montes Claros, MG, Brazil

D. Q. Freitas
Department of Oral Diagnosis, Division of Oral Radiology, State University of Campinas, Avenida Limeira 901, Areião, 13414-903 Piracicaba, SP, Brazil

Nabil Khzam
DBDental, BDS, MPhil, DClinDent, MRACDS (Perio), Perth, WA 6159, Australia

Adam Fell
DBDental, BSc, BDent, MJDF RCS, Perth, WA 6011, Australia

Anthony Fisher
PerioHEALTH and Implants Practice, BDSc, DClinDent, Brisbane, QLD 4059, Australia

Paul Kim
Benowa Mansions Periodontal Practice, BPharm, BDSc, DClinDent, Gold Coast, QLD 4217, Australia

Usman A. Khan
Dalby Dental Clinic, BDS, MDS, PhD,Western Downs, QLD 4405, Australia

Mahmoud M. Bakr
General Dental Practice, School of Dentistry and Oral Health, BDS, MDS, Griffith University, Gold Coast, QLD 4222, Australia

Selma Sano Suga, Paula de Castro Kruly, Talissa Mayer Garrido, Marise Sano Suga Matumoto, Uhana Seifert Guimarães Suga and Raquel Sano Suga Terada
State University of Maringá, Avenida Mandacaru, 1550 Bairro Mandacaru, 87080-000 Maringá, PR, Brazil

Priyanka Kant and Neelkamal Sharda
Department of Oral Medicine and Radiology, Manav Rachna Dental College, Sector 43, Aravalli Hills, Delhi-Surajkund Road, Faridabad, Haryana 121001, India

Rahul R. Bhowate
Department of Oral Medicine and Radiology, Sharad Pawar Dental College and Hospital, Sawangi,Wardha, Maharashtra 442001, India

Nilton Alves
CIMA ResearchGroup, Faculty of Dentistry, La Frontera University, 1145 Francisco Salazar Avenue, P.O. Box 54-D, 4780000 Temuco, Chile

Reinaldo José de Oliveira and Denise Takehana
Faculty of Sciences of Guarulhos (FACIG), 1844 Guarulhos Avenue, 7196 Guarulhos, SP, Brazil

Naira Figueiredo Deana
Private PhysicalTherapist, 1171 Pasaje Frankfurt, 4780000 Temuco, Chile

Ezgi Atik and Ilken Kocadereli
Department of Orthodontics, Faculty of Dentistry, Hacettepe University, 06100 Ankara, Turkey

Index

A
Ameloblastic Fibroma, 18-19, 21
Atrophic Alveolar Ridge, 155, 179
Autosomal Dominant Osteopetrosis, 206-207, 209-213

B
Bilateral Radix Entomolaris, 84
Biocompatibility, 97, 155
Bluegrass Appliance, 10-11
Bone Window Creation, 176

C
Calcifying Epithelioma, 5-7, 9
Calcium Phosphate, 22-24, 26
Casein Phosphopeptide, 22
Central Incisor, 60-61, 73-74, 82-83, 106, 121-123, 125, 169, 173, 186
Central Mucoepidermoid Carcinoma (cmec), 50
Cephalometric Measurements, 222
Complex Root Canal, 70, 72, 84
Computed Tomography (ct), 28, 33, 115, 148
Condylar Aplasia, 147-148
Cone Beam Computed Tomography (cbct), 32, 168, 191
Crestal Osteotomy, 175-176
Crown Fractures, 59-63

D
Deafness Syndrome, 137, 141
Decayed Mandibular Molar, 162
Dens Invaginatus, 168, 170-173

E
Early Childhood Caries (ecc), 44, 141
Endodontic Phase, 162-163
Endodontic Surgery, 32-33, 35, 37, 40-41, 43
Erupted Odontoma, 73
Extraoral Assessment, 80

F
Fatigue Resistance, 220

G
General Anesthesia, 5, 64, 99, 110, 137-140, 142, 203
Glandular Odontogenic Cyst (goc), 50

H
Histopathological Diagnosis, 32, 37, 43, 132
Hutchinson-gilford Progeria Syndrome, 88, 90-91
Hydrogen Peroxide, 22-24, 26
Hypohidrotic (anhidrotic) Ectodermal Dysplasia (hed), 1
Hypomineralization, 22, 26

I
Ichthyosis, 137, 140-141
Idiopathic Orofacial Granulomatosis, 131-133
Implant-prosthetic Rehabilitation, 174
Implantology, 115, 126, 130, 155, 160, 175, 199
Incisional Biopsy, 152, 215
Intraductal Papilloma, 134-136
Intrafamilial Genetic Transmission, 1

K
Keratitis, 137, 139-141
Keratocystic Odontogenic Tumour (kcot), 98, 100

L
Large Periapical Lesions, 32-33, 35, 38, 43, 171
Laugier-hunziker Syndrome, 14-15, 17

M
Malocclusion, 10, 74, 81, 113, 122, 148, 201, 214-215, 220-221, 225-226
Mandibular Canines, 76-77, 105, 110-111
Maxillary First Molar, 69-72
Maxillofacial And Oral Surgery, 191
Mesioangular, 196-198
Microdontia, 143-144, 146
Monostotic Fibrous Dysplasia, 214-215, 218
Mucoepidermoid Carcinoma, 50-51, 54, 186-189
Multidisciplinary Management, 121, 125
Multiple Pulp Stones, 76, 78

N
Neuroleptic Malignant Syndrome, 64, 66-68
Nonpunitive Therapy, 10
Nonsyndrome Patient, 102
Nonsyndromic Concomitant, 80

O
Occlusal Vertical Dimension (ovd), 55-56
Ocular Dystopia, 27-30
Oral Radiology Principles, 78, 213
Orbital Roof Fractures, 30-31
Orthokeratinized Odontogenic Cyst, 98-101
Osteodistraction, 176
Osteonecrosis, 180, 184-185, 218-219
Osteonecrosis of the Jaw Related to Bisphosphonate (bronj), 180

P
Panoramic X-ray, 214-216
Papilliferous Keratoameloblastoma, 151, 153-154
Partial Pulpotomy, 59-63
Pathological Findings, 6-8, 138
Pathophysiology, 30, 64, 66
Pediatric Patients, 10, 44, 46, 48, 189
Preoperative Orthopantograph, 197

R
Radiographic Assessment., 81
Radiographic Imaging, 5, 41
Radiological Findings, 147, 184, 186, 206
Root Fracture, 92-93, 95, 97, 130

S
Sequential Supernumerary Teeth, 200, 204
Single Buccal Canal, 69
Sinus Lift, 126-127, 129-130, 157
Split Crest, 174-175, 178
Spondyloepiphyseal Dysplasia, 143
Symptomless, 5, 110

T
The Temporomandibular Joint (tmj), 147
Tongue Cancer, 64
Transantral Approach, 126
Transmigration, 105-108, 110-111
Treatment Alternatives, 55, 221

V
Vertical Dimension of Occlusion (vdo), 55

W
Wisdom Teeth, 196